SVU CME

PURCHASE AT: insideultrasound.com/VRG_CME   **PASSWORD: Doppler**

Purchasing the Exam

1. Purchase online and enter the password (above).
2. Upon receiving your order, you will get an email receipt.
3. Your login, password, and link to the exam will be emailed **within two business days.**

About the Exam

- The exam contains 100 multiple-choice questions.
- The passing grade is 70%.
- You will be allowed several attempts to complete the exam successfully.
- If you need to exit before completion, you can return later, and your work will be saved.

Upon Successful Completion

- You will be able to download your certificate.
- You will earn 20 hours of CME awarded from the Society of Vascular Ultrasound (SVU). These CMEs are not category 1.
- This program meets the criteria for SVU-CMEs, which are accepted by:
  » American Registry of Diagnostic Medical Sonographers® (ARDMS®).
  » Cardiovascular Credentialing International (CCI).
  » American Registry of Radiologic Technologists (ARRT) for Category A credit.
  » Intersocietal Accreditation Commission (IAC - Vascular) for laboratory accreditation.
  » American College of Radiology (ACR) for laboratory accreditation.

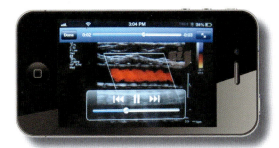

QR codes can be found throughout this book, which will allow you to view video clips of various pathology or duplex findings using your smartphone or tablet. To access these files, use the camera on your device and a QR code reader. Your device must have internet to use this feature.

If your camera does not open the clip automatically after clicking the link on your screen, please check your app store as there are many free QR code readers available for download.

TABLE OF CONTENTS

Dedications..ii

Lists of Tables vi

Authors/Editors x

Contributors xi

Acknowledgements xii

ANATOMY

1. **Extracranial and Intracranial**..1
   - *Extracranial Anatomy* 2
   - *Intracranial Anatomy* 6
2. **Abdominal Venous** 10
3. **Abdominal Arterial** 15
4. **Lower Extremity Venous** 18
5. **Lower Extremity Arterial** 25
6. **Upper Extremity Venous** 27
7. **Upper Extremity Arterial** 31

HEMODYNAMICS AND PHYSIOLOGY

8. **General Principles**...33
9. **Venous** 36
10. **Arterial** 42

DISEASES

11. **Venous Diseases** 55
    - *Chronic Venous Disorders* 55
    - *Iliac Vein Compression* 60
    - *Lymphedema* 61
    - *Pelvic Venous Disorders* 62
    - *Phlegmasia Alba Dolens* 63
    - *Phlegmasia Cerulea Dolens*.......................................63
    - *Portal Hypertension* 64
    - *Pulmonary Embolism (PE)* 65
    - *Superior Vena Cava (SVC) Syndrome* 66
    - *Thoracic Outlet Compression Syndrome* 66
    - *Varicose Veins*...67
    - *Venous Insufficiency (Postphlebitic Syndrome)*............68
    - *Venous Malformations* 69
    - *Venous Thrombosis* 70
12. **Arterial Diseases** 74
    - *Adventitial Cystic Disease*...74
    - *Aneurysm* 74
    - *Aortic Coarctation*..77
    - *Arterial Dissection* 77
    - *Atherosclerosis*..78
    - *Cerebrovascular Events (Transient Ischemic Attack, Stroke)*.............................81
    - *Carotid Body Tumor (CBT)* 84
    - *Fibromuscular Dysplasia (FMD)* 86
    - *Mesenteric Ischemia*...86
    - *Neointimal and Intimal Hyperplasia*............................88
    - *Pseudoaneurysm*..89
    - *Popliteal Artery Entrapment Syndrome* 90
    - *Raynaud's Syndrome* 90
    - *Renovascular Hypertension* 92
    - *Subclavian Steal Syndrome* 93
    - *Thoracic Outlet Compression Syndrome (TOS)* 94
    - *Vasculitis*..95

CEREBROVASCULAR TESTING

13. **Carotid Artery Duplex Ultrasound**..................................98
14. **Carotid Intima-Media Thickness**...................................113
15. **Intracranial Cerebrovascular Testing**.............................116

ARTERIAL TESTING

16. **ABI and Analog Pedal Artery Waveforms** 132
17. **Lower Extremity Segmental Pressures and Doppler Waveforms**...137
18. **Volume Pulse Recording**...142
19. **LE Digital Evaluations: TBI and PPG** 146
20. **Exercise and Stress Testing of the Extremities** 150
21. **Lower Extremity Arterial Duplex** 155
22. **Bypass and Stent Surveillance Duplex Ultrasound**.........164
23. **Upper Extremity Segmental Pressures and Doppler Waveforms**...173
24. **UE Digital Evaluations: DBI and PPG** 177
25. **Cold Immersion Testing for Raynaud's Phenomenon**...........181
26. **Upper Extremity Arterial Duplex Ultrasound**..................185

VENOUS TESTING

27. **Venous Photoplethysmography (PPG)**............................193
28. **Lower Extremity Venous Duplex Ultrasound**...................198
29. **Lower Extremity Venous Insufficiency Duplex** 208
30. **Venous Ablation Duplex Ultrasound**..............................214
31. **IVC and Iliac Venous Duplex Ultrasound**........................219
32. **Venous Stent Duplex**...226
33. **Upper Extremity Venous Duplex Ultrasound**...................234
34. **Upper and Lower Extremity Venous Duplex Mapping** 243

ABDOMINAL ARTERIAL TESTING

35. **Aorto-Iliac Duplex Ultrasound** 249
36. **Aortic Stent Graft (Endograft) Duplex Ultrasound**..................261
37. **Renal Duplex Ultrasound** 269
38. **Renal Transplant Duplex** 277
39. **Celiac and Mesenteric Artery Duplex Ultrasound**..................287
40. **Hepatoportal Duplex Ultrasound**..................................296
    - *TIPS (Transjugular Intrahepatic Portosystemic Shunt)* 301

ADDITIONAL TESTING

41. **Hemodialysis Access Duplex Evaluation**........................303
42. **Pseudoaneurysm Duplex Ultrasound**.............................316
43. **Thoracic Outlet Testing**...321
44. **Penile Testing**..327

TABLE OF CONTENTS

CARDIAC

45. Effects on Spectral Doppler 333
- High Cardiac Output 334
- Low Cardiac Output 334
- Aortic Stenosis (AS) 334
- Aortic Regurgitation (AR) 335
- Mitral Stenosis (MS) 336
- Mitral Regurgitation (MR) 337
- Tricuspid Regurgitation (TR) 337
- Tricuspid Stenosis (TS) 338
- Pulmonary Regurgitation (PR) 338
- Pulmonic Stenosis (PS) 339
- Cardiac Tamponade 339
- Constrictive Pericarditis 339
- Cardiac Arrhythmias 339

RESOURCES

46. Ergonomics 342

47. Correlation Modalities 348
- Computed Tomography (CT) 348
- Magnetic Resonance Imaging (MRI) 349
- Angiography (Arteriogram/Venogram) 351
- Intravascular Ultrasound 354
- VQ Scan 355
- D-dimer 357
- Caprini DTV Risk Score 357

48. Vascular Pharmacology 358
- Aneurysm 358
- Aortic Coarctation 358
- Arterial Dissection 358
- Arteritis (see Vasculitis) 358
- Atherosclerosis 358
- Carotid Body Tumor 358
- Cerebrovascular Events (TIA/Stroke) 358
- Fibromuscular Dysplasia 358
- Iliac Vein Compression Syndrome (previously May-Thurner Syndrome) 358
- Lymphedema 359
- Mesenteric Ischemia 359
- Neointimal Hyperplasia 359
- Phlegmasia Alba or Cerulea Dolens (see Venous Thromboembolism) 359
- Popliteal Artery Entrapment Syndrome 359
- Popliteal Cystic Disease 359
- Portal Hypertension 359
- Postphlebitic Syndrome/Venous Insufficiency 359
- Pseudoaneurysm 359
- Raynaud's Syndrome 359
- Renovascular Hypertension 359
- Subclavian Steal Syndrome 359
- Superior Vena Cava Syndrome 359
- Thoracic Outlet Compression Syndrome 359
- Varicose Veins 360
- Vasculitis 360
- Venous Thromboembolism/Pulmonary Embolism 360

49. Testing Optimization 361

50. Math Used in Sonography 365
- Math Symbols 365
- Order of Operations 365
- Variables 365
- Integers 366
- Fractions 366
- Conversions 366
- Exponents 368
- Formulas 368
- Decibels 368
- Cosine 369
- Manipulating Equations 369

51. Statistics 371
- Formulas 371
- Protocol for Gathering Statistical Correlation 371
- Statistical Correlation 372
- Reporting on QA Studies 374

52. Measurements and Calculations 375
- Lower Extremity Arterial 375
- Upper Extremity Arterial 376
- Penile Arterial Penile 377
- Velocity Ratio 377
- Lumenal Reduction 377
- Pulsatility Index 378
- Peripheral Venous 378
- Renal 378
- Extracranial Cerebrovascular 379
- Hemodialysis AVF/Prosthetic Graft 380

53. Glossary 381
- Prefixes 387
- Suffixes 387
- Acronyms 387

54. Index 390

LIST OF TABLES

ANATOMY

Extracranial and Intracranial
2   1-1   Artery Classification

Lower Extremity Venous
19   4-1   Nomenclature of the Lower Extremity Deep and Superficial Veins
24   4-2   Nomenclature of the Perforating Veins

HEMODYNAMICS AND PHYSIOLOGY

Venous Hemodynamics and Physiology
37   9-1   Flow/Pressure and Volume Relationships
37   9-2   Pressure and Flow Relationships During Inspiration and Expiration
37   9-3   Inspiration/Expiration Flow Changes

Arterial Hemodynamics and Physiology
42   10-1   Pressure/Velocity Relationship
42   10-2   Kinetic/Potential Energy Relationship

DISEASES

Venous Diseases
55   11-1   CEAP Summary of Clinical (C) Classifications
57   11-2   Venous versus Arterial Ulceration

CEREBROVASCULAR TESTING

Carotid Artery Duplex Ultrasound
99   13-1   B-mode and Plaque Morphology
102   13-2   Identification of ICA vs ECA Vessels
104   13-3   Carotid Artery Examination Protocol Summary
105   13-4   Extracranial Vessels Characteristics
109   13-5   IAC Updated Recommendations for Carotid Stenosis Interpretation Criteria
110   13-6   University of Washington Diagnostic Criteria for Classification of Internal Carotid Artery Disease
110   13-7   University of Chicago Diagnostic Criteria for Classification of Internal Carotid Artery Disease
110   13-8   Bluth Diagnostic Criteria for Classification of Internal Carotid Artery Disease
110   13-9   Velocity Criteria Defining Stenoses in the Stented Carotid Artery Compared to Criteria for the Native Carotid Artery

Carotid Intima-Media Thickness
115   14-1   Carotid Intima Media Thickness Protocol at a Glance
115   14-2   CIMT Diagnostic Criteria
115   14-3   Risk for CVD Based on CIMT Values

Intracranial Cerebrovascular Testing
120   15-1   Windows Used for Visualization of the Intracranial Arteries
122   15-2   Intracranial Artery Mean Diameter and Length
124   15-3   Collateral Pathways of Intracranial Flow (Direction and Mean Velocity)
126   15-4   Transcranial Waveforms and Velocities
128   15-5   MCA Vasospasm Criteria
128   15-6   BA Vasospasm Criteria
130   15-7   SLS Grading System (Spencer Logarithmic Scale)
130   15-8   International Consensus Criteria
130   15-9   Quantification of RLS Shunts
131   15-10   Protocol and Diagnostic Criteria Summary for Intracranial Cerebrovascular Techniques

ARTERIAL TESTING

ABI and Analog Pedal Artery Waveforms
134   16-1   ABI Protocol Summary
135   16-2   Diagnostic Criteria for ABI
135   16-3   University of Chicago Diagnostic ABI Criteria
135   16-4   ABI Symptoms

LIST OF TABLES

Lower Extremity Segmental Pressures and Doppler Waveforms

139   **17-1**   Lower Extremity Segmental Pressures Protocol Summary
141   **17-2**   Findings of the Lower Extremities and Level of Disease
141   **17-3**   Diagnostic Criteria for ABI Severity
141   **17-4**   Diagnostic Criteria for Occlusive Disease by Segmental Arterial Pressure Indices

Volume Pulse Recording

143   **18-1**   Typical VPR Settings for Upper Extremities
143   **18-2**   Typical VPR Settings for Lower Extremities
143   **18-3**   Volume Pulse Recording Protocol Summary
144   **18-4**   Normal Amplitudes for Lower Extremity VPR
144   **18-5**   Lower Extremity VPR Waveforms Based on Location of Disease

Lower Extremity Digital Evaluations TBI and PPG

147   **19-1**   Lower Extremity Digital Protocol Summary
148   **19-2**   Lower Extremity TBI Symptoms
148   **19-3**   Diagnostic Criteria for Lower Extremity Digital Testing
148   **19-4**   University of Chicago Lower Extremity TBI Diagnostic Criteria

Exercise and Stress Testing of the Extremities

151   **20-1**   Treadmill Testing Protocol Summary
152   **20-2**   Post-Occlusive Reactive Hyperemia Protocol Summary
153   **20-3**   Lower Arterial Exam with Exercise Report
153   **20-4**   Diagnostic Criteria for Post-Treadmill Exercise Ankle-Brachial Indices and Recovery Times
153   **20-5**   Diagnostic Criteria for Post-Reactive Hyperemia Ankle-Brachial Index

Lower Extremity Arterial Duplex

157   **21-1**   Lower Extremity Arterial Duplex Protocol Summary
159   **21-2**   Normal PSV of Lower Extremity Arteries
161   **21-3**   University of Chicago Arterial Duplex Diagnostic Criteria
161   **21-4**   Duplex Imaging Diagnostic Criteria
161   **21-5**   University of Washington Arterial Duplex Diagnostic Criteria

Bypass and Stent Surveillance Duplex Ultrasound

168   **22-1**   Arterial Bypass Graft or Stent Surveillance Protocol Summary
171   **22-2**   Duplex Diagnostic Criteria for In-Stent Restenosis of the Superficial Femoral Artery
172   **22-3**   Diagnostic Criteria for Prosthetic Graft Surveillance
172   **22-4**   Diagnostic Criteria for Vein Graft Surveillance
172   **22-5**   Diagnostic Criteria for Femoropopliteal Arterial Duplex After Endovascular Intervention

Upper Extremity Segmental Pressures and Doppler Waveforms

175   **23-1**   Upper Extremity Segmental Pressures and Doppler Waveforms Protocol Summary

Upper Extremity Digital Evaluations DBI and PPG

179   **24-1**   Upper Extremity Digital Protocol Summary
180   **24-2**   Diagnostic Criteria for Upper Extremity Digital Testing

Cold Immersion Testing for Raynaud's Phenomenon

183   **25-1**   Cold Immersion Protocol Summary
184   **25-2**   Cold Immersion Thermometry Worksheet

Upper Extremity Arterial Duplex Ultrasound

188   **26-1**   Upper Extremity Arterial Protocol Summary
189   **26-2**   Normal PSV of Upper Extremity Arteries
190   **26-3**   Diagnostic Criteria for Arterial Stenosis

VENOUS TESTING

Venous Photoplethysmography (PPG)

196   **27-1**   Photoplethysmography Protocol Summary
197   **27-2**   Diagnostic Criteria for PPG

LIST OF TABLES

Lower Extremity Venous Duplex Ultrasound
203   28-1   Lower Extremity Venous Protocol Summary
205   28-2   Thrombosis Descriptions and Characteristics
206   28-3   Venous Duplex Diagnostic Criteria

Lower Extremity Venous Insufficiency Duplex
210   29-1   CEAP Summary of Clinical (C) Classifications
212   29-2   Lower Extremity Venous Insufficiency Examination Protocol Summary
213   29-3   Venous Reflux Diagnostic Criteria

Venous Ablation Duplex Ultrasound
217   30-1   Protocol Summary for Venous Ablation Duplex Imaging
218   30-2   Diagnostic Criteria for Post-Venous Ablation Venous Duplex
218   30-3   Post Ablation Superficial Thrombus Extension (PASTE)

IVC and Iliac Venous Duplex Ultrasound
222   31-1   IVC and Iliac Venous Duplex Protocol Summary
224   31-2   Thrombosis Descriptions and Characteristics

Venous Stent Duplex
227   32-1   Areas of Iliac Vein Compression
233   32-2   Diagnostic Criteria for Iliac Vein and Stent Duplex Scan Obstruction

Upper Extremity Venous Duplex Ultrasound
237   33-1   Upper Extremity Venous Protocol Summary
240   33-2   Thrombosis Descriptions and Characteristics
240   33-3   Venous Duplex Diagnostic Criteria

Upper and Lower Extremity Venous Duplex Mapping
246   34-1   Upper and Lower Extremity Venous Duplex Mapping Protocol Summary
248   34-2   Thrombosis Descriptions and Characteristics
248   34-3   Diagnostic Criteria for Venous Duplex Mapping

ABDOMINAL ARTERIAL TESTING

Abdominal Aorto-Iliac Duplex Ultrasound
254   35-1   Abdominal Aortolliac Duplex Protocol Summary
256   35-2   Normal Arterial Diameters and Peak Systolic Velocities

Abdominal Aortic Stent Graft (Endograft) Duplex Ultrasound
265   36-1   Abdominal Aortic Stent Graft Protocol Summary
267   36-2   Endoleak Classification

Renal Duplex Ultrasound
273   37-1   Renal Duplex Protocol Summary
274   37-2   Normal Renal-Aortic PSV
275   37-3   Diagnostic Criteria for Renal Artery Stenosis
276   37-4   Diagnostic Criteria for Significant Renovascular Resistance Within the Kidney

Renal Transplant Duplex
280   38-1   Renal Transplant Duplex Protocol Summary
282   38-2   Resistive Index (RI) Severity for Renal Transplant

Celiac and Mesenteric Artery Duplex Ultrasound
291   39-1   Celiac and Mesenteric Artery Duplex Protocol Summary
293   39-2   Normal Celiac and Mesenteric Waveforms
293   39-3   Normal Celiac and Mesenteric Peak Systolic Velocities (PSV)
294   39-4   Diagnostic Criteria of Celiac for Mesenteric Artery Stenosis

Hepatoportal Duplex Ultrasound
298   40-1   Hepatoportal Duplex Protocol Summary
299   40-2   Normal Hepatoportal Doppler Waveform Analysis
299   40-3   Normal Hepatoportal Velocity Ranges Reported in the Literature
300   40-4   Normal Hepatoportal Interpretation Summary
301   40-5   Diagnostic Criteria for Abnormal Hepatoportal Disease

LIST OF TABLES

ADDITIONAL TESTING

Hemodialysis Access Duplex Evaluation

310   **41-1**   Protocol Summary for Dialysis Arteriovenous Fistula/Prosthetic Dialysis-Loop Graft

314   **41-2**   University of Chicago Diagnostic Criteria for ≥50% Stenosis in a Hemodialysis AVF

315   **41-3**   Diagnostic Criteria for Prosthetic Hemodialysis Grafts

Pseudoaneurysm Duplex Ultrasound

318   **42-1**   Pseudoaneurysm Duplex Protocol Summary

319   **42-2**   Ultrasound-Guided Pseudoaneurysm Injection Protocol Summary

Thoracic Outlet Testing

324   **43-1**   Thoracic Outlet Examination Protocol Summary

326   **43-2**   Diagnostic Criteria for TOS Disease

Penile Testing

330   **44-1**   Penile Artery Duplex Protocol Summary

330   **44-2**   Penile Pressures Protocol Summary

330   **44-3**   Penile VPR Protocol Summary

331   **44-4**   Diagnostic Criteria for Penile Brachial Index

CARDIAC

Effects on Spectral Doppler

333   **45-1**   Summary of Cardiac Effect on Cardiac Output

341   **45-2**   Effects of Cardiac Diseases on the Spectral Doppler Waveform

RESOURCES

Correlation Modalities

356   **47-1**   Pioped Criteria (Prospective Investigation of Pulmonary Embolism Diagnosis)

357   **47-2**   Clinical Prediction Criteria for Pulmonary Embolism

Vascular Pharmacology

358   **48-1**   Anticoagulants and Thrombolytics

359   **48-2**   Pharmacological Agents used for Raynaud's

359   **48-3**   Anti-inflammatory Agents

360   **48-4**   Recommendations for Treatment of DVT and PE

Math Used in Sonography

367   **50-1**   Fraction to Decimal Conversion/Equivalent

367   **50-2**   Prefix Definitions

367   **50-3**   American-Metric Conversion

369   **50-4**   Decibel Chart

369   **50-5**   Commonly Used Cosines

369   **50-6**   Circular Formulas

370   **50-7**   Additional Formulas

Measurements and Calculations

375   **52-1**   Disease Categorization for ABI and TBI

376   **52-2**   Diagnostic Criteria for Post-Treadmill Exercise Ankle-Brachial Indices and Recovery Times

376   **52-3**   Diagnostic Criteria for WBI and DBI

377   **52-4**   Diagnostic Criteria for Penile Brachial Index (PBI)

377   **52-5**   Velocity Ratio vs. Diameter Reduction

378   **52-6**   Pulsatility Index and Resistance Relationship

378   **52-7**   Diagnostic Criteria for Venous Reflux by Duplex

378   **52-8**   Venous Refill Time (VRT)

379   **52-9**   Diagnostic Criteria for Disease According Renal-to-Aortic-Ratio (RAR)

379   **52-10**   Resistive Index (RI)

379   **52-11**   Interpretation of End-Diastolic Ratio (EDR)

380   **52-12**   Ratio Correlation to Diameter Reduction

380   **52-13**   Diagnostic Criteria for Hemodialysis AVF

380   **52-14**   Diagnostic Criteria for Prosthetic Hemodialysis Graft (AVG)

AUTHORS

Gail P. Size BS, RPhS, RVS, RVT, FSVU, LAVALS
Founder and President / Inside Ultrasound, Inc.
Vail, AZ

Gail Size has over 40 years of technical and managerial experience in both clinical and private vascular laboratories. She is the Founder and President of Inside Ultrasound, Inc., a provider of Basic Training in Non-invasive Vascular Testing and Vascular Interpretation for Physicians and vascular accreditation.

Gail has served on the Board of Trustees and then as the President of Cardiovascular International (CCI) Testing, Board of Directors of the Society of Vascular Technology (SVU), Co-Chair and Chairman of the Society's Education Committee, Midwest regional Chapter Advisor, Southwest Regional Chapter Advisor, and President of the Chicago Area Vascular Association. In 1998, Gail received the Distinguished Service Award; in 2004, she was awarded the Professional Achievement Award from SVU. In 2004, Gail was awarded the Fellow status in the SVU. In 2022, Gail was elevated to a laureate member of the American Vein & Lymphatic Society. Gail has served as an IAC-Vascular Reviewer.

Laurie Lozanski BS, RVS, RVT, FSVU
Technical Director / Non-Invasive Vascular Laboratory,
University of Chicago Medicine
Bachelor of Science Program in Vascular Ultrasound,
Rush University College of Health Sciences
Chicago, IL

Laurie Lozanski has 33 years of technical and managerial experience in a dedicated vascular laboratory. Currently, Laurie is the Technical Director of the Non-Invasive Vascular Laboratory at the University of Chicago Medicine. Laurie is also an Adjunct Faculty member of the Bachelor of Science Program in Vascular Ultrasound at Rush University in Chicago, IL.

ILLUSTRATION AND DESIGN

Denise Eggman
Medical Illustrator
Pearce, AZ

Denise has been a freelance graphic designer since 1987. Her first main client, Abbott Northwestern Hospital (now called Allina Health) in Minneapolis, MN, served as a gateway to her medical illustrations. Denise continues to work as a medical illustrator as well as an artist with a passion for pastels. She has won numerous awards for her artwork.

Chellie Buzzeo
Graphic Designer
Scottsdale, AZ

Chellie Buzzeo is the greatest graphic designer in the northern hemisphere, yet she has been saddled working on this yahoo of a project for 20 years. Her greatest desire is for one of the authors of this text to stop with the rabbit holes and, just once, send the pdf back with no comments. In her little free time, Chellie and her husband, Buzz, enjoy quiet time and just being together.

CHIEF EDITORS

Eileen French-Sherry MA, RVT, FSVU
Retired Assistant Professor and Program Director /
Bachelor of Science Program in Vascular Ultrasound, Rush University
College of Health Sciences
Chicago, IL

Eileen French-Sherry has over 35 years of technical, managerial, consulting, and educational experience in vascular ultrasound. Eileen is the retired Program Director of the Vascular Ultrasound Program at Rush University, Chicago, IL and served as Vice Chair of the Joint Review Committee on Education in Diagnostic Medical Sonography (JRCDMS) under the Commission on Accreditation of Allied Health Education Programs.

Christopher L. Skelly MD, RPVI, FACS
Professor / Vascular Surgery and Endovascular Therapy
Medical Director / Noninvasive Vascular Lab
Associate Program Director for the Vascular and Endovascular Surgery
Fellowship / University of Chicago Medicine
Chicago, IL

Christopher Skelly, MD RVPI trained at the University of Chicago for General Surgery, and the University of Pennsylvania for Vascular Surgery. He joined the faculty at the University of Chicago in 2005 and is currently a Professor of Surgery and Endovascular Therapy. Since 2011, he has been the Medical Director of the Chicago Medicine Non-invasive Vascular Lab. He has received funding from NIH, AHA and SVS to investigate vascular biology and hemodynamics. He has publications in PNAS, Gene Therapy, JVS, and PLOS ONE. Additionally, he has taken on numerous leadership roles in his department and within the University of Chicago. He is a recognized field expert and national leader in the treatment of median arcuate ligament syndrome with patients from across the country and the world seeking his clinical expertise in this challenging diagnosis. During his tenure as faculty, Dr. Skelly has embodied the career trajectory of an academic surgeon at the University of Chicago by having a productive research career, being recognized as an inspired educator, and cultivating an international clinical practice.

AUTHORS/EDITORS/CONTRIBUTORS

CONTRIBUTORS

Matthew Allen MHA, RPhS, RVT, RVS
Department Chair / Allied Program Allied Health Programs
Santa Fe College
Gainesville, FL

Linda Antonucci RPhS, RVT, RDCS
President / Linda Antonucci Veins, LLC
Technical Director / Non-Invasive Vascular Laboratories / New York
Comprehensive Cardiology and Vein Center, Body Contour and Veins
West Milford, NJ

James Brorson MD
Associate Professor of Neurology / University of Chicago Medicine
Chicago, IL

Joseph A. Caprini MD, MS, FACS, RVT
Retired / NorthShore University HealthSystem / Evanston IL
Retired / Clinical Professor of Surgery / The University of Chicago Pritzker
School of Medicine
Chicago, IL

Robert De Jong RDMS, RDCS, RVT
Previously Radiology Technical Manager, Ultrasound
The Johns Hopkins Medical Institutions
Baltimore, MD

Brian Funaki MD
Professor of Radiology / Section Chief / Vascular and Interventional Radiology
University of Chicago Medicine
Chicago, IL

Marybeth Georges BS, RVT
Vascular Technologist / University of Chicago Medicine
Clinical Instructor / Rush University College of Health Sciences

Robert N. Gibson MB, BS, MD, FRANZCR, DDU
Professor / Department of Radiology / University of Melbourne
Royal Melbourne Hospital
Australia

Paula Heggerick RVT, RDMS, RPhS, FSVU
Vascular Consultant
Sarasota, FL

Laura Humphries BS, RVT, RPhS
Director of Accreditation / Vein Center
Intersocietal Accreditation Commission (IAC)
Ellicott City, MD

Marge Hutchisson LPN, RVT, RDCS
Director of Accreditation / IAC Vascular Testing
Ellicott City, MD

Jane Keating B.App.Sci Grad.Dip.US
Senior Sonographer / Department of Radiology; Royal Melbourne Hospital
Parkville, Victoria, Australia

Besnike Kashtanjeva MHS CDS, BS, RVT, Ced
Vascular Technologist / University of Chicago Medicine
Clinical Instructor / Rockford Career College, Diagnostic Medical Sonography
Program

Donna Kelly RPhS, RVT, RDMS
Ultrasound Coach / SonoCoach
Technical Director / Non-Invasive Vascular Laboratory
Middlesex Surgical Associates
Winchester, MA

Nicos Labropoulos PhD, DIC, RVT
Professor of Surgery and Radiology
Director, Vascular Laboratory
Department of Surgery
Stony Brook University Medical Center
Stony Brook, NY

Francis Loth PhD
Professor / Northeastern University
Boston, MA

Susan McCormick PhD
Former Assistant Professor / Vascular Research
University of Chicago Medical Center & Biological Sciences
Chicago, IL

Richard Palma BS, ACS, RCCS, RCS, RDCS, FACVP, FSDMS, FASE
Program Director and Clinical Coordinator
Duke School of Medicine Cardiac Sonography
Durham, NC

Donald Ridgway BA, RVT
Professor Emeritus / Grossmont College Cardiovascular Technology Program
El Cajon, CA

Heather Roberts RPh
Pharmacy Manager, Walgreen's
Prescott Valley, AZ

Troy Russo RVT, RVS, RDCS, RDMS
Director / Cardiology and Vascular
Flushing Hospital
Flushing, NY

Janice Hickey Scharf CRGS, RDMS, BSc. MRT
Chairperson / Canadian Association of Registered Diagnostic Ultrasound
Professionals (CARDUP)
Clinical Applications Specialist, Ultrasound
Philips Healthcare
Canada

Robert Scissions RVT, FSVU
Technical Director / Jobst Vascular Laboratory
Toledo, OH

Rita Shugart RN, RVT, FSVU
President, Shugart Consulting
Greensboro, NC

Faye Temple Grad. Dip. U/S (RMIT)
Sonographer in charge / Sonographer tutor at Royal Melbourne Institute of
Technology and Monash University
St. Vincent's Public Hospital
Fitzroy, Melbourne
Australia

Patrick Washko BSRT, RDMS, RVT
Technical Director / Rex Hospital (UNC Healthcare)
Vascular Diagnostic Center
Raleigh, NC

ACKNOWLEDGEMENTS

I wish to thank some of my mentors, those who saw something in me and took the time and energy to help me grow. First, thanks to Dr. Fileno Nicoletti, who in the early 80's asked me to open the hospital's first "Blood Flow Lab." I was consequently honored to be trained in my hometown of Chicago by Donna Blackburn and Drs. John Bergan and James Yao at Northwestern University's Blood Flow Lab. Secondly, my thanks to Dr. Morris Bernstein, one of my great teachers, who insisted I stay at his side through every vascular surgery and every follow-up visit; it was at that time that I received my intense education and training on the vascular patient. The third person I would like to thank is Dr. Joseph Caprini, who had the confidence to allow me to open his vascular laboratory and be a part of his research team along with Dr. Juan Arcelus.

Finally, thanks to my dear friend Dr. Nicos Labropoulos, who made it all fun and connected the loose ends for me.

I am grateful to all my colleagues through the years, especially the excellent medical and technical staff members at the University of Chicago Vascular Laboratory; without their help and guidance, this project could not have become a reality. This reference guide "took a village" to complete, and I am so blessed to have so many wonderful people in my village. Thank you to Laurie Lozanski for your amazing mind and hard work, and Chellie Buzzeo, our graphic designer whose endless dedication and energy made this project happen. Thank you to Denise Eggman, our medical illustrator who created the beautiful medical anatomy and expressive drawings, and the Scott women, who continually devote their lives to my continued lung transplant recovery.

A special thank you to my family and my dear husband, John, who unconditionally loved and encouraged me through the years, especially through this project.

– Gail

ANATOMY
1. Extracranial and Intracranial

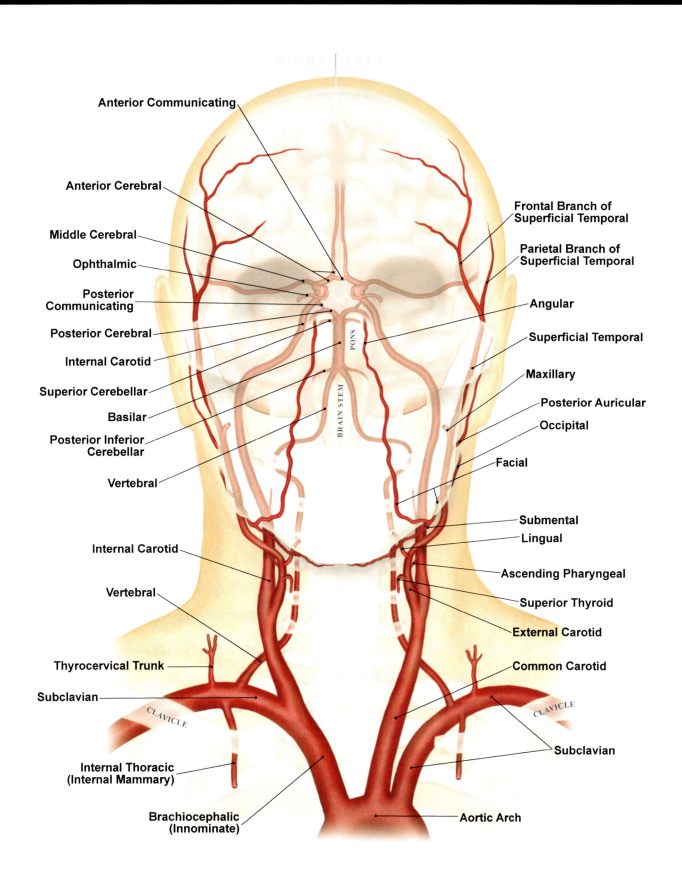

Fig. 1-1: *Frontal view of the extracranial and intracranial arterial system*

Extracranial Anatomy

Within the cerebrovascular arterial system, arteries are considered extracranial or intracranial. The extracranial vessels lay outside the skull or cranium. The intracranial vessels lay within the skull or cranium.

Table 1-1: Artery Classification

Common Carotid Artery	Extracranial Vessel
External Carotid Artery	Extracranial Vessel
Internal Carotid Artery	Extracranial & Intracranial Vessels
Vertebral Artery	Extracranial & Intracranial Vessels

Aortic Arch and Great Vessels

Three arteries supply the extracranial and intracranial arteries originating off the aortic arch:

- The first vessel and largest branch originating off the aortic arch is the brachiocephalic trunk (innominate artery), which is sometimes referred to as the brachiocephalic artery.
  - » The brachiocephalic trunk travels upward, bifurcating into the right subclavian and right common carotid arteries.
  - » The right brachiocephalic trunk and the proximal segments of the right common carotid and subclavian arteries are often rather tortuous. [1]
  - » The brachiocephalic trunk is approximately 4-5cm in length, branching off the aortic arch at the level of the upper border of the second right costal cartilage.
- The second vessel originating off the aortic arch is the left common carotid artery and the third vessel is the left subclavian artery.
- The brachiocephalic trunk, left common carotid and subclavian arteries are commonly referred to as the "great vessels." This is one of the very few places where there is an anatomical variation between the right and left sides of the body.
- The right subclavian can be tortuous and can mimic aneurysmal dilatation. This condition is often seen in elderly hypertensive females, sometimes referred to as a "buckling artery." [2]

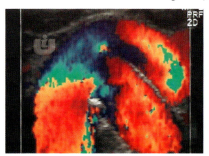

Fig. 1-3: *Buckled subclavian color flow displaying a disturbed flow pattern, due to a change in direction of the vessel rather than a hemodynamically significant stenosis.*

Fig. 1-2: *Internal and external carotid anatomy*

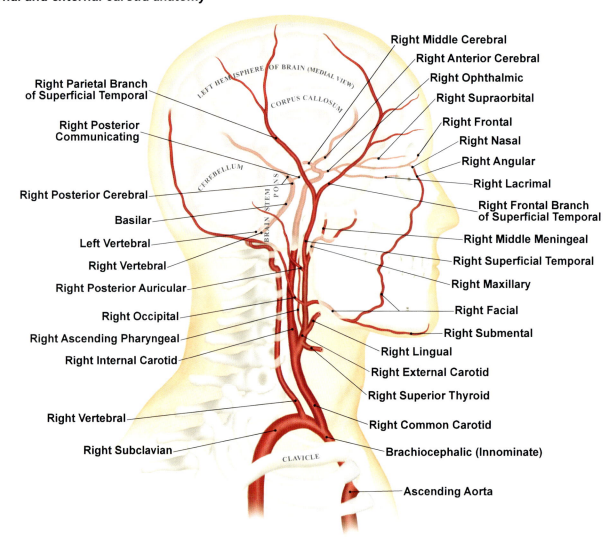

Subclavian Arteries
- The brachiocephalic trunk travels upward, bifurcating into the right subclavian and right common carotid arteries.
- The left subclavian artery originates from the aortic arch.
- Both subclavian arteries pass just above the dome of the pleural cavity (space surrounding the lungs).
- Branches of the subclavian arteries include the vertebral, thryocervical, dorsal scapular, mammary (internal thoracic) and costocervical. All of these branches are capable of providing collateral circulation to the arm in the event of an arterial occlusion.
- The subclavian arteries have three segments traveling:
  1) From its origin to the medial border of the anterior scalene (scalenus) muscle.
  2) Behind the anterior scalene muscle.
  3) From the lateral margin of the scalene muscle to the first rib's outer border.
- Due to the close proximity of the subclavian artery to the clavicle, first rib and scalene muscle, a compression syndrome (known as "thoracic outlet syndrome") can occur.
- The normal diameter of the subclavian is 3 to 5mm.

Common Carotid Artery
- The right common carotid artery (CCA) typically originates from the brachiocephalic trunk. The left CCA arises directly from the aortic arch.
- The CCA moves upward on the anterolateral aspect of the neck to the level of the thyroid cartilage (vertebrae C2-C3), where it bifurcates into the internal carotid artery (ICA) and external carotid artery (ECA).
- The normal diameter of the CCA is 0.75 to 1.25cm.

Note: Many labs have different definitions of location and configuration of the carotid bulb.

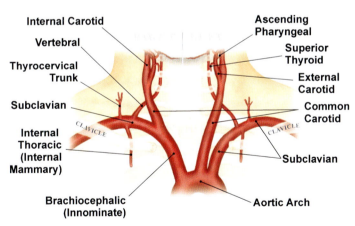

Fig. 1-4: *Common carotid artery and adjacent anatomy*

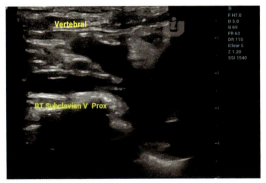

Fig. 1-5: *B-mode image of subclavian artery*

Carotid Bifurcation
- At the level of the carotid bifurcation the vessel becomes enlarged. This area, referred to as the *carotid bulb* or sinus, contains sensory nerve endings acting as baroreceptors. The *carotid body* (a baroreceptor) lies behind the artery and has a chemoreceptor function, making it sensitive to changes in pH, O_2 and CO_2 levels, so it can actually decrease the heart rate during an exam.

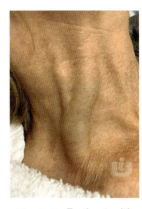

Fig. 1-6: *Patient with distension of the carotid vessels.*

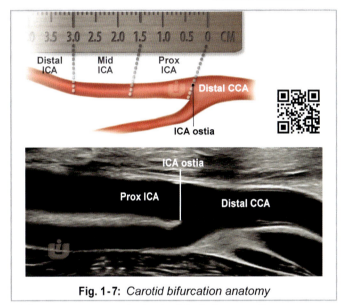

Fig. 1-7: *Carotid bifurcation anatomy*

- There is variation in the level of the bifurcation from side-to-side: [1]
  » 28% of carotid arteries bifurcate at the same level.
  » 50% of left neck bifurcations are higher than the right.
  » 22% of right neck bifurcations are higher than the left.
- Anatomical variations can occur at the level of the carotid bifurcation and can include the CCA, ICA, ECA or any combination of these arteries.
  » The usual anatomical configuration is that the ECA lay more medial and anterior to the ICA artery.
  » The most common variation is the ECA artery laying posterior and lateral to the ICA.
  » The second most common variation is the ECA laying posterior and medial to the ICA.
  » The third most common is the ECA and ICA lay side-by-side.
- The bifurcation is the most common location for atherosclerotic lesions to occur due to the complicated flow patterns associated with the configuration.

External Carotid Artery
- The external carotid artery (ECA) begins at the carotid bifurcation and travels upward terminating as the superficial temporal artery (STA).
- The ECA is smaller than the ICA and usually takes an anterior and medial course after the carotid bifurcation.

Fig. 1-8:
Variations of the external carotid artery [4]

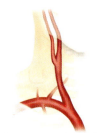
ECA runs anterior medial to the ICA.

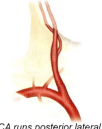
ECA runs posterior lateral to the ICA.

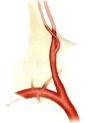
ECA runs posterior medial to the ICA.

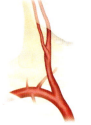
ECA runs medial anterior to the ICA.

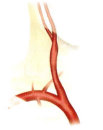
ECA and ICA side-by-side. Then the ECA runs lateral to the ICA.

Variations taken from Gerlock, A. et al. 1988 Applications of Non-invasive Vascular Techniques. Philadelphia Saunders p126.

- The ECA has several branches which supply the face, neck and skull:
  » **Anterior branches:**
    - **Superior thyroid:** branches off the anterior portion and near the origin of the ECA then courses downward to the thyroid.
    - **Lingual:** branches off the anterior ECA
    - **Facial:** branches off the anterior ECA, above the lingual artery.
  » **Posterior branches:**
    - **Occipital:** branches off the posterior portion of the ECA opposite the facial artery.
    - **Posterior auricular:** branches off the posterior portion of the ECA just distal to the maxillary artery.
  » **Ascending pharyngeal branch:**
    - Branches off the posterior ECA and supplies the pharynx.
  » **Terminal branches:**
    - **Superficial temporal artery (STA)** is the terminal ECA and divides into the frontal branch of the STA (anterior branch) and the parietal branch of the STA (posterior branch). The STA courses up the face just in front of the ear.
    - **Internal maxillary** is the terminal anterior branch of the STA.

The first major branch of the ECA is the superior thyroid artery. It helps distinguish the ECA from the ICA.

- ECA branches are important sources of collateral blood supply in carotid and vertebral disease. Common collateral pathways include:
  » Facial, maxillary and orbital branches
  » Superficial temporal artery and branches of the ophthalmic artery.
  » Ascending pharyngeal branches and muscular branches of the vertebral artery
- The normal ECA diameter ranges from 0.25 to 0.70cm.

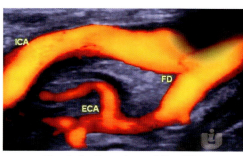
Fig. 1-9: *Branches of the ECA*

Internal Carotid Artery
- The ICA begins at the carotid bifurcation and moves upward as a single vessel until it enters the cranium and terminates, bifurcating into the middle cerebral artery (MCA) and anterior cerebral artery (ACA).
- The ICA is classified as both an extracranial and intracranial vessel.
- The ICA usually takes a posterior and lateral course after the carotid bifurcation.
- The ICA has no branches within the neck area.

Fig. 1-10: *External carotid artery anatomy*

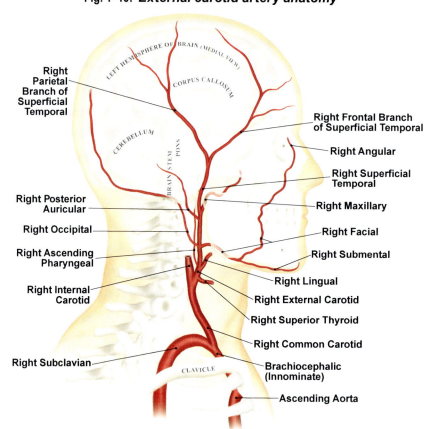

- Approximately 75% of the blood supply to the brain flows through the internal carotid arteries (200-400ml/min).
- The ICA supplies most of the anterior circulation of the cerebrum.
- The vessel's course can be described as tortuous, kinked, coiled, s-shaped, c-shaped, z-shaped, and u-shaped.
- The ICA diameter ranges from 0.5 to 1.0cm
- Variations result from embryologic, pathologic, and aging effects. [2] The three most common distortions are:
  » **Tortuosity:** multiple turns or twists of the vessel, s-shaped elongation or curvature. Typically congenital and asymptomatic.
  » **Kinking:** reveals a sharp angle of 90º or less usually located 2-4cm above the carotid bifurcation.
  » **Coiling:** occurs when the arterial segment forms a complete circle from its longitudinal axis.
- The most important difference between a tortuous, coiled and kinked vessel is that the kinked vessel is most often associated with symptoms of cerebral ischemia.
- The ophthalmic artery is considered the first branch of the ICA supplying the eye. This branch occurs at the level of the carotid siphon.
- The ICA is divided into four major segments:
  » **Cervical:** begins at the carotid bifurcation and terminates when the internal carotid artery enters the skull. This is the longest segment of the ICA.
  » **Petrous:** begins once the ICA enters the carotid canal and courses vertically and then anteromedially through the canal.
  » **Cavernous:** located between the two dural layers that form the floor and roof of the cavernous sinus. The ICA bends forward along the sphenoid sinus and then turns backward; this is the S-shaped curve known as the *carotid siphon*. The ophthalmic artery is located in this segment. The proximal portion of the ICA siphon is the parasellar segment, followed by the genu and the supraclinoid segments.
  » **Cerebral:** short segment which divides into the anterior and middle cerebral arteries.

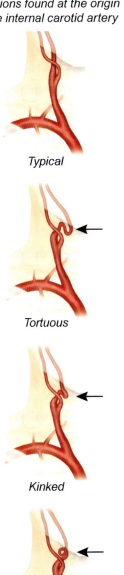

Fig. 1-11: Common variations found at the origin of the internal carotid artery

Typical

Tortuous

Kinked

Coiled

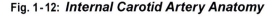

Fig. 1-12: *Internal Carotid Artery Anatomy*

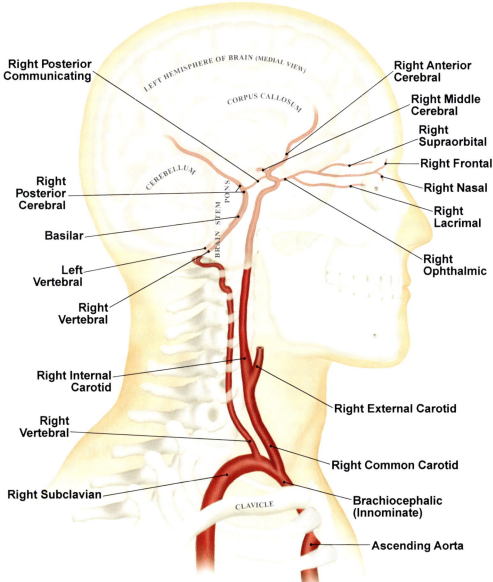

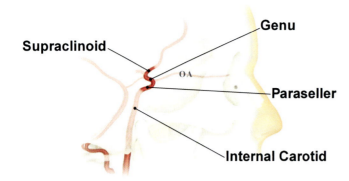

Fig. 1-13: *Anatomy of the carotid siphon*

Vertebral Artery

The cervical portion of the vertebral artery has several small branches to the spinal cord, vertebrae and adjacent muscles which are potential collateral channels in carotid or vertebral occlusive disease. These branches include:

» Posterior meningeal
» Anterior spinal
» Posterior spinal
» Posterior inferior cerebellar
» Bulbar

- The vertebral artery (VA) is the first branch of the subclavian artery and moves superiorly and posteriorly toward the cervical vertebrae through the foramina in the transverse process of the upper C6 vertbrae. [6]
- The right VA may arise as part of a trifurcation (vertebral, subclavian and common carotid arteries) of the brachiocephalic trunk. [7]
- The vertebral arteries are asymmetric in size with the left being dominant (larger) in approximately 50% of patients and the right being dominant in 25% of patients. There are equally sized vertebrals in the remaining 25% of patients. [9]
- The VA can be divided into four segments:
  » Extracranial
  » Intravertebral
  » Horizontal
  » Intracranial
- The vertebrals carry approximately 25% of the blood to the brain.

Intracranial Anatomy

The Circle of Willis includes: the internal carotid, middle cerebral, anterior cerebral and anterior communicating arteries. The vertebral arteries, basilar arteries, posterior cerebral arteries, and the posterior communicating arteries are also part of the Circle of Willis.

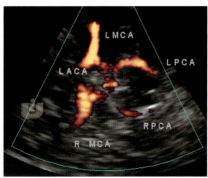

Fig. 1-14: *Circle of Willis*
Courtesy of Philips Healthcare

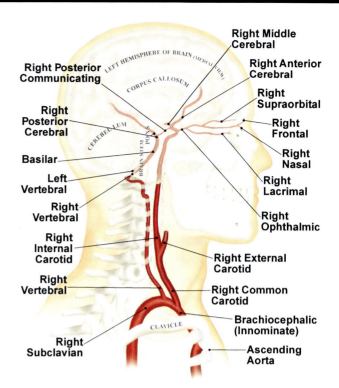

Fig. 1-15: *Anatomy of the Intracranial Circulation*

Ophthalmic Artery (OA)

- The ophthalmic artery is considered the first branch of the ICA and supplies the eye.
- Occurs at the level of the carotid siphon, and travels anterior through the optic canal to the orbit
- Can anastomose with the following branches of the ECA for collateral flow if the ICA becomes occluded:
  » Supraorbital artery
  » Frontal artery (supratrochlear artery)
  » Nasal artery
  » Laychrymal artery
- Collateral blood supply to the orbit is adequate to prevent blindness in the presence of an occluded ICA.[5]
- The normal OA diameter is approximately 1.4mm.

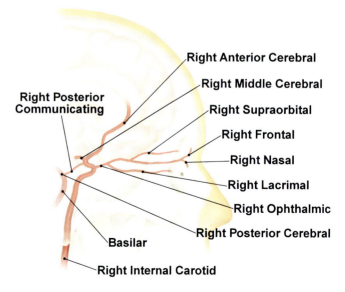

Fig. 1-16: *Anatomy of the Ophthalmic Artery (OA) with terminal branches*

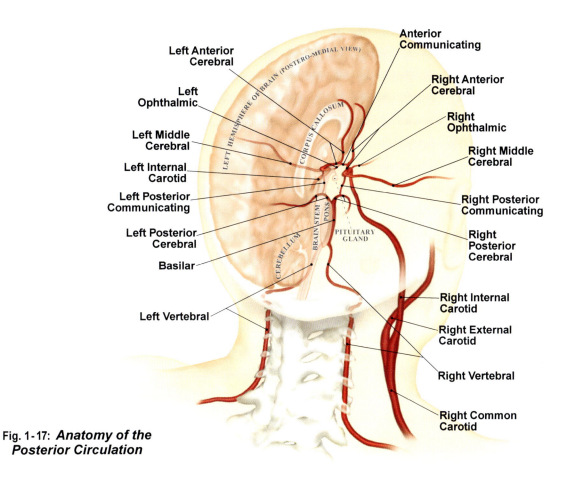

Fig. 1-17: *Anatomy of the Posterior Circulation*

Vertebral Artery

- The right and left vertebral arteries enter the skull through the foramen magnum and join to form a singular basilar artery. Together these arteries form the vertebrobasilar circulation, which then supplies the Circle of Willis.
- The largest branch of the VA is the posterior inferior cerebellar artery (PICA).
- The vertebral arteries supply most of the posterior circulation.
- The vertebral diameter ranges from 3 to 5mm.

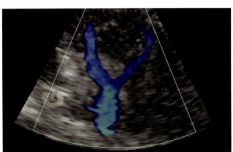

Fig. 1-18: *Vertebrobasilar arteries*

Basilar Artery

- Formed by the joining of the right and left vertebral arteries.
- Approximately 4mm in diameter and courses anteriorly and superiorly until its bifurcation into the right and left posterior cerebral arteries.
- Has many branches including the anterior inferior cerebellar, internal auditory and the superior cerebellar arteries.
- Can be tortuous, which is common in the elderly.
- The basilar diameter ranges from 2.9 to 3.4mm.

Circle of Willis

- Refers to the intracranial arteries which are in a polygonal shape.
- Located at the base of the brain and provides potential for collateral flow between the right and left cerebral hemispheres and the anterior (internal carotid) and posterior circulation (vertebrobasilar) to the brain.
- The anterior portion of the Circle of Willis includes the internal carotid arteries, middle cerebral arteries, anterior cerebral arteries and anterior communicating artery.
- The posterior portion of the Circle of Willis includes the vertebral arteries, basilar arteries, posterior cerebral arteries, and the posterior communicating arteries.
- A complete Circle of Willis is found in 20% of the population. [9]

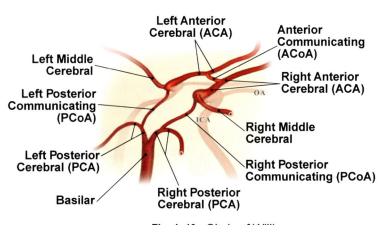

Fig. 1-19: *Circle of Willis*

Anterior Cerebral Artery

- The anterior cerebral artery (ACA) originates off the internal carotid artery and is divided into several segments:
  - » The A-1 segment of the ACA is the proximal, horizontal segment which connects to the contralateral A1 segment. This segment is sometimes referred to as the *precommunicating segment.*
  - » The A-2 segment is distal to the junction with the anterior communicating artery and courses into the cerebral hemispheres. A2 segment joins branches of the PCA. This segment is sometimes referred to as the *postcommunicating segment.*
- Distal segments include segments A-3 to A-5. Approximately 25% of the time, the anterior cerebral artery is found to be hypoplastic.
- The ACA (A-1) is absent in approximately 6% of patients.
- The normal anterior cerebral is approximately 2.6mm in diameter and is the smaller of the two terminal branches of the internal carotid artery.

Anterior Communicating Artery

- The anterior communicating artery (ACoA) is a short artery connecting the right and left A-1 segments of the anterior cerebral arteries.
- This artery runs medially and slightly anteriorly toward the middle of the brain.
- Tortuosity and kinking is noted in longer anterior communicating arteries.
- The ACoA is a potential collateral between the two sides of the anterior circulation.
- The ACoA is the most common site for intracranial aneurysm.
- The normal ACoA is approximately 1.5mm in diameter and can be duplicated.

Middle Cerebral Artery

- The largest terminal branch of the ICA supplies much of the lateral surface of the brain.
- The MCA courses horizontally, laterally and slightly anteriorly.
- The most proximal segment is referred to as the M-1 segment and bifurcates or trifurcates into the M2 and M3 segments.
- The M-2 segment is distal to the bifurcation and courses superior and posterior within the Sylvian fissure.
- The terminal branches of the middle cerebral artery anastomose with the terminal branches of the anterior cerebral and posterior cerebral arteries.
- The third most common site for congenital intracranial aneurysms is the MCA, accounting for about 25% of all intracranial aneurysms.
- The normal MCA is approximately 3.9mm in diameter and is the larger of the two terminal branches of the ICA. There are several perforators off the M1 segment.

Posterior Cerebral Artery

- The right and left posterior cerebral arteries originate off the basilar artery.
- The proximal portion of the posterior cerebral artery joins with the PCoA and is referred to as the P-1 segment.
- The P-1 courses anteriorly and laterally. This segment is sometimes referred to as the *precommunicating segment.*
- The P-2 segment begins distal to the junction with the posterior communicating artery (PCoA). The vessel then travels posteriorly around the lateral surface of the brain.
- The PCA (P-1) is absent in approximately 9% of patients.
- The normal P-1 segment is approximately 2.6mm in diameter.

Posterior Communicating Artery

- Originates from the ICA and courses posteriorly to join the posterior cerebral artery.
- The size of the PCoA can be variable and blood flow through this segment can be in either direction, depending on the configuration of the Circle of Willis and if the blood supply is from the ICA or VA. [8]
- The PCoA anatomy is variable and is often hypoplastic. A complete segment is only found in a small percentage of the population.
- The posterior communicating artery is the second most common site for intracranial aneurysm.
- The PCoA is an important collateral in cases of extensive bilateral occlusive disease.
- PCoA and contralateral PCA are absent in 9% of patients.
- The normal PCoA diameter is 1.9 to 2.1mm.

Anatomic Variations of the Circle of Willis and Collateral Pathways

- Anatomical variations of the Circle of Willis are common. Only 20% of the population is thought to have a "normal" Circle of Willis. [8, 9]
- The most common missing segments are the anterior communicating artery (ACoA), posterior communicating artery (PCoA), anterior cerebral artery (ACA) and the posterior cerebral artery (PCA). These vessels can be hypoplastic, aplastic or atretic. [8]
- The ACA has several possible variations:
  - » The A1 segment of the ACA has variable courses; horizontal, ascending or descending and can be tortuous. [1]
  - » Complete absence of the A1 segment is not uncommon. This condition is reported in the literature to occur in approximately 6% - 25% of patients and is also known as a "hypoplastic" or "atretic" A1 segment. [2]
  - » The size of the A1 segment and the ACoA should be inversely proportionate, (e.g., a hypoplastic A1 segment exists with a larger ACoA). [2]
  - » The Artery of Huebner is commonly a major branch of the A2 segment (80% of cases), but can also originate from the distal A1 segment. [9]
  - » The ACoA may be duplicated or have multiple channels.
- The PCA can be supplied from the ICA, instead of the BA. This is known as a "fetal origin" of the PCA. The prevalence of this variation is approximately 15-22%. [9]
- The vertebral arteries vary in length. In approximately 90% of cases, one VA is larger than the other.[8] The left VA is often the larger or dominant vertebral artery.[10]

Collateral Pathways

- There are three categories of intracranial collateral circulation: the Circle of Willis, ICA-ECA network and the small interarterial communications.
- The primary collateral circulation is via the Circle of Willis and the meningeal anastomoses. (compensatory circulation)[8]
- The most common collateral connection between the left and right hemispheres is the ACoA.[8]
- The PCoA is a common collateral pathway, connecting the carotid and basilar vessels.[8]
- The second most common collateral pathway is the ICA-ECA network (prewillisian anastomoses), in which branches of the internal and external carotid arteries can join to provide blood flow.

- Examples of the ICA-ECA pathways are:
  » Back-front pathway would be vertebrobasilar arteries via the posterior cerebral and posterior communicating arteries (between basilar and right or left common carotid artery).
  » The ophthalmic artery is the common collateral pathway in the event of internal carotid artery obstruction via the ICA-ECA pathway.
  » Supraorbital and/or frontal arteries to superficial temporal artery; usually on or across the forehead.
  » Nasal artery to facial or angular artery.
  » Nasal artery via the angular artery or infraorbital artery.
  » Ophthalmic artery (ICA) to middle meningeal artery (ECA).
- The third category of intracranial collateral circulation is the small interarterial communications called the Rete Mirabile or the "*wonderful net.*" This network runs across the subdural space from the dural arteries to arteries on the surface of the brain.

REFERENCES

1. Cronenwett J, Johnston, K., (2005) in Rutherford's Vascular Surgery Saunders; 7 edition. Philadelphia Saunders Elsevier.
2. Cronenwett J, Johnston, K., (2010) in Rutherford's Vascular Surgery Saunders; 7 edition. Philadelphia Saunders Elsevier.
3. Size, G, Laubach, M et al. Color Flow Imaging For Diagnosis Of Innominate And Carotid Artery Buckling, Video Journal of Color Flow Imaging; Vol 2, No. 3; pp 124-128, 1992.
4. Gerlock, A. et al. (1988) Applications of Non-invasive Vascular Techniques. Philadelphia Saunders p.126.
5. Uflacker, R. (1997) Arteries of the head and neck. In Atlas of Vascular Anatomy: An angiographic Approach P. 11. Baltimore Wolters Kluwer Lippincott Williams & Wilkins
6. Uflacker, R. (2007) Arteries of the head and neck. In Atlas of Vascular Anatomy: An angiographic Approach pp 18-19. Baltimore Wolters Kluwer Lippincott Williams & Wilkins.
7. Uflacker, R. (1997) Arteries of the head and neck. In Atlas of Vascular Anatomy: An angiographic Approach (5-79). Baltimore Wolters Kluwer Lippincott Williams & Wilkins
8. The Handbook of Transcranial Doppler McCartney JP, Lukes-Thomas KM, Gomez CR. (1997). Handbook of Transcranial Doppler. New York. Springer-Verlag
9. Naylor AR, Markose G. (2010) Cerebrovascular disease: diagnostic evaluation, In Cronenwett J, Johnston, K., (2005) in Rutherford's Vascular Surgery Saunders; (7 edition) (Chapter 93) Saunders Elsevier.
10. Cronenwett J, Johnston, K., (2010) in Rutherford's Vascular Surgery Saunders; 7th edition. Philadelphia Saunders Elsevier.

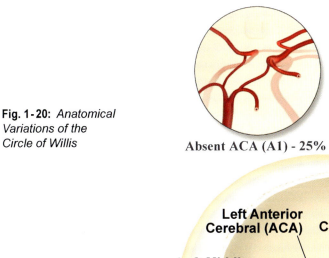

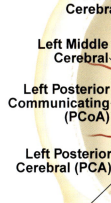

Fig. 1-20: *Anatomical Variations of the Circle of Willis*

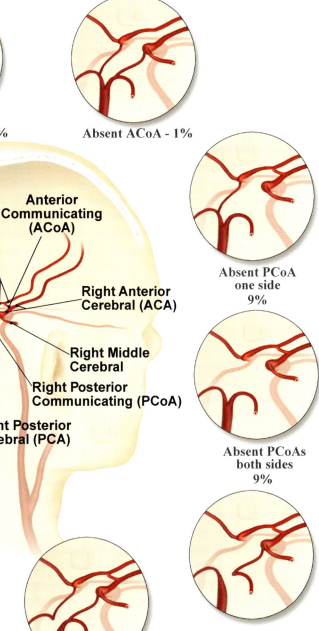

ANATOMY
2. Abdominal Venous

Fig. 2-1: *Abdominal Venous System*

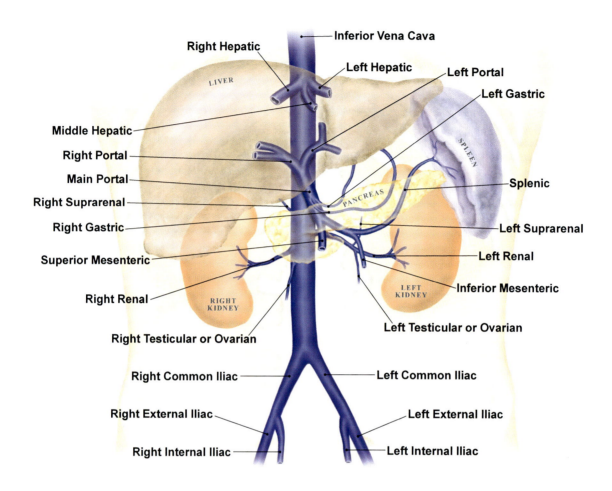

This anatomy is described from the pelvis to the abdomen.
Note: The iliac veins are described in detail later in this chapter.
- The external iliac vein (EIV) drains the inferior portion of the abdominal wall, as well as the legs.
- The internal iliac vein (IIV) drains the pelvis and joins the EIV to form the common iliac vein (CIV).
- The right and left CIV join to form the inferior vena cava (IVC). The left iliac vein is usually longer. [10]
- The IVC is the largest vein of the body; approximately 17.2mm (infrarenal) in diameter during quiet respiration and returns blood flow from the lower extremities and abdomen back to the heart (right atrium).
- For the purposes of the ultrasound examination, the inferior vena cava is divided into three regions:
  » **Suprahepatic**: superior to the liver
  » **Intrahepatic**: includes tributaries from the liver
  » **Infrahepatic**: inferior to the liver and to the level to the iliac bifurcation

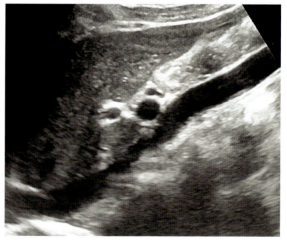

Fig. 2-2: *Longitudinal view of the IVC.*

The IVC has numerous tributaries including:

- **Hepatic veins**: return blood flow from the liver. Each hepatic vein drains different portions of the liver:
  » Right hepatic
  » Middle hepatic
  » Left hepatic
- **Portal veins**: deliver deoxygenated blood from the stomach, pancreas, spleen, gallbladder and intestines to the hepatic venous system. There are several branches. The main portal vein divides into the:
  » Right portal vein
  » Left portal vein
- **Gastric veins:** return blood flow from the stomach
- **Splenic vein:** returns blood flow from the spleen and receives blood from the stomach, pancreas and inferior mesenteric vein
- **Phrenic veins**: return blood flow from the diaphragm
- **Suprarenal veins**: return blood from the adrenal glands (Note: the right suprarenal vein terminates in the IVC and the left suprarenal vein terminates in the left renal vein).
- **Superior mesenteric vein:** returns blood flow from the intestines and stomach
- **Renal veins:** (right and left) return blood flow from the kidneys. The right and left renal veins (RV) drain into the inferior vena cava.
- **Inferior mesenteric vein**: returns blood flow from the colon
- **Testicular or ovarian veins:** return blood from either the testes or the ovaries.
- **Lumbar veins:** return blood flow from the posterior abdominal wall.

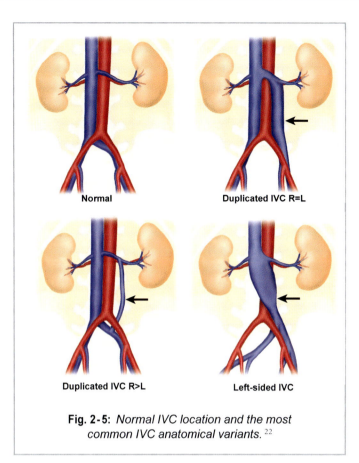

Fig. 2-5: *Normal IVC location and the most common IVC anatomical variants.* [22]

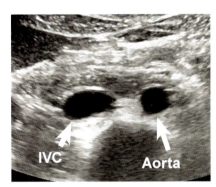

Fig. 2-3: *Transverse view of the IVC and the aorta.*

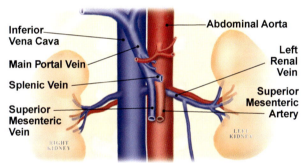

Fig. 2-6: *Longitudinal view demonstrating the LRV coursing between the SMA and aorta.*

Renal Veins

- The course of the left and right renal veins is highly variable in patients. There are many anatomical variants possible as these veins travel away from the kidneys draining the blood flow from the kidney and other organ systems, including the gonads, adrenal glands, and diaphragm. [10]
- The average length of the right renal vein is 2-2.5cm which is much shorter than the average length of the left, about 8.5cm. [10]
- One difference between the right and left renal veins is that the left rein vein usually communicates with other veins like the gonadal or adrenal [10]
- The left renal vein (LRV) drains the kidney. The LRV runs between the abdominal aorta and superior mesenteric artery.
- Tributaries of the LRV include:
  » Left gonadal vein
  » Left adrenal vein
  » Left inferior phrenic vein
- In the majority of the population, the LRV drains into the IVC.

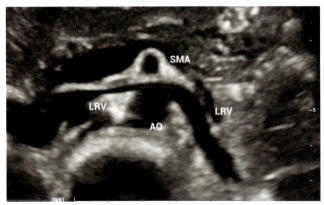

Fig. 2-4: *Mid visceral anatomy. Note how the LRV courses between the aorta and SMA.*

Left renal vein: possible points of extrinsic compression and anatomical variants

- SMA/aorta
  - » Most left renal veins course between the SMA and the aorta, which could create compression of the LRV between the SMA and the aorta.

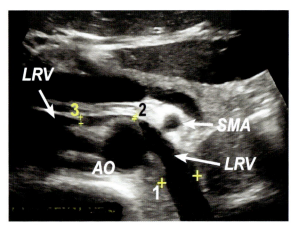

Fig. 2-7: *LRV coursing between the aorta and SMA to its confluence with the IVC appears to be compressed at points #2-3.*

- Aorta/spine
  - » In a small population, the LRV courses posterior to the aorta and anterior to the spine. This could create compression of the LRV between the aorta and spine.
- Left kidney/spine
  - » Stretching of the LRV over the aorta can occur due to the left kidney position. This could create a narrowing of the LRV and cause stenosis.
- The renal hilum may act as a venous reservoir for the left renal vein.

Left renal vein anatomical variants [11]

- » Circumaortic LRV: Where two or more renal veins form a ring around the aorta before entering the IVC. (-3.5% prevalence)
- » Retroaortic LRV: The LRV courses between the aorta and vertebra before entering the IVC. (3% prevalence) This variant is the easiest to appreciate with ultrasound.
- » Multiple left renal veins entering the IVC. (2.1% prevalence)

Left Renal Vein Anatomical Variants

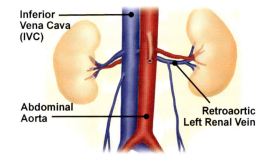

Fig. 2-8: *LRV coursing posterior to the aorta*

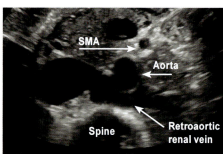

Fig. 2-9: *Retroaortic LRV, where the vein is located between the aorta and the spine.*

Hepatoportal

- The liver can be divided into right and left lobes.
- The splenic vein and superior mesenteric veins converge to form the main portal vein.
- Nutrient rich blood is delivered from the splenic and mesenteric veins.

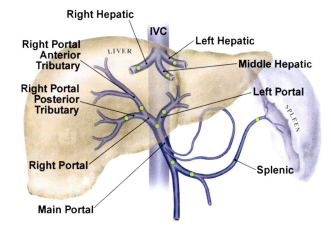

Fig. 2-10: *Hepatoportal veins*

The normal diameter of the main portal vein is 8-12mm in diameter. The hepatic veins can measure up to 10mm in diameter.

- The blood flow from the liver drains through the hepatic veins (right, left, and middle) and into the IVC.
- The liver has a dual blood supply.
  - » 80% is delivered via the main portal vein (nutrient rich/oxygen poor).
  - » 20% is delivered via the hepatic artery (oxygen rich).
- Portal and hepatic blood mix within the portal sinusoids of the liver.
- Each hepatic vein drains different portions of the liver.
- The main portal vein divides into the right and left portal vein branches at the edge of the liver. These branches then further divide in order to feed each segment of the liver.

Abdominal Venous 13

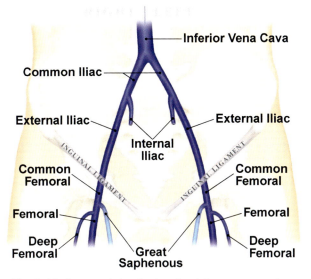

Fig. 2-11: *Lower abdominal and pelvic venous system*

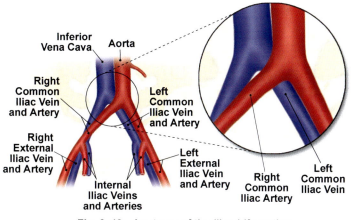

Fig. 2-13: *Anatomy of the iliac bifurcation*

- The tributaries of the EIV are:
  » Inferior epigastric
  » Deep iliac circumflex

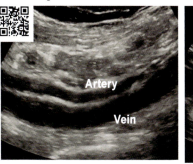 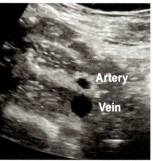

Fig. 2-14: *EIV in longitudinal and transverse views demonstrating pulsatile, repetitive compression of the EIV by the overlying external iliac artery. This repetitive compression can cause damage to the walls of the vein, disrupting flow.*

Iliac Veins
Common Iliac Veins
- The CIV is formed at the level of the sacroiliac joint where the IIV confluences with the EIV.
- The CIVs pass upward to the fifth lumbar vertebra to come together to form the IVC. [5]
- Tributaries of the CIVs include the: [6]
  » Iliolumbar veins
  » Lateral sacral (sometimes)

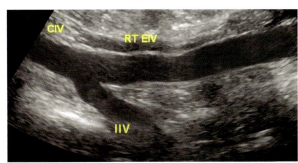

Fig. 2-12: *The confluence of the IIV and EIV to form the CIV on B-mode image.*

Internal Iliac Veins (IIV) [10]
- Runs medially or laterally in the pelvis.
- Drains blood from the parietal and visceral plexus (intrapelvic venous system)
- There are no venous valves typically in the IIV.
- The tributaries of the IIV include the:
  » Middle rectal veins   » Inferior vesical veins
  » Pudendal veins   » Superior vesical veins
  » Obturator veins

External Iliac Veins (EIV): [7]
- Begin above the level of the inferior margin of the inguinal ligament.
- Return blood from the lower extremities and the inferior section of the abdominal wall.
- The EIV may have 1-2 venous valves. [10]

Iliac vein anatomical landmarks and points of possible extrinsic compression:
- Umbilicus (landmark)
  » The right CIV can be identified by placing the ultrasound transducer just to the right of the umbilicus.
  » The left CIV can be identified by placing the transducer at an oblique angle just below the umbilicus. [9]
- Spine/aorta
  » The left CIV courses just anterior to the spine at the level of the aortic bifurcation.
- Iliac arteries
  » The common and external iliac arteries can be a source of extrinsic compression on the underlying iliac veins. These forms of extrinsic compression are referred to as Nonthrombotic Iliac Vein Lesions (NIVLs).

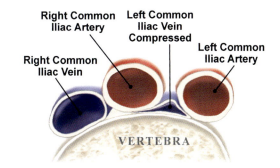

Fig. 2-15: *Cross section view of the left CIV being compressed by the right and left CIAs.* Adapted from www.scgvs.com

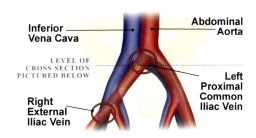

Fig. 2-16: *Most Frequently Occurring NIVLs.*

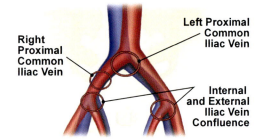

Fig. 2-17: *Less Frequently Occurring NIVLs.*

Note the slight shift in the position of the aorta and the IVC creating additional sites of potential obstruction.

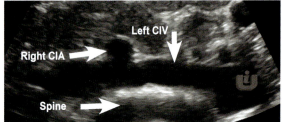

Fig. 2-18: *Left CIV as it courses between the right CIA and the spine.*

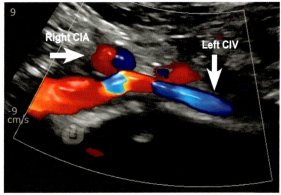

Fig. 2-19: *Color flow showing CIV coursing beneath the right and left CIA.*

Veins Associated with Pelvic Vein Disorders

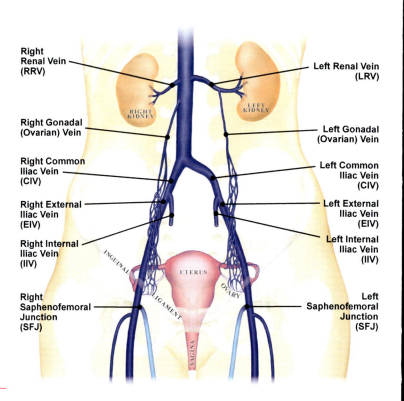

Fig. 2-20: *Primary venous anatomy of the pelvis. Note: Gonadal is a general term for the ovarian or testicular vein.*

Pelvic venous disorders are a collection of venous pathologies including obstruction and/or reflux within the venous system of the pelvis.

It is essential to have a detailed knowledge of pelvic venous anatomy and physiology to have a complete understanding of pelvic venous disorders. For more information, see the *Inside Ultrasound Venous Vascular Reference Guide, 2nd Edition.*

insideultrasound.com

REFERENCES

1. Gray, H. (1977). The portal system of veins. In Pick TP & Howden R. (Eds.), *Gray's Anatomy* (617-619). New York: Bounty Books
2. Netter FH. (2003). Abdomen. In *Atlas of Human Anatomy 3rd ed.* (239-338). Terterboro: Icon Learning Systems.
3. Netter FH. (2003). Pelvis and perineum. In A*tlas of Human Anatomy 3rd ed.* (339-400). Terterboro: Icon Learning Systems.
4. Tortora, G. J., & Anagnostakos, N.P. (Eds.). (1990). The cardiovascular system: vessels and routes. In *Principles of Anatomy and Physiology, 6th ed.* (605-650) New York, NY: Harper & Row Publishers.
5. Uflacker R. (1997). Abdominal aorta and branches. In *Atlas of Vascular Anatomy: An Angiographic Approach.* (405-604). Baltimore: Wolters Kluwer Lippincott Williams & Wilkins.
6. Uflacker R. (1997). Arteries of the pelvis. In *Atlas of Vascular Anatomy: An Angiographic Approach.* (605-634). Baltimore: Wolters Kluwer Lippincott Williams & Wilkins.
7. Uflacker R. (1997). Veins of the abdomen and pelvis. In *Atlas of Vascular Anatomy: An Angiographic Approach.* (635-729). Baltimore: Wolters Kluwer Lippincott Williams & Wilkins.
8. Meissner, M. H., Khilnani, N. M., Labropoulos, N., et al (2021). The Symptoms-Varices-Pathophysiology classification of pelvic venous disorders: A report of the American Vein & Lymphatic Society International Working Group on Pelvic Venous Disorders. Journal of Vascular Surgery. Venous and Lymphatic Disorders, 9(3), 568–584. https://doi.org/10.1016/j.jvsv.2020.12.084
9. Labropoulos N. (2017). *A standardized ultrasound approach to pelvic congestion syndrome. Phlebology.* Oct;32(9):608-619. doi: 10.1177/0268355516677135. Epub 2016 Oct 31. PMID: 27799418
10. Dao DPD, Le PH. Anatomy, Abdomen and Pelvis: Veins. [Updated 2023 Mar 5]. In: StatPearls [Internet]. Treasure Island (FL): StatPearls Publishing; 2023 Jan-. Available from: https://www.ncbi.nlm.nih.gov/books/NBK554574/

ANATOMY
3. Abdominal Arterial

- The abdominal aorta begins as the descending aorta and crosses the diaphragm.
- For the purposes of the ultrasound examination, the abdominal aorta is divided into three regions:
  » **Proximal aorta:** Diaphragm to the origin of the superior mesenteric artery
  » **Mid aorta:** Superior mesenteric artery to the renal arteries
  » **Distal aorta:** Renal arteries to the aortic bifurcation
  » add a bullet missing from the original bible on page 10
- The aorta normally decreases (tapers) in diameter from the diaphragm to the aortic bifurcation.

Some labs use alternative terms, dividing the aorta into the suprarenal, juxtarenal and infrarenal aorta.

- The abdominal aorta has five main branches:
  » **Celiac artery:** (also known as the celiac trunk or celiac axis) supplies the liver, gallbladder, stomach, intestines and pancreas. There are three branches of the celiac artery:
    • Splenic artery
    • Common hepatic artery
    • Left gastric artery
  » **Superior mesenteric artery** (SMA): Supplies the intestines and pancreas.
  » **Renal arteries (right and left):** Supplies the kidneys and adrenal glands.
  » **Inferior mesenteric artery** (IMA): Supplies the colon and rectum.

Celiac Artery
The celiac artery (CA) and the superior mesenteric artery (SMA) originate from the anterior wall of the suprarenal aorta. The CA is the first branch off the abdominal aorta.

Abdominal Arterial System

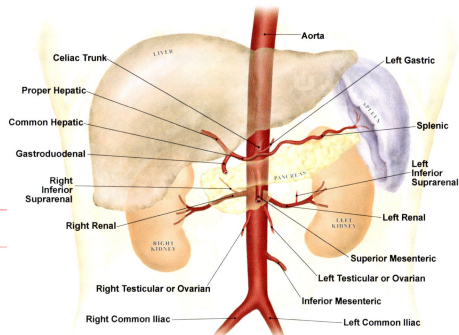

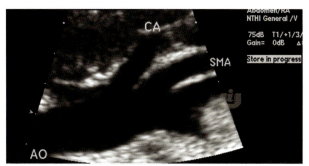

Fig. 3-1: *Celiac and superior mesenteric arteries-origin off the proximal aorta with B-mode.*

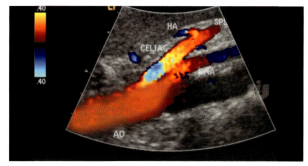

Fig. 3-2: *Celiac and superior mesenteric arteries-origin off the proximal aorta with and color.*

The term "splanchnic" is sometimes used to refer to the visceral arteries.

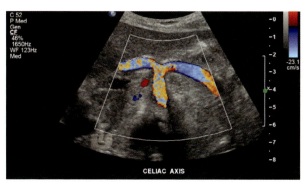

Fig. 3-3: *Transverse celiac trunk with common hepatic and splenic arterial branches.*

Courtesy of Philips Healthcare

- The celiac trunk or celiac artery (CA) divides into the common hepatic (HA) and the splenic (SA) arteries. This division occurs 1-2cm from the celiac artery origin. A third branch, the left gastric artery, is usually too small to visualize on duplex, but may be documented if noted.

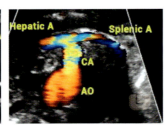

Fig. 3-4: *Transverse celiac trunk with common hepatic and splenic arterial branches (left). Shown also with color flow (right).*

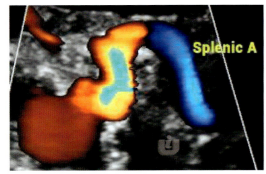

Fig. 3-5: *Transverse images of the splenic artery.*

Superior Mesenteric Artery (SMA)
- The superior mesenteric artery (SMA) originates from the anterior wall of the suprarenal aorta about 1-2cm distal to the celiac trunk.
- Several of the areas the CA and SMA supply blood to the duodenum and small bowel (intestines).
- There is normally an extensive network of collaterals between the mesenteric vessels which enlarge when there is a stenosis or occlusion present.
  » The main collateral channel between the CA and SMA is the gastroduodenal artery to the pancreaticoduodenal arteries.
  » The Arc of Riolan can connect the SMA and IMA and is an important pathway when there is a stenosis or occlusion in either artery.

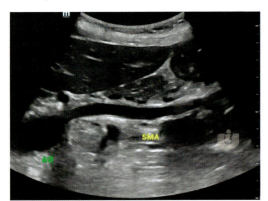

Fig. 3-6: *The SMA course parallel to the abdominal aorta in the longitudinal plane.*

Anatomic Variations of the Celiac/Mesenteric Arteries
- The CA and SMA may share a common origin or trunk.
- Hepatic artery origin off the SMA
- Hepatic artery originating off the abdominal aorta

Renal Arteries (right and left)
- The right and left main renal arteries (RA) originate laterally from the abdominal aorta, immediately inferior to the superior mesenteric artery.

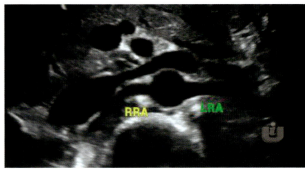

Fig. 3-7: *The right and left RA originate inferior to the SMA.*

- The right RA is longer than the left and is posterior to the inferior vena cava and right RV.
- The left RA lies posterior to the left renal vein.
- The renal artery divides into the segmental arteries at the origin of the kidney.
- The segmental arteries give rise to the interlobar arteries in the kidney parenchyma.
- The parenchyma is divided into the medulla and cortex. The medulla is adjacent to the renal sinus and pyramids and the cortex is the most peripheral portion of the parenchyma, located between the medulla and renal capsule.
- Near the medulla and cortex junction, the arcuate arteries come off at right angles. As the arcuate arteries pass around the pyramids, they give rise to the interlobular arterioles.

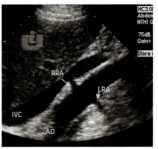 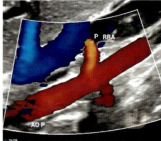

Fig. 3-8: *The right and left renal arteries can sometimes be visualized from the back of the patient.*

Anatomic Variations of the Kidney and Renal Arteries
- A "horseshoe kidney" is a congenital abnormality which results in the fusion of both kidneys. Beginning the scan with a midline abdominal approach is suggested for this situation.
- In 20-30% of patients, one to three accessory renal arteries may be present, especially on the left side. They usually originate from the aorta below the main renal artery and often enter the kidney directly.
- A renal artery may also branch anywhere before entering the kidney.

The right kidney is lower than the left kidney due to the R-lobe of the liver.

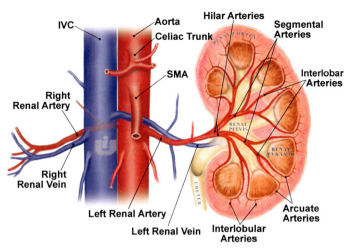

Fig. 3-9: *Renal vessel anatomy*

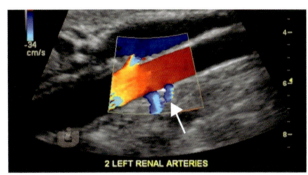

Fig. 3-10: *Left accessory renal artery (Note second left-sided branch off the aorta)*

Image courtesy of GE Healthcare-Ultrasound Division

Inferior Mesenteric Artery (IMA)

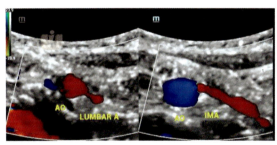

Fig. 3-11: *The IMA and lumbar arteries both branch off the distal aorta; be careful not to confuse the lumbar arteries for the IMA (left). The IMA is located approximately 3-5cm above the iliac artery bifurcation (right).*

- The inferior mesenteric artery (IMA) originates below the renal arteries at the left anteriolateral abdominal aorta, 3-5cm above the iliac bifurcation.
- In transverse, the artery comes off at approximately the 1-2 o'clock position.
- The IMA has multiple collateral pathways: middle colic branch of the SMA to the marginal artery of Drummond or the middle hemorrhoidal artery (branch of the internal iliac).
- The SMA and IMA supply blood to the colon and proximal rectum.

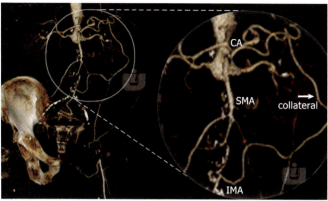

Fig. 3-12: *Collateral pathway: marginal artery of Drummond*

Iliac Arteries

- The abdominal aorta bifurcates into the right and left common iliac arteries (CIA) at the level of the umbilicus.
- The common iliac arteries travel distally and bifurcate into the internal iliac artery (IIA) and external iliac artery (EIA).
- The EIA travels laterally and enters the thigh at the inguinal ligament where it becomes the common femoral artery (CFA).

The right common iliac artery may compress the left iliac vein.

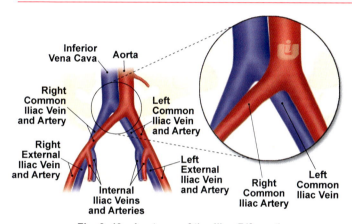

Fig. 3-13: *Anatomy of the Iliac Bifurcation*

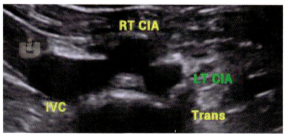

Fig. 3-14: *The aorta bifurcates into the CIAs at the level of the umbilicus.*

REFERENCES

1. Gray, H. (1977). The portal system of veins. In Pick TP & Howden R. (Eds.), *Gray's Anatomy* (617-619). New York: Bounty Books
2. Netter FH. (2003). Abdomen. In *Atlas of Human Anatomy 3rd ed.* (239-338). Terterboro: Icon Learning Systems.
3. Netter FH. (2003). Pelvis and perineum. In *Atlas of Human Anatomy 3rd ed.* (339-400). Terterboro: Icon Learning Systems.
4. Tortora, G. J., & Anagnostakos, NP. (Eds.). (1990). The cardiovascular system: vessels and routes. In *Principles of Anatomy and Physiology, 6th ed.* (605-650) New York, NY: Harper & Row Publishers.
5. Uflacker R. (1997). Abdominal aorta and branches. In *Atlas of Vascular Anatomy: An Angiographic Approach.* (405-604). Baltimore: Wolters Kluwer Lippincott Williams & Wilkins.
6. Uflacker R. (1997). Arteries of the pelvis. In *Atlas of Vascular Anatomy: An Angiographic Approach.* (605-634). Baltimore: Wolters Kluwer Lippincott Williams & Wilkins.
7. Uflacker R. (1997). Veins of the abdomen and pelvis. In *Atlas of Vascular Anatomy: An Angiographic Approach.* (635-729). Baltimore: Wolters Kluwer Lippincott Williams & Wilkins.
8. Meissner, M. H., Khilnani, N. M., Labropoulos, N., et al (2021). The Symptoms-Varices-Pathophysiology classification of pelvic venous disorders: A report of the American Vein & Lymphatic Society International Working Group on Pelvic Venous Disorders. Journal of Vascular Surgery. Venous and Lymphatic Disorders, 9(3), 568–584. https://doi.org/10.1016/j.jvsv.2020.12.084
9. Labropoulos N. (2017). A standardized ultrasound approach to pelvic congestion syndrome. Phlebology. Oct;32(9):608-619. doi: 10.1177/0268355516677135. Epub 2016 Oct 31. PMID: 27799418

ANATOMY
4. Lower Extremity Venous

Fig. 4-1: Comprehensive Venous Anatomy

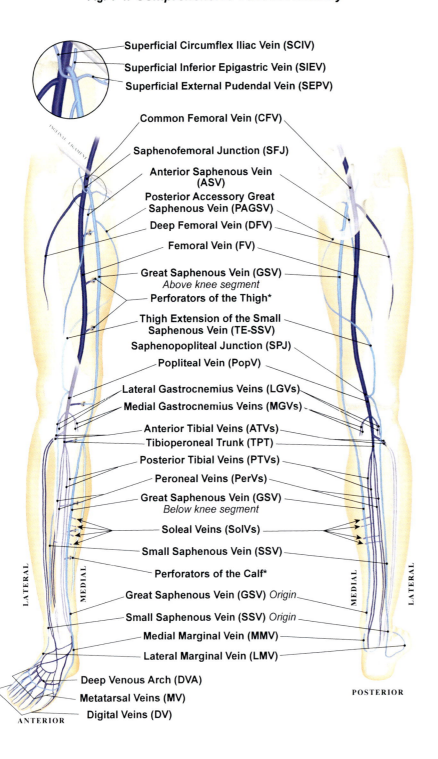

*The perforating veins are too numerous to illustrate. For a more comprehensive list and a schematic representation of the topography see: Caggiati et al [2]

Lower Extremity Venous System [1-3,8,10-13,17]

Three major components of the lower extremity venous system:
- Deep system
- Superficial system
- Communicating system

These systems are located in two main compartments:
- Deep compartment, which is confined by the muscular fascia and contains the deep veins.
- Superficial compartment, which is confined by the muscular fascia and superficially by the dermis.

The term tributary is used to describe a vein that joins with a superficial vein. Superficial veins refer to the main trunk of the GSV, ASV, and SSV.

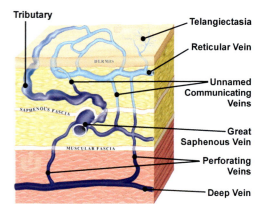

Fig. 4-1: Named and unnamed veins of the superficial compartments.

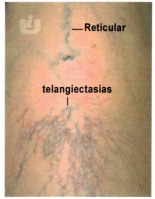

Fig. 4-2: Reticular vein feeding a cluster of Telangiectasias. *Photos courtesy of Linda Antonucci*

Reticular veins are larger than spider veins and are below the skin.

Telangiectasias are also known as spider veins.

Table 4-1: **Nomenclature of the Lower Extremity Deep and Superficial Veins** [1-5, 7, 10, 14, 15, 18, 21, 23, 31, 32]	
Deep Veins	**Superficial Veins**
Thigh • Common Femoral Vein (CFV) • Femoral Vein (FV) • Deep Femoral Vein (DFV)	• Great Saphenous Vein (GSV) • Anterior Saphenous Vein (ASV) • Posterior Accessory Great Saphenous Vein (PAGSV) • Anterior Thigh Circumflex Vein (ATCV) • Posterior Thigh Circumflex Vein (PTCV) • Small Saphenous Vein (SSV) • Thigh Extension of the Small Saphenous Vein (TE-SSV)
Knee • Popliteal Vein (PopV)	
Calf • Anterior Tibial Veins (ATVs) • Tibial Peroneal Trunk (TPT) • Posterior Tibial Veins (PTVs) • Peroneal Veins (PerVs)	

Sural Veins
• Soleal veins (SolVs)
• Gastrocnemius veins (GVs)
  » Medial gastrocnemius veins (MGVs)
  » Lateral gastrocnemius veins (LGVs)	

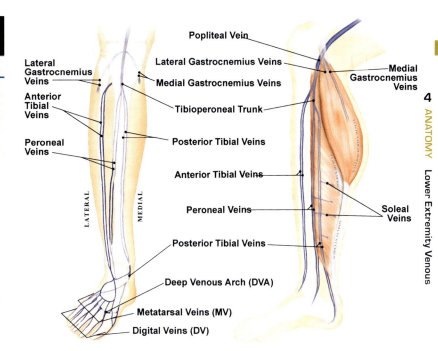

Deep Veins

Venous return or drainage begins at the foot. When describing the lower extremity venous anatomy, it will be described from the foot to the pelvis.
- Deep veins have an accompanying artery.
- Deep calf veins are paired.

Deep Veins of the Foot and Calf [8, 14, 15, 16, 28, 51]

- The deep plantar digital veins drain into the deep plantar metatarsal veins.
- The medial and lateral plantar veins cross the foot to form the deep plantar arch.
- The deep dorsal digital veins drain into the deep dorsal metatarsal veins from which the pedal vein originates.
- Anterior tibial veins (ATVs) are a continuation of the pedal vein. They travel superiorly between the tibia and fibula.
- The peroneal veins (PerVs) originate in the foot and ascend behind the fibula along the lateral aspect of the calf.
- The PTVs join to form a common tibial trunk. The PerVs join to form a common peroneal trunk. The common tibial and common peroneal trunks unite to form the origin of the tibioperoneal trunk. The TPT is a short segment of vein in the upper third of the calf.
- ATVs join to form a common anterior tibial trunk that unites with the tibioperoneal trunk to form the popliteal vein (PopV).

The term confluence is used when two or more veins join together to form a single vein.

Fig. 4-3: *Deep and intramuscular veins of the calf and foot. The gastrocnemius and soleal veins are intramuscular veins of the calf. The gastrocnemius veins are paired with an artery and drain into the popliteal vein. The soleal sinuses are not paired, do not have accompanying arteries and vary in size and extent.*

Gastrocnemius veins (GVs)

- Located within the medial and lateral heads of the gastrocnemius muscle.
- The gastrocnemius veins also referred to as the sural veins are paired or may be seen in triplicate sets.
- There are multiple sets of gastrocnemius veins:
  » Medial gastrocnemius veins: located in the medial head of the gastrocnemius muscle. The medial gastrocnemius veins are typically larger than the lateral gastrocnemius veins.
  » Lateral gastrocnemius veins: located in the lateral head of the gastrocnemius muscle.

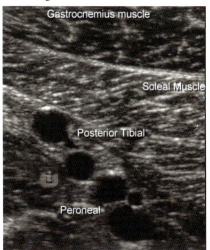

Fig. 4-4: *Gastrocnemius and soleal muscles along with the peroneal and posterior tibial veins*

Soleal veins (SolVs)

- Located within the soleal muscle.
- Typically, soleal veins only have valves where they connect with other veins. These valves will frequently stop functioning (valvular incompetence).
- Blood pooling in the soleal veins cause dilation and possibility of thrombosis.
- Drain into the posterior tibial and peroneal veins.

Deep Venous System of the Thigh and Pelvis

- As the PopV enters the adductor canal in the distal thigh, the vein becomes the femoral vein (FV).
- The FV is a deep vein that travels the length of the thigh. The FV joins the deep femoral (DFV) approximately 9cm below the inguinal ligament to become the common femoral vein (CFV).
- The FV was formerly known as the superficial femoral vein (SFV). The term "superficial" caused confusion, suggesting that the SFV was not a deep vein.
- The DFV was formerly known as the profunda femoral vein (PFV).

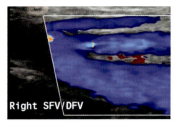

Fig. 4-5: Longitudinal view of femoral vein branches at the femoral junction.

- The CFV is approximately 2 to 4cm in length and continues as the external iliac vein (EIV) at the inferior margin of the inguinal ligament. The EIV dives deep at the inguinal ligament and drains the legs and the inferior part of the abdomen.
- The internal iliac vein (IIV) drains the pelvis, and joins the EIV to form the common iliac vein (CIV).
- The right and left CIV join to form the inferior vena cava (IVC).
- The IVC is the largest vein of the body and drains the lower extremities and the abdomen.

Compression of the left common iliac vein (CIV), by the right common iliac artery (CIA), increases the risk for deep vein thrombosis and can result in left CIV stenosis and left leg swelling.

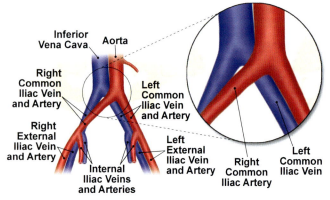

Fig. 4-6: Anatomy of the iliac bifurcation

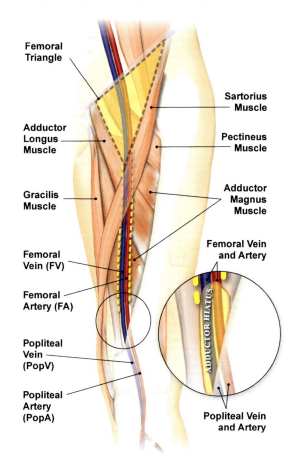

Fig. 4-7: The adductor canal is a "tunnel" in the middle of the thigh. It extends from the apex of the femoral triangle to the adductor hiatus.

Femoral Triangle [29, 30]

- An anatomical wedge-shaped region located in the upper third of the thigh. It appears as a triangular depression below the inguinal ligament when the limb is flexed, and the hip is externally rotated. It acts as a conduit for structures entering and leaving the anterior thigh.
- The femoral triangle consists of three borders (superior, lateral, medial)

Labs refer to this area as "NAVL." (Nerve, Artery, Vein, Lymphatic)

Structures of the femoral triangle (lateral to medial):
- Femoral nerve
- Femoral artery
- Femoral vein
- Lymphatic
- The femoral artery, vein and canal are contained within a fascial compartment, known as the *femoral sheath*.
- The great saphenous vein drains into the femoral vein within the triangle.

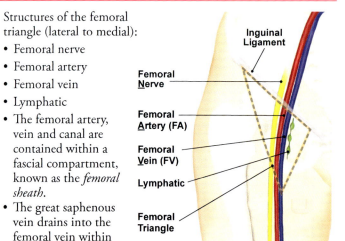

Fig. 4-8: NAVL illustration (Nerve, Artery, Vein, Lymphatic)

Superficial Veins [1, 2, 5, 8, 37]

Superficial venous anatomy is highly variable.

- The superficial system is composed of the great and small saphenous veins, the accessory great saphenous veins and their tributaries.
- Superficial veins do not have a corresponding artery, which allows them to be easily distinguished from deep veins.
- Saphenous veins are located within the saphenous compartment.
- Saphenous tributaries travel in the superficial compartment above the saphenous fascia.

Saphenous Eye [1, 2, 4, 5, 6, 8, 18, 49]

- The compartment, where saphenous trunks course, resembles an eye when scanning in the transverse view. The saphenous lumen is the iris, the superficial fascia the upper eyelid, and the deep fascia the lower eyelid. The "eye sign" allows the saphenous vein to be clearly identified.

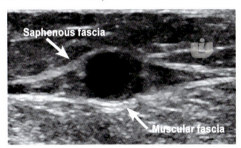

Fig. 4-9: *The saphenous compartment is bound superiorly by the saphenous fascia and inferiorly by the muscular fascia. The GSV is bound within this compartment which resembles an eye.*

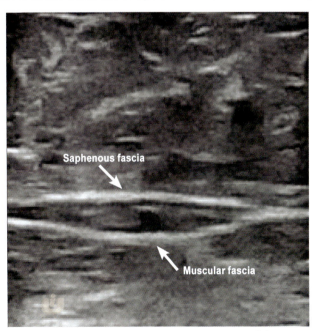

Fig. 4-10: *The saphenous compartment and GSV are deeper in this image due to the patient's BMI.*

- The saphenous compartment will vary in size depending on the BMI of the patient.

Saphenofemoral Junction [8, 9, 25]

The saphenofemoral junction includes the valves of the deep vein central and peripheral to the ostium and the terminal segment of the great saphenous vein from the preterminal valve to the ostium.

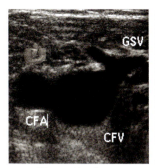 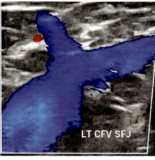

Fig. 4-11: *Cross-sectional and longitudinal views of the saphenofemoral junction (SFJ).*

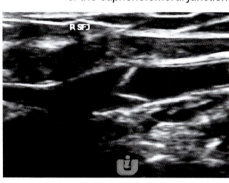

Fig. 4-12: *Valve at the saphenofemoral junction*

The first valve of the saphenofemoral junction is located directly at the confluence of the common femoral and great saphenous veins and may consist of only a single leaflet.

Great Saphenous Vein (GSV) [1, 2, 8, 13]

- The great saphenous vein is the longest vein in the body.
- The GSV originates on the medial aspect of the dorsum of the foot where it is a continuum of the medial marginal vein.
- The GSV courses anteriorly over the medial malleolus, ascends the medial side aspect of the calf and thigh, until draining into the CFV and terminating at the inguinal crease just inferior to the inguinal ligament.
- The GSV is an interfascial vein that lies within the saphenous compartment.
- The superficial veins are prone to dilatation because they have less muscle support than deep veins.
- The *saphenous hiatus* is an opening in the deep fascia. The GSV travels through the hiatus (approximately 3 to 4cm below the inguinal ligament) where it joins the CFV.
- The area where these veins join is known as the *saphenofemoral junction* (SFJ). The SFJ is located 1 to 4cm lateral to and 0 to 3cm below the pubic tubercle.
- The average diameter of the GSV is 3 to 5mm at the level of the saphenofemoral junction and 1 to 3mm at the level of the ankle.
- Familiarizing yourself with the course of the GSV is crucial. Many patients may have had prior interventions and the GSV compartment will still require interrogation.

The great saphenous vein (GSV) was formerly known as either the greater saphenous vein or the long saphenous vein.

Additional Pelvic Veins [1, 2, 7]

- Superficial circumflex iliac vein
- Superficial inferior epigastric vein: GSV tributary that drains the anterior abdominal wall.
- Superficial external pudendal vein: Drains the pelvis and empties into the GSV or femoral vein.

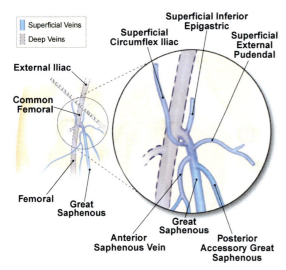

Fig. 4-13: Several superficial inguinal veins drain into the GSV near the saphenofemoral junction.

Some of these veins, or all of these veins, may or may not be present.

The small saphenous vein (SSV) was formerly known as either the lesser saphenous vein (LSV) or the short saphenous vein.

Anterior Saphenous Vein (ASV) [1,2,5,6,7,8,21,31,32]

- The ASV (formerly the anterior accessory great saphenous vein or AAGSV) is an interfascial superficial vein, present in approximately 50% of patients. Anterior accessory saphenous vein (AASV) was another former term for this vein.
- The termination point is variable, but the ASV usually joins the GSV between 0.5cm and 2cm peripheral to the SFJ.
- The ASV lays lateral to the great saphenous vein as it ascends the thigh and aligns itself over the deep system. This "alignment" sign distinguishes the ASV from the GSV.

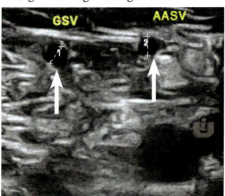

Fig. 4-14: The alignment of the ASV lateral to the GSV and directly above the deep system (CFV/CFA) is a helpful way to identify the superficial veins near the SFJ.

Accessory Veins [1, 2, 3, 5, 8]

- Accessory veins are venous segments that course in a plane parallel to the saphenous veins. They may be anterior, or posterior to the main trunk.

Posterior Accessory Great Saphenous Vein (PAGSV) [1, 2, 5, 8, 18]

- The PAGSV is an interfascial superficial vein.
- The origin is variable, most commonly arising from the thigh extension of the small saphenous vein.
- It joins the great saphenous vein about 5-10cm peripheral (away from) to the saphenofemoral junction.

The PAGSV is not present as often as the ASV.

Circumflex Veins [1, 2, 5, 18, 32]

Circumflex veins are tributaries that course obliquely to the GSV/ASV.

- The anterior thigh circumflex vein is a tributary of the ASV that ascends obliquely in the anterior thigh. It may originate from the lateral venous system.
- The posterior thigh circumflex vein is a tributary of the PAGSV that ascends obliquely in the posterior thigh. It may originate in the SSV, its thigh extension, or the lateral venous system.

At times the posterior thigh circumflex vein forms a connection between the great saphenous vein and the small saphenous. This intersaphenous connection is often referred to as Giacomini's anastomosis.

Small Saphenous Vein (SSV) [1, 2, 8, 34]

- The small saphenous vein is an interfascial vein that lies within the saphenous compartment.
- The SSV is the primary superficial vein of the posterior aspect of the lower limb.
- The SSV originates on the lateral aspect of the dorsum of the foot where it is a continuum of the lateral marginal vein.
- The SSV originates posterior to the lateral malleolus, ascends along the posterolateral aspect of the calf between the two heads of the gastrocnemius muscle at the popliteal crease where it can drain into the popliteal vein. But the termination point of the small saphenous vein is highly variable as the SSV often extends into the thigh as the thigh extension of the small saphenous vein (TE-SSV).
- The average diameter of the SSV is 2 to 4mm at the level of the saphenopopliteal junction and 1 to 2mm at the level of the ankle.

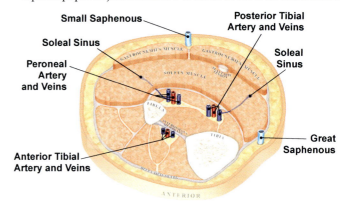

Fig. 4-15: Deep, superficial, and intramuscular veins of the calf.

Intramuscular Veins of the Calf [8, 14, 15, 16]

Valves [8, 9, 10, 11, 12, 13, 17, 19, 20, 22, 25, 26, 27, 33]

- Venous valves are bicuspid, containing two luminal leaflets.
- Both luminal leaflets or valve cusps are crescent in shape.
- These crescent shaped leaflets are formed by a reduplication of the intima.
- The vein wall is thicker at the base of the valve cusps making it sturdier in this area.
- The lumen is enlarged in the area where the cusps sit, and when closed, creates a pouched appearance. This area is known as a *valvular sinus*.

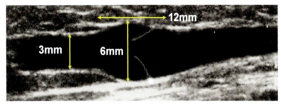

Fig. 4-16: *Valve sinus and adjacent segment of vein: diameter and length relationship.*

- Valves are meant to be unidirectional or one-way and are designed to prevent the backwash of blood.
- Deep, superficial and perforating veins contain valves.
- Perforating veins contain one-way valves that allow blood to flow inward from the superficial veins to the deep veins.
- There are more venous valves in the calf than in the thigh.
- Lower extremity veins have more valves than upper extremity veins. The number of valves is higher in the more distal portions of the extremities and decreases centrally.
- Valves can withstand retrograde pressures up to 300mmHg.

The diameter in the area of the valve sinus is usually two times the diameter of the adjacent segment of vein. The vertical length of the valve sinus is approximately twice its diameter.

Competent Valves [8-13,17,19,20,22,25,35,38]

- In healthy leg veins, these unidirectional valves allow blood to move in one direction: towards the heart. When walking, the foot, calf and thigh muscles squeeze the veins, pushing non-oxygenated blood back to the heart. As blood moves toward the heart, it pushes the cusps open.
- When the leg muscles relax, the valves inside the veins close, preventing the backwash of blood flow down the legs.
- Valve closure time in the femoropopliteal veins is <1sec or <1000ms, and <0.5sec or <500ms in the superficial, perforating and deep calf veins. [24]

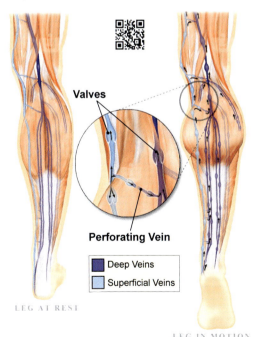

Fig. 4-17: *The calf muscle pump drives venous flow. While walking, muscle contractions squeeze the veins and open the venous valves allowing the blood to flow towards the heart. As the muscle relaxes, valves close to prevent the backward flow of blood (reflux).*

Antegrade flow opens the valves. The valves close to prevent retrograde flow. This is known as unidirectional flow.

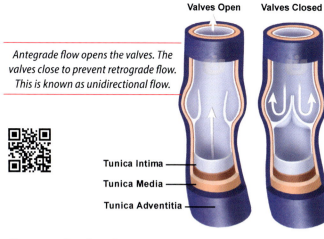

Communicating Systems

- Communicating veins connect two different points of the venous system. They can communicate with the great saphenous vein, small saphenous and deep veins.
- Perforating veins cross the muscular fascia, connecting the superficial and deep systems.
- Tributaries cross the saphenous fascia, connecting interfascial superficial veins to epifascial superficial veins.
- The term *tributary* is used when describing a vein; the term *branch* is used when describing an artery.

Perforating Veins (PVs) [1, 2, 3, 8, 26, 27]

- Perforating veins pierce the muscular fascia as they travel from the superficial compartment to the deep compartment.
- PVs are variable in size, distribution, connection and arrangement.
- PVs are located in the foot, calf and thigh.
- There are approximately 100-150 perforators in each leg, most are located below the knee.
- The function of perforating veins is to return venous blood from the superficial venous system to the deep venous system, except in the foot where the blood typically flows from the deep to the superficial venous system.

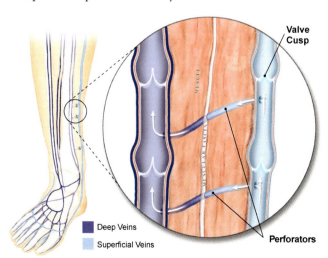

Fig. 4-18: *Blood flows from the superficial to the deep system under normal circumstances.*

Table 4-2: Nomenclature of the Perforating Veins
1, 2, 3, 6, 10, 11

Inguinal PV
- Medial thigh PV
- Anterior thigh PV
- Posterior thigh PV
- Lateral thigh PV

Knee Perforators
- Popliteal fossa PV
- Medial knee PV
- Lateral knee PV
- Suprapatellar PV
- Infrapatellar PV

Medial Calf Perforators
- Medial leg PV
- Paratibial PV
- Posterior tibial PV

Posterior Calf Perforators
- Medial gastrocnemius PV
- Lateral gastrocnemius PV
- Intergemellar PV

Ankle Perforators
- Medial ankle PV
- Lateral ankle PV

Nerves [8,24,27,34,36]

Saphenous Nerve
- The saphenous nerve and the great saphenous vein merge approximately 8-10cm below the popliteal fossa.
- The saphenous nerve is responsible for the sensitivity of the distal inner calf and the inside of the foot.

Sural Nerve
- The medial sural cutaneous nerve is a branch of the tibial nerve that adheres to the small saphenous vein in the lower third of the calf at the descent of the tail end of the gastrocnemius muscle.
- This nerve is responsible for the sensitivity of the back of the distal calf and the outer side of the foot.

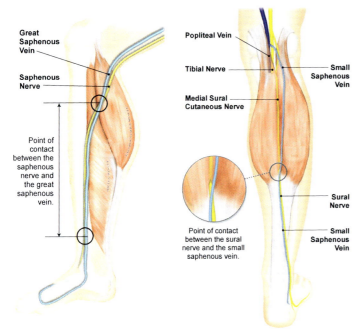

Fig. 4-19: Nerve locations of the tibial and short saphenous veins.

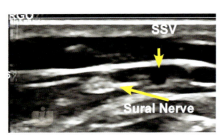

Fig. 4-20: SSV and sural nerve displayed using B-mode.

REFERENCES

1. Caggiati A, Bergan JJ, Gloviczki P, Eklof B, Allegra C, Partsch H; International Interdisciplinary Consensus Committee on Venous Anatomical Terminology. Nomenclature of the veins of the lower limb: extensions, refinements, and clinical application. *J Vasc Surg.* 2005 Apr;41(4):719-24.
2. Caggiati A, Bergan JJ, Gloviczki P, Jantet G, Wendell-Smith CP, Partsch H; International Interdisciplinary Consensus Committee on Venous Anatomical Terminology. Nomenclature of the veins of the lower limbs: an international interdisciplinary consensus statement. *J Vasc Surg.* 2002 Aug;36(2):416-22. doi: 10.1067/mva.2002.125847. PMID: 12170230
3. Caggiati A. The nomenclature of the veins of the lower limbs, based on their planar anatomy and fascial relationships. Acta Chir Belg. 2004 Jun;104(3):272-5. doi: 10.1080/00015458.2004.11679553. PMID: 15285536
4. Coleridge-Smith P, N, Partsch H, Myers K, Nicolaides A, Cavezzi A. (2006). Duplex ultrasound investigation of the veins in chronic venous disease of the lower limbs: UIP consensus document. Part I. Basic principles. Eur *J Vasc* Endovasc Surg .31, 83–92.
5. Cavezzi A, Labropoulos N, Partsch H, Ricci S, Caggiati A, Myers K. Nicolaides A. Smith PC. (2006). Duplex ultrasound investigation of the veins in chronic venous disease of the lower limbs: UIP consensus document. Part II. Anatomy. Eur *J Vasc* Endovasc Surg 31, 288–299.
6. Ricci S, Moro L, Ferrini A, Rossi Bartoli I, Antonelli Incalzi R. The E point: A New Echographic great saphenous identification sign in specific anatomical variants and applications. Phlebology. 2017 Mar;32(2):120-124. doi: 10.1177/0268355516633381. Epub 2016 Jul 9. PMID: 26908639
7. De Maeseneer M. (2019). What a phlebologist should know about the anterior accessory saphenous vein? Phlebolymphology. 26(2):68–72.
8. Caggiati, Alberto & Mendoza, Erika & Murena-Schmidt, Renate & Lattimer, Christopher. (2014). Anatomy of the Superficial Veins. 10.1007/978-3-642-40731-4_2.
9. D. Mühlberger, L. Morandini, E. Brenner. (2008). An anatomical study of femoral vein valves near the saphenofemoral junction. J Vasc Surg, 48, 994-999.
10. Caggiati A, Mendoza E, Murena-Schmidt R, Lattimer CRMendoza E, Lattimer CR, Morrison N. (2014). Duplex Ultrasound of Superficial Leg Veins. (19–47). USA Salmon Tower Building New York City Springer.
11. Uhl, JF, Gillot C. (2020). Atlas of venous anatomy. Anatomieunesco.org. https://anatomieunesco.org/3155/atlas-of-venous-anatomy-by-j-f-uhl/
12. Almeida JI. (2019). Venous Anatomy. In J.I. Almeida (Ed.), Atlas of Endovascular Venous Surgery (2nd ed., pp.1-20). Elsevier.,https://doi.org/10.1016/B978-0-323-51139-1.00001-2
13. Lo Vuolo, M.L.(2014). Venous Ultrasound: A Comprehensive Approach; Lower Extremities and Pelvis; Atlas and Texts. 9789873343599 https://books.google.com/books?id=akPksw EACAAJ
14. Akayo R, Kageyama N. (2016). Clinical Significance of the Soleal Vein and Related Drainage Veins, in Calf Vein Thrombosis in Autopsy Cases with Massive Pulmonary Thromboembolism. Annals of vascular diseases, 9(1), 15–21. https://doi.org/10.3400/avd.oa.15-00088
15. Aragão JA, Reis FP, Pitta G, Miranda F, Poli de Figueiredo LF. (2006) Anatomical Study of the Gastrocnemius Venous Network and Proposal for a Classification of the Veins, *European Journal of Vascular and Endovascular Surgery, 31*(4), Pages 439-442, ISSN1078-5884, https://doi.org/10.1016/j.ejvs.2005.10.022. (https://www.sciencedirect.com/science/article/pii/S1078588405006556)
16. Kageyama N., Ro A., Tanifuji T., Fukunaga T. (2008). Significance of the soleal vein and its drainage veins in cases of massive pulmonary thromboembolism. *Annals of vascular diseases*, 1(1), 35–39. https://doi.org/10.3400/avd.AVDoa07004
17. Parsi, K. (2007). Anatomy for the Phlebologist. Retrieved October 7, 2022, from http://www.conferencematters.co.nz/pdf/ParsiAnatomy%20and%20physiology%202007.pdf
18. Georgiev M, Myers KA, Belcaro G. (2003). The thigh extension of the lesser saphenous vein: From Giacomini's observations to ultrasound scan imaging, Journal of Vascular Surgery, Volume 37(3), 558-563. ISSN 0741-5214, https://doi. org/10.1067/mva.2003.77
19. Caggiati A. (2009) International Interdisciplinary Consensus Committee on Venous Anatomical Terminology. Regarding "Venous valves and major superficial tributary veins near the saphenofemoral junction." *J Vasc Surg. Dec;* 50(6):1547; author reply 1547-8. doi: 10.1016/j.jvs.2009.07.125. PMID: 19958997
20. Dickson, R., Hill, G., Thomson, I. A., & van Rij, A. M. (2013). The valves and tributary veins of the saphenofemoral junction: ultrasound findings in normal limbs. Veins and Lymphatics, 2(2), e18. https://doi.org/10.4081/vl.2013.e18
21. Laredo J, Lee BB, Neville RF. (2010). Endovenous Thermal Ablation of the Anterior Accessory Great Saphenous Vein. Endovascular Today. Retrieved October 7, 2022, from https://assets.bmctoday.net/evtoday/pdfs/et0310_SF_laredo.pdf
22. Caggiati A, Rippa Bonati M, Pieri A, Riva A. (2004). 1603-2003 Four centuries of valves. Eur *J Vasc* Endovasc Surg. 2004 Oct;28(4):439-41. doi: 10.1016/j.ejvs.2004.04.004. PMID: 15350570
23. Caggiati, A. (2015). Clinical Anatomy of the Venous System of the Lower Extremity. In Lanzer, P. (Ed.) PanVascular Medicine. Springer, Berlin, Heidelberg. https://doi.org/10.1007/978-3-642-37078-6_158
24. Labropoulos N, Tiongson J, Pryor L, Tassiopoulos AK, Kang SS, Mansour MA, Baker WH. (2001). Nonsaphenous superficial vein reflux. *J Vasc* Surg. Nov;34(5):872-7. doi: 10.1067/mva.2001.118813. PMID: 11700489
25. Mühlberger D., Morandini L., Brenner E. (2007). Frequency and exact position of valves in the saphenofemoral junction. Phlebologie. 36. 3-7. 10.1055/s-0037-1622161
26. Labropoulos N. (2020). Current Views on the Management of Incompetent Perforator Veins. Ann Phlebology. 18:1-3. https://doi.org/10.37923/phle.2020.18.1.1
27. Meissner MH. (2005). Lower extremity venous anatomy. Semin Intervent Radiol. Sep;22(3):147-56. doi: 10.1055/s-2005-921948. PMID: 21326687; PMCID: PMC3036282
28. Ricci S., Moro L., Antonelli IR. (2014). The foot venous system: anatomy, physiology and relevance to clinical practice. Dermatol Surg. Mar;40(3):225-33. doi: 10.1111/dsu.12381. Epub 2013 Dec 23. PMID: 24372905
29. Pellerito, J., & Polak, JF. (2019). Introduction to Vascular Ultrasonography (7th Edition). Elsevier - OHCE. https://bookshelf.health.elsevier.com/books/9780323625258
30. Basinger H., Hogg JP. Anatomy, Abdomen and Pelvis, Femoral Triangle. [Updated 2021 Jul 26]. In: StatPearls [Internet]. Treasure Island (FL): StatPearls Publishing; 2022 Jan-. Available from: https://www.ncbi.nlm.nih.gov/books/NBK541140/
31. Schul MW., Vayuvegula S., Keaton TJ. (2020). The clinical relevance of anterior accessory great saphenous vein reflux. *J Vasc* Surg Venous Lymphat Disord. Nov;8(6):1014-1020. doi: 10.1016/j.jvsv.2020.02.010. Epub 2020 Mar 21. PMID: 32205127.
32. Welch HJ., (2022). Combined Treatment of the Anterior Accessory Saphenous Vein and the Great Saphenous Vein, Vascular & Endovascular Review;5:e01. https://doi.org/10.15420/ver.2021.07
33. Labropoulos N., Tiongson J., Pryor L., Tassiopoulos AK., Kang SS., Mansour MA., Baker WH. (2003). Definition of venous reflux in lower-extremity veins. *J Vasc* Surg. Oct;38(4), 793-8. doi: 10.1016/s0741-5214(03)00424-5
34. Caggiati A. (2001) Fascial relationships of the short saphenous vein. *J Vasc* Surg 34:241–246.
35. Labropoulos N., Tiongson J., Pryor L., Tassiopoulos AK., Kang SS., Mansour MA., Baker WH. (2003). Definition of venous reflux in lower-extremity veins. *J Vasc Surg. Oct;*38(4), 793-8. doi: 10.1016/s0741-5214(03)00424-5
36. Hyland S., Sinkler MA., Varacallo M. Anatomy, Bony Pelvis and Lower Limb, Popliteal Region. [Updated 2021 Jul 31]. *In: StatPearls [Internet]*. Treasure Island (FL): StatPearls Publishing; 2022 Jan.
37. Caggiati A., Ricci S., (1997). The Long Saphenous Vein Compartment. *Phlebology, 12.* 107-111. 10.1177/026835559701200307
38. Schul MW., Vayuvegula S., Keaton TJ. (2020). The clinical relevance of anterior accessory great saphenous vein reflux. *J Vasc* Surg Venous Lymphat Disord. Nov;8(6):1014-1020. doi: 10.1016/j.jvsv.2020.02.010. Epub 2020 Mar 21. PMID: 32205127

ANATOMY
5. Lower Extremity Arterial

Lower Extremity Arterial System

The vessel anatomy is described from the pelvis to the foot:

- The abdominal aorta bifurcates into the right and left common iliac arteries (CIA) at the level of the umbilicus.
- The common iliac arteries travel distally and bifurcate into the internal iliac artery (IIA) and external iliac artery (EIA).
- The EIA travels laterally and enters the thigh at the inguinal ligament where it becomes the common femoral artery (CFA).

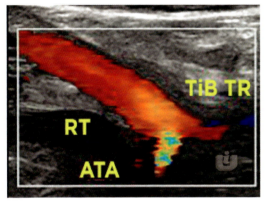

Fig. 5-1: *Bifurcation of the popliteal artery into the anterior tibial artery and tibioperoneal trunk*

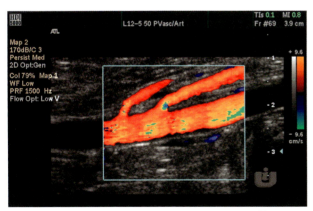

Fig. 5-2: *Gastrocnemius artery branches off the popliteal*
Courtesy of Philips Healthcare

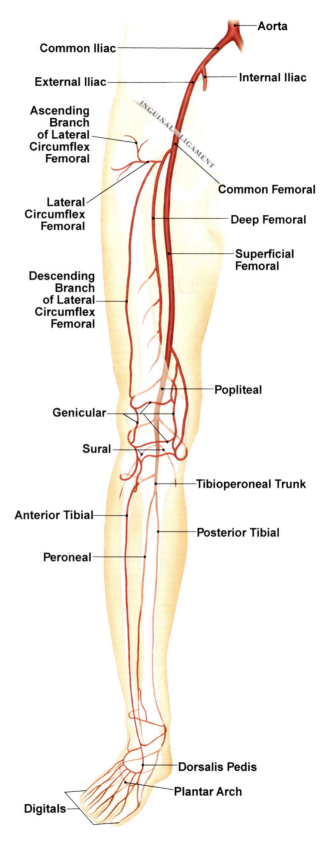

Fig. 5-3: *Lower Extremity Arterial System*

- The CFA travels for approximately 4cm and bifurcates into the superficial femoral artery (SFA) and the deep femoral artery (DFA). The profunda femoral artery (PFA) is an older, alternative term for the DFA.
- The DFA travels laterally and medially to supply the deep muscles of the thigh. Distal branches of the DFA communicate with popliteal artery tributaries.
- The SFA travels distally in the thigh entering the adductor canal (Hunter's Canal) then into the popliteal fossa behind the knee to become the popliteal artery (PopA).
- The PopA has numerous branches including the gastrocnemius, medial and lateral superior genicular, medial and lateral inferior genicular and middle genicular arteries.
- The PopA bifurcates into the anterior tibial artery (ATA) and the tibioperoneal trunk (TPT).
- The ATA travels anteriorly and laterally between the tibia and fibula. The vessel name changes to the dorsalis pedis artery (DPA) as it travels across the foot.
- The DPA crosses the dorsal aspect of the foot and bifurcates into the metatarsal arteries.
- The TPT bifurcates into the posterior tibial artery (PTA) and the peroneal artery (Per A).
- The PTA travels posterior to the medial malleolus and the Per A travels down the mid line of the calf.
- The PTA bifurcates into the medial plantar and lateral plantar arteries in the foot.

Fig. 5-6: *Lower Extremity Digital Arterial Anatomy*

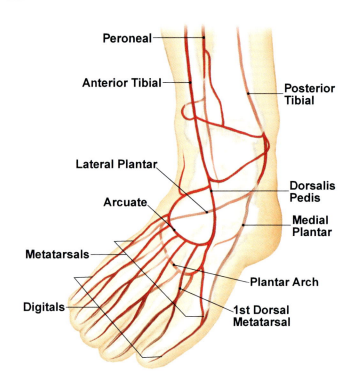

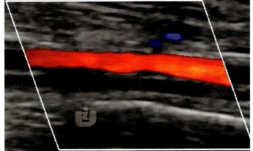

Fig. 5-4: *Color Doppler of the posterior tibial artery*

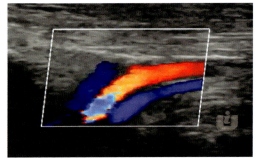

Fig. 5-5: *Color Doppler of the anterior tibial artery with two veins on each side of the artery*

- The lateral plantar artery and four plantar metatarsal arteries join to form the plantar arch.
- The plantar digital arteries run along the sides of the second through fourth toes. The fifth toe receives blood on its medial side from a plantar digital branch and on its lateral side from the lateral plantar artery.
- The great toe receives blood on its medial side from the first dorsal metatarsal artery.

Fig. 5-7: *Cross Section of the Calf*

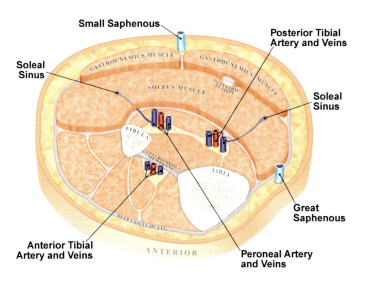

REFERENCES

1. Gray, H. (1977). The blood-vascular system. In Pick TP & Howden R. (Eds.), Gray's Anatomy (551-592). New York: Bounty Books.
2. Keck GM, Zwiebel, WJ (2005). Arterial anatomy of the extremities. In Zwiebel WJ, Pellerito JS (Eds.), *Introduction to Vascular Ultrasonography 5th ed.* (261-274). Philadelphia: Elsevier Saunders.
3. Netter FH. (2003). Lower limb. In Atlas of Human Anatomy 3rd ed. (467-528). Terterboro. Icon Learning Systems.
4. Thrush A, Hartshorne, (2005). "Duplex assessment of lower limb arterial disease" in Peripheral Vascular Ultrasound, How Why and When, 2nd ed. (112-131). Edinburgh. Elsevier Churchill Livingstone.
5. Tortora, G. J., & Anagnostakos, NP. (Eds.). (1990). The cardiovascular system: vessels and routes. In *Principles of Anatomy and Physiology*, 6th ed. (605-650) New York, NY: Harper & Row Publishers.
6. Uflacker R. (1997). Arteries of the lower extremity. In Atlas of Vascular Anatomy: An Angiographic Approach. (743-778). Baltimore: Wolters Kluwer Lippincott Williams & Wilkins.

ANATOMY
6. Upper Extremity Venous

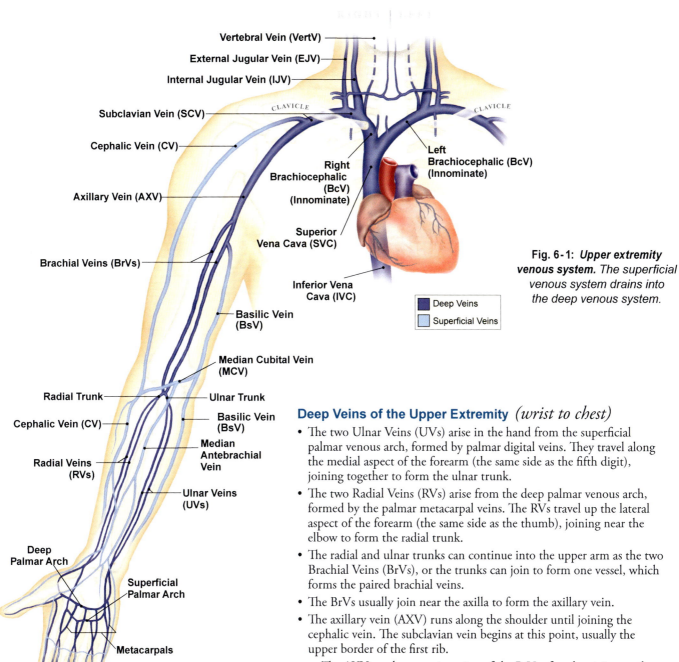

Fig. 6-1: *Upper extremity venous system.* The superficial venous system drains into the deep venous system.

Deep Veins of the Upper Extremity *(wrist to chest)*

- The two Ulnar Veins (UVs) arise in the hand from the superficial palmar venous arch, formed by palmar digital veins. They travel along the medial aspect of the forearm (the same side as the fifth digit), joining together to form the ulnar trunk.
- The two Radial Veins (RVs) arise from the deep palmar venous arch, formed by the palmar metacarpal veins. The RVs travel up the lateral aspect of the forearm (the same side as the thumb), joining near the elbow to form the radial trunk.
- The radial and ulnar trunks can continue into the upper arm as the two Brachial Veins (BrVs), or the trunks can join to form one vessel, which forms the paired brachial veins.
- The BrVs usually join near the axilla to form the axillary vein.
- The axillary vein (AXV) runs along the shoulder until joining the cephalic vein. The subclavian vein begins at this point, usually the upper border of the first rib.
  » The AXV can be a continuation of the BrVs after they join together near the axilla.
  » The basilic vein drains into the BrVs at the mid-arm or more proximal to form the AXV.
- The subclavian vein (SCV) joins the internal jugular vein to form the brachiocephalic vein (or innominate vein) at the clavicular level.
- The internal jugular vein (IJV) runs adjacent to the common carotid artery and receives blood from the face and neck. As mentioned, the IJV joins the SCV to form the brachiocephalic (innominate) vein.
- The right and left brachiocephalic veins (BCV), also known as the innominate veins (INV), join to form the superior vena cava (SVC).
- The SVC enters the heart at the right atrium.

Upper Extremity Venous System
- Veins return blood back to the heart.
- Deep veins have an accompanying artery.
- Forearm and brachial veins are duplicated.
- Axillary veins may also be duplicated.
- Tributaries usually correspond to the AXV: thoracoacromial, lateral thoracic, scapular, anterior circumflex, humeral, and posterior circumflex humeral veins.

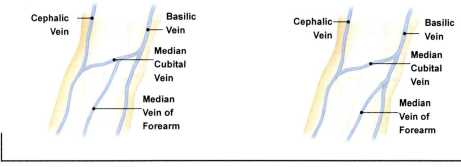

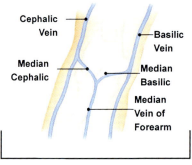

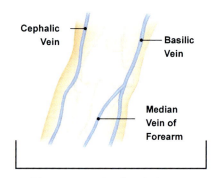

Fig. 6-2: *Typical anatomic variations of the veins at the antecubital fossa.*

H and N-shaped configurations with the MCV terminating in CV and BsV, respectively

M-shaped configuration

No communication between the CV and BsV

Superficial Veins of the Upper Extremity
(wrist to chest)

Superficial veins run within the superficial compartment above the deep fascia.

- The cephalic vein (CV) is the longest vein in the arm. The CV originates from the medial component of the dorsal venous arch in the hand and runs laterally along the arm. As it courses along the upper end of the deltoid muscle, it dives at the clavicular end of the pectoralis muscle to join the axillary-subclavian veins.
- The Basilic Vein (BsV) originates from the ulnar component of the dorsal venous arch in the hand and runs medially along the arm. The BsV joins the axillary vein near the medial border of the biceps muscle.
- Medial Vein (MV) of the forearm, also known as the Median Antebrachial Vein (MAV), arises from a palmar venous plexus.
- The median cubital vein (MCV) crosses the antecubital fossa obliquely, connecting the cephalic and basilic veins. In the antecubital fossa, there are several anatomical variations of the superficial veins including:
  » M-shaped configuration where the MV branches into the median cephalic and median basilic veins, which terminate in the cephalic and basilic veins, respectively, with no MCV present.
  » H and N-shaped configurations where the sides of the letters (H and N) are formed by the CV and BsV. The letter N is created when the MCV connects to the cephalic and basilic veins at oblique angles. The letter H is formed when the connections are at right angles. In both cases, the MV can terminate in either the MCV or the BsV.
- » There can be no communication between the BsV and CV. In this case, there is no MCV, and the MV will terminate in the BsV.
- » CV is hypoplastic, especially after the MCV tributary.
- » Most common are the M-, H-, and N-shaped configurations.

Neck Veins
- The External Jugular Vein (EJV) receives blood from the cranium, face, and neck via the following veins:
  » Anterior jugular vein
  » Posterior jugular vein
  » Suprascapular vein
  » Transverse cervical vein
- The EJV terminates in the SCV.
- The Anterior Jugular Vein (AJV) is highly variable in size and course. The AJV cross-sectional area varies in size inversely with that of the EJV; if the AJV cross-sectional area is large, the EJV cross-sectional area will be small and vice versa.
  » Typically, right and left AJVs connect via the jugular arch, a transverse trunk that runs just superior to the sternum.
  » There can be just one AJV. In this case, the AJV will usually travel along the midline of the neck.
- The anterior jugular venous system is part of a collateral venous network that sustains venous return when the SCV or brachiocephalic veins thrombose or occlude.[14]
- The AJV terminates in either the EJV (46%) or the SCV (54%).[12,13]
- The Internal Jugular Vein (IJV) runs adjacent to the common carotid artery and drains the face and neck.
- The IJV can communicate with the AJV via a large branch from the IJV.

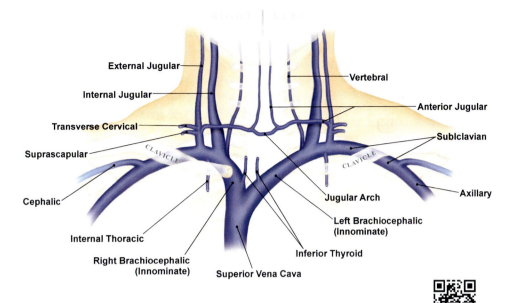

Fig. 6-3: *Neck veins. Venous flow to the heart.*

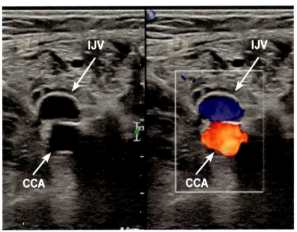

Fig. 6-4: *Internal jugular vein in transverse.* B-mode and color images of a typical normal IJV.

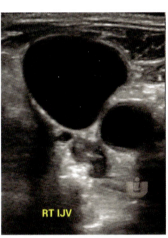

Fig. 6-5: *Transverse image of an enlarged IJV in a patient with congestive heart failure.*

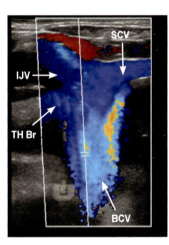

Fig. 6-6: *Confluence of the distal innominate, internal jugular, subclavian and internal thoracic branch.*

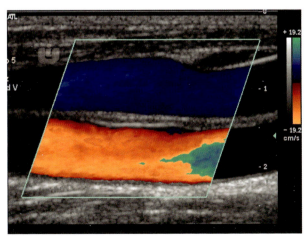

Fig. 6-7: *Longitudinal image of the internal jugular vein using color Doppler (top vessel) and the carotid artery (lower vessel).*

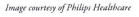

Image courtesy of Philips Healthcare

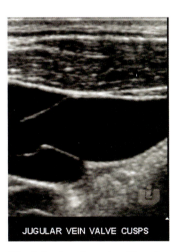

Fig. 6-8: *Jugular vein with valve leaflets extending into the lumen.*

- The SCV is the continuation of the AXV after the lateral border of the first rib joins the IJV at the clavicular level to form the Brachiocephalic/Innominate (BCV/InV).

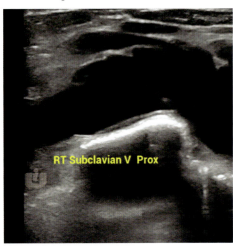

Fig. 6-9: *Longitudinal B-mode image of the subclavian vein near the confluence of the brachiocephalic vein.*

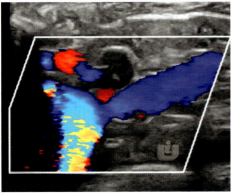

Fig. 6-10: *Color Doppler of the confluence of the subclavian and brachiocephalic vein.*

- The right and left BCVs join to form the SVC.
- The Superior Vena Cava (SVC) terminates at the right atrium of the heart, draining the head, neck, and upper extremities.
- The vertebral vein drains the head and terminates in the posterior aspect of the BCV.
- Veins that drain into the BCVs include:
  » Internal thoracic vein (mammary vein)
  » Inferior thyroid vein
  » Vertebral veins

Venous Valves

- Venous valves are comprised of two leaflets, or cusps (bicuspid valves) formed from the tunica intima. There are bulges at valve sites due to the valve cusps. *(Fig. 6-11)*
- When antegrade flow ceases, you may see a quick period of retrograde flow. However, in competent veins, this retrograde flow quickly ceases as it closes the valve by pushing the valve leaflets together. This flow reversal should not be reported as pathological venous reflux (venous insufficiency).
- Valves can withstand retrograde flow. pressures >200mmHg.
- Upper extremity veins have fewer valves than lower extremity veins.

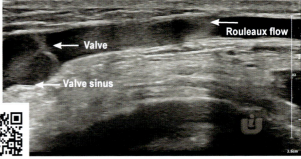

Fig. 6-11: *Valve leaflets in the cephalic vein on B-mode image. Notice how the vein bulges at the valve site and the presence of rouleaux flow.*

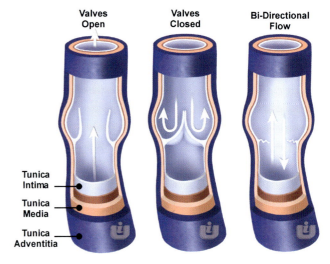

Fig. 6-12: ***Venous valve anatomy.*** *Under normal physiological conditions antegrade flow opens the valves. The valves close to prevent retrograde flow.*

REFERENCES

1. Gray, H. (1977). The blood-vascular system. In Pick TP & Howden R. (Eds.), *Gray's Anatomy* (551-592). New York: Bounty Books.
2. Gray, H. (1977). The veins. In Pick TP & Howden R. (Eds.), *Gray's Anatomy* (593-614). New York: Bounty Books.
3. Netter FH. (2003). Head and neck. In Atlas of Human Anatomy 3rd ed. (1-144). Terterboro. Icon Learning Systems.
4. Netter FH. (2003). Thorax. In Atlas of Human Anatomy 3rd ed. (174-238). Terterboro. Icon Learning Systems.
5. Netter FH. (2003). Upper limb. In Atlas of Human Anatomy 3rd ed. (401-466). Terterboro. Icon Learning Systems.
6. Tortora, G. J., & Anagnostakos, NP. (Eds.). (1990). The cardiovascular system: vessels and routes. In *Principles of Anatomy and Physiology, 6th ed.* (605-650) New York, NY: Harper & Row Publishers.
7. Uflacker, R. (1997). Veins of the head and neck. In Atlas of Vascular Anatomy: An Angiographic Approach. (81-112). Baltimore: Wolters Kluwer Lippincott Williams & Wilkins.
8. Uflacker, R. (1997). Veins of the thorax. In Atlas of Vascular Anatomy: An Angiographic Approach. (189-212). Baltimore: Wolters Kluwer Lippincott Williams & Wilkins.
9. Uflacker R. (1997). Veins of the upper extremity. In Atlas of Vascular Anatomy: An Angiographic Approach. (389-399). Baltimore: Wolters Kluwer Lippincott Williams & Wilkins.
10. Zwiebel, WJ (2005). Extremity venous anatomy, terminology, and ultrasound features of normal veins. In Zwiebel WJ, Pellerito JS. (Eds). *Introduction to Vascular Ultrasonography 5th ed.* (415-429). Philadelphia: Elsevier Saunders.
11. Mikuni, Y., et al. (2013). "Topographical anatomy of superficial veins, cutaneous nerves, and arteries at venipuncture sites in the cubital fossa." Anat Sci Int 88(1): 46-57.
12. Deslaugiers B, Vaysse P, Combes JM, et al. Contribution to the study of the tributaries and the termination of the external jugular vein. Surg Radiol Anat 1994;16:173–7.
13. Von Lanz T, Wachsmuth W. Praktische Anatomie. Berlin, Heidelberg, New York: Springer, 1955
14. Schummer, W., et al. (2004). "The anterior jugular venous system: variability and clinical impact." Anesth Analg 99(6): 1625-1629,
15. Gurarie, M .("The Anatomy of the Axillary Vein. Very Well Health (2021) 1-6.

ANATOMY
7. Upper Extremity Arterial

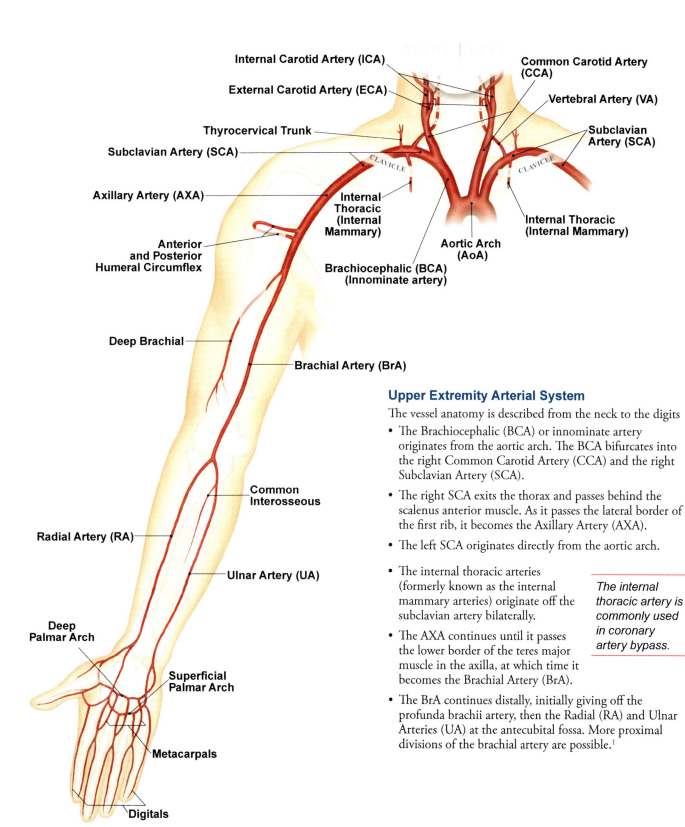

Fig. 7-1: *Upper Extremity Arterial System*

Upper Extremity Arterial System

The vessel anatomy is described from the neck to the digits

- The Brachiocephalic (BCA) or innominate artery originates from the aortic arch. The BCA bifurcates into the right Common Carotid Artery (CCA) and the right Subclavian Artery (SCA).

- The right SCA exits the thorax and passes behind the scalenus anterior muscle. As it passes the lateral border of the first rib, it becomes the Axillary Artery (AXA).

- The left SCA originates directly from the aortic arch.

- The internal thoracic arteries (formerly known as the internal mammary arteries) originate off the subclavian artery bilaterally.

- The AXA continues until it passes the lower border of the teres major muscle in the axilla, at which time it becomes the Brachial Artery (BrA).

- The BrA continues distally, initially giving off the profunda brachii artery, then the Radial (RA) and Ulnar Arteries (UA) at the antecubital fossa. More proximal divisions of the brachial artery are possible.[1]

The internal thoracic artery is commonly used in coronary artery bypass.

- With the palm up, the RA passes along the lateral side of the forearm and the UA passes along the medial side.

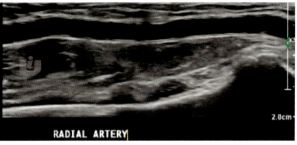

Fig. 7-2: *B-Mode imaging of the radial artery*

- The RA and UA join in the palm of the hand to form the deep and superficial palmar arches. These arches may or may not communicate with each other.[1]
  » The RA becomes the deep palmar arch in the hand.
  » The UA becomes the superficial palmar arch in the hand and runs distal to the deep arch.
- The digital arteries arise from the palmar arches. There are often four palmar common digital arteries in the hand.[2]
- The common digital arteries branch into the proper digital arteries. These proper palmar digital arteries run along each side of the second through fifth fingers.[2]

An early bifurcation of the RA and UA (off the AXA) is possible in up to approximately 3% of the population.[1]

- The thumb receives blood from the first palmar metacarpal artery, radial artery or the palmar arches (anatomy varies).[2]

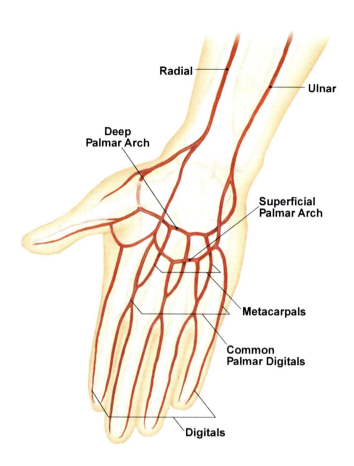

Fig. 7-5: *Digital Arterial Anatomy*

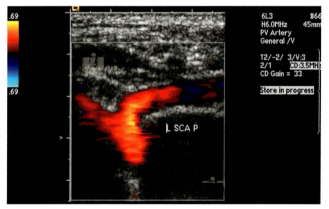

Fig. 7-3: *Left subclavian artery comes off the aortic arch*

REFERENCES

1. Keck GM, Zwiebel, WJ (2005). Arterial anatomy of the extremities. In Zwiebel WJ, Pellerito JS. (Eds). *Introduction to Vascular Ultrasonography 5th ed.* (261-274). Philadelphia: Elsevier Saunders.
2. Chloros, GD, et al. (2008). Non-invasive evaluation of upper extremity vascular perfusion. *J Hand Surg Am.* Apr; 33(4):(591-600).
3. Additional references:
4. Gray, H. (1977). The blood-vascular system. In Pick TP & Howden R. (Eds.), *Gray's Anatomy* (551-592). New York: Bounty Books.
5. Netter FH. (2003). Head and neck. In *Atlas of Human Anatomy 3rd ed.* (1-144). Terterboro. Icon Learning Systems.
6. Netter FH. (2003). Thorax. In *Atlas of Human Anatomy 3rd ed.* (174-238). Terterboro. Icon Learning Systems.
7. Netter FH. (2003). Upper limb. In *Atlas of Human Anatomy 3rd ed.* (401-466). Terterboro. Icon Learning Systems.
8. Uflacker R. (1997). Arteries of the head and neck. In *Atlas of Vascular Anatomy: An Angiographic Approach.* (3-79). Baltimore: Wolters Kluwer Lippincott Williams & Wilkins.
9. Uflacker R. (1997). Arteries of the upper extremity. In *Atlas of Vascular Anatomy: An Angiographic Approach.* (339-338). Baltimore: Wolters Kluwer Lippincott Williams & Wilkins.
10. Tortora, GJ, Anagnostakos NP. (Eds.). (1990). The cardiovascular system: vessels and routes. In *Principles of Anatomy and Physiology,* 6th ed. (605-650) New York, NY: Harper & Row Publishers.

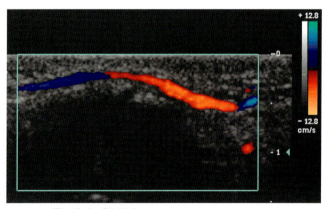

Fig. 7-4: *Digital artery* Courtesy of Philips Healthcare

HEMODYNAMICS AND PHYSIOLOGY
8. General Principles

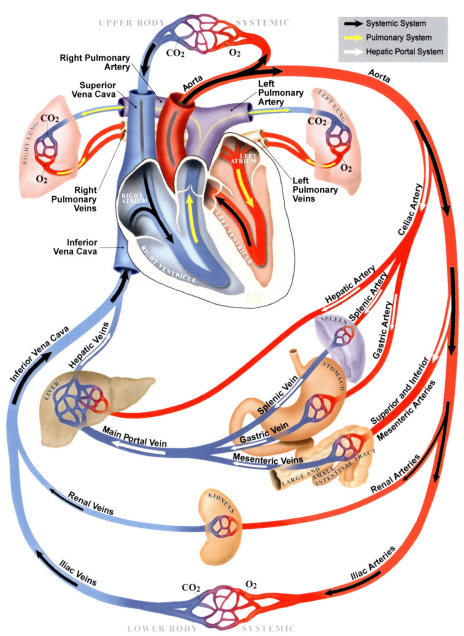

Fig. 8-1: *Blood circulates through the following pathway: from the left ventricle of the heart to the arteries, arterioles, capillaries, venules, veins, right atrium, right ventricle, pulmonary artery, lung capillaries, pulmonary vein, to the left atrium and to the left ventricle.*

Circulation is controlled by the nervous system and the state of the tissue bed.

This chapter offers general knowledge and basic principles that guide the measurements taken and interpreted in the vascular lab. The primary hemodynamic measurements covered are pressure and velocity. Other measurements are covered in each specific chapter.

Why bother understanding hemodynamics?
Without the basic knowledge of hemodynamics and its relationship to physiology, it would be difficult to understand how to use or interpret certain findings or know what else to look for when you come upon reversed flow in a vessel for example, or how a simple ankle/brachial pressure index can indicate proximal obstruction, or what it may mean if a Doppler waveform shows no diastolic flow velocity. Basic knowledge can also assist in understanding unusual findings.

This text starts with basic knowledge of the circulatory system and blood composition to give perspective. Basic principles will also be presented in this chapter regarding some of the more common vascular exam data points and measurements taken in the lab.

Each chapter will explain the measurements necessary for that type of exam in more detail.

Overview of Vascular Systems

The arteries, capillaries, and veins in the body provide a vital tubular transportation system for the blood to provide products required for healthy tissue and to pick up any waste for disposal.

Arteries course from the heart to all of the tissues in the body delivering oxygen and nutrients necessary for the body to function. Veins pick up waste for later disposal as blood flows back toward the heart. In between the arteries and veins, the capillaries provide the opportunity for product delivery and waste pick up since they are narrow and thin-walled for molecular exchanges and directly connect the arteries to the veins.

The circulatory system is a vast transportation system of roads similar to our expressways (freeways), highways, streets, side streets, and alleys. If there is a blockage or damage to one road, there are backup systems to keep the traffic moving.

Blood Circulation [1,2]

The four major systems involved in blood circulation include:

- Systemic
- Pulmonary
- Coronary
- Hepatoportal

Arteries Vs. Veins
Similarities
- Veins, like arteries, are composed of 3 layers:
  » *Tunica Intima* or Interna: Innermost layer composed of endothelial cells.

» *Tunica Media:* Middle layer composed of smooth muscle cells and connective tissue.

» *Tunica Adventitia* or *Externa:* Outermost layer composed of collagen fibers, the vasa vasorum and the sympathetic nerve fibers.

Differences
- Veins are not as structurally robust as arteries.
- Vein media is ten times thinner than the arterial media.
- Vein media has significantly less elastin than the arterial media.

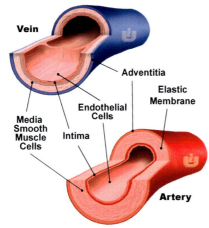

Fig. 8-2: Wall composition: Vein vs. Artery

Systemic Circulation
- The heart muscle is essentially a pump that pushes blood out of the heart and starts it flowing.
- Blood flows from the left atrium and ventricle to the arteries, arterioles, capillaries, venules, veins, and back to the right atrium and ventricle of the heart.
- Arterioles are small arteries that flow into capillaries. They are responsible for regulating flow into each tissue group by controlling resistance to flow.
- At the capillary level, oxygen is delivered to the tissues and waste materials are picked up for later disposal.
- Venules are very small, thin vessels that collect blood from the capillaries.
- The deoxygenated blood flow that returns via the veins to the right atrium of the heart is sent to the pulmonary system from the right ventricle where it cycles back to the left atrium to begin circulating again.

Coronary Circulation
The heart muscle itself is fed by the right and left coronary arteries, which arise from the aorta just outside the aortic valve of the heart. The coronary arteries supply blood to the branches of the outer surface of the heart, the smaller arteries, capillaries, veins and finally the coronary sinus, which is a large vein that collects deoxygenated blood from the coronary veins and feeds it into the right atrium for oxygen/carbon dioxide exchange in the lungs.
- Note that blood does not pass from the chambers of the heart to the heart muscle.
- Blood flows in the coronary arteries differently than it does through the systemic arteries. Coronary flow is greater during diastole since systolic contractions compress the vessels in the heart wall. The amount of coronary flow is determined by the diastolic level of arterial pressure.

Pulmonary Circulation
Blood flows from the right atrium to the right ventricle, pulmonary artery, lung capillaries, pulmonary vein and back to the left atrium and ventricle. The right ventricle pumps blood into the pulmonary artery.
- Deoxygenated blood moves from the pulmonary artery through the pulmonary capillaries where carbon dioxide is excreted and oxygen is absorbed in the lung alveoli.
- The oxygenated blood leaves the alveoli and enters the pulmonary veins. *Pulmonary veins are one of the few veins in the body that contain oxygenated blood;* all other veins contain deoxygenated blood. There are usually four pulmonary veins, two from each lung.

Only the pulmonary and hepatic veins carry oxygenated blood.

- From the pulmonary veins, the oxygenated blood flows into the left atrium and is then pumped into the left ventricle for redistribution to the systemic circulation via the aorta.

Hepatoportal Circulation
Blood flow to the liver is unusual because it is delivered in two forms, 1) as oxygenated blood from the celiac artery and 2) as deoxygenated blood from the portal vein.
- The portal vein collects blood from the veins of the spleen, stomach, intestines, gallbladder and pancreas and actually feeds blood INTO the liver, even though it is a vein.
- Blood is cleansed in the liver before it is collected in the hepatic veins and flows into the inferior vena cava.

It is important to know that the transportation of blood flow that happens within the vascular system is vital to the proper function of the body. The function of the heart will affect pressure and flow characteristics in the arteries and veins. These changes will be described throughout the testing chapters.

Blood Composition
The average human body contains approximately 5 liters of blood that is circulated through the body about once every minute. Blood consists of approximately 55% plasma and 45% formed particles (hematocrit).
- **Plasma**, the liquid component of the blood is:
  » Composed of a mixture of water (90%), sugar, fat, proteins, enzymes nutrients, hormones, gases and salts.
  » Transports blood cells and nutrients, waste products, antibodies, proteins, hormones, and clotting proteins.
  » Maintains the body's fluid balance.
- **Hematocrit** contains three types of blood cells: **red blood cells**, **white blood cells** and **platelets**. The hematocrit level is higher in males than females.

Red Blood Cells (RBC) or Erythrocytes
- RBC function is specifically to transport oxygen to body tissues and transfer carbon dioxide to the lungs.
- RBC are shaped like biconcave disks with a flattened surface.
- RBC do not have a nucleus and can easily change shape for passage through small capillaries.
- RBC measure about 7μ (μ=micron or 1×10^{-6} meter) in diameter. Since this is much smaller than the wavelength of an ultrasound beam, the RBC causes the beam to scatter in every direction, creating a very weak reflection. This reflection pattern is known as "Rayleigh scattering" and the very low strength of the RBC echoes explains why blood is displayed as black on ultrasound images.

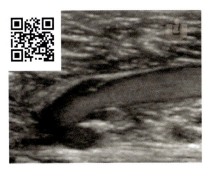

Fig. 8-3: *"Rouleaux flow" (moving smoke-like echoes sometimes noted) are really red blood cells (RBCs) which aggregate to form a larger reflector so they can be seen, whereas a single RBC is too small to be seen on B-mode.*

- Blood appears red because of the large number of red blood cells, which get their color from the hemoglobin.
- RBC survive 120 days on average.
- An increase or decrease in RBC size is usually characteristic of one of the many types of anemia. *Anemia* is a condition when there are not enough healthy red blood cells to carry a sufficient amount of oxygen to the tissues. A common RBC disorder found in the African-American population is *sickle-cell anemia*. In this condition:
  » RBC become malformed and elongated.
  » Clumping and thrombosis commonly occurs in branch vessels causing ischemia and infarction.
  » Stroke is a major concern and occurs in over 10% of children with homozygous sickle cell anemia (HbSS). [1]

White Blood Cells or Leukocytes

- White blood cells are the largest cells, followed by RBC.
- Although white blood cells (WBC) are larger in size, they are fewer in number than RBC, comprising approximately 1% of blood.
- WBC protect the body from infection and can move in and out of capillaries to fight disease, infections or injury.
- The most common type of WBC is the *neutrophil*, accounting for 55 to 70% of the total white blood cell count.
- Another type of WBC is a lymphocyte and there are two kinds:
  » *T-lymphocytes* regulate the function of other immune cells and directly attack infected cells and tumors.
  » *B-lymphocytes* make antibodies, that specifically target bacteria, viruses, and other foreign materials.

Platelets *(also called thrombocytes)*

- Platelets are small fragments of cells. Platelets help the blood clotting process (coagulation) by adhering to the intimal lining of the injured vessel so that blood coagulation can begin.
- A decrease in platelets can cause extensive bleeding.
- *Thrombocytopenia* can result from a decrease in thrombocytes during heparin therapy. (Heparin is an anticoagulant drug used to stop the formation of thrombus.)
- Some patients receiving heparin experience *heparin-induced thrombocytopenia* or HIT, which is a >50% drop in their baseline platelet count following administration of heparin. This is a serious complication of heparin therapy which can be limb/life-threatening. Patient symptoms range from chills, fever, chest pain to skin lesions and venous gangrene. Direct thrombin inhibitors can be used as alternative anticoagulants in such cases.
- An increase in platelets can cause unnecessary clotting, leading to stroke or heart attack.
- Platelets are associated with early stages of atherosclerosis. The interruption of the intima attracts platelets to the site of "injury," causing potential embolic material or further obstruction of the vessel at the site. (See *Atherosclerosis* in the *Arterial Diseases* chapter.)

Hemodynamics Overview

Blood flow is caused by pressure gradients, with blood flowing from higher to lower pressure regions. The contraction of the left ventricle causes blood to flow along the artery in a wave. The contraction increases the pressure within the ventricle, and because the pressure is greater in the ventricle than in the aorta, blood flows from the ventricle into the aorta. This increases the volume of blood in the aorta, causing an increase in aortic pressure. As the pressure increases, it pushes the blood further along the artery, down the pressure gradient. And as the amount of blood increases in a region of the artery, so does the pressure. Thus, as a wave of blood travels along the artery, so does a pressure wave.

As the left ventricle relaxes and fills with blood from the left atrium, blood is again pumped from the left ventricle into the aorta. As the wave of blood flows distally, the amount of blood proximal to the wave decreases. This decrease in blood volume causes the pressure to decrease to a baseline value. Cycling the left ventricle between contraction and relaxation causes pressure waves in the arteries, which propels the blood to travel in a series of waves (pulsatile flow).

As a wave of blood travels through the vessels, it loses energy, and eventually the ability to increase pressure. Energy is lost due to 1) the resistive frictional force caused by the blood flowing along the vessel's surface that must be overcome. 2) the work required to stretch the vessel wall as the wave passes by temporarily increasing local blood volume.

The energy loss and force required to contract the vessel increase as the blood travels distally. [3] As the wave of blood moves through the body, the energy it uses rapidly increases for two primary reasons:

- As the arteries bifurcates, the number of vessels carrying the blood increases, and they become smaller and smaller. This increases vessel surface area per unit volume of blood, increasing the resistant frictional force, which requires more energy to keep the blood moving.
- As the vessels' compliance decreases, energy required by the wave of blood to expand them as they pass through increases.

As a blood wave moves through the vessels, it causes smaller and smaller pressure increases, and the size of the wave decreases. In the arterioles, the wave will cease to exist when it no longer has the energy required to expand the vessel wall. The flow is then no longer pulsatile. The flow pattern in microcirculation is different as blood velocity is significantly reduced. Patients with chronic venous disease may have altered flow patterns in the microcirculation, reflecting, the inflammatory changes in the area. [4,5]

Because the resistance for a unit volume of blood flow in small vessels is greater than in large vessels, the force required to move the same volume of blood through small vessels is greater than the force needed for the aorta and large arteries. Thus, the pressure gradient, the driving force moving the blood, is greater in the arterioles and capillaries than in the aorta and large arteries. The pressure gradient across the arterioles and capillaries is about 15mmHg, while the pressure drops across the aorta and large arteries are approximately 1mmHg.

REFERENCES

1. M Boron, WF and Boulpaep, EL Medical Physiology, A Cellular and Molecular Approach. Elsevier, 2005.
2. Klabunde, Richard E. PhD, (2011) Cardiovascular Physiology Concepts, Chapters 5,7,& 8. Lippincott, Williams and Wilkins.
3. Owen, C, Robers, M. Arterial Vascular Hemodynamics .Journal of Diagnostic Medical Ultrasound 23:129-140, May/June 2007.
4. Labropoulos N. How Does Chronic Venous Disease Progress from the First Symptoms to the Advanced Stages: A Review. Adv Ther. 2019 Mar;36(Suppl 1):13-19.
5. Labropoulos N, Wierks C, Golts E, Volteas SK, Leon M, Volteas N, et al. Microcirculatory changes parallel the clinical deterioration of chronic venous insufficiency. Phlebology. 2004;19(2):81–86.

HEMODYNAMICS AND PHYSIOLOGY
9. Venous

The normal venous system is a compliant, low-pressure, non-pulsatile flow system which is responsive to positional changes, cold, respiratory variation, and muscle contraction. Two-thirds of the blood is within the venous system.

Two primary functions of the venous system are:
- Transporting blood from the capillaries to the heart
- Being the blood reservoir of the body and maintaining the filling pressure of the right heart by increasing or decreasing the volume of blood circulating through the body. [1-7]

Hydrostatic pressure, compliance and capacitance are key components of venous studies that will be discussed in this chapter. The effects of respiration, temperature, vasomotor tone, cardiac and muscular pumps on venous return and the function of venous valves are some of the other topics covered which are important to venous hemodynamics.

Hydrostatic Pressure

Hydrostatic pressure is pressure exerted by a fluid at equilibrium at any point of time due to the force of gravity. [21]

In venous hemodynamics, the hydrostatic pressure caused by gravity upon standing increases venous pressure, which must be overcome for blood to flow back to the heart. Other physiologic forces also facilitate venous return to the heart and reduce the high venous pressure at the ankle, including respiratory changes, skeletal muscle contraction, venous valves, temperature control, and motor tone.

- All fluids need a pressure gradient to flow. Since the pressure in the capillaries is about 15mmHg and the central venous pressure in the heart's right atrium is much lower (2 to 6mmHg), a pressure gradient exists.
- When a person stands upright, gravity resists blood flow from the ankle and wrist to the heart. A 6-foot-tall individual who is standing has a venous pressure of approximately 117mmHg.

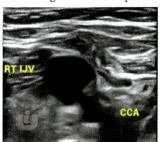 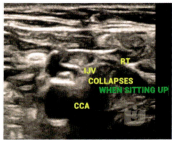

Fig. 9-1: *The effects of hydrostatic pressure will cause the jugular vein to collapse when the patient is sitting.*

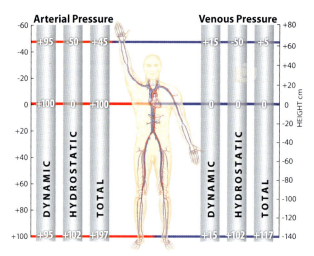

Fig. 9-2: *Hydrostatic pressure within the vascular system*

The vein wall stiffens with standing.

- The additional 102mmHg pressure is an example of hydrostatic pressure, the weight of the column of blood from the ankle to the heart.
- The pressure is highest in the lower portion of the body.
- The further the distance from the right atrium, the greater the force of gravity.
- In an arm that is lifted, the dependent wrist is closer to the heart than the ankle, making the column shorter and the hydrostatic pressure lower. Capillary pressure increases in the arm, so vessels do not collapse.

Compliance and Capacitance [3,4]

- Approximately 2/3 of systemic blood is located in the veins. The vein walls are very compliant and collapse or expand depending on the internal (intramural) and external pressures (tissue pressure) placed on the vein.
- The shape of the venous wall depends upon the pressure, volume, and flow.

Veins act similarly to rubber bands and can be stretched and collapsed in a wide range of sizes.

- This ability to collapse and expand is referred to as *capacitance*, and allows the venous system to easily adapt to variations in blood volumes. Extra fluids can be stored or adjusted for blood loss.
- This compliance allows for a large increase in venous flow without a significant increase in venous pressure. So, a wide range of venous volume changes can occur without changing the central venous pressure.

$$C = \frac{\Delta V}{\Delta P}$$

C = Vessel compliance (mL/mmHg)
(ΔV) = Change in volume (mL)
(ΔP) = Change in pressure (mmHg)

- This variable amount of blood capacitance is dependent upon the limb's position, muscle pump activity, integrity of the venous valves, and blood volume.
- Veins are less elastic than arteries but more compliant.

- Extreme changes that occur with fluid overload or severe blood loss will affect the central venous pressure.

Compliance decreases at higher pressures and volumes.

- By changing the cross-sectional area, the vein can change its resistance. Veins can distend 3-4 times that of the corresponding artery.[1]
- The greatest resistance occurs when the vein is elliptical. The least resistance exists when the vein is distended.

Flow/Pressure and Volume Relationships

- As venous flow increases, pressure and volume decrease and as venous flow decreases, pressure and volume increase.
- The shape of the vein wall depends upon the pressure, volume, and flow.

Table 9-1: Flow/Pressure and Volume Relationships

↑ Blood back to the heart	↓ Blood back to the heart
↓ Venous pressure	↑ Venous pressure
↓ Blood volume	↑ Blood volume

Transmural Pressure

- Different pressure forces surround blood vessels. The force occurring from outside the vein is the *tissue pressure*. The force occurring within the walls of a vessel is called *intraluminal pressure*.
- The pressure difference between the forces pushing on the inside and outside of the vessel wall is called *transmural pressure*.
  - » **Low transmural pressure:** as volume and pressure decrease, the vein wall collapses and becomes elliptical in shape.
  - » **High transmural pressure:** as volume and pressure increase, the vein wall becomes circular and may distend at higher venous pressures.

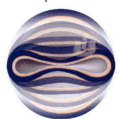

Fig. 9-3: *Transmural pressure. (intraluminal vs. tissue pressure)*

The more blood a vein contains the more pressure within the vein, making the vein more circular in shape.

Pressure While Supine [2,3,4,6]

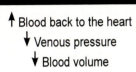
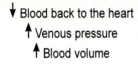

Fig. 9-4: *When supine, the venous pressure (mmHg) is very low*

Arterial Pressure: 90 mmHg, 89 mmHg, 80 mmHg
Venous Pressure: 2 mmHg, 5 mmHg, 10 mmHg

During inspiration, the intrathoracic cavity pressure is less than the abdominal cavity pressure; this causes a pressure gradient in the inferior vena cava. The intrathoracic pressure decreases, the intra-abdominal pressure increases, and blood moves from the abdomen into the chest, but the outflow from the peripheral veins stops. During inspiration, inflow is allowed from the upper extremities.

Table 9-2: Pressure and Flow Relationships During Inspiration and Expiration

Inspiration	Expiration
Intrathoracic pressure decreases ↓	Intrathoracic pressure increases ↑
Diaphragm moves down ↓	Diaphragm moves up ↑
Intra-abdominal pressure increases ↑	Intra-abdominal pressure decreases ↓
Outflow from peripheral veins decreases ↓	Outflow from peripheral veins increases ↑

Venous Return

Respiratory Function at Rest

- Respiration creates large changes in intrathoracic and intra-abdominal pressures.[2]
- During inspiration, intra-abdominal pressure increases by lowering the diaphragm, which causes the vena cava to collapse and reduces or stops the venous flow from the lower extremities.
- During expiration, intra-abdominal pressure decreases by lifting the diaphragm, the vena cava opens, and flow resumes in a phasic pattern from the lower extremities.
- During expiration, venous flow into the thorax decreases.
- The presence of respiratory variation is a major indicator of normal venous flow.
- Respiratory function has a lesser effect on the upper extremity veins than on the lower extremities:
  - » During inspiration, the intra-thoracic pressure decreases, resulting in increased flow from the upper extremity veins. Sometimes we ask the patient to perform a quick sniff, which results in a pressure drop and an increase in venous flow, especially in the central veins.
  - » During expiration, the intra-thoracic pressure increases in the upper extremity veins decreases venous flow.
  - » Upper venous augmentation is less and sometimes difficult to obtain because of the smaller vein size and lower blood volume.
  - » Venous flow in the upper extremities is more pulsatile because of the close proximity to the heart.
  - » Respiration has a small effect on upper venous flow when standing.

Table 9-3: Inspiration/Expiration Flow Changes

Upper Extremities	Lower Extremities
↑ Flow increases with inspiration	↓ Flow decreases with inspiration
↓ Flow decreases with expiration	↑ Flow increases with expiration

- » **Pressure gradient and muscle pumps:** the muscle pumps drive blood into the popliteal and femoral veins.
  - The valves prevent retrograde flow (reflux) during relaxation, generating negative pressure and drawing blood from the superficial to the deep system through perforating veins.
  - Venous pressure is lowered until arterial inflow equals venous outflow.
  - When exercise ceases, the veins slowly fill from the capillary bed, causing a slow return to the resting venous pressure.

Skeletal Muscle Contraction [6]

- During muscle contraction, venous flow in the deep and superficial veins is toward the heart. On relaxation of the muscles, there is a small amount of flow in the perforators, as it moves from the superficial to the deep veins.

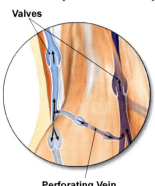

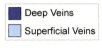

Fig. 9-5: *Blood normally flows from the superficial to the deep system through perforator veins.*

The calf muscle pump is the most important of the three muscle pumps. It is highly efficient, has the most significant capacitance, and generates the highest pressures during muscular contraction. [21, 24, 26]

- Multiple components facilitate effective venous return from the lower extremities. [19-25] Besides cardiac and respiratory pumps, there are three veno-muscular pumps in the leg; the thigh pump, the calf muscle pump and foot (plantar) pump. The calf muscle is the main pump.
  - » **Cardiac pump:** During cardiac contraction and relaxation, there is a passive push from the arterial system and mild suction from the cardiac valves that assist venous blood flow. [11, 19-25]
  - » **Respiratory pump:** During inspiration and expiration pressure changes occur in the thoracic and abdominal cavities. These pressure changes compress the nearby veins and assist blood return to the heart. [11, 19-25]
  - » **Foot pump (plantar pump)** assists with filling the calf with venous flow. When you walk/run and your foot hits the ground, the veins that comprise the plantar venous plexus are flattened and stretched to squeeze blood flow into the calf.
  - » **Calf muscle pump:** contraction of the gastrocnemius and soleus muscles is the most efficient of the pumps. The calf has a high capacitance and generates great pressure (about 200mmHg during contraction), while 40-60% of the venous volume is ejected with a single contraction.
    - The calf muscles act as a venous "heart" when contracted and squeeze the calf veins, propelling the blood in the calf veins toward the heart. The venous valves are very important calf muscle pump efficiency, stopping the blood from flowing toward the foot and directing it to the heart.
    - The calf muscle pump lowers venous pressure, reduces venous volume in the leg, and facilitates venous return to the heart.
  - » **Thigh pump:** Moves blood from the femoral and deep femoral into the common femoral vein by squeezing the veins against the quadricep muscle. It has an ejection fraction of approximately 15%. [5]
- Chronic venous disease occurs from venous hypertension or the failure to reduce venous pressure with exercise.
- There is abnormally high venous pressure on standing with *ambulatory venous hypertension*. When the calf muscle pumps the blood, it is expelled in any direction due to dysfunction of the valves. Subsequently, venous pressures do not decrease normally. [3]

Venous Valves

- Venous valves assist blood flow back toward the heart and prevent retrograde flow (reflux) back down the venous segment. [3]
- The valves are bicuspid and function to divide the column of blood into segments. This reduces hydrostatic pressure.
- There are more venous valves in the calf veins, possibly due to high hydrostatic pressure in the distal limb. The calf has a valve approximately every 2-5cm.
- Valves in the perforating veins prevent deep to superficial venous flow.
- Valves can withstand retrograde pressures up to 300mmHg.
- Venous blood typically flows towards the heart and from the superficial to the deep venous system. [19-25]
- In the perforating veins, blood flows from the superficial to deep veins. [19-25]
- When standing still, with the calf muscle relaxed, the veins in the calf fill with blood. Pressure on the valves from retrograde flow forces the valves to close, preventing blood flow toward the feet. [19-25]

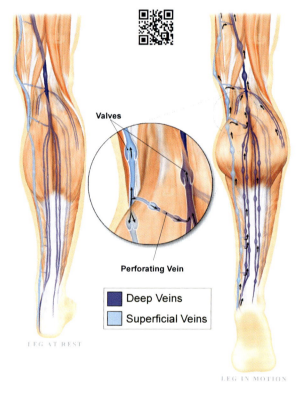

Fig. 9-6: *When the leg is in motion (walking), muscle contractions squeeze the veins, forcing blood past the open valves of the deep, superficial, and perforating veins upward towards the heart. After the muscle relaxes, valves close to prevent backflow (reflux).*

- While walking, muscle contractions squeeze the veins initiating venous blood flow. Venous flow opens the venous valves allowing the blood to flow towards the heart. As the muscle relaxes, the valves close to prevent the backflow of blood (reflux). [19-25]
- UE veins have fewer valves than LE veins. Gravity has a lesser effect on UE flow due to the shorter column of blood and the closer proximity to the heart.
- It is possible for thrombus to form behind a valve cusp.

- Valvular damage and dysfunction (valvular incompetence) result in venous reflux and subsequent venous hypertension. Ambulatory Venous Pressure (AVP) is the "gold standard" test for evaluation of the efficiency of the calf muscle pump. It is performed by placing a small needle into one of the veins of the foot and connecting a needle to a blood pressure unit.
- Air Plethysmography (APG)* has widely replaced the AVP exam by non-invasively measuring absolute volume changes of the calf in response to positional changes and exercise.

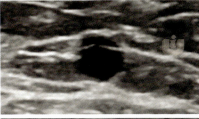

Fig. 9-7: Normal venous valves with no evidence of thrombus.

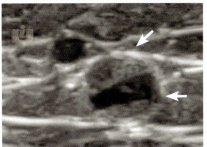

Fig. 9-8: Abnormal venous valves with thrombus behind valve cusps.

Vasomotor Tone

- Veins contain sympathetic-adrenergic constrictor nerves, which control contraction of smooth muscle.[7] Veins will either get bigger or dilate (vasodilation) or shrink/contract (vasoconstriction).
- Vasodilation increases venous blood volume at a lower pressure so that cardiac output can be reduced.[7]
- Veins react to physical and emotional stress, creating vasoconstriction.
- Vasoconstriction increases blood flow to the heart, increasing cardiac output.

Vein diameter varies with muscle contraction (vasomotor tone).

Effect of Cardiac Contraction

- With cardiac contraction and relaxation, there is a suction effect on venous blood flow.
- Because of the strong respiratory variation in the legs, cardiac contraction does not affect the blood flowing from the lower extremities.
- In the presence of congestive heart failure, central venous pressure increases, creating pulsatile waveforms in the lower extremities.

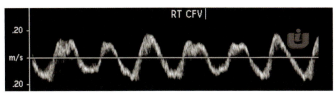

Fig. 9-9: Pulsatile venous flow

Thermal Regulation

- Thermal regulation is controlled by the sympathetic nerves.
- Vasoconstriction occurs in response to cold. Vasodilatation occurs in response to heat.
- Superficial veins are sensitive to cold and vasoconstriction.
- Venous blood flow in the superficial veins is slow, allowing heat to be transferred from the body to the skin to increase heat loss.

Waveform Terminology [22]

What can a waveform tell you about hemodynamics?

- Doppler derived waveforms can add information regarding the proximal, focal, and distal conditions of flow at any given location. A change in a Doppler waveform from one location to the next is helpful diagnostic information.
- Sometimes analysis of Doppler waveforms is described as "what's coming in (inflow), what's going on (focally), and what's going out (outflow.)"

Venous Waveform Terminology

- Venous waveform terminology is agreed upon among professionals more so than terminology used to describe arterial waveforms. A consensus document endorsed in 2020 by the Society of Vascular Ultrasound and the Society for Vascular Medicine addressed the terminology and interpretation of peripheral venous waveforms. This section will describe the important components of the venous waveform.

Components of Normal Venous Waveforms

Flow Direction

- Normal venous flow direction is toward the heart, moving deoxygenated blood toward the heart and lungs.
- Traditionally flow in a vein is displayed below the baseline of a spectral tracing for a Doppler waveform that is "reversed" or "retrograde."
- In certain situations, flow can be "bidirectional" (formerly referred to as "to and fro"). In such cases the antegrade and retrograde parts of the waveform are fairly equal in duration. This occurs when the proximal and distal pressure change with the cardiac cycle so flow moves towards the lower pressure when it changes. This can occur for example in the setting of hypervolemia, when you have too much fluid volume in your system and pulsatile venous flow is noted in the legs.

Flow Description

Spontaneous: Venous flow is observed by color flow or the Doppler signal is heard automatically, (no manual compression or muscular contraction is required).

Normal phasicity with respiration or respirophasic: Cyclical increase and decrease in the venous spectral Doppler waveform is directly associated with respiration and movement of the diaphragm.

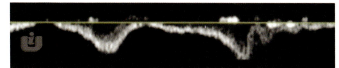

Fig. 9-10: Normal spectral Doppler waveform in a common femoral vein.

Augmentation: A distinct pattern in the spectral Doppler waveform produced by a sudden surge and increased flow through the vein. The augmentation is directly related to the patency of the vein, usually when the limb veins are manually compressed distal to the transducer or upon muscle contraction. The 2020 Consensus paper suggests adding the modifier "Normal augmented."

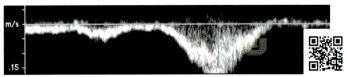
Fig. 9-11: *Distal compression producing augmentation*

Pulsatility: Venous flow increases and decreases cyclically. This finding is expected in the upper extremity veins due to their proximity to the heart and in the upper thigh veins of patients with congestive heart failure (CHF). Venous flow in the lower extremities should normally be non-pulsatile (and respirophasic).

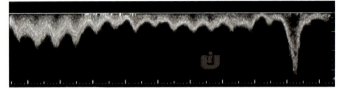
Fig. 9-12: *Pulsatile venous spectral Doppler signal*

Venous Competence: The Valsalva maneuver or proximal compression demonstrates competency of the venous valves. Normal flow will stop on proximal compression of veins or a Valsalva maneuver, returning on release of the maneuver.

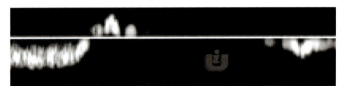
Fig. 9-13: *Normal venous spectral Doppler waveform during a Valsalva maneuver which stops flow momentarily.*

Components of Abnormal Venous Waveforms

Flow Direction

Venous Incompetence can increase venous pressure due to the lack of unidirectional flow back to the heart. While distal augmentation also helps confirm venous patency, this maneuver can also demonstrate venous incompetence and demonstrate the inability of the venous valves to function properly, resulting in retrograde flow, away from the heart and back down the limb.

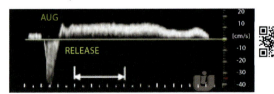
Fig. 9-14: *Venous reflux by spectral Doppler upon release of distal compression. Image courtesy of GE Healthcare*

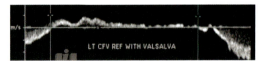
Fig. 9-15: *Venous reflux with a Valsalva maneuver*

Flow Description

- **Decreased spontaneity:** Venous flow is not observed without having to perform manual compression, significantly decreasing the color scale, Doppler baselines and increasing gains.
- **Absent spontaneity:** When flow is not observed at all by color or spectral Doppler after manual compression or transducer and setting adjustments.

- **Abnormal phasicity with respiration:** changes in the expected cyclical venous waveform pattern can indicate an obstruction proximal or at the level of the transducer. Abnormal phasicity can be described as:
  - » **Decreased phasicity:** When the venous waveform demonstrates less variation with the respiratory cycle than normal for that segment. Comparing the contralateral venous segment at the same level can sometimes be helpful. The 2020 consensus paper suggests using "decreased respirophasic" as a descriptor.[22]
  - » **Absent phasicity:** There is no evidence of flow, phasic or otherwise with respiration.
- **Continuous flow** takes on a steady and consistent appearance with little to no variability during normal respiration. It is suggestive of significant proximal obstruction, occlusion, or extrinsic compression, impeding the venous outflow and causing a flat/continuous signal on spectral Doppler.

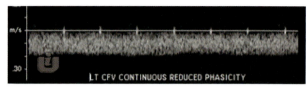
Fig. 9-16: *Continuous venous spectral Doppler flow*

- **Augmentation:** Reduced (or absent) augmentation can indicate an obstruction proximal to the transducer. The 2020 consensus paper suggests using the following terms:
  - » **Reduced augmentation:** Decreased venous flow augmentation in response to compression maneuvers.
  - » **Absent augmentation:** No increase in venous flow in response to compression maneuvers.

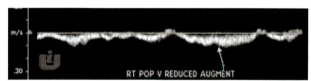
Fig. 9-17: *Reduced augmentaion: no significant increase with compression of the distal limb.*

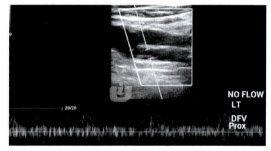
Fig. 9-18: *Absent augmentation: no flow due to thrombosis*

- **Pulsatility:** This finding is abnormal in the lower extremity veins and could suggest congestive heart failure.

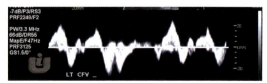
Fig. 9-19: *Pulsatile venous flow demonstrated with spectral Doppler.*

- **Regurgitation:** A term suggested by the 2020 Consensus paper to describe bidirectional venous flow that has similar amplitude in both the forward and reversed direction seen in cases of certain cardiac conditions.

Soft Tissue Edema [3,4]

- **Edema** is a common finding in patients with venous disease and is usually associated with elevated venous pressures.[3] Fluid shifts from intravascular compartments (heart and blood vessels) to the extravascular spaces (interstitial space, cells, and cerebrospinal fluid) with inadequate absorption from the lymphatic vessels leading to edema.[15,16]
- Causes of edema include venous reflux, obstruction (DVT), chronic post-thrombotic changes, compression, and organ failures. Right heart failure, lymphedema, vascular malformations, and drug effects are other common causes.
- Venous hypertension increases fluid filtration leading to edema. Fibrinogen and red blood cells (RBC) escape into the tissues, promoting an inflammatory cascade responsible for skin discoloration and fibrosis. Some patients eventually will develop an ulcer.[3,5,11,12]
- Elevating the legs causes a drop in hydrostatic pressure which will reduce the intracapillary pressure, decreasing the swelling.

The forces between the pressures are usually balanced with any remaining fluid absorbed by the lymphatics.

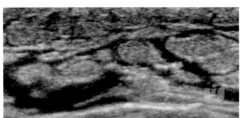

Fig. 9-20: *Soft tissue edema in the lower extremity.*

REFERENCES

1. Owen, C, Robers, M. Arterial Vascular Hemodynamics .Journal of Diagnostic Medical Ultrasound 23:129-140, May/June 2007.
2. M Boron,WF and Boulpaep, EL Medical Physiology, A Cellular and Molecular Approach. Elsevier, (2005)
3. Richard E. Klabunde, Ph.D., Cardiovascular Physiology Concepts, 2011 Chapters 5,7,& 8 Lippincott, Williams and Wilkins.
4. Needham, T, Needham, A. Characteristics of Pressure and Flow in Arteries and Veins: The Application to Noninvasive Peripheral Vascular Testing. The journal for Vascular Ultrasound 35(4):229-236, 2011.
5. Sumner DS, Zierler RE. (2005). Vascular physiology: essential hemodynamic principles. In Rutherford Vascular Surgery 6th edition. Philadelphia. Elsevier Saunders.
6. Kupinski, Anne Marie (2013) In The Vascular System 1st edition (p 66, 81), Philadelphia. Wolters Kluwer
7. Miele, FR: Ultrasound Physics and Instrumentation. 4th edition, Forney, TX, Miele enterprises, 2006
8. Meissner MH. (2010). Chronic venous disorders. In Zierler RE (Ed.), Strandess's duplex scanning. disorders in vascular diagnosis 4th ed. (223-229). Philadelphia Wolters Kluwer Lippincott Williams & Wilkins.
9. Size, Gail, Introduction to Venous testing, Inside Ultrasound, Pearce, AZ, Inside Ultrasound 1995.
10. Gianni Belcaro, Andrew N. Nicolaides, M. Veller, A Manual of Diagnosis and Treatment W.B. Saunders, 1995.
11. Sumner DS, Zierler RE. (2005). Vascular physiology: essential hemodynamic principles. In Rutherford Vascular Surgery 6th edition. (75 - 123). Philadelphia. Elsevier Saunders.
12. Meissner MH. (2010). Chronic venous disorders. In Zierler RE (Ed.), Strandess's duplex scanning disorders in vascular diagnosis 4th ed. (223 - 229).Philadelphia Wolters Kluwer Lippincott Williams & Wilkins. Oklu et al. (2012). J Vasc Interv Radiol; 23:33-39.
13. Labropoulos N. How Does Chronic Venous Disease Progress from the First Symptoms to the Advanced Stages: A Review. Adv Ther. 2019 Mar;36(Suppl 1):13-19.
14. Labropoulos N, Wierks C, Golts E, Volteas SK, Leon M, Volteas N, et al. Microcirculatory changes parallel the clinical deterioration of chronic venous insufficiency. Phlebology. 2004;19(2):81–86.
15. Levick JR, Michel CC. Microvascular fluid exchange and the revised Starling principle. Cardiovasc Res. 2010;87(2):198–210.
16. Mortimer PS, Rockson SG. New developments in clinical aspects of lymphatic disease. J Clin Invest. 2014 Mar;124(3):915-21.
17. Byju's. (n.d.). Hydrostatic Pressures. https://byjus.com/physics/hydrostatic-pressure/#:-:text=Asked%20 Questions%20%E2%80%93%20FAQs-,What%20is%20Hydrostatic%20Pressure%3F,a%20 downward%20force%20is%20applied.
18. Kim ES, Sharma AM, Scissons R, et al. Interpretation of peripheral arterial and venous Doppler waveforms: A consensus statement from the Society for Vascular Medicine and Society for Vascular Ultrasound. Vascular Medicine. 2020;25(5):484-506. doi:10.1177/1358863X20937665
19. Labropoulos, N., et al. (2009). Secondary chronic venous disease progresses faster than primary. Journal of Vascular Surgery, 49(3), 704–710. https://doi.org/10.1016/j.jvs.2008.10.014
20. Venous return. (n.d.). howMed. Retrieved April 1, 2022 from http://howmed.net/physiology/venous-return/#.YdcaV7YJqns
21. Ludbrook, J. (1996) The Musculovenous Pumps of The Human Lower Limb. Am Heart J. 71(5), 635-641.
22. Lejars, F., (1890). Les veines de la plante du pied. Archives de Physiologie. 5ᵉ série.
23. Uhl, J.F., Gillot, C. (2010). The plantar venous pump: Anatomy and physiological hypotheses. Phlebolymphology.org. https://www.phlebolymphology.org/the-plantar-venous-pump-anatomy-and-physiological-hypotheses
24. Meissner, M. H., et al. (2007). The hemodynamics and diagnosis of venous disease. Journal of Vascular Surgery, 46 Suppl S, 4S–24S. https://doi.org/10.1016/j.jvs.2007.09.043
25. Goldman, M.P., Fronek, A. (1989). Anatomy and pathophysiology of varicose veins. J Dermatol Surg Oncol, 15, 138-145.
26. Burnand K.G. (2001). The physiology and hemodynamics of chronic venous insufficiency of the lower limb. In: P. Gloviczki, P & Yao. J.S.T. (Eds.), Handbook of Venous Disorders Guidelines of the American Venous Forum. (2nd ed., pp. 49-57). London Arnold.

HEMODYNAMICS AND PHYSIOLOGY
10. Arterial

Normal Arterial Hemodynamics

What is hemodynamics?
- *Hemo* refers to blood and *dynamics* related to motion. Hemodynamics is the study of the motion of blood flow.
- Hemodynamic measurements are the primary type of data recorded in vascular laboratory exams.
- Hemodynamic measurements are typically related to either pressure or velocity. Each of these is influenced by a variety of physical conditions.

Why measure pressure and velocity?
Pressure and velocity are inversely related. When one increases the other will decrease. Since energy must remain the same: an increase in velocity creates a corresponding decrease of pressure energy.

Table 10-1: Pressure/Velocity Relationship

↑ Increases pressure	↓ Decreases velocity
↓ Decreases pressure	↑ Increases velocity

Energy and The Bernoulli Equation [3,4,5,6]

The *Bernoulli equation* explains how the total energy in a system (like the vascular system) is a combination of potential energy (PE) and kinetic energy (KE). In the circulatory system, potential energy is in the form of pressure and kinetic energy is the velocity. That explains why we measure both pressure and velocity in vascular exams on patients.

- When fluid flows from one point to another, total energy remains constant assuming that flow is steady with no frictional energy losses.
- **Potential energy is stored energy** and represents approximately 98% of the energy in the circulatory system. The vast majority of this stored or potential energy is in the form of pressure. The other major source of PE in the vascular system is hydrostatic pressure from gravity.
- **Kinetic energy is the energy of motion** and represents approximately 2% of the energy in the circulatory system. KE occurs when blood flows and is reflected by density and velocity squared.

In the vascular system, potential energy is primarily pressure, and kinetic energy is primarily velocity.

Table 10-2: Kinetic/Potential Energy Relationship

↑ Increases Kinetic energy	↓ Decreases Potential energy
↓ Decreases Kinetic energy	↑ Increases Potential energy

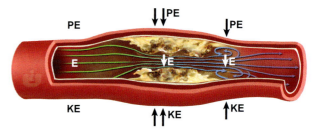

PE = potential energy
KE = kinetic energy
E = energy

Fig. 10-1: *Bernoulli Equation:* Kinetic E + Potential E = Total E

- Since total energy must remain constant, as kinetic energy increases, potential energy must decrease and vice versa.

Pressure [3,4,5,6]

What does pressure have to do with blood flow?
In the circulatory system, pressure is the amount of force that presses on a blood vessel at any point in time and location. This pressure is measured in *millimeters of mercury* (mmHg).

Pressure is supplied primarily from the action of the heart pushing blood into the vessels. Pressure changes within the vessels during the cardiac cycle, with higher pressure during the systolic push and lower pressure during diastole when blood flows on its own momentum.

Pressure Gradients
- Blood flows due to a change in pressure from one location to another.
- Flow will always move from a point of higher pressure toward a point with lower pressure.
- This change in pressure is called a *pressure gradient* and is defined as a reduction in pressure from one point to the next.
- Blood flows from the heart to the arteries, capillaries, venules and veins and back to the heart. A significant pressure gradient (decrease in pressure) must be present for this complete circulation to occur.

Systolic and Diastolic Pressure
- The primary source of pressure to start blood flowing is the contraction of the heart. This contraction period of the cardiac cycle is called *systole*.
- During systole a certain amount of blood is expelled from the left ventricle into the aorta This is known as *stroke volume*.
- The amount of blood that suddenly enters the aorta causes arterial pressure to increase and the arterial walls to expand. The pressure that is placed on the arterial walls during heart contraction is called *systolic pressure*.

As we age, arteries become stiffer, increasing systolic pressure.

- When the heart stops its contraction, the heart chambers fill up with blood again getting ready for the next systolic contraction. This resting phase of the heart is called *diastole*.
- As the heart rests, the arterial blood volume decreases causing a decrease in both the arterial diameter and its pressure. The pressure that occurs during the heart's resting phase is called *diastolic pressure*.

- During diastole the blood continues to flow on its own momentum and is highly affected by the amount of resistance encountered.
- The blood flows because of a pressure gradient from the left ventricle where typically the systolic pressure might be 120mmHg and returns to the right atrium via the veins where the typical pressure is 2-6 mmHg.
- Although systolic pressure rises slightly from the heart to the ankles, diastolic pressure decreases. This results in a mean pressure decrease creating the necessary pressure gradient needed for flow to move from the heart to the ankles.

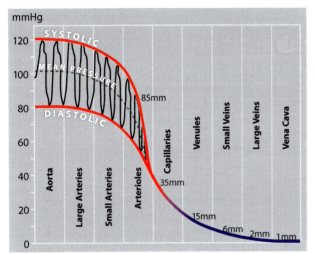

Fig. 10-2: Pressure drops across different levels of the circulation. Note the large drop in pressure seen as flow passes through the arterioles and again through the capillaries.

Flow, Pressure Gradient and Resistance [2,3,4]

- For flow to occur, the pressure gradient must overcome resistance to flow as stated in *Poiseuille's Law:*
  » Resistance occurs from the friction of the blood cells rubbing against the walls of the vessel as well as one layer of blood cells rubbing against other layers of flowing blood. Friction can be increased by the length of a tube that the blood is flowing through as well as the viscosity or stickiness of the blood which will cause more friction.

  $$Q = (P_2 - P_1) \div R$$

  » **Flow (Q)** is the amount of a liquid moving past a point in a given amount of time. Flow units are reported in *volume per time*. (e.g., pouring 5 gallons of milk in a minute (gal/min) or blood flowing in milliliters per minute (ml/min) in the vascular system. Flow should not be confused with velocity (v) which is speed in a certain direction, such as 5mph; eastward.
  » **Pressure (P)** is the amount of force placed on an artery at any given point in time and is measured in millimeters of mercury (mmHg).
  » **Resistance (R)** is a force that must be overcome for flow to occur. Resistance to flow occurs from friction and obstruction.
- Poiseuille's Law, $Q = P/R$ describes the relationship between steady flow (Q), pressure gradient (P), and resistance (R) in a straight tube. This is obviously not the case in the circulatory system where flow is not continuous but instead pulsatile and sometimes turbulent. However, this law helps us to understand the relationship between pressure, resistance, and blood flow. A pressure gradient allows a decrease in pressure. An increase in the pressure gradient means there is a greater difference in pressure from point A to point B. If resistance to flow increases due to obstructions for instance, the pressure gradient must increase to try to maintain flow.
- For blood to flow it must have a pressure gradient AND overcome resistance in its path.

$$Q = \frac{\Delta P}{R}$$

Q = flow
ΔP = pressure gradient or pressure drop where $\Delta P = (P_1 - P_2)$
R = resistance to flow

- **Length:** A longer tube will cause more friction and therefore give more resistance to flow than a shorter tube. As length increases, so does resistance.

A longer vessel has more wall surface for flow to drag on, which can create higher resistance.

- **Viscosity:** Resistance to flow depends on the "stickiness" of the fluid, called *viscosity*. An example of a highly viscous fluid is syrup, while water has a low viscosity. The most important factor affecting viscosity is the concentration of red blood cells (RBC), hematocrit and plasma protein. Friction is caused by the RBC dragging against each other in the layers of flow.
- **Radius:** Resistance to flow in a tube is highly affected by the radius of the tube to the 4th power, *making radius the most influential characteristic of resistance.*

$$Q = \frac{\Delta P}{R} \quad \text{then} \quad Q = \frac{\Delta P \pi r^4}{8 \eta L}$$

Small changes in the vessel's radius can result in large changes in flow volume.

- The radius of an artery changes as the blood flows from larger to smaller vessels and can change as a matter of normal function of the arterioles.
- *Arterioles* are the small arteries that connect larger arteries to the capillaries. Their diameters are measured in micrometers. They act as the gatekeepers controlling the amount of flow allowed to enter the tissues they guard. They have the ability to either contract or expand to control the amount of blood needed by their tissues at any point in time.
  » For example, if more flow is needed by tissues due to exercise or because of flow obstruction to the tissues, the arterioles can open up, increasing the radius, decreasing resistance, and increasing flow.

Resistance Equation

The relationship between resistance, length, viscosity, and radius is demonstrated in this equation:

$$R = \frac{8 L \eta}{\pi r^4}$$

R = resistance to flow
L = length of the tube
η = viscosity of the blood
π = pi (3.14)
r = radius of the tube

- Length and viscosity are directly proportional to resistance. If the length of the tube or the viscosity of the blood increases, it causes an increase in resistance to flow, and vice versa.
- Conversely, the radius of the tube in the denominator indicates it is indirectly proportional to resistance.
- A decrease in radius results in a fourfold increase in flow, and vice versa.

Poiseuille's Law

- If the resistance to flow increases, the pressure gradient must also increase to maintain flow levels. Note that the pressure itself does not increase, it is the pressure gradient that increases as it shows a greater CHANGE in pressure from point A to point B. For example:
  » A pressure change from 120mmHg to 100mmHg results in a pressure gradient of only 20mmHg ΔP = (P1-P2).
  » A pressure change from 90mmHg to 40mmHg is a larger pressure gradient of 50mmHg, despite the lower pressures involved.
- An arterial obstruction will increase resistance to flow, so flow will be reduced. Poiseuille's Law tells us there will be a corresponding increase in the pressure gradient to maintain flow. For instance, if there is normally a pressure drop of 15mmHg from the upper thigh to lower thigh, a significant obstruction in the mid-thigh may result in a pressure gradient of 40mmHg from the upper thigh to the lower thigh.

Combining the Resistance Equation with Poiseuille's Law

When the resistance equation ($R = 8 L \eta \div \pi r^4$) replaces R in Poiseuille's equation ($Q = \Delta P/R$), the result is a summary of factors involving flow, pressure, and resistance.

$$Q = \frac{\Delta P \pi r^4}{8 L \eta}$$

Q = flow
ΔP = pressure gradient
r^4 = radius to the fourth power
L = length
η = viscosity
π = pi

Combining these equations demonstrates how a significant decrease in the arterial radius (r^4) will be balanced by a significant pressure gradient (ΔP) down the limb to try to maintain flow. By measuring pressures and checking the pressure gradient we can detect significant obstruction. Also, multiple obstructions in the arterial system will result in lower pressures than a single obstruction would cause, so pressures are helpful to distinguish the sum total effect of all significant obstructions feeding the distal tissues of the arm or leg. Refer to the interpretation section of each chapter for specific details.

Systemic and Hydrostatic Pressure Within the Vascular System

Effects of Gravity on Pressure = Hydrostatic Pressure

Hydrostatic pressure is the force of gravity on a column of fluid that gives it weight. The effects of hydrostatic pressure are primarily noted when a person is standing, sitting, or raising a limb. Think about the column of blood as a tube from the heart to the ankle while an individual is standing. Gravity increases the pressure especially at the ankle, which is holding most of the weight in that column of blood. When a person is standing, the pressure is the highest at the ankles where the arterial pressure while standing is the sum of the systolic pressure PLUS the hydrostatic pressure from gravity.

- The right atrium is considered the 0-point for hydrostatic pressure. Since the brachial artery in its normal resting location is at the same level or right next to the heart, it is used to represent systemic pressure.

- However, if an arm is raised above the level of the heart, gravity causes blood to rush down to the heart and hydrostatic pressure is negative in that arm. This negative pressure in the raised arm causes the pressure in the arteries and veins to be lower in that position. That is why veins collapse when the arm is raised.

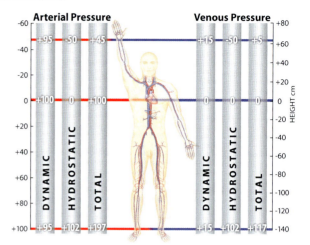

Fig. 10-3: *For a 6 ft. tall person, standing hydrostatic pressure adds ~102mmHg pressure to the existing arterial or venous pressure.* [6]

- Blood pressure measurements are always taken in the lower extremities with the patient in the supine position. This is important in order to negate the effects of hydrostatic pressure (gravity) on the blood pressure. Hydrostatic pressure increases for every centimeter the artery is below the heart; enough so that a 6 ft tall person can have ~102mmHg pressure added to the arterial and venous pressures at the ankle upon standing. Hydrostatic pressure also causes a decrease in pressure in the arms when they are raised above the heart.

When pressures are measured, an individual needs to be in a supine position to negate the effects of hydrostatic pressure. When a person is laying down, hydrostatic pressure is applied fairly equally on all parts of the circulation with very little change in pressure from gravity between one level and the next.

- Hydrostatic pressure is important in the venous system. Hydrostatic pressure acts as resistance to flow going back to the heart while a person is standing. *(See Venous Hemodynamics)*
- To increase pressure, the limb can be positioned lower than the heart. *See the Chronic Venous Insufficiency chapter to see how you can reduce pressure by raising the limb above the level of the heart.*

Effects of Exercise on Pressure, Resistance, and Flow

Exercising muscles demand more blood flow due to the need for more oxygen and nutrients as the muscles work.

- To understand the effect of exercise on blood flow, recall Poiseuille's Law ($Q = \Delta P \div R$).
- Blood flow (Q) during exercise increases 3-5 times over the resting flow in normal vessels.
- Upon exercise, arterioles normally open, decreasing resistance (R) and thereby increasing needed flow.
- Normal post-exercise pressures should remain the same as the pre-exercise pressures OR increase slightly due to decreased peripheral resistance.

During exercise, the flow and pressure gradient increase.

Velocity

The first part of this section explained the role of pressure in arterial hemodynamics. This section explains blood flow velocity and its role in assessing arterial hemodynamics.

Velocity Measurements

- **Flow** is the volume of fluid moving past a point in a certain amount of time (e.g., milliliters per minute).
- **Velocity** is the speed in a certain direction. Velocities are typically measured on Doppler waveforms at peak systole, end diastole, and can be compared as a velocity ratio. These measures are used as the diagnostic criteria to indicate the presence, severity, and location of arterial obstructions to flow.
- Doppler measurements in vascular exams are usually expressed in cm/s or m/s.

Do not confuse velocity with flow.

- Velocity direction is described as either toward or away from the Doppler beam. This is turn is interpreted as either an antegrade, or retrograde direction.
  - » **Antegrade** = in the direction of normal blood flow for that vessel.
  - » **Retrograde** = flow moving backwards or in the opposite direction expected for that vessel.
- Blood flow velocities vary throughout the circulatory system and in response to both normal and abnormal conditions.
- Doppler ultrasound is used to display velocity changes throughout the cardiac cycle over time (waveforms) and to measure peak systolic (PSV) and end diastolic (EDV) velocities.
- The velocity scale is established using a calculation done performed by the equipment based largely on the frequency shift and the Doppler angle used for the Doppler sample displayed.
- Velocities are calculated by the equipment using the Doppler equation. This calculation uses the frequency shifts collected by the equipment from the echoes as well as the Doppler angle established by the sonographer.

Doppler Waveforms

- Doppler waveforms are created by sending an ultrasound beam into the tissue and collecting the echoes. The computer analyzes changes in frequency shifts, which are proportional to velocities. These frequency shifts create the pulsatile arterial flow patterns seen as Doppler waveforms.
- Waveforms display Doppler frequency shifts across time.
- Each "dot" that makes up the waveform represents frequency shifts on the y-axis. The Doppler display shows a velocity scale rather than a frequency shift scale.

Doppler Equations for Frequency Shift and Velocity

$$\Delta f = \frac{2\, v\, f_0 (\cos\theta)}{C} \qquad v = \frac{\Delta f\, C}{2\, f_0\, (\cos\theta)}$$

Δ f = (frequency shift) difference between original and echo frequency

v = velocity of moving reflector (RBC's)

f_0 = frequency of sound source (transducer)

cos θ = cosine of the angle between the ultrasound beam and flow direction (cosine of the Doppler angle)

C = speed of sound in tissue (C = 1540m/s)

- The accuracy of the velocities is highly dependent upon the angle of the Doppler beam (or the Doppler angle). In order to document accurate velocities, the sonographer must set their angle parallel to the direction of flow by steering the Doppler beam on the equipment appropriately. This also helps to obtain the best waveform. The Doppler angle should be kept under 60° and the angle of the cursor should be parallel to the walls of the artery or flow of blood.
- Velocities are measured using calipers placed on the spectral Doppler waveforms. Blood flow velocities are typically measured at peak systolic and end diastolic points within the pulsatile arterial flow pattern.

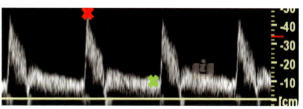

Fig. 10-4: *The Doppler Waveform Explained:*

  - » Peak systolic velocity (PSV) is measured at the height of the waveform during the systolic phase. **(X)**
  - » End diastolic velocity (EDV) is measured at the right before the next systolic uprise. **(X)**

- Flow direction is displayed either as flow toward the Doppler beam or away from it. Flow toward the beam is displayed above the baseline. Flow away from the Doppler beam is displayed below the baseline. Traditionally, normal arterial flow direction is set above the baseline and normal venous flow is set below the baseline.

Why do we measure velocities?

- Both velocities and velocity flow patterns are important elements for accurate interpretation of arterial examinations. Velocities and velocity ratios can indicate stenosis in an artery and its severity, while velocity waveform patterns can yield information about inflow, focal flow, and outflow. This section describes the basic principles behind these uses.
- Mean velocity times area = flow. As the artery narrows, velocity increases and if the artery widens, velocity will decrease.

Flow Velocity Equation

$$Q = \text{mean } V \times A$$

(Flow = mean velocity × area)

Basic Circle Measurements

Area (A) = π r²

Diameter (d) = 2 r

Radius (r) = d ÷ 2

- Arteries have natural areas of widening and narrowing causing natural changes in velocities and flow patterns.
- Disease will cause abnormal areas of narrowing and widening such as stenosis or aneurysm. A widened area (e.g., aneurysm) will display lower velocities than the non-aneurysmal area.
- Velocity measurements and/or velocity ratios are typically used to suggest areas of narrowing using velocity thresholds for that particular artery.

Normal Velocities and Velocity Ratios

Velocities

- Normal velocities are typically much higher in the arteries than in the veins due to the systolic push of blood from the heart.
- Normal velocities vary from one artery to the next throughout the circulatory system, from patient to patient, and depend on the hemodynamic conditions of the patient at the time.

- » Velocities normally decrease as blood flows from the groin to the ankles. For example, a PSV of 100cm/s in the common femoral artery may lower to 60cm/s in the popliteal segment.
- » Obviously if arterial velocities differ throughout the body, a normal arterial velocity in one area of the body is not necessarily normal in another area. Each technical chapter will address the typical, normal velocity ranges as appropriate.

Velocity Ratios

- Velocity ratios often compare proximal velocity (V_1) to one just distal (V_2). The useful ratio helps to assess how much the velocity changes at a stenosis.
- Due to the variations in normal velocities, velocity ratios (V_2/V_1) are often used as an additional diagnostic velocity tool in vascular exams.
- Peak systolic velocities typically do not increase more than two-times the proximal velocity in vessels similar in wall-to-wall size (i.e., proximal vessel is not aneurysmal.) A PSV ratio <2.0 is typically normal.

$$\text{PSV ratio} = \frac{\text{PSV of the distal segment or at site of stenosis } (V_2)}{\text{PSV of the proximal segment or before stenosis } (V_1)}$$

Velocity Waveform Terminology [1,2,3,4,5,6]

- Doppler derived velocity waveforms can add information regarding the proximal, focal, and distal conditions of flow at any given location. A change in a Doppler waveform from one location to the next is helpful diagnostic information.
- Sometimes analysis of Doppler waveforms is described as "what's coming in (inflow), what's going on (focally), and what's going out (outflow.)"
- Arterial Doppler waveforms can be described in terms of flow direction, phasicity, and resistance. Other modifiers exist for Doppler waveforms created from specific flow conditions encountered in the arterial system.

Arterial Waveform Terminology

Although interpretation of arterial waveforms is usually agreed upon among professionals, the terminology used to describe these waveforms is not consistent. A consensus document was endorsed in 2020 by the Society of Vascular Ultrasound and the Society for Vascular Medicine regarding the terminology and interpretation of peripheral arterial waveforms. This section will describe the important components of the arterial waveform.

- To begin, arterial flow is pulsatile due to the contribution of the heart as its source of energy.
- The pulsatile segments of the Doppler velocity waveform that make up the interpretation of the waveform are its *upstroke, peak,* and *downstroke* into diastolic flow. In addition, blood flow moves in a certain *direction*.

Components of Arterial Velocity Waveforms
Direction

- Normal arterial flow direction is away from the heart, moving oxygenated blood toward a set of tissues or an organ.
- Normal direction is termed *antegrade*.
- Traditionally antegrade flow in an artery is displayed above the baseline of a spectral tracing for a Doppler waveform. "Reversed" or "retrograde" arterial flow direction is displayed below the Doppler baseline.

In certain situations, flow can be *"bidirectional"* (formerly referred to as "to and fro.") In this case the antegrade and retrograde parts of the waveform are fairly equal in duration. This occurs when the proximal and distal pressure changes with the cardiac cycle so flow moves towards the lower pressure when it changes. This can occur for example at the neck of pseudoaneurysm, where flow moves out of a hole in the artery into a contained space during systole, and then flow returns to the artery during diastole.

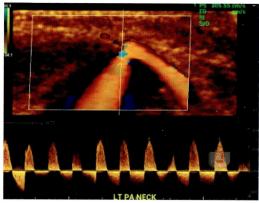

Fig. 10-5: *Bidirectional waveform pattern typically observed when sampling the neck of a pseudoaneurysm with spectral Doppler.*

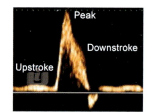

Fig. 10-6: *Normal, triphasic Doppler waveform*

Upstroke

- The upstroke of the Doppler waveform is formed by the influence of both the heart contraction and any significant obstructions proximal to the Doppler sample site (between the Doppler transducer and the heart.)
- Normally during the systolic push, there is a quick increase in flow volume and velocity in the arteries. A normal upslope in the waveform is a quick rise from the end of the prior cardiac cycle to the systolic peak.

Peak

- The systolic peak is the highest point you would measure on the waveform.
- The systolic peak is normally sharp rather than broad or blunted.

Downstroke into Diastolic Flow

- Diastolic flow is highly influenced by resistance because the power from the systolic push has ended and blood is flowing on its own momentum.
- After the systolic push is completed, velocities slow down rapidly, normally creating a quick initial downslope in the velocity waveform.
- The shape of the downstroke into diastolic flow is highly dependent upon the resistance and flow demand of the distal vascular bed that artery is feeding.
- Tissues such as brain, kidneys, and liver require constant forward flow to meet the demand of their function. This allows the arterioles to stay open wide, reducing resistance, so continuous forward flow is seen in the diastolic segment of the arterial waveforms feeding them.

» Conversely, some tissues vary in their need for flow depending on if they are at rest or highly functioning at the time. For example, when leg muscles are at rest, the arteries feeding them do not need constant forward flow. Instead, they demonstrate waveforms with a short period of reversed flow at late systole/early diastole that recovers to forward flow after that short duration of reversed flow. The reversed flow phase is due to the flow resistance set by distal arterioles holding a smaller diameter at rest.

» When the distal vascular bed changes to an active state, for example when walking, there is higher flow demand than at rest so the arterioles open to reduce resistance and increase flow as needed. The waveform that demonstrated high resistance at rest becomes low resistance during and immediately after exercise reflecting constant forward flow in diastole.

- Waveforms can be described as high, intermediate, or low resistance in nature depending on the shape of the waveform and downslope through diastole, after the peak. As the distal resistance changes, the diastolic portion of the waveform will reflect that change.

Resistance in Arterial Waveform Patterns

- Velocity profiles in Fig. 10-7 correspond to the waveform phases observed during spectral analysis.
- 90% of total vascular resistance results from flow through the arteries and capillaries and 10% results from venous flow.
- The large and medium sized arteries are responsible for 15% of the total resistance.
- The arterioles and capillaries are responsible for over 60% of the total resistance.

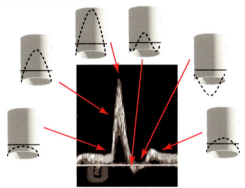

Fig. 10-7: *The Doppler waveform reflects various phases encountered as the blood flows through the artery. In this example from an artery feeding a high resistant bed, blood flow moves forward during systole, reverses for a moment in early diastole before continuing forward again in late diastole.*

High, Intermediate, and Low Resistance Waveforms

- Normal waveforms can have different shapes depending on the resistance of the distal vascular bed and the conditions at the time, i.e., at-rest versus post exercise.

High Resistance Waveform

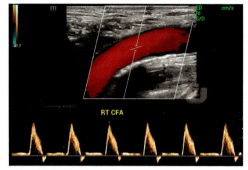

Fig. 10-8: *High resistance spectral Doppler waveform (Note the reversed flow below the baseline at end systole/early diastole).*

- A quick downstroke that ends with a short period of reversed flow direction (below the baseline) at end systole/early diastole is termed a *high resistance waveform*. This reversed flow segment in the waveform may or may not be followed by a third segment with a low, short segment of forward flow This waveform can also be referred to as *triphasic*.
- The reversed flow segment is due to the antegrade flow hitting resistance at the smaller arterioles. Flow is being "sent back" at that particular point in the cardiac cycle because the systolic push has ended and resistance to flow is lower proximally for a moment. Remember: flow moves toward areas that offer lower resistance to flow or lower pressure.
- Waveforms that have this reversed flow period are normal for certain arteries at rest such as the peripheral arteries of the lower extremities and superior mesenteric arteries prior to eating, when constant forward flow is not necessary.
- Examples of high resistance vessels:
  » External carotid artery   » Aorta
  » Pre-prandial mesenteric artery   » Upper/Lower extremity peripheral vasculature

Intermediate Resistance Waveform

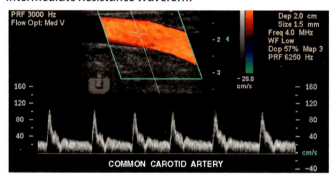

Fig. 10-9: *CCA spectral Doppler waveforms are an example of intermediate resistance (Note the notch in the downslope at late systole/early diastole).* Courtesy of Philips Healthcare

- A waveform with a quick downstroke without reversed flow direction below the baseline may demonstrate a short period of acceleration in the downstroke called a "notch." A waveform with a notch in the downstroke in late systole instead of the reversed flow period is considered an *intermediate resistance waveform*[11] (also referred to as biphasic).
- A waveform with a downslope notch is typically noted in normal forearm arteries and the external carotid artery.

Low Resistance Waveform

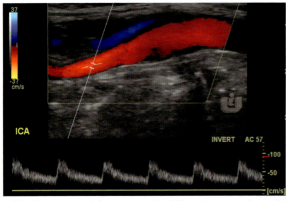

Fig. 10-10: *Low resistance spectral Doppler waveform (Note the continuous forward flow throughout the cardiac cycle).*

- If the downstroke decelerates into continuous forward flow throughout the cardiac cycle with no reversed flow phase or notch, it demonstrates low resistance flow and is described as a *low resistance waveform*.
- When the distal vascular bed requires constant flow, the arterioles are wide open, reducing resistance and increased flow.
- This constant forward flow with no reversed flow phase or notch is normally seen in the internal carotid and vertebral arteries that feed the brain, the celiac artery which feeds the liver and spleen, and renal arteries feeding the kidneys.
- A low resistance waveform is also seen in normal conditions requiring more flow to function, such as lower extremity arteries during and after exercise or in the superior mesenteric artery after eating.
- Examples of low resistant vessels:
  » Internal carotid artery
  » Vertebral arteries
  » Renal arteries
  » Splenic artery
  » Post-prandial mesenteric artery
  » Celiac artery
  » Hepatic artery

Vascular resistance to flow is highly affected by the arterioles in the distal vascular bed being fed by the assessed artery.

Arterial Waveform Phasicity

- According to the waveform consensus paper, a waveform can also be termed *multiphasic or monophasic*.[11] The particular descriptor used is dependent on the presence or absence of the reversed flow phase at end systole.
- A *multiphasic waveform* displays a short-reversed flow segment (below the baseline) at end-systole whether or not there is a short recovery flow phase after it.

Multiphasic Waveforms

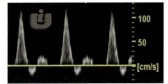

Fig. 10-11: *Waveform with reversed flow and recovery phase.*

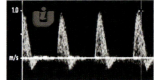

Fig. 10-12: *Waveform displays only the reversed flow phase with no recovery phase.*

- Both waveforms above are considered multiphasic. Most labs would consider the left waveform triphasic, but the waveform on the right was described differently with some labs using the term triphasic due to the reversed flow and some calling it biphasic due to the lack of the recovery segment.

Monophasic Waveforms

- A monophasic waveform shows blunted, continuous flow into diastole with no flow reversal phase throughout the cardiac cycle.

A monophasic waveform can be either intermediate resistance or low resistance.

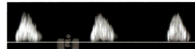 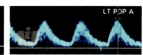

Fig. 10-13: *Monophasic waveform: Note the flow is in a single direction and does not cross the zero baseline at any part of the cardiac cycle.*

Fig. 10-14: *Monophasic waveforms that are low resistant: Note the continuous forward flow throughout the cardiac cycle.*

The waveform on the right demonstrates a deceleration/acceleration notch in the downslope at late systole/early diastole. The waveform on the left displays no notch. Both can be considered monophasic due to the constant flow above the baseline with no reversed flow at late systole/early diastole.[11] Some labs might term the waveform on the left biphasic to distinguish it from the waveform on the right which most labs would term monophasic due to the broader peak and possibly lower velocity.

Arterial Flow Patterns and Interpretation

- The interpretation of the waveform as normal or abnormal is highly dependent on understanding the hemodynamic flow patterns found in both normal abnormal conditions.
- A normal waveform in one part of the body may be considered abnormal in another location or under different conditions. For example, a normal waveform in the internal carotid artery would be considered abnormal in a lower extremity artery. Doppler waveforms are dependent upon the physiological conditions.
- This next section includes an overall view of some common flow patterns and the waveform characteristics expected. *Refer to each chapter for normal and abnormal hemodynamics and waveform characteristics commonly associated with different types of vascular exams.*

Normal Flow Patterns [1,3,5,7]

Normal flow patterns are different in straight arterial segments, branches, widenings, curves, and after exercise.

Normal Straight Artery

Laminar Flow with Parabolic Flow Profile

- Laminar flow is referred to as "parabolic flow" because of the velocity profile; in the shape of a parabola.
- Normally blood flows in *layers (laminar flow)* with a faster flow layer in the center of the vessel and slower flow in each layer along the vessel walls (this is known as a *parabolic flow profile*). The flow is slowest along the walls primarily due to friction between RBCs and the wall, as well as between RBCs themselves.
- Each layer travels at a different velocity with the fastest in the center of the stream, creating a normal spectral Doppler waveform with a clear spectral window.
- With the sample volume placed in the center of the normal lumen, the Doppler velocity waveform will typically demonstrate the highest velocities at the systolic peak.

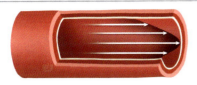

Fig. 10-15: Laminar– faster flow center stream

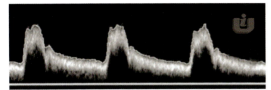

Fig. 10-16: Laminar flow in the internal carotid artery

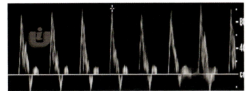

Fig. 10-17: Laminar flow in a peripheral artery

- Under normal flow conditions, flow is travelling at the same velocity so there is a narrow range of velocities at peak systole. This leaves a black triangular area under the waveform peak where no "slow" velocities are demonstrated. This triangular black area is termed the *spectral window* and is indicative of laminar flow.
- Note that the spectral window depends on multiple crystals used to obtain the Doppler data. Each crystal will have a similar but different Doppler angle, which can result in a wider range of frequency shifts. It is also important to understand that this spectral window may be filled in due to non-laminar flow, technical issues with sample volume placement and size, over-gain, and abnormal flow conditions.

Laminar Flow

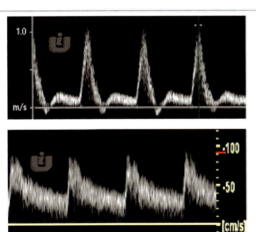

Fig. 10-18: Spectral window: the dark area under the peak indicates a narrow range of velocities.

Normal Flow in Branches

Blunt Flow (plug flow) and Disturbed flow

- Blunt flow also referred to as "plug flow" is when blood travels at generally the same speed across a tube rather than having faster velocities moving mid-stream. This creates a flow profile that is flat at the center (not parabolic) and slower along the walls. Blunt flow profiles normally occur in large arteries like the aorta as well as branch points.

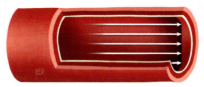

Fig. 10-19: Blunt: uniform flow across the vessel

- When an artery branch point is encountered, the flow layers become disrupted as they split between the two arteries causing a disturbed flow pattern (think about traffic when an expressway splits and cars choose which route to travel).
- The flow patterns at bifurcations differ depending on the angulation and size of the vessel. The angle and anatomy at bifurcations determine the flow disturbances and loss of energy. The greater the angle, the greater the flow disturbance. The less the angle of the artery branching off, the less flow disturbance that occurs.
- Disturbed flow is a slight change in the laminar flow pattern. There is some spectral broadening filling in the spectral window, or waveform differences across the vessel diameter at a widening, but no significant increase in velocity. Disturbed flow can occur at branches or in arterial vessels with a small amount of plaque.

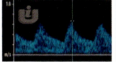 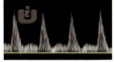 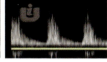

Fig. 10-20: Examples of spectral broadening where the spectral window is filled in. Spectral broadening indicates a wide range of velocities at a specific point in time due to disturbed or turbulent flow conditions.

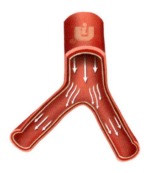

Fig. 10-21: Disturbed flow occurs at branching/bifurcations and at bypass anastomotic sites. The disturbed flow can predispose the artery to new or recurrent disease.

Normal Flow at Arterial Widening

Flow Separation

- *Flow separation* is a disrupted flow pattern that occurs naturally at the carotid bifurcation and frequently at the end of a stenotic narrowing where the lumen widens just past the plaque.
- Flow separation is distinguished by an area of reversed flow direction typically along one wall at a widening. At the carotid bifurcation the wall opposite the reversed area typically demonstrates antegrade flow. The mid lumen between each side has a combination of low velocity and a disturbed flow pattern, combining each pattern near the walls.

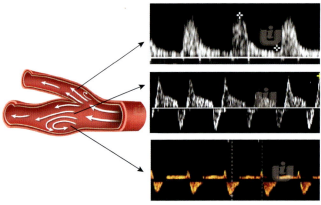

Fig. 10-22: *Flow separation at the carotid bulb. Depending on where the sample gate is placed, Doppler waveforms will vary.*

- When blood flows into an artery that has widened, the flow must move out of its layered pattern to fill the space. This causes the flow current on one side to first move past the widening and then reverse to fill the gap or move in a helical (spiral) flow pattern with one side moving away from the Doppler beam.
- Flow on the opposite side of the reversed flow, typically moves in an antegrade direction. This normal phenomenon is called flow separation.

Flow Along Curved Vessels
- As blood flows around a curve, fluid in the center of the vessel flows toward the outer wall and is replaced by the slower flow located near the inner wall, resulting in a type of helical flow pattern.
- **Flow on a curve:** Fluids flow faster on the outside of a curve and as the fluid makes the turn, the flow ends up in a spiral motion (think about a curve on a water slide). The helical motion may result in some flow moving toward the Doppler beam and some moving away along the opposite wall.
- It is typically best to avoid measuring velocities directly on a curve if possible. Instead, sample the artery mid-stream to avoid the higher velocity artifact encountered along the outer wall since it's not elevated due to stenosis.

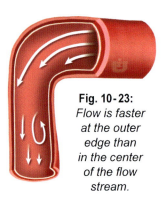

Fig. 10-23: *Flow is faster at the outer edge than in the center of the flow stream.*

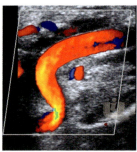

Fig. 10-24: *Note the brighter color on the curve of the vessel indicating faster flow.*

Abnormal Arterial Hemodynamic Characteristics [1,3,4,5,6]

Atherosclerosis is the most common disease in the arterial system. Atherosclerotic plaque, made up of fat, cholesterol, smooth muscle cells and other substances, first forms in the walls of arteries. Over many years plaque can encroach upon the arterial lumen and block flow as described in the *Vascular Diseases* chapter. In addition, it may break apart and send pieces called emboli to other parts of the body where they can become lodged in a smaller branch and block flow at that level.

Hemodynamics of Atherosclerosis

This section will focus on the general hemodynamic effects of atherosclerotic plaque as assessed by pressure, velocity, and velocity waveforms. Each technical chapter will describe the specific abnormalities for each measurement in that particular exam including other conditions such as volume changes. In addition, each technical chapter will describe abnormalities encountered from other vascular diseases.

Definitions

- When the plaque encroaches the lumen and results in a narrowing of the artery, it is called a *stenosis*. (Fig. 10-25) If a stenosis narrows the lumen by <50% its diameter, the body adjusts and flow, velocity, and pressure are not significantly affected.
- Each part of the body has a unique set of velocity criteria to grade the severity of stenosis. For instance, velocity criteria used for grading internal carotid artery stenosis will be different than the velocity criteria for renal arteries. The technical chapters will outline common velocity criteria used along with supporting waveform and image data.
  » Calculating % stenosis on duplex:

$$\frac{\text{narrowest residual lumen (mm)}}{\text{true lumen same location (mm)}} - 1$$

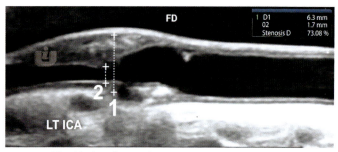

Fig. 10-25: *Stenosis measurement of the ICA*

The true/residual lumen can be measured at the point of stenosis on B-mode. Note: Angiographic calculation of diameter reduction uses the distal normal vessel where walls are parallel for the true lumen because the true walls are not visible on arteriograms.

- An occlusion is when plaque blocks the entire diameter of the artery (100%) and allows no flow to get through.
- The word "obstruction" refers to a hemodynamically significant stenosis and/or an occlusion.

Abnormal Pressures

- Recall that systolic blood pressure normally increases slightly from the groin to the ankles and from the arm to the forearm when the patient is supine.
- When there is a stenosis of <50% diameter, there is no significant change in pressure distally.
- If there is a hemodynamically significant obstruction (>50% stenosis or occlusion), a significant decrease in pressure occurs distal to the obstruction.
- Pressure ratios are often used to define the amount of pressure decrease from the systemic pressure. Normal ratios are typically 1.0 or greater comparing limb to brachial pressure. This varies slightly with cuff size and in the digits. Each chapter will specify the normal/abnormal pressure ratios.
- In general, a pressure difference >20-30mmHg between adjacent pressure cuffs on a limb indicates a hemodynamically significant obstruction.

Exercise [5]

Exercise will normally result in an increase or no change in systolic pressure. Hemodynamically significant obstructions will a decrease in systolic pressure distal to the obstruction.

Normal Response
- Recall that during exercise muscles require more flow to work. This increase in flow is achieved by the action of the arterioles opening to reduce resistance to flow. A reduction in resistance results in an increase in flow. (Poiseuille's Law: $Q = \Delta P \div R$)

Abnormal Response
- When arterial obstruction is present, resting pressures are often already decreased and arterioles are frequently already dilated to maintain adequate resting flow to the tissues according to Poiseuille's Law.
- When exercise is attempted and there is an obstruction present, the body may not be able to reduce the resistance any further, so the pressures decrease even more to expand the pressure gradient and increase flow. This explains why a drop in post-exercise pressure is an abnormal response and indicates a significant obstruction.
- When adequate flow cannot be reached during exercise, the patient experiences pain in the muscle area.
- In some patients, proximal obstruction does not decrease ankle pressures at rest because it is either of borderline hemodynamic significance or there is excellent compensation of flow from collaterals.
- Patients are sometimes referred for stress-testing when studies are normal at rest. Exercise increases the demand for blood flow, which will exaggerate a pressure gradient according to Poiseuille's Law ($Q = \Delta P \div R$) and decrease post-exercise pressures, uncovering the flow blockage that was unable to be appreciated at rest.

Abnormal Velocity Ratios and Velocity Waveforms
Inflow, focal, and outflow conditions can change the configuration of Doppler waveforms. This section presents an overall analysis of commonly encountered abnormal waveforms and the hemodynamic situations they represent. Each exam chapter has more detail on this topic.

Non-hemodynamically Significant Stenosis
Velocity
Plaque that blocks the artery by <50% its diameter may demonstrate a slight increase in velocity particularly if the stenosis is close to 50%, but the change in PSV is less than double the velocity 1-2cm immediately proximal. The velocity ratio is <2.0.

Waveforms
- The spectral window may be lost due to the disruption of the layers of blood moving out toward the walls in order to fill in the widened area past a narrowing.
- Spectral broadening can be seen at and just distal to a developing stenosis, but the primary shape of the peri-stenotic waveform is intact.

Hemodynamically Significant Stenosis
Velocity
- Once a stenosis blocks the artery >50% its diameter, velocities will increase significantly at the stenosis and pressure and flow will decrease distally. This is called a *hemodynamically significant stenosis*.
  » In general terms throughout the body, a hemodynamically significant stenosis will yield a peak systolic velocity within the stenosis that is at least two times the velocity in the proximal segment. So, in general a velocity ratio >2.0 is typically related to a hemodynamically significant stenosis.
  » Peak Systolic Velocity (PSV) Ratio:

$$\frac{\text{PSV within the stenosis}}{\text{PSV pre-stenosis within the normal lumen}}$$

- Stenoses at the high end of the 50-99% range also demonstrate a significant increase in end diastolic velocities.
- Flow (Q) = mean velocity times area (A). When a stenosis reaches at least 50% diameter reduction (mathematically equivalent to a 75% reduction in area,) the peak systolic velocity is noticeably increased.
- Specific ranges of normal and abnormal velocities vary greatly from one artery to the next.
- Once the artery reaches approximately a 90-95% diameter stenosis, the open lumen is so narrow that velocities start decreasing towards zero as the stenosis moves toward total occlusion. Think of it as covering almost the entire opening of a garden hose with your thumb so that the water barely comes out. This is sometimes called a "string sign." It is important to check velocities against the image to confirm that they agree.

Waveforms
Just proximal to a significant stenosis
- The waveform can have any type of configuration depending on what obstructions lie proximally, if any.

Within the stenosis
- There is an increase in the height of the systolic peak representing the increase in velocity.
- There may or may not be associated spectral broadening at the proximal end of the stenosis, however, there will certainly be spectral broadening observed distal to its tightest point.
- Frequently, the stenotic waveform includes reversed flow directly under the systolic peak *(Fig. 10-26)*, extending the range of velocities seen as spectral broadening.

Distal to the stenosis
- Turbulence increases distal to the hemodynamically stenosis and is known as *post-stenotic turbulence*.
- In addition to the velocity increase and spectral broadening, post-stenotic turbulence is an important marker of a hemodynamically significant stenosis.
- Turbulence is markedly chaotic flow with eddies and whirls moving blood in many directions just past the stenosis.
- Turbulence is much more chaotic than disturbed flow.
- The turbulent velocity pattern typically has marked spectral broadening and a "feathered" appearance along the upper border of the waveform. The feathering makes the upper border of the waveform difficult to trace, unlike the smooth upper border of the normal laminar or disturbed waveform pattern.

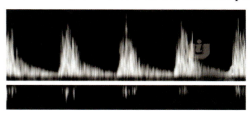

Fig. 10-26: *As the sample volume is moved distally beyond the stenosis the velocity will decrease and the waveform will eventually lose its feathered, turbulent appearance.*

More on Turbulence

In a hemodynamically significant stenosis, velocities increase within the stenosis and are typically at least double the pre-stenotic PSV. Post-stenotic flow is turbulent, chaotic flow moving in multiple directions immediately distal to the stenosis. Turbulence lessens as blood flows distally.

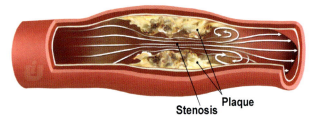

Fig. 10-27: *Flow changes around a hemodynamically significant stenosis.*

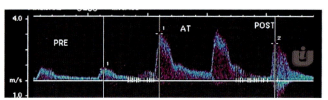

Fig. 10-28: *"Walking" through a significant stenosis: pre-stenosis, tightest point of the stenosis, and post-stenosis. In this example, the pre-stenosis velocity was 75cm/s, at stenosis: 305cm/s and post-stenosis: 242cm/s. The velocity ratio is 4.07 and post-stenotic turbulence is clearly seen with marked spectral broadening, reverse flow under the peak, and feathered outline at the early downslope of the peak.*

- Turbulence occurs when the flow velocity is so high that laminar flow is disrupted. Blood flow becomes chaotic and energy and pressure losses occur. The point where flow breaks up is defined by the *Reynolds' number*.
- The Reynolds' number (Re) predicts when turbulence will occur. [5,8]
- The Reynold's number describes the variables in blood flow that will cause the flow to become disrupted and disturbed.
- The Reynolds number is dimensionless.

Turbulence occurs when the critical Reynolds number (Re) is exceeded.

$$Re = \frac{Vq2r}{\eta}$$

Re = Reynold's Number
V = Velocity
q = Fluid Density
r = Radius
η = Viscosity

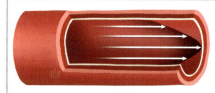

Laminar: faster flow center stream

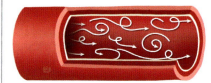

Eddy current: flow displayed after a stenosis

Fig. 10-29: *Laminar flow occurs at a low Re and is smooth, constant fluid motion. Turbulent flow occurs at a high Re producing flow instabilities, e.g., flow eddies and vortices.*

- The Reynold's number is typically <2000. Below 2000, there is laminar flow. Between 2000-3500, transitional flow is displayed by a mixture of both laminar and turbulent flow, and a Re >3500 creates turbulent flow. Some references use 2000-4000 as transitional and 4000 as the critical number for turbulence.
- Most importantly, Re increases as velocity or radius increases and decreases as viscosity increases.
  » Turbulence is more likely in large vessels with high flow/ high velocities (e.g., dialysis fistulas.)
  » Patients with sickle cell anemia may be more likely to show increased viscosity usually causing turbulent flow.

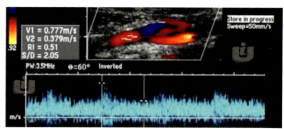

Fig. 10-30: *Turbulent post-stenotic waveform pattern displays marked spectral broadening and a "feathered" appearance along the upper border of the waveform.*

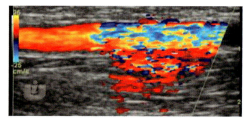

Fig. 10-31: *Turbulence creates a color Doppler bruit by causing vibrations radiating into the tissues surrounding the stenosis.*

- In the circulatory system, flow disturbances and turbulence can occur at lower Re values because of body movement, pulsatile flow, vessel diameter changes and diseased endothelium.
- Turbulence can create vessel vibrations called *bruits*. Bruits are vibrational sounds that can be heard using a stethoscope or seen in color images or within spectral Doppler waveforms. The turbulence causes the nearby tissues to vibrate which is motion that can be picked up by Doppler as echoes within the tissue during each cardiac cycle.

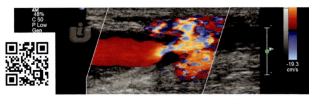

Fig. 10-32: *Turbulence creates a color Doppler bruit by causing vibrations in the tissue surrounding a highly turbulent area of flow.* Courtesy of Philips Healthcare

- **Occlusions:** An occluded artery must be proven with spectral Doppler even when no color flow is noted.
- Spectral Doppler, color, and B-mode will be used along with pre- and post-occlusion waveforms to indicate an occluded vessel.
- Waveforms proximal and close to an occlusion will typically demonstrate a loss of end diastolic flow.
  » A waveform with no diastolic flow is not a diagnostic sign of occlusion, only a marker that an occlusion may be encountered distally.
  » When there is a lack of end diastolic velocity and there is a change in the waveforms recorded proximally, these findings are good indicators of a distal occlusion or possibly an extremely tight stenosis.
  » Diastolic flow may be seen in a waveform proximal to an occlusion where a branch is present.
  » If no branches are present, the waveform may show a very low velocity, short duration waveform with an equally short duration reversed flow segment known as a "staccato" waveform proximal to an occlusion.
- Post-occlusion waveforms can be captured past the re-entry point of collateral flow. Post-occlusion waveforms are nearly always monophasic, blunted with a slow upstroke and wide peak (formerly referred to as *parvus tardus.*)

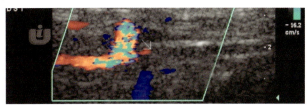

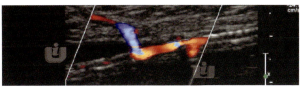

Fig. 10-33: *Collateral vessels known as "stem" and "re-entry" arteries" route flow around an occluded arterial segment. Re-entry arteries (lower image) signify the distal end of the occluded segment.*

Note the perpendicular takeoff of the collateral from the artery proximal to an occluded segment. Some collateral branches are only seen from a transverse view.

Collateral Blood Flow

- Collateral vessels are pre-existing pathways that enlarge in the presence of obstructions.
- Collateral pathways are routes for blood to flow around an occlusion or very tight obstruction in an artery.
- The collateral takes over the supply of blood when needed. Collateral routes are typically seen with chronic obstructions and develop more efficiency over time.

- Some collateral pathways in the circulatory system cause reversed flow in a short segment of the artery acting as a collateral. For example, if the origin of the subclavian artery is occluded, flow often reverses in the ipsilateral vertebral artery to feed the arm.
- Collateral arteries develop as numerous small and longer vessels compared to the native artery.
- There is very little vasodilation in response to vasodilator drugs in collateral vessels which have a relatively fixed vasomotor tone.
- Collateral vessels do not respond to exercise the same as native arteries.
- Collateral systems have three components:
  » **Stem arteries:** Large branches which can often be seen just proximal to an occlusion. Often found coming from the main artery at a perpendicular angle, so a transverse view may be helpful to identify all of the arteries.
  » **Mid zone collateral arteries** are smaller intramuscular channels. These channels cannot typically be followed on duplex due to their small size and vast number.
  » **Re-entry arteries** are branches that join the main artery distal to the disease. These are often seen at the site of reconstitution of flow in the main artery past the occluded segment.

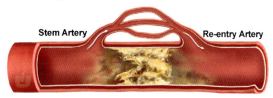

Fig. 10-34: *Stem and Re-entry collateral Arteries*

- The total resistance in the circuit takes into account the principle surrounding the collective resistance beds:
  » Flow, like current, always takes the path of "least resistance."
  » In a diseased patient, the flow would predominantly pass through the "lowest resistance" bed available.
  » Collaterals are generally less efficient. Due to their smaller diameter, collaterals would have higher resistance than an efficient, non-diseased main vessel; but they may be a lower resistance route when compared to a diseased main vessel.

Doppler samples should be taken with the smallest sample volume and center stream as opposed to along the walls to avoid these branches.

Tandem Lesions

- As blood flow passes a hemodynamically significant stenosis there is a great loss of energy as it flows distally. When this lower energy flow encounters a second stenosis, there is even more energy lost after the second lesion.
- If two hemodynamically significant stenoses run tandem to each other in the same artery, the actual velocity measurement in the first stenosis will be higher than the velocity in the second stenosis because of the loss of energy entering the second stenosis. This can cause an underestimation of the degree of stenosis at the second site unless other parameters are also used, i.e., image measurement, velocity ratio.
- Multiple stenoses in the same vessel *(a.k.a. stenoses in series)*, will increase the total resistance and have a greater effect on flow compared to two stenoses in two arteries running parallel to each other *(a.k.a. stenoses in tandem)*.

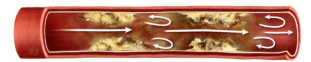

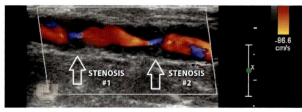

Fig. 10-35: *Velocities in stenosis #1 will have greater incoming energy, typically producing higher velocities than stenosis #2 which is approximately the same percent stenosis but has less energy coming in, so velocities will be lower.*

Bernoulli Principle Revisited [1,3,4,7]

Remember the Bernoulli Principle describes the relationship between area, velocity, and pressure at a stenosis.

Kinetic E + Potential E = Total E

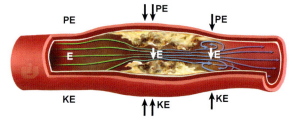

Fig. 10-36: *PE = potential energy*
KE = kinetic energy
E = energy

- Since energy must remain the same; an increase in velocity (KE) creates a corresponding decrease in pressure energy (PE). When fluid flows from one point to another, its total energy remains constant; assuming that flow is steady with no frictional energy losses.
- Proximal to a stenosis, the velocity and pressure are used as the baseline.
- Velocity and pressure are inversely related within a stenosis. As velocity increases in a stenosis, pressure decreases.
- As flow leaves the significant stenosis, velocity will decrease again and pressure will increase, but neither returns to the pre-stenotic baseline values due to the energy lost.

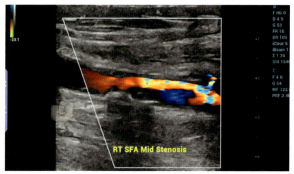

Fig. 10-37: *Flow at a higher velocity has a higher ratio of kinetic to potential energy. Due to the resistance of the stenosis and post-stenotic turbulence, the post-stenosis potential energy and overall energy will fall.*

REFERENCES

1. Owen, C, Robers, M. Arterial Vascular Hemodynamics. Journal of Diagnostic Medical Ultrasound 23:129-140, May/June 2007.
2. M Boron, WF and Boulpaep, EL Medical Physiology, A Cellular and Molecular Approach. Elsevier, 2005.
3. Klabunde, Richard E. PhD, (2011) Cardiovascular Physiology Concepts, Chapters 5,7,& 8. Lippincott, Williams and Wilkins.
4. Needham, T, Needham, A. Characteristics of Pressure and Flow in Arteries and Veins: The Application to Noninvasive Peripheral Vascular Testing. The journal for Vascular Ultrasound 35(4):229-236, 2011.
5. Sumner DS, Zierler RE. (2005). Vascular physiology: essential hemodynamic principles. In Rutherford Vascular Surgery 6th edition. Philadelphia. Elsevier Saunders.
6. Kupinski, Anne Marie (2013) In The Vascular System 1st edition (p 66, 81), Philadelphia. Wolters Kluwer/Miele, FR: Ultrasound Physics and Instrumentation. 4th edition,. Forney, TX, Miele enterprises, 2006.
7. Miele, FR: Ultrasound Physics and Instrumentation. 4th edition,. Forney, TX, Miele enterprises, 2006
8. Meissner MH. (2010). Chronic venous disorders. In Zierler RE (Ed.), Strandess's duplex scanning. disorders in vascular diagnosis 4th ed. (223-229). Philadelphia Wolters Kluwer Lippincott Williams & Wilkins.
9. Size, Gail, Introduction to Venous testing, Inside Ultrasound, Pearce, AZ, Inside Ultrasound 1995.
10. Kim, Gianni Belcaro, Andrew N. Nicolaides, M. Veller, A Manual of Diagnosis and Treatment W.B. Saunders, 1995.
11. Kim, ESH, et.al. Interpretation of Peripheral Arterial and Venous Doppler Waveforms: A Consensus Statement From the Society for Vascular Medicine and Society for Vascular Ultrasound. Journal for Vascular Ultrasound 44(3)118-143, September, 2020.

Chronic Venous Disorders

The term "Chronic Venous Disorder (CVD) includes the full spectrum of morphologic and functional abnormalities of the venous system, from telangiectasias to venous ulcers.[1,2] Varicose veins, venous insufficiency and venous thrombosis which are some of the venous diseases that lead to chronic venous disorder, will each be discussed separately later in this chapter.

The term "chronic venous insufficiency" implies a functional abnormality of the venous system and is usually reserved for more advanced diseases, including edema (C3), skin changes (C4), or venous ulcers (C5-6).[2]

CEAP Classification System [3,4,5]

The CEAP classification system is used to distinguish the different manifestations of CVD. The fundamentals of the CEAP classification include a description of the limb based on the following terms:

- (C) Clinical class based upon objective signs
- (E) Etiology (cause of the condition)
- (A) Anatomical distribution of reflux and obstruction in the superficial, deep, and perforating veins
- (P) Pathophysiology (whether due to reflux or obstruction)

For more in-depth interpretation, refer to the *Inside Ultrasound Venous Vascular Reference Guide, 2nd Edition.* insideultrasound.com

- To further define the clinical class (C), a subscript can be added indicating the presence of symptoms (subscript s) or the absence of symptoms (subscript a).[5]
- Symptoms include aching, pain, tightness, skin irritation, heaviness, muscle cramps, and other complaints attributed to venous dysfunction.
- For example, a patient with:
  » Varicose veins with symptoms would be classified as $C2_s$
  » Telangiectasias without symptoms would be classified as $C1_a$

Table 11-1: CEAP: Summary of Clinical (C) Classifications	
C0	No visible or palpable signs of venous disease
C1	Telangiectasias or reticular veins
C2	Varicose veins
$C2_r$	Recurrent varicose veins
C3	Edema
C4	Changes in skin and subcutaneous tissue secondary to CVD
$C4_a$	Pigmentation or eczema
$C4_b$	Lipodermatosclerosis or atrophie blanche
$C4_c$	Corona Phlebictatica
C5	Healed venous ulcer
C6	Active venous ulcer

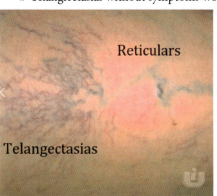

Fig. 11-1: *C1 Telangiectasias and Reticulars:* Telangiectasias are multiple dilated intradermal venules of <1mm in diameter joined together. Reticulars are dilated intradermal veins that are often 1-3mm in diameter.

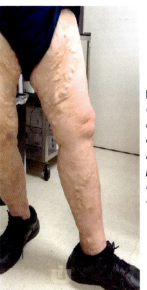

Fig. 11-2: *C2 and C2r:* Subcutaneous dilated veins that are >3mm in diameter. Varicose veins occur because of a degenerative process of the vein wall leading to venous dilation and valvular incompetence.

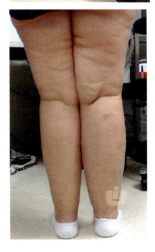

Fig. 11-3: *C3 Edema:* Caused by increased capillary hydrostatic pressures secondary to venous hypertension leading to extraction of fluid and proteins.

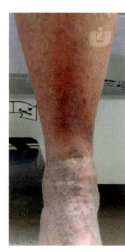

Fig. 11-4: C4a Pigmentation: A brownish pigmentation (hemosiderin deposition) that typically occurs in the gaiter area resulting from extravasation and breakdown of the red blood cells, which have escaped from the capillaries into the surrounding tissue in response to high venous pressure.

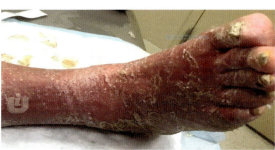

Fig. 11-5: C4a Eczema: As capillary fluid leaks into the skin, oxygen is blocked from reaching the skin surface, causing dry, itchy, sensitive skin, which appears as scaly patches.

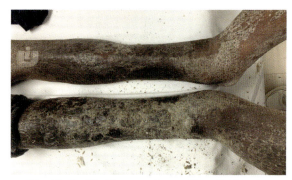

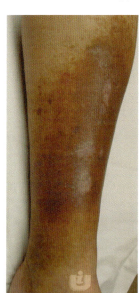

Fig. 11-6: C4b Lipodermatosclerosis: Localized chronic inflammation and fibrosis of the skin and subcutaneous tissues as fibrin escapes into the tissue.

Photo courtesy of Nicos Labropoulos PhD

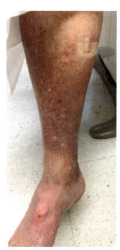

Fig. 11-7: C4b Atrophie Blanche: Localized, often circular whitish, and atrophic skin areas surrounded by dilated capillaries and sometimes hyperpigmentation caused by thrombosis within dermal blood vessels and endothelial proliferation.

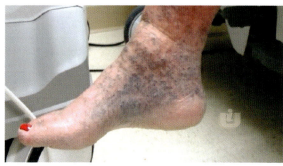

Fig. 11-8: C4c Corona Phlebectatica: Abnormally visible fan-shaped pattern of numerous small intra-dermal veins on medial or lateral aspects of the ankle and foot where deoxygenated blood flows upstream toward the heart.

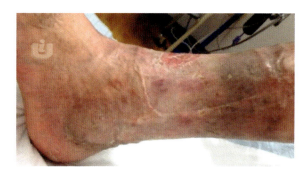

Fig. 11-9: C5 Healed Ulcer: A healed venous leg ulcer usually leaves skin damage around the ankle or lower leg typical of CEAP C4. This patient presents with a history of an open ulcer (C6) in the area. *Photo courtesy of Dr. Joseph Caprini*

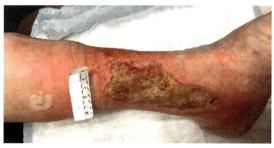

Fig. 11-10: C6 and C6r Active Ulcer: Ulcers appear as open sores with no skin covering the underlying tissue. Local tissue hypoxia results in an open, draining wound and redness of the limb.[6]

Table 11-2: Venous versus Arterial Ulceration [6,7,8]

	Venous	Arterial
Cause	Venous hypertension	Arterial obstruction
Location	Between the knee and the ankle. The medial or lateral malleoli are the most common sites, but other sites can be involved.	Prominent bony areas between the toes, tips of the toes, over phalangeal heads, lateral malleolus, and points subjected to repetitive trauma
Ulcer appearance	Variable ulcer bed appearance	Even sharply demarcated and punched-out ulcer margins
Surrounding tissue appearance	Eczematous, presenting with erythema, scaling, weeping, induration, and crusting	Blanched or purpuric skin that is often shiny and tight
Symptoms	Itchy, painful if infected	May be localized to the ulcer or more generalized to the foot

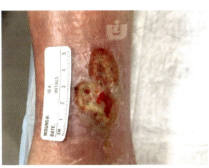

Fig. 11-11:
Venous ulcer lateral malleolus

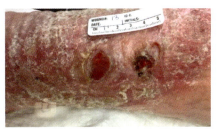

Fig. 11-12:
Venous ulcer lateral malleolus with stasis dermatitis and eczema

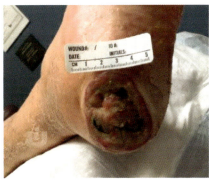

Fig. 11-13:
Arterial ulcer of the heel

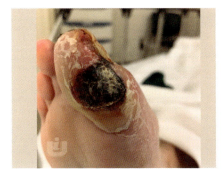

Fig. 11-14:
Arterial ulcer-toe

Etiology (Divided into three categories)

Primary
- The most common causes of venous insufficiency are often under-recognized or poorly defined. [9]
- The pathogenesis remains unclear. Initially, it was thought that varicose veins were due to valvular incompetence.
- A current hypothesis states that the structural changes of the vein wall as they become varicosed cause valvular dysfunction. [10]

Secondary
- DVT (deep venous thrombosis) is the most common cause of chronic deep venous obstruction or valvular insufficiency. [9]
- Post-thrombotic valvular damage may result from initial thrombus adherence to the valve cusp or trauma to the vein wall. [11]
- Valvular insufficiency may also develop following venous recanalization or pregnancy and progesterone-induced venous wall and valve weakness. [9]
- Congenital causes include venous malformations. Examples include Klippel-Trenaunay variants and avalvulia (absence of valves). [9]

An estimated 40% of people in the United States have CVD: [24]
» *Occurring more often in women than in men.* [24]
» *Occurring more frequently in people over age 50*
» *Approximately 50% of people over the age of 50 have VVs* [24]

Varicose veins can occur anywhere in the body, though most often occur in the legs.

Dilatation of the lower extremity venous system can be due to venous or portal hypertension.

Studies estimate that 69% of patients with a history of DVT will develop chronic venous insufficiency within one year. [26]

Risk Factors

- Age (greater with advanced age)
- Previous DVT
- Female
- Pregnancy
- Obesity
- Family history
- Occupations requiring extended periods of standing or sitting
- Congenital abnormalities (e.g., Klippel-Trenaunay)
- Birth control pills can increase the risk of varicose/spider veins. [28]

Mechanism of Disease

Normal Venous Valve Function [11-18]

- Venous blood typically flows towards the heart and from the superficial to the deep venous system.
- In the perforating veins, blood flows from the superficial to deep veins.
- When standing still, with the calf muscle relaxed, the veins in the calf fill with blood. Pressure on the valves from retrograde flow forces the valves to close, preventing blood flow toward the feet.
- While walking, muscle contractions squeeze the veins initiating venous blood flow. Venous flow opens the venous valves allowing the blood to flow towards the heart. As the muscle relaxes, the valves close to prevent the backflow of blood (reflux).
- Multiple components facilitate effective venous return from the lower extremities.
  - » Cardiac pump: During cardiac contraction and relaxation, there is a passive push from the arterial system and mild suction from the cardiac valves that assist venous blood flow.
  - » Respiratory pump: During inspiration and expiration pressure changes occur in the thoracic and abdominal cavities. These pressure changes compress the nearby veins and assist blood return to the heart.
  - » Peripheral muscle pumps:
    - Foot: During flexion, the plantar venous plexus is compressed and primes the calf muscle pump.
    - Calf: Gastrocnemius and soleus muscles eject 40-60% of venous volume with a single contraction.
    - Thigh: Although the thigh-level veins are surrounded by muscle, the contribution to venous return is less when compared to the calf.

The calf muscle pump is the most important of the three muscle pumps. It is highly efficient, has the most significant capacitance, and generates the highest pressures (mmHg during muscular contraction) [14,17,19]

  - » Pressure gradient and muscle pumps: the muscle pumps drive blood into the popliteal and femoral veins.
    - The valves prevent retrograde flow (reflux) during relaxation, generating negative pressure and drawing blood from the superficial to the deep system through perforating veins.
    - Venous pressure is lowered until arterial inflow equals venous outflow.
    - When exercise ceases, the veins slowly fill from the capillary bed, causing a slow return to the resting venous pressure.
  - » **Competent venous valves:**
    - Are unidirectional
    - Function to divide the hydrostatic column of blood into segments
    - Prevent retrograde venous flow

The manifestations of chronic venous disease result from a complex interaction of anatomy and hemodynamic failure. [10]

Venous Obstruction [20, 21]

- The theory of Virchow's Triad states that three factors are responsible for the formation of venous thrombosis. A combination of any of these events may result in venous thrombosis.
  - » Vein wall injury
  - » Hypercoagulability
  - » Stasis of blood flow
- Obstruction of the iliac veins can directly affect the lower extremities. This should be considered when assessing the lower extremities for venous disease, particularly when the signs and symptoms are out of proportion with the lower extremity ultrasound findings.
- Compression, although most often found in the left common iliac vein, may be observed in the right common iliac and both external iliac veins.
- There can also be a combination of obstruction and reflux.

Terms used to describe venous issues are sometimes misused. The correct terminology is:

- *Thrombophlebitis: An inflammation of a vein associated with a thrombus.*
- *Phlebitis: Venous inflammation which can occur in the absence of a thrombus.*
- *Superficial venous thrombosis: Thrombosis within a superficial vein which can occur with or without inflammation.*

Venous Reflux

- Reflux is defined as the retrograde flow of blood caused by incompetent valves and, in rare cases, absent valves.
- Reflux or pathologic retrograde flow occurs when the valves are absent or rendered incompetent either by degenerative processes (primary venous disease) or an episode of DVT (secondary venous disease). [10]
- Along with reflux, there can also be a component of obstruction.

Dysfunction of the Muscular Pump

- Retrograde flow during calf muscle relaxation prevents the usual reduction in pressure, and rapid venous refilling occurs from the retrograde flow of blood, as well as slow capillary inflow. [10]
- Normally, when walking (contracting and relaxing the calf muscles), the calf muscle pump is activated and propels blood upwards toward the heart, reducing blood volume and venous pressure.
  - » When venous valves are incompetent, blood flows backward during calf muscle relaxation, which can cause a significant increase in venous pressure.
- Increased venous pressure may also be transmitted from the deep to the superficial veins through incompetent perforators. [10]

The function of the calf muscle pump may be impaired in patients with chronic venous disease, an observation that is at least partially related to reduced ankle range of motion. [10]

Less Common Venous Disorders

- Malformations
- Aneurysms

Location of Disease
Incompetent valves may be located anywhere within the deep, superficial, or perforating venous systems, including:
- Common femoral vein
- Femoral vein
- Popliteal vein
- Saphenofemoral Junction (SJF)
- Saphenopopliteal Junction (SPJ) if present
- Saphenous veins
- Superficial tributaries
- Perforating veins, most commonly those in the gaiter area

If both parents had VVs, their children are estimated to have a 90% chance of developing varicosities.

Differential Diagnosis
- Deep venous thrombosis
- Stasis dermatitis
- Contact dermatitis
- Nerve compression
- Arterial disease
- Lymphedema
- Cellulitis
- Skin cancer
- Inguinal hernia

Correlation
- Duplex ultrasonography
- Air plethysmography
- Descending venography
- Intravascular Ultrasound (IVUS)
- MR venogram
- CT venogram

Medical/Conservative Treatment
Elastic Compression (graduated compression stockings)
- Elastic compression therapy conforms to leg size changes and thus sustains compression during activity and at rest.
- The most common type of elastic compression is graduated compression stockings. These stockings work by exerting the greatest degree of compression at the ankle, with the level of compression gradually decreasing up the garment.
- The pressure gradient ensures that blood flows upward toward the heart instead of refluxing downward to the foot or laterally into the superficial veins.
- Different degrees of compression are available, and the level of compression is chosen based on the severity of the venous disease.

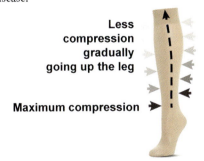

Fig. 11-15: *Compression stockings are used to decrease distal swelling.*

Inelastic Compression (bandages, Velcro wraps)
- Inelastic compression therapy does not conform to leg size changes; the degree of compression is not sustained at rest.
- Provides a high working pressure with muscle contraction, and during ambulation, but no resting pressure
- Inelastic bandages do not accommodate changes in leg volume if edema increases during prolonged standing or decreases when the legs are elevated.
- The most common type of inelastic compression, particularly for patients with venous ulcers, is the Unna boot. It is an inelastic single-component moist bandage that is impregnated with zinc oxide or calamine (with or without glycerin) that hardens after application.
- A Velcro wrap is another type of inelastic compression
  » A series of overlapping, interlinked straps are fastened using Velcro.

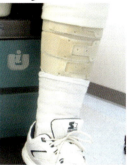 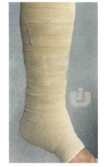

Fig. 11-16: Velcro wrap   Fig. 11-17: Unna boot

Photos courtesy of Dr. Caprini

Non-compression, Conservative Treatment Options
- Periodic elevation of legs during the day
- Anti-inflammatory medication

Surgical Treatment
- Ligation and Stripping
  » The proximal portion of the vein is ligated
  » Stripping of the vein may be performed with ligation
- Ambulatory Phlebectomy
  » The removal of large tortuous varicose veins through small incisions in the skin.

Endovascular Treatment
- **Thermal Ablation:** A procedure using heat to remove tissue or destroy its function. Two types of thermal ablation methods are used:
  » Endovenous LASER Ablation
  » Radiofrequency Ablation (RFA)
- **Chemical Ablation:** A procedure using a chemical to remove tissue or destroy its function. Sclerotherapy is the targeted chemical ablation of a varicose vein by intravenous injection of a liquid or foam sclerosant. [22]
- **Adhesive Ablation:** A procedure using cyanoacrylate to close a vein. Cyanoacrylate (Superglue) is a strong, biodegradable tissue adhesive that polymerizes upon contact with tissues. [23]

For more detailed descriptions of treatment for chronic venous disorders refer to the Venous Ablation chapter.

There are multiple options available for the treatment of chronic venous disorders.

A complete understanding of the disease process and the treatment options are needed to make a well-informed decision when choosing a treatment modality.

Iliac Vein Compression
(Previously May-Thurner Syndrome)

- **Iliac vein compression syndrome** is the pathologic compression of an iliac vein by an overlying iliac artery causing lower extremity venous hypertension and/or the development of pelvic varices.
- This syndrome was previously known as May-Thurner syndrome and was specific to the compression of the left common iliac vein by the overlying right common iliac artery.
- The left common iliac vein is the most likely to have obstructive pathology. However, compression of the right common iliac and bilateral external iliac veins has been documented. *(Table 11-3)*
- These iliac vein lesions are referred to as *nonthrombotic iliac vein lesions* (NIVLs).
- Obstruction of the iliac veins results in high outflow resistance, venous claudication, and a higher deep vein thrombosis recurrence. It also causes more prevalent and severe post-thrombotic symptoms, impairing the quality of life for patients. [21]
- Symptomatic iliocaval obstruction of NIVL or thrombotic etiology can present with a wide range of clinical features, including all clinical CEAP classes. Specific correction is seldom warranted unless patients present with advanced symptoms (CEAP clinical class 3 or greater) or significant pain. [29]

It is critical that anatomic stenosis alone not be considered a criterion for intervention and that any measurement of stenosis be interpreted in the context of the patient's clinical presentation. [7]

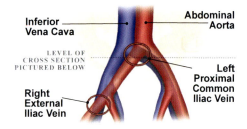

Fig. 11-18: *Most frequently occurring NIVLs typical mid-line anatomy.*

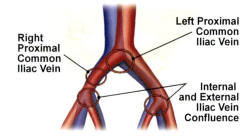

Fig. 11-19: *Less frequently occurring NIVLs. Notice that a slight shift in the mid-line anatomy will create additional areas of potential extrinsic compression.*

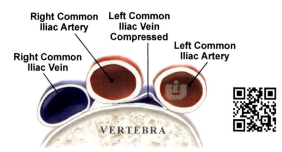

Fig. 11-20: *Cross-sectional view of the left common iliac vein being compressed by the right and left common iliac arteries* Adapted from www.scgvs.com

Table 11-3: Areas of Iliac Vein Compression*

Common Iliac Veins
- Right common iliac artery on left common iliac vein
- Right common iliac artery on right common iliac vein
- Left common iliac artery on left common iliac vein

External Iliac Veins
- Right external iliac artery on right external iliac vein
- Right internal iliac artery on right external iliac vein
- Left external iliac artery on left external iliac vein
- Left internal iliac artery on left external iliac vein
- Inguinal ligament on right external iliac vein
- Inguinal ligament on left external iliac vein

More than one type of compression may exist.

Labropoulos N. (2018). Diagnosis of iliac vein obstruction with duplex ultrasound criteria used during duplex ultrasound examination to identify iliac vein obstruction. Endovascular Today, 17(7), 3.

Etiology
- Congenital
- A traumatic etiology from pulsations of the adjacent artery [29]

Mechanism of Disease
Extrinsic obstruction
- Compression of an iliac vein by an overlying artery (NIVL). NIVL is defined as venous reflux or obstruction arising from complex lesions involving not only external compression of an iliac vein but also wall fibrosis and intraluminal changes caused by the pulsations of an overlying artery. [7,29]
- Could be a partial compression or a complete occlusion of the vein.
- Anatomical structures surrounding the veins, including the inguinal ligament may also cause obstruction of a vein. [21]

Symptomatic iliocaval obstruction of NIVL or PTS etiology can present with a wide range of clinical features, including all clinical CEAP classes [29]

Intrinsic obstruction
- Wall fibrosis and intraluminal changes caused by the pulsations of an overlying artery. (NIVL) [7, 29]

Location of Disease
- Common iliac vein
- External iliac vein

Iliac vein compression can involve the bilateral common and external iliac veins.

Differential Diagnosis
- Unilateral DVT not caused by iliac compression
- Lymphedema
- Cellulitis
- Hematoma
- Adenopathy
- Vascularized mass

Correlation
- Duplex ultrasonography
- CT venography
- MR venography
- IVUS
- Venography

Medical Treatment
- Anticoagulation
- Thrombolysis

Surgical Treatment
With the improvement of endovascular procedures to treat iliac vein obstruction, these surgical procedures are rarely utilized:
- Iliocaval bypass
- Transposition of the right CIA
- Iliac vein disobliteration (opened to remove webs/spurs)

≥50% iliac stenosis may be present in 25-33% of the general population; it is critical that anatomic stenosis alone not be considered a criterion for intervention and that any measurement of stenosis be interpreted in the context of the patient's clinical presentation.[7]

Endovascular Treatment
- Iliac vein angioplasty
- Iliac vein stenting (common and external)
- Vena cava filters (in cases of thrombus and risk of PE)

Lymphedema [30,31,32]

An accumulation of interstitial fluid develops due to obstruction or abnormal lymphatic system development (vessels or lymph nodes). The lymphatic system serves to balance intracellular and extracellular environments. Some of the components of this system include lymph nodes, spleen, thymus, nasopharyngeal tonsils, lymphocytes, and macrophages. This unidirectional system transports fluid throughout the tissues and collects bacteria, viruses, and waste products. There are numerous communications between the blood and lymph streams.

For example, lymph from the upper extremities enters the bloodstream at the junction of the subclavian and jugular veins.

There are two types of lymphedema:
- **Primary lymphedema:** Occurs independently (less common).
- **Secondary lymphedema:** Secondary to a disease or another condition (most common).

Etiology
- Congenital
- Surgery (post-op complication)
- Infection
- Cancer
- Radiation
- Trauma

Risk Factors
- Family history
- Female
- Cancer, with a history of surgery or radiation for the condition (e.g., breast cancer with mastectomy)
- History of lymph node dissection
- Exposure to infectious bacteria, especially in tropical regions
- Trauma

Mechanism of Disease
- Primary lymphedema: An inherited condition that affects the development of the lymph vessels. During the embryonic stage, there is a malformation of lymph nodes or an absence of valves in the lymph vessels. This can occur during infancy (Milroy disease), in childhood or puberty (Meige disease), or later, after the age of 35 (lymphedema tarda).
- Secondary lymphedema: Certain conditions or interventions can damage your lymph vessels and cause lymphedema. Lymph nodes are often removed during surgery to biopsy and assess for the spread of cancer. If the remaining lymph nodes/vessels do not compensate for this loss, the limb will swell.
- Scarring and inflammation of the lymph nodes/vessels after radiation treatment can restrict flow in the lymphatic system.
- Cancerous tumors can block lymphatic pathways and prevent flow. Infections and parasites can access the lymphatic system and restrict lymphatic flow.

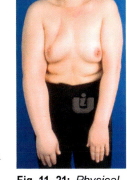

Fig. 11-21: Physical presentation of secondary lymphedema after breast surgery
Image courtesy of Byung-Boong Lee MD PhD FACS

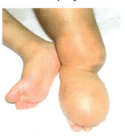 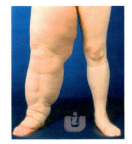

Fig. 11-22: Physical presentation of primary lymphedema

Fig. 11-23: Physical presentation of secondary lymphedema

Images courtesy of Byung-Boong Lee MD Ph.D. FACS

Location of Disease
- Lower and upper extremities

Differential Diagnosis
- Vascular conditions such as venous insufficiency, congenital malformation, or arteriovenous fistula
- Infection
- Cardiac failure (edema is usually bilateral in such cases)
- Insect bites
- Renal failure
- Liver failure
- Rheumatoid arthritis
- Side effects of certain drugs, hormones

Lymphedema *is a common differential diagnosis for lower extremity edema and is aggravated by repetitive attacks of cellulitis, which scar the existing lymphatic channels.*

Elephantitis *is a complication of lymphedema where the skin becomes extremely hard and thick. These patients are at risk for chronic ulcers and infection.*

Lymphangiosarcoma *is a rare soft tissue cancer resulting from severe cases of untreated lymphedema that originate in the lymph nodes and vessels.*

Correlation
- Duplex ultrasonography
- CT angiogram
- MR angiography
- Contrast lymphangiography
- Lymphoscintigraphy

Medical Treatment
- Leg elevation
- Compression stockings
- Manual lymph drainage
- Intermittent pneumatic compression
- Prompt treatment of cellulitis
- Exercise

Surgical Treatment
- Microsurgical lymphatic reconstruction (lymphatic grafting)
- Liposuction (reduce edema)

Pelvic Venous Disorders
(Previously Pelvic Congestion Syndrome)

The term Pelvic Venous Disorders (PeVD) describes a group of related clinical findings with overlapping clinical presentations ultimately leading to venous hypertension or high pressure within the pelvic veins and/or other peripheral venous beds. The signs and symptoms of PeVD may vary depending on the venous bed(s) affected by the underlying venous hypertension. The symptoms may include chronic pelvic pain, pelvic, lower extremity and genital varices, lower extremity pain, swelling, and left flank pain and hematuria. [33]

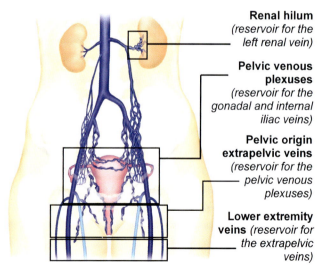

Fig. 11-24: *Diagram depicting the venous reservoirs affected by venous hypertension of the abdominal and pelvic veins.*

Labels: Renal hilum *(reservoir for the left renal vein)*; Pelvic venous plexuses *(reservoir for the gonadal and internal iliac veins)*; Pelvic origin extrapelvic veins *(reservoir for the pelvic venous plexuses)*; Lower extremity veins *(reservoir for the extrapelvic veins)*

Etiology [7,33]
- **Thrombotic**
  - » Reflux arising from a previous DVT
  - » Obstruction arising from a previous DVT
- **Nonthrombotic**
  - » Reflux arising from a degenerative process of the vein wall
  - » Reflux arising from a proximal obstruction due to an extrinsic compression
- **Congenital**
  - » Venous malformation
  - » Mixed vascular malformation

Mechanism of Disease
Increased central venous pressure of the pelvic veins leads to the development of peri-uterine and trans-uterine varicosities. [7] This increased pressure occurs due to a more central obstruction and/or reflux. These may occur concurrently or independently.

Obstruction
Obstruction is most likely to occur in the left renal vein and the left common iliac vein.
- **Extrinsic pathology** Non-thrombotic iliac vein lesions (NIVL)
  - » Mechanical compression of a vein due to an overlying artery or other anatomic structure, which results in obstruction.
- **Intrinsic pathology** Development of an obstruction within the vein.
  - » Chronic pulsatile compression of an iliac vein by an overlying iliac artery stimulates the formation of fibrotic adhesions that can cause partial or complete iliac vein obstruction over time. This finding is associated with NIVLs. [34,35,36]
  - » Changes associated with previous DVT

Reflux
Reflux is most likely to occur in the following:
- Gonadal veins
- Internal iliac veins and their tributaries

Nonsaphenous origin lower extremity varicose veins are often caused by pelvic varicose veins via the pelvic escape/pelvic leak points.

Based upon anatomic patterns and patients' symptoms, reflux within the pelvic veins has been described as compensated or uncompensated. [37]

- **Compensated reflux** [7,33,37]
  - » Venous pressure is decompressed via collaterals into more peripheral venous reservoirs.
  - » Will result in the development of symptoms in the peripheral venous reservoir, not at the direct site of the pathology.
- **Uncompensated reflux** [7,33,37]
  - » Venous pressure is transmitted directly to the peripheral venous reservoirs (renal hilar, pelvic venous plexus, pelvic origin extrapelvic veins, and the lower extremity).
  - » Will result in the development of symptoms at the location of the pathology.

 For a complete list of reflux patterns and associated symptoms, refer to the Inside Ultrasound Venous Vascular Reference Guide.
insideultrasound.com

Location of Disease
- Gonadal vein, left more often than right
- Left renal vein
- Iliocaval
- Pelvic venous plexus (peri-uterine and/or trans-uterine)
- Extrapelvic tributaries of the IIVs. These tributaries originate outside of the pelvis and then join the IIV in the pelvis.

It is useful to consider the venous circulation of the pelvis to consist of multiple interconnected venous systems—the left renal and ovarian veins, the iliac veins (common, external, and internal), and the lower extremity veins.

Communications between these three systems frequently allow for crossover from one side to the other within the pelvis.

Differential Diagnosis
- Endometriosis
- Adhesions
- Adenomyosis
- Malignancy
- Uterine prolapse
- Ovarian cysts
- Cystitis
- Irritable bowel

Correlation
- Duplex ultrasonography
- CT venography
- MR venography
- IVUS
- Venography

Medical/Surgical Treatment
Left Renal Vein
- Nephropexy
- External renal vein stenting
- Aortomesenteric transposition
- Renal autotransplantation
- Gonadal vein transposition
- Left renal vein transposition

Ovarian and Iliac Veins
- Endovascular approaches to primary ovarian and internal iliac venous reflux have largely replaced medical and surgical approaches.

Endovascular Treatment
- Coil embolization of the refluxing trunk (gonadal)
- Combination of coil embolization and sclerotherapy
- Sclerotherapy of the pelvic venous plexus
- Iliac vein angioplasty
- Iliac vein stenting (common and external)
- Left renal vein stenting (not considered the gold standard for treatment, more research is needed)

Phlegmasia Alba Dolens [38,39]

Decreased venous drainage due to thrombosis of extremity deep veins, without collateral vein involvement. Phlegmasia alba dolens can progress to phlegmasia cerulea dolens.

Etiology
- Hypercoagulable state
- Massive venous thrombosis

Risk Factors
- Female > male
- Middle-aged
- Pregnancy (esp. during the last trimester)

Mechanism of Disease
- Extensive edema (usually due to iliofemoral thrombosis) obscures capillary circulation causing a "white" discoloration of the skin.
- Arterial spasms similar to those in phlegmasia cerulea dolens may also be a contributing factor.

Location of Disease
- Iliofemoral deep veins; iliac, common femoral, deep femoral, and femoral veins
- Upper extremity deep veins (rare)

Differential Diagnosis
- Arterial embolism
- Aortic dissection
- Lymphedema

Correlation
- Duplex ultrasonography
- Arteriography
- Venography

Medical Treatment
- IV heparin and Coumadin
- Graduated compression stockings

Surgical Treatment
- Venous thrombectomy
- Compartment fasciotomy
- Cross pubic vein-vein reconstruction with PTFE
- Creation of an arteriovenous fistula between the femoral artery and great saphenous vein
- Amputation

Endovascular Treatment
- Mechanical thrombectomy
- Thrombolytic therapy

Phlegmasia Cerulea Dolens [38,39]

Massive venous occlusion due to multi-segment thrombosis of extremity deep veins; iliofemoral, lower leg veins, and collaterals. Venous gangrene can occur with phlegmasia cerulea dolens because of substantial venous outflow and arterial inflow obstructions. All toes and part of the foot will be gangrenous, instead of only one or two toes, as typically occurs in cases of gangrene caused by arterial disease.

Etiology
- Malignancy
- Hypercoagulable state
- Trauma

Risk Factors
- Female > male
- Middle-aged
- Post-operative
- Vena cava insertion
- Ulcerative colitis
- Gastroenteritis
- Heart failure
- Mitral valve stenosis
- Iliac vein compression syndrome

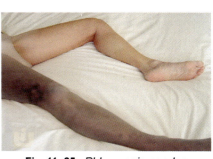

Fig. 11-25: *Phlegmasia cerulea dolens of the right leg.*

Mechanism of Disease
- Massive obstruction of venous outflow reduces arterial inflow to the limb and causes arterial vasoconstriction, and may cause arterial thrombosis.
- Venous congestion results from significant iliac vein thrombosis and causes a "blue" discoloration of the skin.

Location of Disease
- Iliofemoral deep veins; iliac, common femoral, deep femoral, and femoral veins (along with their collaterals).
- Upper extremity deep veins (only 2-5% of cases)

Differential Diagnosis
- Arterial ischemia/thrombosis
- Aortic dissection
- Toxic shock syndrome
- Superficial phlebitis of the upper extremity

Correlation
- Duplex ultrasonography
- Arteriography
- Venography

Medical Treatment
- Maximize limb elevation
- Correct any hypovolemia
- Aggressive anticoagulation
- Graduated compression stockings

Surgical Treatment
- Venous thrombectomy
- Compartment fasciotomy
- Cross pubic vein-vein reconstruction with PTFE
- Creation of an arteriovenous fistula between the femoral artery and great saphenous vein
- Amputation

Endovascular Treatment
- Mechanical thrombectomy
- Thrombolytic therapy

Portal Hypertension

Increased blood pressure within the portal venous system. The normal portal venous pressure is 5mmHg. Portal hypertension is defined as pressures >12mmHg.[101] Complications from portal hypertension include varices and ascities.[102]

A serious complication associated with varices is the risk of rupture which may be fatal due to internal bleeding.[102,110]

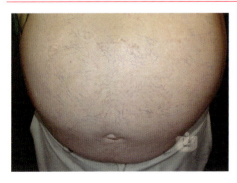

Fig. 11-26: Typical presentation of portal hypertension with abdominal varices

Etiology
- Cirrhosis (scarring of the liver)
- Hepatitis
- Alcohol abuse
- Portal splenic vein thrombosis
- Schistosomiasis

Risk Factors
The theory of Virchow's triad explains portal splenic thrombosis; venous thrombosis is caused by venous stasis, vein wall (intimal) injury or a hypercoaguable state.

Additional risk factors for portal hypertension include:
- Hepatocellular disease (acute or chronic)
- Liver disease (e.g., cirrhosis)
- Tricuspid regurgitation: Backflow of blood through the tricuspid valve resulting in increased pressures within the IVC and hepatic circulation.
- Heart disease causing increased right-heart pressures (e.g., congestive heart failure)
- *Schistosomiasis:* Parasitic disease found in Asia, Africa and South America
- Constrictive pericarditis
- Trauma
- Family history
- Cancer
- Appendicitis
- Diverticulitis

Mechanism of Disease
- Pressure is affected by changes in volume or resistance. Portal hypertension refers to the elevation of portal pressure within the portal circulation caused by an increased resistance to flow, usually within the hepatic parenchyma.[102]
- Changes in resistance are affected by the radius of the blood vessel which can be significantly decreased when liver disease, liver fibrosis, thrombosis or tumor are present. A decrease in vessel radius increases hepatic resistance.[102,110]
- Nitric oxide (NO) levels are believed to affect portal hypertension in cirrhosis cases. An increase in NO levels causes vasodilatation and increased portomesenteric blood flow. Decreased NO causes vasoconstriction and increased portal pressure.[101]
- In response to increased pressure within the portohepatic system, the body attempts to reduce pressure by diverting blood away from the liver through collaterals, varices or shunts. This dilatation of veins may progress to causes esophageal, gastric, and anal varices.[102] Rupture of these varices can result in life threatening hemorrhage.[102,110]
- Other consequences of portal hypertension are encephalopathy[101] and *splenomegaly* (enlarged spleen).[110]

Location of Disease
- Portal veins
- Main portal vein
- Right portal vein
- Left portal vein

The portal vein receives blood from the stomach, intestines, spleen, gallbladder and pancreas.

Differential Diagnosis
- Budd-Chiari syndrome
- Tuberculosis
- Polycystic kidney disease
- Cirrhosis
- Pericarditis
- Congestive heart failure
- Tricuspid regurgitation
- Sarcoidosis
- Vitamin A toxicity

Budd-Chiari syndrome results from obstruction to hepatic venous outflow. The syndrome presents with ascites, abdominal pain and can result in liver necrosis. [101]

Correlation
- Duplex ultrasonography
- Upper GI series
- CT angiography
- MRI or MRA
- Endoscopy
- Angiography

Medical Treatment
- Managing complications of portal hypertension (e.g., variceal hemorrhage, ascites)
- Managing the cause of portal hypertension (e.g., anticoagulation for hepatic vein thrombosis, treating any identified cause of liver disease).
- Beta-blockers can reduce portal pressure
- Dietary changes

Surgical Treatment
- Paracentesis
- Liver transplant
- Splenectomy
- Transjugular intrahepatic portosystemic shunt (TIPS)

TIPS involves placing a stent to connect the hepatic vein to the portal vein (usually right portal to right hepatic). [101]

- Distal splenorenal shunt (DSRS) (connects the splenic vein to the left renal vein in order to reduce varices and bleeding). [101]
- Portocaval shunt (main portal blood shunted to the IVC)
- Mesocaval shunt (blood from the superior mesenteric vein shunted to the IVC)

Endovascular Treatment
Endoscopic treatments/banding/sclerotherapy all are treatment modalities for esophageal varices, not direct treatment of portal hypertension.

Pulmonary Embolism (PE) [40-43]

The occlusion of a pulmonary artery by a thromboembolism. Pulmonary embolism (PE) is a complication of venous thrombosis. The source of emboli is usually iliofemoral thrombus. Calf thrombi rarely result in pulmonary emboli, though they often propagate above the knee, becoming a greater risk for embolus.

PE is the third most common cause of death in the US, with approximately 630,000 cases/per year. It is one of the top causes of "unexpected death" in any age group.

Etiology
- Venous sites that may thrombose and be the source of the embolus include:
  - » Lower extremity deep veins (90%)
  - » Pelvic deep veins
  - » Upper extremity deep veins

Risk Factors
- Age (greater with advanced age)
- Immobilization (e.g., long-distance air travel, paraplegia)
- Genetic prothrombotic conditions (clotting disorders, such as Factor V Leiden)
- Post-operative phase (especially after orthopedic surgery)
- Central venous or femoral catheters
- Cancer/malignancy
- Pregnancy
- Medications (e.g., oral contraceptives)
- Estrogen replacement therapy
- Previous DVT
- Heart complications
- Obesity
- Family history
- Smoking
- Chronic Obstructive Pulmonary Disease (COPD)
- Blood type (highest risk with type-A, the lowest risk with type-O)
- Trauma
- Antiphospholipid antibodies (lupus, etc.)
- Varicose veins
- Inflammatory bowel disease

Studies have indicated that approximately one-third of PE cases are asymptomatic.

Mechanism of Disease
- Embolization occurs when a piece of a blood clot (embolus) breaks free from a venous thrombus and travels centrally to the pulmonary arterial circulation.
- An embolus can pass through the right side of the heart to the lungs, where it obstructs one of the pulmonary arteries. As a result, lung tissue is deprived of blood, which can be fatal.

Location of Disease
- Pulmonary artery
- Pulmonary artery branches

Differential Diagnosis
- Bronchitis pneumonia
- Pleurisy
- Myocardial ischemia (MI)

Correlation
- CT angiography
- Ventilation-perfusion (VQ) scan
- Chest x-ray
- Pulmonary angiogram

A normal, negative VQ scan excludes PE. False positive VQ results may occur in patients for other reasons, such as lung disease.

Medical Treatment
- Heparinization
- Long-term anticoagulation

Surgical Treatment
- Caval filter placement
- Pulmonary embolectomy

To decrease the risk of a PE, an IVC filter is placed via a catheter (typically using CFV, EIV, or jugular access). This procedure aims to "catch" any thrombi floating in the bloodstream, lowering the risk of PE.

Endovascular Treatment
- Thrombolytic therapy
- Pulmonary suction embolectomy

Venous duplex exams do not rule out a pulmonary event; they can only suggest a source of emboli for an episode of PE.

Superior Vena Cava (SVC) Syndrome [44,45]

Obstruction of the superior vena cava due to thrombosis or extrinsic compression.

Etiology
- Central venous interventions (e.g., central catheters, pacemakers)
- Malignancy, with or without lymphadenopathy (esp. of lung and thorax) is the chief cause of SVC syndrome.
- Histoplasmosis (fungal disease)
- Genetic prothrombotic conditions (clotting disorders, such as Factor V Leiden)
- Radiation therapy to the thorax

Risk Factors
- Cancers/lymphoma of the head, neck, and thorax regions
- Central catheterization
- Cardiac pacemaker

Mechanism of Disease
- Decreased venous return from the head, neck, and upper extremities can result in extremity edema, headaches, facial swelling, dilated torso veins, and in extreme cases, respiratory "embarrassment" or difficulty.

The severity of symptoms depends on the degree of collateral circulation.

Location of Disease
- Superior vena cava

Differential Diagnosis
- Acute respiratory distress
- COPD/emphysema
- Aortic dissection
- Mediastinitis (tissue inflammation in the mid-chest or mediastinum)
- Pericarditis
- Pneumonia
- Syphilis
- Tuberculosis

Correlation
- X-ray
- Duplex ultrasonography
- CT angiography
- MRI
- Venography
- IVUS

Medical Treatment
- Elevation of patient's head during night-time hours
- Limit daily episodes of bending over
- Clothing: wear loose collars
- Diuretics to reduce edema
- Anticoagulation

Chemotherapy and radiotherapy may relieve symptoms in patients suffering from SVC syndrome caused by malignancies (extrinsic compression).

Surgical Treatment
- SVC reconstruction (using femoral vein, spiral saphenous, PTFE, allograft, or cryopreserved homografts)
- Removal of external compression (e.g., tumor resection)

Endovascular Treatment
- Thrombolysis
- Angioplasty and stenting

Thoracic Outlet Compression Syndrome

Compression of the brachial plexus, subclavian artery or subclavian vein in the thoracic outlet or space between the collarbone and first rib of the upper extremity, resulting in symptoms of pain or neurologic deficit.

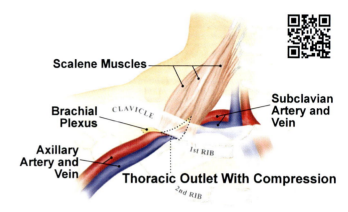

Fig. 11-27: Arteries/veins can be compressed in the space known as the thoracic outlet.

Etiology
- Congenital (cervical rib, costoclavicular tendon)
- Trauma
- Occupational related injury
- Sports related injury
- Vasculitis
- Atherosclerosis
- Thrombus
- Embolization from the subclavian or axillary arteries
- Aneurysm
- Pseudoaneurysm
- Intimal hyperplasia
- Traumatic occlusion
- Extrinsic compression
- Radiation arteritis

Risk Factors
- Age (young)
- Males > females
- Athletic, active lifestyle
- Family history
- Obesity
- History of radiation

Mechanism of Disease
- There are three types of thoracic outlet syndrome (TOS): neurogenic, venous and arterial.[58] All result from mechanical compression of the subclavian vein, artery or brachial plexus in the thoracic outlet region. One cause may be an anatomical defect such as congenital abnormalities of the first rib or fracture of the clavicle, which would be a source of compression. Weight training can result in muscle enlargement significant enough to cause compression in the thoracic outlet.[59]

The cause of TOS is neurogenic in 93% of cases. A venous cause is present in 5%, while an arterial cause is present in only 1% of cases.[60]

- Types of thoracic outlet syndrome include:[58,60]
  » **Neurogenic** (most common): compression of the brachial plexus from the cervical ribs, first rib, anterior scalene muscles, congenital myofascial bands and ligaments.
  » **Venous:** also known as *effort thrombosis* or *Paget-Schroetter* syndrome results from repetitive trauma to the subclavian vein (SCV). Arm abduction causes the SCV to be compressed against the first rib and scalenus anticus muscle,

resulting in this trauma. Venous trauma may result in venous thrombosis.[61] In cases of venous compression, the severity of symptoms relates to the length of the thrombosed segment and activity level of the patient.

» **Arterial** (least common): The head of the humerus can cause arterial compression when the arm is abducted and externally rotated. Due to such repetitive extrinsic compression of the SCA, post-stenotic dilatation or frank aneurysm develops. The typical pathogenesis then is focal compression, dilation, ulceration, and thrombus formation.[62]

- Most of these patients will present with thromboembolic symptoms.
- Patients also present with ischemic complications secondary to repeated episodes of embolization.
- "White-finger syndrome" resulting in small artery vasospasm can occur with the repetitive use of vibrating tools.[59]

• Venous or arterial compression results in:

» **Stenosis:** significant narrowing of the artery or vein decreasing the vessel lumen and possibly resulting in decreased blood flow.

» **Occlusion:** plaque, thrombus, or external compression of the artery completely blocking blood flow in that arterial segment.

» **Embolization:** contents of a plaque and/or fragments of an organized thrombus become lodged in a distant blood vessel.

» **Swelling:** significant compression of the subclavian vein causes limb swelling.

Location of Disease
- Subclavian vein
- Subclavian or axillary artery
- Brachial plexus

Differential Diagnosis
- Spinal stenosis
- Carpal tunnel syndrome
- Nerve impingement (herniated disc)
- Raynaud's disease
- Venous thrombosis
- Neuropathy
- Muscle/tendon strains or tears
- Arthritis
- Tumors, including *Pancoast's tumors* (lung tumor which grows in the thoracic area)
- Degenerative spinal chord diseases (MS)
- Orthopedic shoulder problems
- Angina pectoris

Correlation
- Non-invasive arterial vascular testing
  » UE including volume pulse recording and digital testing
  » Duplex ultrasonography
- X-ray (chest, cervical spine)
- Electromyography
- Nerve conductivity testing
- CT angiography
- MRI
- MR angiography
- Arteriography
- Positional venography

Medical Treatment
- Modify risk factors
- Anti-inflammatory medication (e.g., aspirin)
- Muscle relaxants
- Physical therapy
- Nerve block treatments
- Anticoagulation (warfarin)
- Thrombolytic therapy (acute blockage)

Surgical Treatment
- Thoracic outlet decompression
- Removal of the first rib or cervical rib
- Dividing scalene muscle attachments and fibromuscular bands
- Cervical sympathectomy
- Resection of aneurysmal disease with bypass grafting
- Embolectomy
- Bypass grafting

Endovascular Treatment
- Thrombolysis
- Angioplasty
- Stent

Varicose Veins

Elongated, dilated, tortuous veins which are most commonly found in the extremities. Although varicose veins can occur anywhere in the body, they are usually located in the leg.

- **Primary varicosities** occur without deep venous incompetence
- **Secondary varicosities** caused by vein thrombosis or deep valvular incompetence

Etiology
- Genetic
- History of venous thrombosis

Risk Factors
- Age (greater with advanced age)
- Female
- Pregnancy
- Obesity
- Occupations requiring long periods of standing
- Family history
- Congenital abnormalities (e.g., Klippel-Trenaunay)
- Arteriovenous fistula (acquired or congenital)

Mechanism of Disease
- The pathogenesis of primary varicose veins remains unclear. Initially it was thought that varicose veins are due to valvular incompetence.[63] However, a current hypothesis states that alterations in vein wall structure (cells and extracellular matrix) cause weakness and altered tone, leading to valvular dysfunction.
- There is a decrease in the elastin content of varicose vein walls. There is also a change in the ratio of type I to type III collagen, with an increase in type I (rigid, provides tensile strength) and a decrease in type III (compliant, increases elasticity).
- Interspersed in varicose veins are thick (2-fold thicker than normal veins) and thin regions (2-fold thinner than normal veins).[64] In the thick regions, smooth muscle cells are no longer organized in circumferential and longitudinal bundles but disrupted by an increased amount of fibrous tissue. The intima is thickened with an increase in smooth muscle cells. In the thin regions, there is a decrease in cell number. The adventitia is thin and lacks vasa vasorum. These regions correspond to areas of dilatation.
- Varicose veins demonstrate decreased ability to contract normally[65] and the valves of varicosed veins become stretched.[12]
- Branches of the great saphenous vein (GSV) are thought to varicose before the main trunk of the GSV[12] because they contain fewer smooth muscle cells in their vessel walls and lack support in the subcutaneous fat layer under the skin, where they are commonly located.[66]

- Pregnancy increases the amount blood circulating in the cardiovascular system and causes veins to enlarge. The pressure of the gravid uterus on veins decreases the blood flow back through the pelvic venous system because as the uterus gets larger, it moves from the pelvis into the abdomen. [12,7,67]
  » Varicose veins can improve post-partum. The number and severity of varicose veins can increase with each additional pregnancy. [12,67]

Birth control pills can increase the risk of varicose veins or telangiectasias (spider veins).[67]

- If both parents had VV, there are estimates that there is a 90% chance of developing them. If you are male and only one parent had VV, the chances of developing VV is 25%. If you are female, the chances of developing VV is 62%. Even if neither parent had VV, there is still a 20% chance of developing VV.[65]
- Approximately 20-25% of American women and 10-15% of American men suffer from some type of varicose veins (VV). Higher estimates have been reported. [70,71]
- Approximately 50% of those over 50 years of age have VV.[67]
- Klippel-Trenaunay syndrome is a congenital condition characterized by port-wine stains on the skin, varicosed veins and excessive limb growth. Either one limb or multiple limbs may be affected. In some cases, deep veins are abnormal (absent segments, smaller diameters or dilated veins and/or lack of venous valves). [68,69]

Telangiectasias are not true varicose veins and are oftentimes thought to be related to hormonal changes.[67]

Location of Disease *(in order of typical occurrence)*
- Below-knee great saphenous vein and its tributaries
- Above-knee great saphenous vein
- Saphenofemoral junction
- Any other superficial or deep venous segment

Differential Diagnosis
- Nerve compression
- Arthritis
- Deep venous thrombosis
- Peripheral neuritis
- Stasis dermatitis
- Klippel-Trenaunay
- Lymphatic obstruction

Correlation
- Duplex ultrasonography
- Continuous-wave Doppler
- Plethysmography
- Venography

Medical Treatment
- Compression stockings
- Injection sclerotherapy
- Ultrasound-guided sclerotherapy

Varicose veins may return after treatment.

Surgical Treatment
- Ligation/stripping (of saphenofemoral junction, for example)
- Stab avulsion phlebectomy
- Transverse repair of incompetent valves
- Subfascial ligation of perforators
- Ambulatory phlebectomy
- Ultrasound-guided sclerotherapy

Endovascular Treatment
- Radiofrequency ablation
- Laser ablation
- Transilluminated power phlebectomy

Venous Insufficiency (Postphlebitic Syndrome)

Inadequate venous return resulting in an increase in ambulatory venous pressure. Symptoms range from varicose veins to swelling and ulceration.

Etiology
- Venous hypertension, caused by valve damage or dysfunction
- History of venous thrombosis
- Genetic factors

Risk Factors
- History of venous thrombosis
- Occupations requiring long periods of standing or sitting
- Female
- Family history
- Pregnancy
- Obesity
- Smoking
- Age (greater with advanced age)

Studies estimate than 80% of patients with a history of DVT will develop chronic venous insufficiency.[127]

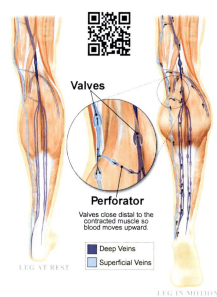

Fig. 11-28: When the leg is in motion, (walking) muscle contractions squeeze the veins, forcing blood past the open valves of the deep, superficial and perforating veins upward towards the heart. After the muscle relaxes, valves close to prevent backflow (reflux).

Mechanism of Disease
- The calf muscle pump functions to move blood from the superficial to the deep venous system through *perforators* or communicating veins.
- Venous valves serve to propagate blood flow back toward the heart and prevent retrograde flow (*reflux*) back down the venous segment.

- Valvular damage and dysfunction (*valvular incompetence*) results in venous reflux and subsequent venous hypertension.[17]
  - » When one suffers from *ambulatory venous hypertension*, there is an abnormally high venous pressure on standing.
  - » When the calf muscle pumps the blood, it is expelled in multiple directions due to dysfunction of the valves. Subsequently, venous pressures do not decrease normally.[17]
- Venous hypertension increases pressures within the venules and capillaries.
  - » Local edema results in a decrease in fluid and protein reabsorption.
  - » Fibrinogen and red blood cells (RBC) escape into the tissues.
  - » Proteins organize and form tissue fibrosis.
  - » The RBCs breakdown and cause hyperpigmentation. This fibrotic, hyperpigmented condition is known as *lipodermatosclerosis*.
  - » Oxygen intake is decreased in the tissues causing tissue malnutrition/hypoxia. Ulceration may follow.[17]

Approx. 2-5% of Americans suffer from venous insufficiency.[132]
Approx. 500,000 suffer from venous ulceration.[127,132]

Location of Disease
- Gaiter area (most common): medial aspect of the leg, just above the medial malleolus
- Lateral or posterior calf

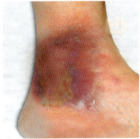

Fig. 11-29: *Venous ulcerations in the gaiter area can result from venous insufficiency*

Differential Diagnosis
- Arterial disease
- Lymphedema
- Cellulitis
- Collagen vasculitis
- Skin cancer

Correlation
- Duplex ultrasonography
- Plethysmography
- Continuous-wave Doppler
- Descending venography

Medical Treatment
- Compression stockings
- Periods of leg elevation
- Proper skin care
- Compression bandaging (ulceration)
- Sclerotherapy

Surgical Treatment
- GSV or SSV stripping/ligation
- Subfascial endoscopic perforator vein surgery
- Transverse repair of incompetent valves
- Subfascial ligation of perforators
- Stab avulsion phlebectomy
- Ambulatory phlebectomy
- Sclerotherapy

Endovascular Treatment
- Thermal venous ablation
- Mechanico-chemical ablation
- Transilluminated power phlebectomy (TIPP)

Venous Malformations [46-49]

Venous Malformations (VM) are developmental anomalies (birth defects) of the venous system. Together with arterial, capillary, and lymphatic malformations, they are a part of a large group of Congenital Vascular Malformations (CVM), which are developmental anomalies of the peripheral vascular system.

Etiology
- Congenital

Mechanism of Disease
Arrested development of the venous system during the various stages of embryogenesis may result in venous malformation.

Extratruncular Lesions
- Developmental arrest occurring before the main vascular trunks are formed.
- May produce symptoms due to compression of the surrounding structures (muscles, nerves).
- May have a significant hemodynamic impact on the involved vascular system.
- There is a high risk of re-occurrence after treatment.

Truncular Lesions
- Defects affecting fully formed and often named vessels
- Developmental arrest occurs during the "later" stages of vascular trunk formation
- Associated with more serious hemodynamic consequences. Incomplete, abnormal development of the main axial veins results in:
  - » Aplasia, hypoplasia, or hyperplasia of the vessel (e.g., agenesis/rudimentary femoral vein)
  - » Obstruction (e.g., vein web, spur, annulus, or septum)
  - » Dilation (e.g., popliteal or iliac vein ectasia or aneurysm)
- Klippel-Trenaunay Syndrome (KTS) affects the development of blood vessels, soft tissues, and bones. This syndrome has three characteristic features: a red birthmark called a port-wine stain, overgrowth of soft tissues and bones, and vein malformations such as varicose veins or malformations of deep veins in the limbs.[46]
- These lesions also manifest as persistent embryonic veins (marginal or sciatic) when a fetal (truncal) vessel fails to develop normally.

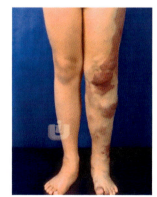

Fig. 11-30: *Klippel-Trenaunay Syndrome (KTS)* Courtesy of Byung-Boong Lee MD Ph.D. FACS

  - » A **persistent marginal vein** courses along the lateral aspect of the thigh and calf just under the skin.
    - Incompetent along its entire length because it lacks valves.
    - Drainage is either into a lateral branch of the deep femoral vein or the internal iliac vein.
    - The vein sometimes crosses anterior in the thigh and joins the femoral vein next to the great saphenous vein.

» A **persistent sciatic vein** may either:
  • Run within the main trunk of the nerve, surrounded by the nerve fibers
  • Or have a spiral course around the main trunk of the nerve, inside the epineurium.
• Risk of re-occurrence after treatment is minimal to none.

Prior to treatment of any superficial veins, it is essential to include a complete duplex ultrasound assessment of the deep venous system to ensure that it is intact. In patients with venous malformations, the superficial system may act as the primary outflow for the lower extremity.

Location of Disease
• Venous Malformations (VMs) most commonly appear on the skin but can be present in other tissues and organs as well.
• Lateral lower extremity with the appearance of a varicosity (persistent marginal vein)
• Posterior thigh along the sciatic nerve (persistent sciatic vein)

Differential Diagnosis
• Hemangioma (vascular tumors that have a distinctly different etiology, genetics, presentation, prognosis, and treatment)
• Peripheral nerve sheath tumors
• PTEN hamartoma syndrome
• Fibroadipose vascular anomaly
• Spindle cell hemangioendothelioma
• Congenital fibrosarcoma

Venous malformations should be differentiated from hemangiomas. Hemangiomas are vascular tumors that present on ultrasound as a soft tissue mass. A venous malformation is a collection of abnormal vessels.

Correlation
• Duplex ultrasound
• CT
• MRI
• Angiogram/Venogram

Medical Treatment
• Compression stockings [56]

Surgical Treatment
• Surgical removal of the malformation [56]

Endovascular Treatment
• Sclerosant injections [57]

Venous Thrombosis

The obstruction of venous outflow within a deep or superficial vein by thrombus.

Etiology
The theory of Virchow's Triad states that venous thrombosis is caused by: venous stasis, vein wall injury, or a hypercoagulable state. Varicose veins and extrinsic compression can lead to one or more of these.

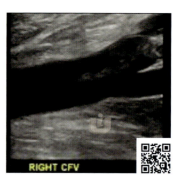

Fig. 11-31: *Free-floating tail of thrombus located in the common femoral vein.*

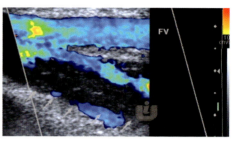

Fig. 11-32: *Free-floating tails (here in the deep femoral vein) are an acute event.*

Risk Factors
• Age (greater with advanced age)
• Immobilization
• Prothrombotic gene mutations (clotting disorders such as Factor V Leiden)
• Post-operative phase (especially after orthopedic surgery)
• Central venous or femoral catheters
• Female
• Pregnancy
• Oral contraceptives
• Estrogen replacement
• Cancer/malignancy
• Previous DVT
• Heart complications (myocardial infarction, congestive heart failure, etc.)
• Obesity
• Family history
• Smoking
• COPD
• Covid-19
• Blood type (highest risk with type-A lowest risk with type-O)
• Trauma
• Antiphospholipid antibodies (e.g., lupus, etc.)
• Occupations requiring extended periods of standing or sitting
• Varicose veins
• Congenital abnormalities (e.g., Klippel-Trenaunay)
• Inflammatory bowel disease
• Drug abuse
• Cerebrovascular events (stroke, TIA)
• Iliac vein compression syndrome

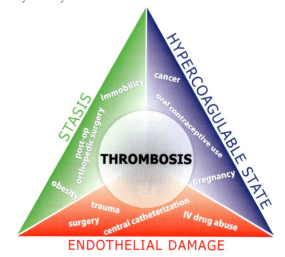

Fig. 11-33: *Virchow's Triad with examples of risk factors that can lead to thrombosis*

Mechanism of Disease

- There are three factors responsible for the formation of venous thrombosis, as outlined in Virchow's Triad: vein wall injury, hypercoagulability, and stasis of blood flow. A combination of any of these events may result in venous thrombosis.
- In blood, coagulation factors are balanced by anticoagulation factors. This allows blood coagulation to occur where and when vessels are severed to stop bleeding and prevent exsanguination (bleeding to death) and blood coagulation in the lumens of blood vessels that leads to blood flow obstruction.
- Endothelial cells line the lumen of blood vessels and provide the antithrombotic surface which normally inhibits blood coagulation, thrombus formation and prevents the adhesion of platelets to the vessel's wall.
- The body is designed so that when a blood vessel is severed or cut, a fibrin clot will form to plug the hole. In a severed vessel, endothelial cells are injured, exposing the thrombotic surface below them. Platelets can now attach to the vessel wall where they will aggregate, forming a platelet plug that stops the bleeding. Blood coagulation pathways are also instantly activated by the injury, leading to fibrin formation. The fibrin will be incorporated into the platelet plug, forming a fibrin clot.
- The coagulation pathways are a series of reactions requiring the sequential activation of numerous enzymes. Anticoagulation factors work by inhibiting these reactions and thus blocking the pathway. At the end of the coagulation pathway, the plasma protein prothrombin is converted to thrombin by the enzyme "prothrombin activator." The enzyme thrombin then converts fibrinogen to fibrin. Once bleeding has ceased, and the fibrin clot has formed, the coagulation pathway is blocked by anticoagulation factors. If the pathways are not blocked, the clot will continue to obstruct blood flow.
- Hypercoagulable states result from genetic mutations or acquired deficiencies in anticoagulation factors that accompany certain diseases (e.g., liver disease). In such cases, naturally occurring anticoagulants (antithrombin, protein C, protein S, etc.) are deficient or unable to function. For example, a genetic mutation in the gene encoding coagulation factor V results in the synthesis of factor V Leiden instead of factor V. Factor V Leiden functions like factor V in the coagulation pathway. However, protein C, the anticoagulation factor that inhibits factor V, cannot inhibit factor V Leiden. Therefore, once factor V Leiden is activated, it functions when it should not, producing a hypercoagulable state. Individuals with this mutation are at increased risk for venous thromboembolism (VTE).
- There are several mechanisms through which blood stasis can increase one's risk of thrombosis. Although stasis never actually occurs in normal blood vessels, the velocity can become extremely low and the flow very sluggish.

> "Economy class syndrome," where travel passengers have been exposed to cramped positions for extended periods, can result in venous thrombosis. Venous stasis during travel may increase the incidents of clot formation for those already at risk for venous thrombosis due to other risk factors. [51]

- Under very low blood flow conditions, the tendency for platelets to become trapped behind valve cusps is believed to increase. Behind the valve cusps is a small region in which blood flow is turbulent. This is where venous thrombi form in the valve. It is thought that the turbulent flow injures the local endothelial cell layer activating the coagulation pathway and leading to venous thrombosis. These two factors, (an increased number of platelets and injured endothelial cells due to turbulent flow) combine to increase the risk of pathological thrombosis in these regions.
- Cancer is thought to increase the formation of venous thrombi by activating coagulation factors and decreasing the levels of coagulation inhibitors (e.g., proteins C and S) in the blood.
- Thrombosis in pregnancy is attributed to a prothrombotic state,[50] along with decreased venous outflow due to the weight of the fetus.[51]
- The use of estrogen (in replacement therapy or contraceptives) alters coagulation and may predispose an individual to thrombosis.[51]
- Once a thrombus is formed, it can remain stable, propagate, or shed/embolize:
  » **Stabilize:** Stabilized thrombi firmly adhere to the vessel wall and do not move, change location or propagate. If a thrombus has formed, the most favorable occurrence would be stabilization. This reduces the risk of embolization for the individual.
  » **Propagate:** Propagation includes "growth of thrombus" in size or location. Likely examples of propagated thrombi are:
    - Thrombus starting in the superficial system and "growing" into the deep venous system.
    - A thrombus that extends from a calf vein into the popliteal vein. It probably first formed in the calf vein and grew into the popliteal vein.
  » **Embolize:** A portion of a thrombus breaks free and is carried by the flowing blood through the vessel until it becomes lodged in a smaller vessel, causing obstruction. Because emboli can and do become wedged in pulmonary vessels, a thrombus releasing emboli is an extremely high-risk factor for pulmonary embolism.
- A pulmonary embolism can occur when a portion or an entire thrombus breaks loose and travels to the lungs.
- Von Willebrand Factor (vWF) is a blood protein activated by thrombin early in the coagulation process to help promote clotting by binding with platelets.[50,53] Patients with vWF deficiency or dysfunction (von Willebrand Disease) have bleeding complications (GI bleeds, nosebleeds, etc.). This disease can be inherited or acquired and occurs in approximately 1-2% of the population.[53]
- The Covid-19 virus is said to increase a patient's risk for excessive blood clotting in the body for 6-12 months after diagnosis. Possible reasons for this increase in hypercoagulability include inflammation and disruption of the coagulation process.[54,55]

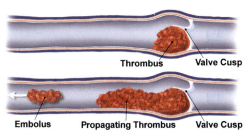

Fig. 11-34: *Venous thrombosis and propagation. In the top vessel, a thrombus has formed behind the valve cusp. This thrombus can stabilize, or as depicted in the bottom vessel, it can propagate. A piece of the thrombus can break off and cause a pulmonary embolism.*

Location of Disease

A thrombus frequently originates at a valve cusp site or in the soleal veins. [51]

Although a thrombus can develop at any venous site, the more common sites are the:

- Muscular veins (gastrocnemius and soleal sinus)
- Behind venous valves
- Venous confluences
- Deep venous system (common femoral, deep femoral, femoral, popliteal, peroneal, posterior tibial, anterior tibial, jugular, innominate, subclavian, axillary, brachial, radial, ulnar, inferior vena cava and iliac veins)
- Superficial venous system (great saphenous, small saphenous, basilic, cephalic, median cubital veins)
- A thrombus frequently originates at a valve cusp site or in the soleal veins. [51]

The length of the thrombosed segment, the number of veins involved, and the degree of collateralization all affect the presentation of venous symptoms. [52]

Physical Examination

- Clinical diagnosis of DVT based on patient's symptoms and history is not very reliable (<50%). [52]

Differential Diagnosis

- Arterial disease
- Lymphedema
- Cellulitis
- Cysts (popliteal, Baker's, etc.)
- Extrinsic compression
- Hematoma
- Muscle tear
- Joint effusion
- Adenopathy
- Arteriovenous fistula
- Heart failure (edema)
- Direct injury to an extremity
- Vascularized mass
- Collagen vasculitis
- Abscess

Correlation

- Duplex ultrasonography
- Venogram
- MRI
- CT angiography
- IVUS

Medical Treatment

- Serial venous duplex exams to monitor for change
- Anticoagulation therapy (e.g., heparin, low-molecular-weight heparin, or warfarin)
- DVT prophylaxis (e.g., intermittent pneumatic cuff compression)
- Limit long periods of inactivity
- Promote venous drainage (e.g., elevate legs, wear elastic stocking/support hose)

Differentiation of chronic DVT versus acute DVT may be difficult.

Surgical Treatment

- IVC filter
- Iliofemoral venous thrombectomy
- Bypass grafting (caval occlusion)
- SVC reconstruction (using femoral vein, spiral saphenous, PTFE, or cryopreserved grafts)

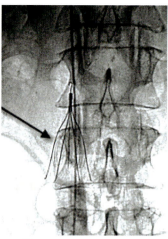
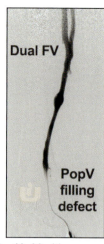

Fig. 11-35: *Inferior vena cavagram showing an IVC filter*

Fig. 11-36: *Venogram of popliteal vein thrombosis*

Endovascular Treatment

- Catheter-directed thrombolysis with Urokinase, etc. (acute DVT)
- Balloon venoplasty and stenting (chronic iliofemoral DVT)
- Mechanical catheter-directed thrombectomy (acute DVT)
- Percutaneous transluminal angioplasty and stenting (SVC syndrome)

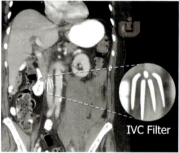
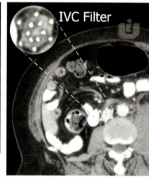

Fig. 11-37: *IVC filter on CT angiograms*

REFERENCES

1. Partsch, H. Varicose veins and chronic venous insufficiency. (2009). Vasa. 38. (4), 293-301. doi: 10.1024/0301-1526.38.4.293. PMID: 19998250
2. Eklof, B., Perrin, M., Delis, K. T., Rutherford, R. B., Gloviczki, P., American Venous Forum, European Venous Forum, International Union of Phlebology, American College of Phlebology, & International Union of Angiology (2009). Updated terminology of chronic venous disorders: the VEIN-TERM transatlantic interdisciplinary consensus document. Journal of Vascular Surgery, 49(2), 498–501. https://doi.org/10.1016/j.jvs.2008.09.014
3. Eklof et al., (2004). Revision of the CEAP classification for chronic venous disorders: Consensus statement. J Vasc Sur. 40, 1248-1252.
4. Porter, J.M., Moneta, G.L. (1995). Reporting standards in venous disease: an update. International Consensus Committee on Chronic Venous Disease. J Vasc Surg, 21, 635-645.
5. Fedor Lurie, M., De Maeseneer, G.R., (2020). The 2020 Update of the CEAP Classification: What is New? European Journal of Vascular and Endovascular Surgery, 59(6), 859-860.
6. Singer, A. J., Tassiopoulos, A., & Kirsner, R. S. (2017). Evaluation and Management of Lower-Extremity Ulcers. *The New England Journal of Medicine*, 377(16), 1559–1567. https://doi.org/10.1056/NEJMra1615243
7. Meissner, M.H., et al. (2021). The Symptoms-Varices-Pathophysiology Classification of Pelvic Venous Disorders: A Report of the American Vein & Lymphatic Society International Working Group on Pelvic Venous Disorders. Journal of Vascular Surgery: Venous and Lymphatic Disorders, 9(3), 568-584.
8. Moneta, G. (2021). Classification of Lower Extremity Chronic Venous Disorders. UpToDate. https://www.uptodate.com/contents/classification-of-lower-extremity-chronicvenous-disorders#
9. Lew, W.K., (2021, August 19). Varicose Vein Surgery. eMedicine. https://emedicine.medscape.com/article/462579-overview
10. Meissner, M.H. (2005). Lower extremity venous anatomy. Semin Intervent Radiol. 22(3), 147-156. https://doi:10.1055/s-2005-921948
11. Labropoulos, N., et al. (2009). Secondary chronic venous disease progresses faster than primary. Journal of Vascular Surgery, 49(3), 704–710. https://doi.org/10.1016/j.jvs.2008.10.014
12. Sumner, D.S., Zierler, R.E. (2005). Vascular physiology: essential hemodynamic principles. In Rutherford Vascular Surgery (6th ed., pp.75-123). Philadelphia. Elsevier Saunders.
13. Venous return. (n.d.). howMed. Retrieved April 1, 2022 from http://howmed.net/physiology/venous-return/#.YdcaV7YJqns
14. Ludbrook, J. (1996) The Musculovenous Pumps of The Human Lower Limb. Am Heart J. 71(5), 635-641.
15. Lejars, F., (1890). Les veines de la plante du pied. Archives de Physiologie. 5° série.
16. Uhl, J.F., Gillot, C. (2010). The plantar venous pump: Anatomy and physiological hypotheses. Phlebolymphology.org. https://www.phlebolymphology.org/the-plantar-venous-pump-anatomy-and-physiological-hypotheses
17. Meissner, M. H., et al. (2007). The hemodynamics and diagnosis of venous disease. Journal of Vascular Surgery, 46 Suppl S, 4S–24S. https://doi.org/10.1016/j.jvs.2007.09.043

18. Goldman, M.P., Fronek, A. (1989). Anatomy and pathophysiology of varicose veins. J Dermatol Surg Oncol, 15, 138-145.
19. Burnand K.G. (2001). The physiology and hemodynamics of chronic venous insufficiency of the lower limb. In: P. Gloviczki, P & Yao. J.S.T. (Eds.), Handbook of Venous Disorders Guidelines of the American Venous Forum. (2nd ed., pp. 49-57). London Arnold.
20. Kushner, A., West, W.P., Pillarisetty, L.S. (Updated 2021 Sep 14). Virchow Triad. StatPearls Publishing, Treasure Island FL. https://www.ncbi.nlm.nih.gov/books/NBK539697/
21. Labropoulos N. (2018). Diagnosis of iliac vein obstruction with duplex ultrasound: Criteria used during duplex ultrasound examination to identify iliac vein obstruction. Endovasc Today, 17(7), 50–52.
22. F. Rabe et al. (2014). European guidelines for sclerotherapy in chronic venous disorders. Phlebology, 29(6), 338–354
23. Calık, E.S. et al. (2019). Ablation therapy with cyanoacrylate glue and laser for refluxing great saphenous veins – a prospective randomized study. Vasa, 48, 405–412.
24. Joseph, D. (2019, May 14). Chronic Venous Insufficiency (CVI). Cleveland Clinic. https://my.clevelandclinic.org/health/diseases/16872-chronic-venous-insufficiency-cvi
25. Cornu-Thenard, A., et al. (1994). Importance of the familiar factor in varicose disease. Clinical study of 134 families. J Dermatol Surg, 20(5), 318-326.
26. Labropoulos, N., Leon, L.R. (2005) Evaluation of chronic venous disease. In Mansour MA & Labropolos N. (Eds.), Vascular Diagnosis, (pp. 447-461). Philadelphia: Elsevier Saunders.
27. Size, G.P., et al. (2013). Cardiac Effects on Spectral Doppler. In C. L. Skelly & E.F. Sherry (Eds.), Inside Ultrasound Vascular Reference Guide (pp. 336-344). Inside Ultrasound Inc.
28. Min, R.J., Rosenblatt, M. (2010). Varicose Veins and Spider Veins. US Department of Health and Human Services, Office on Women's Health. Retrieved April 23, 2022 from http://www.womenshealth.gov/faq/varicose spider veins.cfm
29. Raju, S. (2013). Best management options for chronic iliac vein stenosis and occlusion. J Vasc Surg, 57, 1163-1169.
30. Gloviczki, P., Wahner, H.W. (2005). Clinical diagnosis and evaluation of lymphedema. In Rutherford Vascular Surgery (6th ed., pp. 2396-2415). Philadelphia. Elsevier Saunders.
31. Jobst Publication. (2002). Lymphedema; its cause and how to manage it. Charlotte. BSN-Jobst, Inc. Retrieved May 2022
32. Witte, C.L., Witte, M.H. Lymph circulatory dynamics, lymphangiogenesis and pathophysiology of the lymphovascular system. In Rutherford Vascular Surgery (6th ed., pp. 2379-2396). Philadelphia. Elsevier Saunders.
33. Khilnani, N.M., et al. (2021). Clinical Presentation and Evaluation of Pelvic Venous Disorders in Women. Tech Vasc Interventional Rad, 24(1), 100730. https://doi.org/10.1016/j.tvir.2021.100730
34. Brinegar, K.N., et al. (2015). Iliac vein compression syndrome: Clinical, imaging and pathologic findings World J Radiol, 7(11), 375-381.
35. McDermott, S., et al. (2013). May-Thurner Syndrome: Can It Be Diagnosed by a Single MR Venography Study? Diagn Interv Radiol, 19, 44-48. 22801870 https://doi.org/10.4261/1305-3825.DIR.5939-12.1
36. Heijmen, R.H., Bollen, T.L., Duyndam, D.A., Overtoom, T.T., Van Den Berg, J.C., Moll, F.L. (2001). Endovascular venous stenting in May-Thurner Syndrome. *The Journal of Cardiovascular Surgery*, 42(1), 83–87.
37. Meissner, M.H., Gloviczki, P. (2019). Pelvic venous disorders. In J.L. Almeida (Ed.), Atlas of Endovascular Venous Surgery. (2nd ed., pp.567-599). Philadelphia (PA), Elsevier.
38. Dardik, A., Rahhal, D. (2009-9-10). Phlegmasia alba and cerulea dolens. eMedicine. Retrieved December 10, 2021, from http://emedicine.medscape.com/article/461809-overview.
39. Browse, N.L., Burnand, K.G., Thomas, M.L. (1988). Disease of the Veins; Pathology, Diagnosis and Treatment, (pp. 674). London. Edward Arnold, a division of Hodder & Stoughton.
40. Tortora, G.J., Anagnostakos, N.P. (1990). The respiratory system. In Principles of Anatomy and Physiology (6th ed., pp. 689-730). New York. Harper Row Publishers.
41. Feied, C.F., Handler, J.A. (2004-12-23). Pulmonary Embolism. eMedicine. Retrieved (4-22-2022) from http://www.blueguitar.org/new/misc/pe_copd.pdf.
42. Stein, P.D., Matta, F., Musani, M.H., Diaczok, B. (2010). Silent pulmonary embolism in patients with deep venous thrombosis: A systematic review. Am J Med. 123(5), 426-431.
43. Torbicki, A., et al. (2000). Guidelines on diagnosis and management of acute pulmonary embolism. European Heart Journal. 21, 1301-1336.
44. Gloviczki, P., et al. (2005). Surgical treatment of superior vena cava syndrome. In Rutherford Vascular Surgery (6th ed., pp. 2357-2371). Philadelphia. Elsevier Saunders.
45. Dake, M.D. (2005). Endovascular treatment of vena caval occlusions. In Rutherford Vascular Surgery (6th ed., pp. 2352-2344). Philadelphia. Elsevier Saunders.
46. Lee, B. B., et al. (2015). Diagnosis and Treatment of Venous Malformations. Consensus Document of the International Union of Phlebology (IUP): International angiology: A Journal of the International Union of Angiology, 34(2), 97–149.
47. Huegel, U., & Baumgartner, I. (2019). Implementation of new endovenous treatments in therapy for lateral embryonic veins. Journal of vascular surgery cases and innovative techniques, 5(3), 243–247. https://doi.org/10.1016/j.jvscit.2018.12.016
48. Olivieri, B., White, C. L., Restrepo, R., McKeon, B., Karakas, S. P., & Lee, E. Y. (2016). Low-Flow Vascular Malformation Pitfalls: From Clinical Examination to Practical Imaging Evaluation--Part 2, Venous Malformation Mimickers. AJR. American journal of roentgenology, 206(5), 952–962. https://doi.org/10.2214/AJR.15.15794
49. Klippel-Trenaunay Syndrome. (2021, February 1). National Center for Advancing Translational Services. Retrieved April 22, 2022, from https://rarediseases.info.nih.gov/diseases/3122/klippel-trenaunay-syndrome
50. Fareed J., et al. (2005). Normal and abnormal coagulation. In Rutherford Vascular Surgery (6th ed., pp. 493-511). Philadelphia. Elsevier Saunders.
51. Meissner, M.H., Strandess, D.E. (2005). Pathophysiology and natural history of acute deep venous thrombosis. In Rutherford Vascular Surgery (6th ed., pp. 2124-2142). Philadelphia. Elsevier Saunders.
52. Cook J., Meissner, M.H. (2005). Clinical and diagnostic evaluation of the patient with deep venous thrombosis. In Rutherford Vascular Surgery (6th ed., pp. 2143-2156). Philadelphia. Elsevier Saunders.
53. Eagleton, M., Ouriel, K. (2005). Perioperative considerations: coagulation and hemorrhage. In Rutherford Vascular Surgery (6th ed., pp. 545-567). Philadelphia. Elsevier Saunders.
54. Knight, R., Walker, V., Ip, S., Cooper, J. A., Bolton, T., Keene, S., Denholm, R., Akbari, A., Abbasizanjani, H., Torabi, F., Omigie, E., Hollings, S., North, T. L., Toms, R., Jiang, X., Angelantonio, E. D., Denaxas, S., Thygesen, J. H., Tomlinson, C., Bray, B., ... CVD-COVID-UK/COVID-IMPACT Consortium and the Longitudinal Health and Wellbeing COVID-19 National Core Study (2022). Association of COVID-19 With Major Arterial and Venous Thrombotic Diseases: A Population-Wide Cohort Study of 48 Million Adults in England and Wales. Circulation, 146(12), 892–906. https://doi.org/10.1161/CIRCULATIONAHA.122.060785
55. Kollias, A., Kyriakoulis, K. G., Lagou, S., Kontopantelis, E., Stergiou, G. S., & Syrigos, K. (2021). Venous thromboembolism in COVID-19: A systematic review and meta-analysis. *Vascular medicine* (London, England), 26(4), 415–425. https://doi.org/10.1177/1358863X21995566
56. Venous malformation. UChicago Medicine. (n.d.). https://www.uchicagomedicine.org/comer/conditions-services/vascular-anomalies/venous-malformation
57. Burrows PE, (2013), Endovascular Treatment of Slow-Flow Vascular Malformations, *Techniques in Vascular and Interventional Radiology*, 16 (1), 12-21.ISSN 1089-2516, https://doi.org/10.1053/j.tvir.2013.01.003.
58. Kreienberg PB, Shah, DM, Darling III, RC, Change BB, Paty SK, Roddy SP, Ozsvath KJ, Manish,, (2005). Thoracic Outlet Syndrome: In Mansour MA, Labropoulos N. (Eds.), Vascular Diagnosis, (517-522). Philadelphia,: Elsevier Saunders.
59. Eskandari MK, Yao JST. (2005). Occupational vascular problems. In Rutherford Vascular Surgery 6th edition. (1393-1401). Philadelphia. Elsevier Saunders.
60. Thompson RW, Bartoli MA. (2005). Neurogenic thoracic outlet syndrome. In Rutherford Vascular Surgery 6th edition. (1347-1365). Philadelphia. Elsevier Saunders.

61. Green RM. (2005). Subclavian-axillary vein thrombosis. In Rutherford Vascular Surgery 6th edition. (1371-1392). Philadelphia. Elsevier Saunders
62. Zarins CK, Xu C, Glagov S. (2005). Artery wall pathology in atherosclerosis. In Rutherford Vascular Surgery 6th edition. (123-148). Philadelphia. Elsevier Saunders.
63. Oklu et al. J Vasc Interv Radiol 2012; 23:33–39, Lim and Davies 2009 Pathogenesis of primary varicose veins British Journal of Surgery 2009; 96: 1231–1242
64. Badier-Commander et al. J Pathol 2001; Smooth muscle cell modulation and cytokine overproduction in varicose veins. An in situ study"193: 398-407
65. Pappas PJ, Lal BK, Cerveira JJ, Duran WN. (2005). The pathophysiology of chronic venous insufficiency. In Rutherford Vascular Surgery 6th edition. (2220-2229). Philadelphia. Elsevier Saunders.
66. Caggiati A. (2000). Fascial relations and structure of the tributaries of the saphenous veins. Surg Radiol Anat. 22(3-4):191-6.
67. Min RJ, Rosenblatt M. US Department of Health and Human Services, Office on Women's Health (2010). Varicose Veins and Spider Veins. Retrieved from http://www.womenshealth.gov/faq/varicose-spider-veins.cfm. (7-7-2010).
68. Janniger CK. (3-17-2010). Klippel-Trenaunay-Weber Syndrome. eMedicine. Retrieved from http://www.emedicine.com/article/1084257-overview. (12-5-2010).
69. Connors JP, Mulliken JB. (2005). Vascular tumors and malformations in childhood. In Rutherford Vascular Surgery 6th edition. (1626-1645). Philadelphia. El sevier Saunders.
70. Callam MJ. (1994). Epidemiology of varicose veins. British Journal of Surgery, 81:167-173.
71. Varicose veins and venous insufficiency: Interventional radiology nonsurgical outpatient procedure treats varicose veins. (2010). Society of Interventional Radiologists. http://www.scvir.org/patients/varicose-veins/. (12-9-2010).

12. Arterial Diseases

Adventitial Cystic Disease

Presence of a cyst within the wall of the artery that extends into the arterial lumen causing focal stenosis or occlusion. Adventitial cystic disease (ACD) often occurs in the popliteal fossa. ACD is a rare condition. When it does occur, popliteal cystic disease is the most common type of ACD.

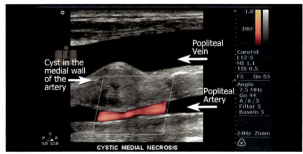

Fig. 12-1: *Arterial cyst narrowing the arterial lumen*
Courtesy of Philips Healthcare

Etiology
- Developmental
- Trauma
- Occupational arterial injury
- Unknown

Risk Factors
- Young males
- Certain occupations (involving heavy manual leg work or repetitive kneeling)
- Males are affected by ACD 15:1 more than females.

Mechanism of Disease
There are several theories on how this disease develops: [87]
- **Repetitive trauma theory**: The adventitial layer of the popliteal artery is thought to degenerate due to repetitive stretch injuries. Small tears between the adventitial and medial layers result in the formation of mucinous cyst(s) within the vessel wall. Joint capsule degeneration may also contribute to cyst development.
- **Embryonic (developmental) theory**: Cells which would normally synthesize connective tissue in the knee joint migrate into the adventitial layer of the artery during limb bud development. These cells secrete mucin which eventually forms a cyst within the vessel wall.
- **Ganglion theory**: Cysts which form due to joint capsule degeneration extend and invade the adventitia of the adjacent artery where they grow and coalesce. This theory stems from the finding that adventitial cysts closely resemble ganglion cysts in chemical composition.

Location of Disease
- Popliteal artery (most common)
- Femoral artery
- External iliac artery
- Upper extremity: ulnar, radial, brachial, axillary artery (rare) [82]

Differential Diagnosis
- Atherosclerosis
- Aneurysm
- Extrinsic compression
- Deep vein thrombosis
- Venous entrapment
- Compartment syndrome
- Muscle strain/tendonitis
- Arterial embolism

Correlation
- Duplex ultrasonography
- CT angiography
- Arteriography

Medical Treatment
- Ultrasound guided cyst aspiration

Surgical Treatment
- Resection with vein or prosthetic bypass (end-to-end anastomosis)
- Intraoperative aspiration/evacuation
- Venous patch angioplasty

Duplex findings of ACD include: focal stenosis or occlusion or compression on the arterial lumen by the cyst (Scimitar sign). [82,87]

Aneurysm

Localized dilatation of a blood vessel of at least 1.5x the normal diameter.

Etiology
- Atherosclerosis
- Trauma
- Dissection
- Infection
- Inflammation
- Congenital abnormalities
- Connective tissue disorders (e.g., Marfan's syndrome, Ehler-Danlos syndrome)

The predicted expansion rate of AAA is 0.2-0.5cm per year. Many AAA cases present without symptoms (asymptomatic). [25]

Risk Factors
- Smoking
- Male
- Hypertension
- Age
- Atherosclerosis
- Caucasian
- Immediate relative with a history of abdominal aortic aneurysm (AAA)
- Family history (other than an immediate relative)
- Dyslipidemia
- COPD

Family history of AAA increases risk 4-fold. The risk increases to 12-fold if an immediate family member develops an AAA. [25]

Multiple pregnancies can induce degenerative changes in specific arterial segments and increase the risk of rupture of any pre-existing visceral artery aneurysms. [33]

Types of Aneurysm

Multiple aneurysms can be present. The terms "bilobed" (two aneurysms) or "multilobed" are sometimes used for multiple dilatations in the same area.

- **True aneurysm**: wall is made up of all arterial layers
  - » **Fusiform**: shaped like a spindle
  - » **Saccular**: round, berry-like or shaped like a sac
- **Pseudoaneurysm**: a hole in the arterial wall which allows blood to escape into the surrounding tissue (essentially a hematoma, in which blood continues to circulate). Because the wall of a pseudoaneurysm does not contain all three layers of a blood vessel, they are not true aneurysms. [25]

Mechanism of Disease

- Aneurysms are most commonly caused by atherosclerotic or inflammatory processes. Inflammatory aneurysms are diagnosed 5-10 years earlier than atherosclerotic. [32] The average age at diagnosis is 66 years for inflammatory and 71 years for atherosclerotic aneurysms.
- The exact cause of degenerative (atherosclerotic) aneurysms, which comprise 90-95% of aneurysms and contain atherosclerotic plaques, is unknown.
- A variant of the common degenerative (atherosclerotic) aneurysm is the inflammatory aneurysm which accounts for 5-10% of all abdominal aortic aneurysms. [32]
- Whether atherosclerosis has an active role in the formation of aneurysms, simply co-exists or if it develops as a result of aneurysms is still debated. [11] The factors that determine if a vessel will proceed towards occlusion or dilatation in the presence of atherosclerosis have yet to be identified. However, several of the processes that contribute to aneurysm formation have been identified and hypotheses for the development of this disease have been proposed.
- Aneurysms are caused by the breakdown of the vessel wall by a multifactorial process involving: connective tissue metabolism, nutrient and oxygen levels, chronic inflammation and biomechanical wall stress.
  - » Connective tissue metabolism: Elastin and collagen are important structural components of the vascular wall. Elastin is a regulator of smooth muscle cell function. Collagen is a protein responsible for providing structural support to the tissues.
  - » There is increased degradation of elastin and collagen in aneurysmal arteries. An increase in enzymes, such as matrix metalloproteinases (MMPs) is one cause. Inflammatory and smooth muscle cells are responsible for the increase in protease levels. [27,28]
    - Elastin degradation plays a key role in aneurysmal dilatation whereas the degradation of collagen leads to rupture.
    - It has been suggested that the infrarenal abdominal aorta is at greater risk for aneurysm compared to the thoracic aorta because the infrarenal abdominal aorta has fewer vasa vasorum per medial lamellar unit. Vasa vasorum are the primary source of nutrients and oxygen for media smooth muscle cells. [2,25]
  - » Reduced nutrient and oxygen levels: The thickened intima could significantly decrease the diffusion of nutrients and oxygen from the lumen to the media. This would presumably cause smooth muscle cells to become dysfunctional and a significant number to undergo *apoptosis*, programmed cell death. [2,25]
  - » Chronic inflammation: Aneurysms are characterized as a chronic inflammatory condition.

The primary disease sites in aneurysms are the media and adventitia, whereas in occlusive atherosclerosis it is the intima.

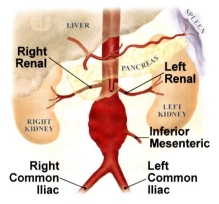

Fig. 12-2: *Fusiform aneurysm of the abdominal aorta*

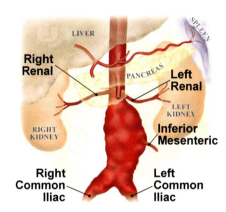

Fig. 12-3: *Fusiform aneurysm of the abdominal aorta with iliac artery involvement*

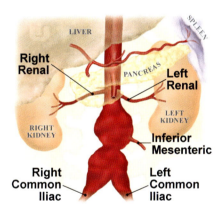

Fig. 12-4: *Bilobed aneurysm involving the aortoiliac arteries*

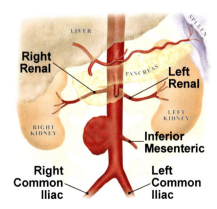

Fig. 12-5: *Saccular aneurysm of the infrarenal abdominal aorta*

- There is an increase in inflammatory cells (neutrophils, macrophages and lymphocytes) especially in the media and adventitial layers of the blood vessels.[4]
- There is significant degradation and thinning of the media during the progression of aneurysms which mediate connective tissue destruction. Smooth muscle cell apoptosis increases and may be mediated by inflammatory cells which secrete death-promoting proteins in aneurysms.[4] Smooth muscle cell density is 74% less in the media of aneurysm tissue than in healthy vessels.[3]
    - » Biomechanical wall stress: Tangential stress is directly proportional to vessel radius and lumenal pressure, and inversely proportional to wall thickness.
    - » Loss of elastin and especially collagen fibers decreases the tensile strength of the arterial wall.
    - » The tension applied to the vessel by the luminal pressure is first resisted by elastin. As elastin breaks down the force is transferred to the collagen fibers. When the collagen fibers no longer have the strength to resist the wall tension, the vessel bursts. Large aneurysms are more likely to rupture than small aneurysms.[6,7,8]
- Inflammatory aneurysms are differentiated from atherosclerotic aneurysm by three gross pathological differences.[9] Inflammatory aneurysms have:

Hypertension: high luminal pressure correlates more with rupture than initial aneurysm formation.

    - » A thickened aneurysm wall measuring approximately 0.5-3.0cm (primarily the thickening involves the adventitia, but some thickening of the intima will occur).
    - » Perianeurysmal and retroperitoneal fibrosis.
    - » Extensive adhesion of adjacent abdominal organs.
- *Ehler-Danlos syndrome* is a group of over 10 distinct diseases in which genetic mutations cause the inhibition of collagen synthesis and fiber formation, as well as a decrease in stability.[37]
- Destruction of the arterial wall may also be caused by virulent gram-negative organisms or fungal infections resulting in atypical aneurysms.[27]
- Aortic and peripheral aneurysms are associated with mural thrombosis.[31] Patients may present with "blue toe syndrome" due to an embolization secondary to a peripheral or abdominal aortic aneurysm.[32]

The "Screening Abdominal Aortic Aneurysms Very Efficiently (SAAAVE) Act" as part of the Deficit Reduction ACT (DRA) of 2005 calls for CMS to cover a one-time abdominal aortic aneurysm ultrasound screening test for men ages 65-75 with a history of smoking, and men and women ages 65-75 with a family history of AAA. Reimbursement began January 1, 2007.[36]

Location of Disease
- The majority of AAA are degenerative (atherosclerotic) and occur below the renal arteries (infrarenal).[2,25]
- The infrarenal abdominal aorta is at greater risk for an aneurysm than the thoracic aorta with an annual rupture incidence of 9.2 and 2.7 per 100,000 persons, respectively.[34]

The primary complication of visceral aneurysms is rupture. Ruptured abdominal and thoracic aortic aneurysms have mortality rates of 50 and 94%, respectively.[29] Peripheral aneurysms are more likely to have complications involving distal emboli.

Rupture, regardless of aneurysm size is always an indication for intervention.[5]

- *Note*: Although aneurysmal disease can occur anywhere in the body, typical locations are:
    - » Infrarenal abdominal aorta (most common)
    - » Thoracoabdominal
    - » Iliac artery
    - » Femoral artery
    - » Popliteal artery
    - » Mesenteric artery
    - » Cerebral artery
    - » Subclavian artery
    - » Superficial or deep venous segments (rare)

62% of individuals with a popliteal artery aneurysm will have an AAA and between 36-38% will have an iliofemoral arterial aneurysm.[30]

Correlation
- CT angiography
- MR angiography, with or without contrast
- Duplex ultrasonography

The anterior-posterior diameter measurement taken perpendicular to the flow channel is more reliable than the transverse diameter.[5]

Aneurysms Identified by Duplex Ultrasound Scans

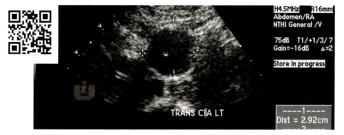

Fig. 12-6: *B-mode image of a common iliac artery aneurysm*

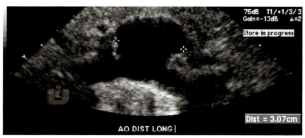

Fig. 12-7: *B-mode image of a saccular aneurysm off the distal aorta-longitudinal view*

The incidence of AAA in the general population is 5-7%. 1

Medical Treatment
- Serial imaging exams to monitor for changes in diameter or disease progression

Surgical Treatment
- Open repair for aneurysm diameter >5.0 cm and/or for aneurysms rapidly increasing in size (>1.0 cm per year)
- Aortic rupture is a surgical emergency

Endovascular Treatment
- Endolumenal graft

Smaller aneurysms may require intervention. Rapidly expanding symptomatic aneurysms is another indication for intervention.

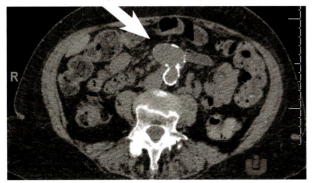

Fig. 12-8: *CT angiogram image of the same saccular aneurysm detected by duplex exam in previous figures.*

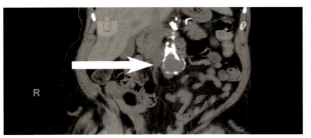

Fig. 12-9: *CT angiogram – saccular aneurysm*

Aortic Coarctation

A segmental narrowing of the aorta which increases blood flow resistance. This leads to hypertension and the left ventricle must pump harder to overcome this resistance and maintain adequate blood flow.

Aortic coarctation typically occurs with other heart defects.[77]

Coarctation is a part of *Shone's complex* (supravalvular mitral valve ring, parachute mitral valve, discrete subaortic stenosis, bicuspid aortic valve and coarctation).[78]

Etiology
- Congenital
- Takayasu's arteritis
- Neurofibromatosis

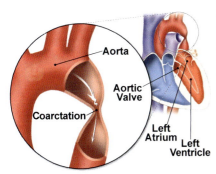

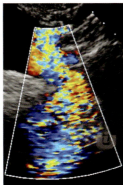

Fig. 12-10: *Aortic coarctation*
Image courtesy of Brad Roberts, RDCS, RCS

Risk Factors
- Hypertension
- Turner's syndrome (females)
- Heart defects
- Bicuspid aortic valve
- Ventricular septal defect
- Patent ductus arteriosus
- Valvular aortic stenosis
- Subaortic stenosis
- Family history

Mechanism of Disease
- During fetal development, the *ductus arteriosus* is a shunt between the pulmonary artery and aortic arch, allowing blood from the right ventricle to bypass the fetus' fluid-filled lungs. The ductus arteriosus functionally closes during the first three hours after birth.
- Aortic coarctations are classified based on their position relative to the ductus arteriosus and can occur preductal, postductal or at the ductus arteriosus (juxtaductal).
- Aortic coarctations are caused by congenital defect or abnormality that occurs during fetal development of the aortic arch. According to one theory, the abnormality is caused by migration of smooth muscle cells from the ductus arteriosus to the periductal aorta. There they synthesize an extensive amount of extracellular matrix narrowing the lumen. Another theory credits diminished left ventricular and aortic isthmus fetal blood flow for the development of coarctation.[79]

Location of Disease
- Thoracic aorta (most common)
- Abdominal aorta (rare; 2% of cases)

> *Coarctation of the aorta may occur at the level of the abdominal aorta and present with symptom of claudication.[79]*

Differential Diagnosis
- Takayasu's arteritis
- Neurofibromatosis
- Fibromuscular dysplasia

Correlation
- Electrocardiogram (EKG)
- Chest x-ray
- MRI
- Transesophageal echocardiography
- Angiography
- Cardiac catheterization

Medical Treatment
- Treatment for heart failure
- Antihypertensive medication

Surgical Treatment
- Synthetic graft insertion (Dacron)
- Dacron patch
- Bypass
- Resection of the coarctation site with end-to-end anastomosis
- Subclavian arterial flap angioplasty

Endovascular Treatment
- Angioplasty
- Stent

> *Symptoms vary according to the severity of the narrowing.[77]*

Arterial Dissection

A tear in the intimal lining of an artery, with or without outer medial wall involvement. Blood enters the media of the vessel through this tear creating a "false lumen." Simultaneously, blood is also flowing through the original or "true lumen."

The false lumen may have one or more "*fenestrations*" which are additional openings to the true lumen allowing blood to flow through the false lumen and back to the true lumen (*fenestrated dissection*).

Dissections can occur spontaneously without a clear cause.[44] Carotid artery dissection is a significant cause of ischemic stroke.[44]

Etiology
- Iatrogenic (caused by medical exam or treatment)
- Collagen vascular diseases (such as Marfan's and Ehlers-Danlos syndromes)
- Trauma
- Atherosclerosis
- Uncontrolled hypertension
- Fibromuscular dysplasiav

Risk Factors
- Abdominal aortic aneurysm
- Age (40-70 years)
- Connective tissue disorders (e.g., Marfan's syndrome)
- Hypertension
- Smoking
- Pregnancy
- Drug abuse

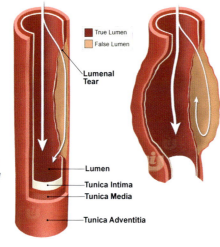

Fig. 12-11: *A fenestrated arterial dissection (left) and a non-fenestrated dissection within an aneurysmal artery (right)*

Mechanism of Disease
- The breakdown of collagen and elastin fibers within the arterial wall (cystic medial necrosis) due to aging or connective tissue disorders, such as Marfan's syndrome causes degenerative changes, rendering the arterial wall weak and at risk for tears.[42]
- Tears in the intimal layer of the arterial wall allow blood flow to access the media.
- Pulsatile flow and high blood pressure cause propagation of a dissection.[42]
- Blood flows through the tear in the intimal layer and sometimes clots.
- Dissection between the medial layers may result in a false lumen.[34] A false lumen can progressively dilate into a pseudoaneurysm.[35]
- Expansion of the false lumen that develops during a carotid dissection can narrow the carotid lumen.[44]
- Malperfusion or end organ ischemia can be caused by occlusion or transient occlusion of a branch vessel or the aortic lumen due to the motion of the dissection flap.
- Arterial dissection can result in rupture of the aorta.

Location of Disease
- Left subclavian artery (most common site for origin of aortic dissection)
- Ascending aorta or arch (2nd most common site for origin of aortic dissection)
- Extracranial carotid arteries
- Intracranial carotid arteries
- Vertebral arteries
- Renal arteries
- Brachiocephalic vessels
- Infrarenal abdominal aorta (rare)

Extracranial internal carotid artery (ICA) dissection is more common than intracranial ICA dissection.[81]

Types of Dissection
- **Stanford Classification** [43]
  - » **Type A**: dissections involve the area from the heart (aortic valve) up to the left subclavian artery
  - » **Type B**: dissections from the left subclavian artery and beyond, not involving the ascending aorta

Differential Diagnosis
- Myocardial infarction
- Acute abdominal conditions (e.g., appendicitis, diverticulitis, pancreatitis, perforated ulcer of the stomach)
- Chronic diseases of the digestive tract
- Urinary tract infections

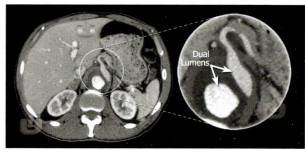

Fig. 12-12: *Dissecting aneurysm at the celiac axis level imaged by CT angiogram*

Correlation
- Duplex ultrasonography
- Echocardiography
- CT angiography
- MR angiography with contrast
- Angiography
- Aortography
- Intravascular ultrasound (IVUS)

Medical Treatment
- Serial imaging exams to monitor changes

Surgical Treatment
- Resection and bypass grafting

Endovascular Treatment
- Stenting

The mortality rate of an acute aortic dissection within the first week is high when left untreated.[42]

Atherosclerosis

Atherosclerosis is a type of "arteriosclerosis," though the terms are often used incorrectly and in place of each other.

Process involving accumulation of fatty substances (cholesterol, triglycerides, oxidized lipids) extracellular matrix, inflammatory cells and calcific regions in the intima of medium and large sized arteries.

- **Atheroma**: derived from the Greek word for porridge or gruel.
- **Sclerosis**: hardening

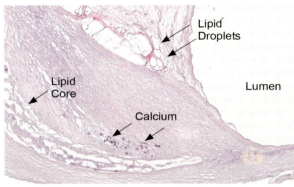

Fig. 12-13: *Calcium deposits develop within atherosclerotic plaques*

Etiology
- Endothelial cell dysfunction
- Hemodynamic forces (oscillatory flow, turbulent flow, low shear stress)
- Inflammation

Risk Factors
- Hypertension
- Diabetes
- Hypercholesterolemia
- Smoking
- Obesity
- Physical inactivity
- Renal failure
- Genetic predisposition
- Homocysteinemia

Mechanism of Disease
Plaque Evolution
- An artery consists of three layers: the intima, media and adventitia.

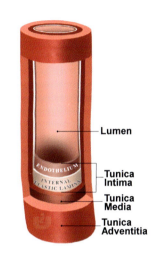

Fig. 12-14: *Three layers of an artery*

- The intimal layer (tunica intima) consists of a confluent monolayer of endothelial cells residing on a thin basement membrane. The endothelial cells, by their regulation of smooth muscle cells, regulate vascular tone (degree of vessel constriction) and the intima plays a role in platelet aggregation and formation of surface thrombi.[1] The intimal and medial layers are separated by a thin layer of elastic fibers known as the *internal elastic lamina*.
- The medial layer (tunica media) is composed of smooth muscle cells, surrounded by extracellular matrix consisting primarily of elastin, collagen and proteoglycans. The collagen and elastin fibers provide structural support for the artery.
- The smooth muscle cells constrict and dilate the vessel to maintain vascular tone and blood flow rates.[1,2,11]
- The adventitial layer (tunica adventitia) consists primarily of fibroblast cells and collagen. Vasa vasorum (small arteries, capillaries and venous channels) enter the vascular wall through the adventitia and may extend into the outer layers of the media. They are usually present in vessels with more than 29 layers of cells and lumens >0.5mm in diameter. They provide nutrients and oxygen to cells in the adventitia and outer layers of the media in large vessels, as these regions are too distant for diffusion from the luminal surface. Vasa vasorum are also present in the plaques of atherosclerotic vessels and it has been postulated that they play a role in atherogenesis.[10]

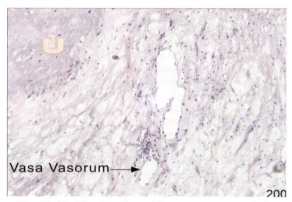

Fig. 12-15: *The function of the vasa vasorum is to provide nutrients and oxygen to the cells*[1]

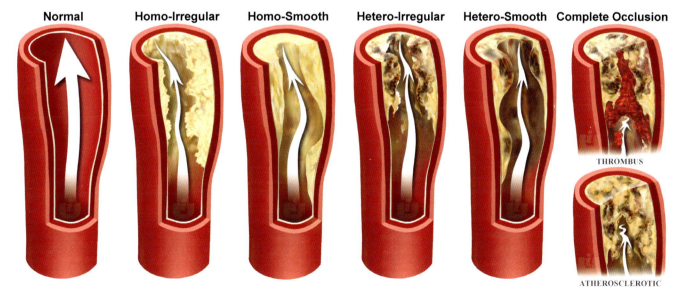

Fig. 12-16: *Presentations of atherosclerosis within an artery. Plaque composition determines whether the terms homogenous, heterogeneous, irregular or smooth are used as descriptors.*

- Damage to the endothelium is caused by various risk factors such as those listed, resulting in dysfunctional endothelial cells. As a result, there is an increase in the adhesion of *monocytes* (a white blood cell) to endothelial cells, which is required for their migration across the endothelial cell barrier, into the intima and medial layers of the artery. In the medial layer and in the "neointima," which forms below the endothelial cells, the monocytes will differentiate into macrophages. [1,11]
- Macrophages take up cholesterol and oxidized lipids that have accumulated in the vessel wall, and become macrophage foam cells. This is one of the initial microscopically detectable cellular events in the formation of lesions. Later, smooth muscle cells will also contain lipid droplets and a "fatty streak," the precursor to atherosclerotic plaque. [1,12]

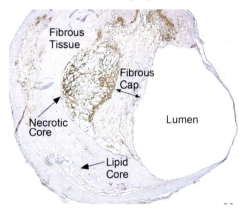

Fig. 12-17: *Plaque development narrows the arterial lumen*

Fatty streaks can appear in infants, although many of these may regress. They will continue to form during childhood and early adulthood.

- Initially, arteries dilate and the arterial wall remodels to increase the diameter of the lumen (**Glagovian remodeling**). This is in response to an increase in wall *shear stress* (frictional force due to blood flow) acting on the endothelial cells, as the arterial lumen narrows due to plaque growth. Eventually, the artery will reach a threshold and will no longer be able to increase in lumenal diameter. Additional plaque growth will cause significant stenosis, defined as a greater than 50% reduction in lumenal area. [1,13]

The various stages of atherosclerotic lesions are:
- **Early lesions**: Consists of lipid-laden macrophages or "foam cells" that go from being dispersed to forming organized layers. Also present are smooth muscle cells with lipid droplets, although at a lower density and a "fatty streak" may be visible. [12] Early lesions can be reversed by exercise and risk factor modification. These lesions can also progress depending on an individual's risk factors.
- **Atheroma**: Characterized by a lipid core, with displacement of smooth muscle cells and extracellular matrix by lipid particles and a proteoglycan matrix between the core and luminal surface of the intima. This is the first stage of disease where the lesion has the potential to become clinically significant. Ischemic events may occur as a result of the formation of fissures or tears, which expose thrombogenic surfaces to the blood.
- **Fibrous plaques** (or *fibroatheromas*): Typically appear after 40 years of age. They are characterized by a lipid core that is separated from the lumenal surface by the "fibrous cap," a layer of fibrous connective tissue, consisting primarily of collagen and elastin. [1,14]

Additional terms related to atherosclerosis include:
- **Fibrous cap**: Organized layers of smooth muscle cells and connective tissue fibers which provides a barrier between the necrotic core and the blood. Once the fibrous cap forms, the lesion is called a *fibroatheroma* which can project into the intima and cause lumenal reduction. Disruption of the fibrous cap can cause thrombosis, which can lead to vessel occlusion or embolization. [1]

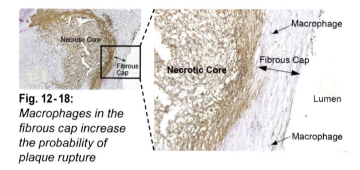

Fig. 12-18: *Macrophages in the fibrous cap increase the probability of plaque rupture*

- **Necrotic core**: Deep region of a plaque containing primarily dead, macrophage foam cells. [1]
- **Complicated lesions:** Complex plaques that contain areas of hemorrhage, necrosis, ulceration and/or thrombosis. [24]
    » **Hemorrhage:** Bleeding into or within a plaque. Occurs either due to the breakdown or tearing of the fibrous cap *(plaque hemorrhage)* or the breakdown of defective microvessels within the plaque *(intraplaque hemorrhage)*.

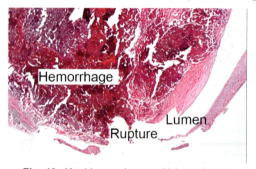

Fig. 12-19: *Hemorrhage within a plaque*

    » **Necrosis:** Dead cells
    » **Ulceration:** Loss of the non-thrombogenic intimal surface, plus a portion of the plaque, which results in the exposure of a thrombogenic substrate and thus a risk of thrombosis.
    » **Embolization/Thrombosis:** Due to disruption of the fibrous cap and endothelium, plaque content is shed into the bloodstream leaving behind a thrombogenic surface. A blood clot *(thrombosis)* then forms on this surface.
        - After a thrombus forms, part may break off *(embolus)* and travel through the blood stream. This is carried distally where it may occlude an artery *(embolization)* resulting in an ischemic event (e.g., stroke, myocardial infarction, etc.).

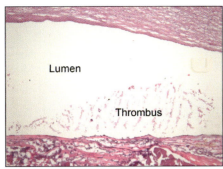

Fig. 12-20: *Thrombus on the surface of an ulcerated plaque*

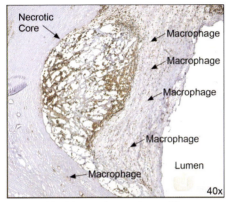

Fig. 12-21: *Macrophage dense fibrous cap*

Location of Disease

- Disease can be focal or diffuse and affect any level or multiple levels of the vasculature.
- Atherosclerosis primarily occurs in regions where the endothelial cells are dysfunctional due to shear stress exposure. Pathological shear stresses, (low, oscillatory or turbulent flow) occur at the outer wall of arterial bifurcations, the inner wall of curved arteries and at the ostia. Typical locations for disease include:
  » Carotid arteries
  » Coronary arteries
  » Infrarenal abdominal aorta and the iliac bifurcation
  » Distal femoral/popliteal arterial segment
  » Tibial arteries

Correlation

- Non-invasive vascular testing, including physiological exams and duplex ultrasonography
- CT angiography
- MR angiography
- Arteriography

Please refer to individual disease/testing sections for Differential Diagnosis, Medical, Surgical and Endovascular Treatments on this topic.

Cerebrovascular Events (Transient Ischemic Attack, Stroke)

A cerebrovascular event is when brain tissue is damaged due to disruption of blood flow. Traditionally a cerebrovascular event is considered a transient ischemic attack (**TIA**) if the neurological deficit (motor, sensory, speech deficit, etc.) lasts less than 24 hours. However, neuroimaging informed operational definitions have been proposed, which state that there should be no evidence of an acute infarction.[15] Deficits lasting longer than 24 hours are considered a completed stroke (**CVA**).

Previously, an episode where symptoms lasted longer than 24 hours, but eventually completely resolved, was classified as a reversible ischemic neurological deficit (**RIND**). However, this is now considered obsolete as it was realized that events lasting between 24 hours and 7 days are associated with infarctions.[15]

The two types of stroke are *ischemic* and *hemorrhagic*:[16,17]

- **Ischemic stroke** (most common, approximately 85% of all strokes): due to a decrease in blood flow to the brain caused by an arterial narrowing or blockage. The five widely accepted sub classifications of ischemic stroke based on etiology are:
  » **Cardioembolic (embolic):** an embolus from a cardiac or pericardiac source causes a territorial infarction. Most common cause is atrial fibrillation, where there is pooling of the blood in the heart which can lead to the formation of blood clots. Note: Some classifications will include emboli that originate from peripheral arteries, (such as the carotid arteries) under this sub-category and then use the term embolic stroke for this sub-classification. Others will place them under the classification "large vessel atherosclerosis."
  » **Large vessel atherosclerosis:** (Atherothrombotic) Occlusion or stenosis greater than 50% of the major intra- and extracranial arteries supplying the vascular territory of the stroke (internal carotid, common carotid, vertebral, basilar, middle cerebral, anterior cerebral or posterior cerebral). There is a decrease in the lumenal area due to atherosclerosis and/or thrombosis.
  » **Lacunar:** (Small vessel disease) accounts for approximately 25% of all acute ischemic strokes.[16,17] Lacunar infarcts are small infarcts (3 - 20mm in diameter) in the deeper noncortical parts of the cerebrum and brainstem. They result from occlusion or stenosis of penetrating branches of the large cerebral arteries. Dementia and cognitive decline are associated with silent lacunar infarcts, infarcts that are not associated with obvious acute clinical stroke symptoms.[21]
  » **Stroke of other determined etiology:** These rare cases normally occur in the young patients who have no stroke risk factors. Causes include coagulopathies, vasculopathies, genetic disorders and metabolic disorders.
  » **Stroke of undetermined etiology**: In a significant number of cases (≤40%), no clear explanation can be found for an ischemic stroke despite an extensive diagnostic evaluation.
- **Hemorrhagic stroke:** (Approximately 15% of all strokes) due to arterial rupture or venous malformation in the brain. Blood accumulates and compresses the surrounding brain tissue. In addition, there is no or little blood flow distal to the rupture site. Hemorrhagic strokes are classified as either subarachnoid hemorrhage or intracerebral hemorrhage.
  » **Subarachnoid hemorrhage:** Most commonly due to trauma, but can also occur due to rupture of a cerebral aneurysm. In 10-20% of spontaneous, nontraumatic cases, no cause is found.
  » **Intracerebral hemorrhage:** (*Parenchymatous*) Rupture of a blood vessel within the parenchyma, often the result of chronic hypertension or an intrinsic vessel problem such as amyloid angiopathy or other vascular malformation. May also be caused by a brain tumor.

- There has been research conducted on what makes a plaque vulnerable to rupture or stable and how to identify these plaques, as a plaque's vulnerability is a major determinant in whether or not it should be removed. There are many theories on what makes a plaque vulnerable to rupture and thus likely to cause a TIA or stroke. Both the plaque's hemodynamic environment and composition need to be considered. Considerations include:
  - » **Active plaques:** Plaques with a large number of macrophages. Their presence is thought to increase the likelihood of plaque rupture as they degrade the fibers in the extracellular matrix decreasing the structural integrity of the plaque, increasing its susceptibility to rupture. The destruction caused by macrophages in the fibrous cap is especially harmful, as it increases the risk of plaque rupture the most.
  - » **Fibrous cap thickness:** The thinner the fibrous cap, the more vulnerable the plaque. The thicker the cap, the more stable the plaque is thought to be. Smooth muscle cells are important for the maintenance of fibrous caps as they synthesize collagen and elastin. Macrophages are detrimental to fibrous caps as they secrete enzymes, such as metallomatrix proteases which degrade the fibrous cap.

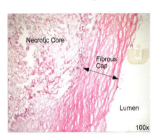 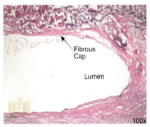

Fig. 12-22: *Histological images of a thick (left) and thin (right) fibrous cap.*

  - » **Calcium:** The effect depends upon size, location and type of artery. In carotid arteries calcium is believed to stabilize the plaque, with stability increasing as the percentage of calcium increases. The effect of calcium in coronary arteries is debated with many studies showing a negative effect on plaque stability. Micro-deposits of calcium near the surface of the plaque have been suggested to increase the vulnerability of plaques. Calcium is used as an indication of plaque stability clinically as it can be detected by both ultrasound and CT angiography.

Etiology

- Atherosclerosis
- Embolism
- Thrombus
- Fibromuscular dysplasia
- Arterial kinking
- Arterial dissection
- Traumatic occlusion
- Extrinsic compression
- Radiation-therapy induced carotid stenosis

Risk Factors

- Age
- Hypertension
- Smoking
- Hypercholesteremia
- Diabetes
- Obesity
- Hypercoaguable state
- Cardiac disease (e.g., arrhythmia, heart failure, infection)
- Patent foramen ovale
- Mechanical heart valve
- Family history
- Sedentary lifestyle
- Previous TIA or stroke
- Radiation-therapy
- Hormone therapy or use of birth control pills
- Alcohol abuse

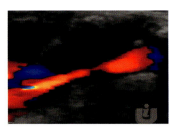

Fig. 12-23: *Duplex scan of a symptomatic ICA stenosis (50-79%)*

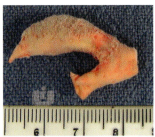 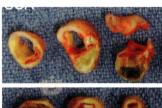

Fig. 12-24: *Atherosclerotic plaque removed from the carotid arteries using the semi-eversion method.*

Fig. 12-25: *Sectioned atherosclerotic carotid plaque (same plaque shown above intact).*

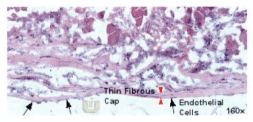

Fig. 12-26: *Histological image of a thin fibrous cap (between red arrows).*

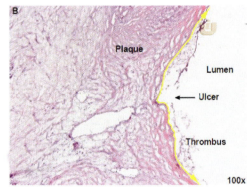

Fig. 12-27: *Plaque ulceration*

Mechanisms of Disease

Ischemic infarcts

- Ischemic infarcts can be separated into three categories based on their pathophysiological mechanism: lacunar, territorial and border zone.
- The mechanisms leading to cortical and subcortical infarcts are likely to be different. Subcortical infarcts have a strong hemodynamic mechanism. Micro-emboli may have more of a causal relationship with isolated cortical border zone infarcts than hemodynamic compromise (low flow). Cortical infarcts in the presence of subcortical infarcts appear to be a result of hemodynamic compromise. [19]
- The prognosis for patients with subcortical infarcts is poor with increased risk for morbidity and a future stroke compared to patients with cortical infarcts. [19]

- **Lacunar strokes:** are caused by the occlusion of a single small perforating cerebral artery.
  - » Due to the stenosis or occlusion of the penetrating arteries of the middle cerebral artery, anterior choroidal artery, anterior cerebral artery, posterior cerebral artery, posterior communicating artery, basilar artery, vertebral artery and the cerebellar arteries. Lacunar strokes result in small infarcts, 3-20mm in diameter in the putamen, caudate, thalamus, pons, internal capsule, and convolutional white matter.
  - » Occlusion is most commonly due to a microatheroma, with or without a superimposed thrombus in an artery that ranges from 400-900μm in diameter resulting in infarcts 5mm in diameter or larger.
  - » Small lacunar infarcts, 2-5mm in diameter are usually the result of occlusion by *lipohyalinosis* (small vessel disease in the brain). This is a hypertensive vasculopathy in which the lumen of arteries 40-200μm in diameter are occluded. There is a loss of normal arterial architecture and the presence of macrophage foam cells.
  - » Rarely will lacunar infarcts be caused by emboli from the heart or atherosclerotic lesions in the carotid artery or aortic arch.
  - » Lacunar infarcts 3mm or less in diameter are usually asymptomatic. Larger lacunar infarcts are normally symptomatic.
  - » Although it is debatable, there is evidence linking hypertension and diabetes with lacunar infarctions, especially with those caused by lipohyalinosis.
  - » The mechanisms described above for lacunar stroke has become known as the "lacunar hypothesis." This hypothesis has been debated. The lacunar hypothesis was formed when hypertension was not as well controlled as it is today. Later studies have suggested that a significant number of lacunar infarcts occur in the absence of hypertension or diabetes. It has been proposed that emboli (cardiac or arterial origin) may be a major cause of these lacunar infarcts.
- **Territorial or embolic infarcts** are most frequently due to an embolus, which originates from a proximal thrombus and occludes a cerebral vessel. The embolus circulates through the vasculature until the vessel becomes too narrow for its passage. The embolus occludes the artery, which blocks blood flow causing ischemia leading to infarction. Territorial infarcts are restricted to territories supplied by major intracerebral arteries, their branches or pial arteries.
  - » If the embolus originates from the heart it is classified as a *cardioembolic infarction*. However, they may originate elsewhere, particularly the carotid arteries.
- **Border zone infarcts** (*watershed infarcts*) 10% of all cerebral infarcts [18] occur in an area between two "neighboring" vascular territories (distal fields of two non-anastomizing arterial systems). [19,20] The two subtypes, based on location are cortical (external) border zones (**cortical watershed areas**) or subcortical (internal) border zones (**internal watershed areas**).
  - » Cortical watershed areas are located between:
    - Anterior and middle cerebral arteries
    - Posterior and middle cerebral arteries.
  - » Internal watershed areas are located between:
    - Lenticulostriate and middle cerebral arteries
- Lenticulostriate and anterior cerebral arteries
- Heubner and anterior cerebral arteries

- Anterior chorodial and middle cerebral arteries indent one level, same as Lenticulostriate and middle cerebral arteries
  - » Pathophysiology of these infarcts is still unclear and debated.
    - The classical theory states that a change in hemodynamics, caused by repeated systemic hypotension in conjunction with occlusion or severe arterial stenosis, primarily of the internal carotid artery, leads to infarction. Hypotension causes a decrease in perfusion pressure, which significantly decreases blood flow within the border zones. Since border zone perfusion pressures are already low at the distal ends of the arterial tree, these areas are highly susceptible to ischemia and infarcts during repeated episodes of hypotension.
    - A recent hypothesis states that microemboli (50-300μm), which may originate from the heart or carotid arteries, occlude the terminal vascular field causing border zone infarcts, rather than the slowing of the cerebral blood flow. This is observed primarily in cortical border zone infarcts that occur in the absence of subcortical border zone infarcts. Since microemboli are small, they tend to circulate to cortical border zones, where the low perfusion rate limits their wash out. Isolated cortical border infarcts have occurred without hemodynamic compromise.
    - Another hypothesis combines the previous two; microemboli and hypoperfusion together have a greater chance of causing border zone infarcts since the microemboli would be more likely to cause micro-infarcts in the presence of chronic hypoperfusion. The hypoperfusion would reduce the clearance of the microemboli and the microemboli, due to their blockage of the vessels, would increase the local hypoperfusion.

Approximately 795,000 cases of new or recurrent stroke occur each year. About 610,000 of these are new events, while 185,000 are recurrent attacks. [89]

Mechanisms of Carotid Artery Stenosis

- **Atherosclerosis** [1] is the most common arterial disease. Atherosclerotic plaque forms in the arterial wall and decreases or stops blood flow by either narrowing the lumen (*arterial stenosis*) or completely blocking the artery (*arterial occlusion*). The term "*hemodynamically significant obstruction*" refers to either a stenosis or an occlusion that results in a significant decrease in blood pressure or flow distal to the obstruction. A stenosis is considered clinically significant, with measurable decreases in pressure and flow velocities distally, when the area is decreased 50% or more. An arterial occlusion is typically seen from one major branch to the next.
- **Kinks**: Blood flow is compromised in kinked arteries and kinks are often associated with plaque and arterial stenosis. Congenital kinks are a result of faulty descent of the vessels during embryonic development. Kinks can be acquired with age; arteries can elongate and at the same time, the medial layer degenerates. [44]
  - » The ICA may be "kinked," which is a sharp angulation of the vessel, usually resulting in stenosis. The kink is typically located 2-3cm from the bifurcation. These patients may present with cerebrovascular symptoms.
  - » Carotid artery kinks occur four times more often in women than men. [44]
  - » The ICA may be coiled or tortuous; creating an "S" or "C" shape or it can be elongated or curved. Either may produce a bruit. Double, complete loops have also been reported. The patient is usually asymptomatic. [44]

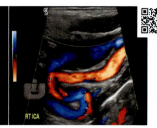 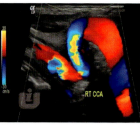

Fig. 12-28: *Duplex image of a tortuous artery-ICA (left) and kinked artery-CCA (right)* Images courtesy of Patrick Washko, BS RT RDMS RVT

- **Fibromuscular dysplasia** (FMD): The internal carotid is a long segment artery without branches that lacks vasa vasorum (which supplies nutrients and oxygen to vessel walls) typically found at branch points. Arterial wall ischemia may result, which is one theory for the development of FMD. [88] This long arterial segment is also thought to be subject to unique mechanical forces (greater axial stress).

Location of Disease
- Brain tissue
- Contributing atherosclerotic or emboli origination sites, include:
  - » Intracranial vessels
  - » Proximal internal carotid artery (ICA)
  - » Origin of the vertebral artery
  - » Basilar artery
  - » Middle cerebral artery
  - » Anterior or posterior cerebral arteries
  - » Aortic arch
  - » Heart

Differential Diagnosis for CVA/TIA
- Vasculitis (e.g. arteritis)
- Fibromuscular dysplasia
- Moyamoya disease
- Cerebral hemorrhage
- Carotid artery dissection
- Seizure
- Lupus
- Metabolic problems (e.g., glucose derangement)
- Migraines
- Cardiac embolization
- Nonatherosclerotic vasculopathy
- Systemic infections
- Mass lesions
- Intracranial tumor
- Primary central nervous system (CNS)
- Metastatic
- Subdural hematoma
- Cerebral abscess
- Multiple sclerosis
- Alcohol or drug abuse
- Cardiac failure
- Syncope
- Positional vertigo

Systemic reasons for low flow states include: hypotension, arrhythmia, heart failure, anemia or pacemaker malfunction.

Correlation
- Duplex ultrasonography
- TEE (transesophageal echocardiography)
- CT angiography
- Brain CT
- MR angiography
- MRI
- Cerebral angiography

Medical Treatment
- Modify risk factors (e.g., smoking cessation, low cholesterol, etc.)
- Statin therapy
- Antithrombotics
- Tissue plasminogen activator (TPA) therapy: to treat ischemic stroke, within three hours of onset of symptoms
- Intra-arterial thrombolysis (within six hours of onset of symptoms)
- Treatments for ischemic and hemorrhagic strokes are very different. [22,23]

Surgical Treatment
- Carotid endarterectomy
- ICA resection and reanastomosis (for kinking)

For occluded ICAs it is important to clearly demonstrate that there is no "trickle" flow present during the duplex scan since carotid endarterectomy is not usually performed on completely occluded ICAs.

- Carotid thrombectomy
- Bypass (subclavian-carotid or carotid-carotid)
- Vertebral artery transposition (to CCA)
- Vertebral artery reconstruction

NASCET (North American Symptomatic Carotid Endarterectomy Trial) demonstrated that the long term-benefit of carotid endarterectomy was significantly greater than medical treatment in symptomatic patients with >70% stenosis. [90] ACAS (Asymptomatic Carotid Atherosclerosis Study) demonstrated marginal benefit of carotid endarterectomy in asymptomatic male patients with >60% stenosis. [91]

Endovascular Treatment
- Carotid angioplasty and stenting

Carotid Body Tumor (CBT)

A highly vascularized tumor of the carotid body. The carotid body is a chemoreceptive organ located in the adventitia of the common carotid artery at the bifurcation. CBTs are also referred to as "Glomus" tumors. [44,64]

The carotid body normally measures 5 x 3 x 2mm in size. [44]

Within the carotid body there are peripheral arterial chemoreceptors that sense arterial partial pressures of oxygen and carbon dioxide as well as blood pH. Through the release of neurotransmitters, they are primarily responsible for hyperventilation during hypoxia and contribute significantly to the hyperventilation associated with respiratory or metabolic acidosis.

The tumor can widen the bifurcation by separating the internal and external carotid arteries.

- CBT types (Shamblin classification)
  - » **Group 1:** small tumors, minimally attached to the carotid vessels.
  - » **Group 2:** moderately-sized tumors, partially encircling the carotid vessels.
  - » **Group 3:** large tumors which encase both carotid arteries and the vagus nerve.

CBTs are benign tumors in 90-95% of all cases. [64]

Etiology
- Genetic mutations: approximately 10-30% of carotid body tumors (CBTs) are inherited. [45]

CBTs are bilateral in 26-33% of hereditary cases and 3-5% of sporadic cases. [61,62,63]

- Sporadic etiology: (70-90% of cases) not predisposed to CBT formation by an inherited genetic mutation.
- Environmental factors

Sporadic CBTs are associated with living at high altitudes. [46]

Risk Factors

- Middle age (occurring during the 5th decade of life on average)
- Female (more common)
- Individuals born/living at high altitudes [45]
- CBTs are more frequent in people living at higher altitudes. [92,93]
- Although much less common, FMD also occurs in young children and infants. [94]

The percent of men and women with hereditary CBTs are similar, whereas women are more likely to have sporadic CBTs. [63]

Mechanism of Disease

- The carotid body is a parasympathetic, extra-adrenal paraganglion, which is a neuroendocrine organ. [47] Parasympathetic paraganglia are clusters of two cell types, chemoreceptive cells (type I cells, chief cells) and supporting cells (type II cells, sustentacular cells) that arise embryologically from neural crest cells. The chemoreceptive cells form nests. Each nest is surrounded by supporting cells and an extensive capillary network making CBTs highly vascularized. [45] CBTs are driven by genetically mutated chemoreceptive cells.
- Inherited CBTs result from a genetic mutation from one generation to the next. Inherited CBTs follow the "two-hit model," first was the inherited genetic mutation in one of the alleles and second hit was the mutation that the second allele acquired in the somatic cell. [45]
- Hereditary CBTs are caused by mutations in the genes encoding subunits and related proteins of the mitochondria enzyme complex *succinate dehydrogenase* (SDH). [48,49,50,51]
  » SDH, also known as complex II, is a component of the Krebs cycle as well as the mitochondrial electron transport chain.
  » Only offspring who inherit a mutated SDHD gene from their father are predisposed to CBTs. Tissue specific epigenetic methylation causes maternal genomic imprinting (suppression) of SDHD alleles in certain tissues. [52] Thus, the expression of mutated SDHD genes is suppressed when they are inherited from the mother. No CBTs have been histopathologically proven in offspring who inherited SDHD mutations from their mother. [53] This results in CBTs skipping a generation making it difficult to assess familial history. The mutated gene continues to be passed down through the generations and when a child inherits it from their father, they are genetically predisposed to develop CBTs. Maternal genomic imprinting also occurs for the SDHAF2 gene. [51,54]
  » In paternal SDHD hereditary cases of CBT, there is a mutation in the germline cells, which results in the somatic cells being heterozygous (paternal allele is inactive but the maternal allele is active) for SDHD. In the tumor cells there is a loss of heterozygosity (the maternal allele is completely lost). [48] The germline loss of function mutation in the paternal allele combined with the loss of the maternal allele in the tumor cells classifies SDHD as a tumor suppressor gene. Furthermore, it shows that SDHD needs *two-hits* for inactivation. The chemoreceptive cells in the carotid body have been identified as the cells containing the required *two-hits*, germline mutation and somatic cell mutation. They are considered the neoplastic proliferating cells of CBTs. [55]

There is evidence that genes other than SDHB, SDHC, SDHD and SDHAF2 have a significant role in the tumorigenesis of a subset of CBTs. [64,65]

» The mechanisms by which mutations in the genes lead to tumorigenesis are unknown. However, it has been postulated that mutations in the genes create a "pseudo-hypoxic" microenvironment that leads to an increase in cell number. [51] For both hypoxia and a lack of SDH activity result in an increase in succinate levels. Plus, there is evidence that suggests SDH mutations activate the same signaling pathways as hypoxia. [56] And hypoxic conditions due to high altitudes or chronic hypoxemia cause hyperplasia (an increase in cell number) of the carotid body. [57,58,59,60]

- There is also an environmental factor in the etiology of CBTs as individuals living at high altitudes in Peru develop CBTs at a frequency ten times greater than individuals living at sea level. [45] It has been postulated that this is due to chronic hypoxia and resulting hyperplasia in carotid bodies. [57,58,59,60]
- In most cases, the external carotid artery supplies blood to the tumor. [44,92] As the tumor grows, blood flow can also be supplied by the internal carotid, vertebral artery or thyrocervical trunk. [44]

Location of Disease

- Common carotid artery bifurcation between the internal and external carotid arteries.

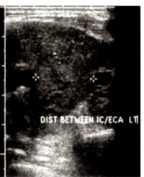

Fig. 12-29: *B-mode ultrasound image with distance measured between the carotid arteries*

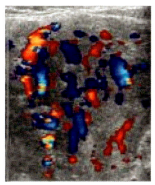

Fig. 12-30: *Color flow duplex ultrasound image of a CBT showing extensive vascularization*

Differential Diagnosis

- Lymphomas
- Metastatic tumors
- Aneurysms of the carotid arteries
- Thyroid lesions
- Brachial cleft cysts
- Salivary gland tumors

Correlation

- Color duplex ultrasonography
- CT scan (with contrast)
- MRI
- MR angiography
- Angiography

Conservative Treatment

- Monitor for changes

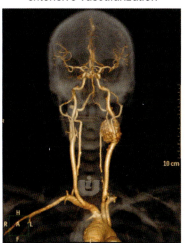

Fig. 12-31: *CT angiogram multiplanar reconstruction of a CBT*

Medical Treatment
- Radiation therapy

Surgical Treatment
- Surgical excision with and without prior transcatheter embolization to decrease vascularity

Endovascular Treatment
- Some tumors are treated with pre-operative transcatheter embolization to reduce blood loss during the surgical excision.

Fibromuscular Dysplasia (FMD)

Non-atherosclerotic arterial disease which affects medium and large sized vessels, especially the renal and internal carotid arteries resulting in either a focal stenosis or multifocal stenoses. In multifocal stenoses of the arterial segment, there appears to be a "string of beads" on imaging studies.

On duplex ultrasound, multifocal FMD is characterized by a series of tandem stenoses and dilatations accompanied by a moderate-significant increase in peak-systolic velocity (a "string of beads"). [43,92,94,95]

The abbreviation FMD is also used to describe another vascular issue, "flow mediated dilatation." Flow mediated dilatation is defined as widening of an artery due to increased blood flow. Make sure everyone is talking about the same "FMD" during any discussion or reporting.

Approximately 25% of individuals with FMD have more than one narrowed artery. [88]

Etiology
- Hormonal
- Mechanical stressors
- Arterial wall ischemia
- Genetics

Risk Factors
- Female
- Younger than 60 years of age (pre-menopausal)
- Family history
- Tobacco use
- Certain medications causing irritation of arterial walls

Mechanism of Disease
- Since the renal, internal and external iliac are long segment arteries without branches, they lack vasa vasorum typically found at these branch points which supply nutrients and oxygen to vessel walls. Arterial wall ischemia results and is one theory for the development of arterial dysplasia. [94]
- According to another theory, long arterial segments, such as the renal and internal carotid arteries, are subject to unique mechanical forces (i.e., greater axial stress) which cause stretching of vessels. [94]
- Although the exact mechanism remains unclear, hormonal influences on smooth muscle cells suggest the prevalence of FMD in women during their reproductive years. [94]

Location of Disease *(can be unilateral or bilateral)*
- Distal renal artery (most common)
- Mid-distal internal carotid artery
- External iliac artery
- Brachial artery
- Abdominal arteries, including the mesenteric

Coexisting FMD in the renal and carotid arteries is a common occurrence. [88]

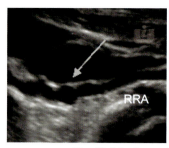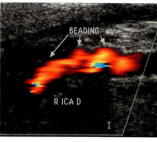

Fig. 12-32: *B-mode and color image of "beading" in the renal artery and ICA*

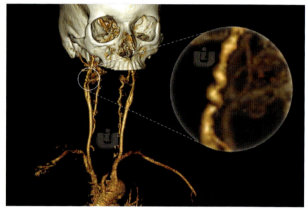

Fig. 12-33: *FMD by CT angiogram: 3D reconstruction*

Fibromuscular dysplasia (FMD) usually occurs in females in the mid-section of the internal carotid artery. [88,95]

Differential Diagnosis
- Atherosclerotic stenosis
- Takayasu's arteritis
- Vasospasm
- Neurofibromatosis
- Moyamoya disease
- Vasculitis
- Neurosyphillis
- Varicella zoster virus

Correlation
- Duplex ultrasonography
- CT angiography
- MRI
- MR angiography
- Angiography

Medical Treatment
- Antiplatelet medication (e.g., aspirin)
- Serial imaging studies to check for disease progression

Surgical Treatment
- Open arterial dilation
- Bypass grafting

Endovascular Treatment
- Balloon angioplasty
- Stenting

Mesenteric Ischemia

Mesenteric ischemia is caused by a significant decrease in blood flow to the small intestines or colon due to a blockage in the mesenteric arteries (celiac, superior and inferior mesenteric arteries), with two out of the three arteries usually being affected. [99,100,101]

- **Chronic mesenteric ischemia**–progressive condition with symptoms developing over a long period of time (e.g., involuntary weight loss). [100]
- **Acute mesenteric ischemia**–symptoms present abruptly and progress quickly over a short period of time.

Etiology
- Embolic
- Thrombosis of pre-existing arterial stenosis
- Atherosclerosis
- Intestinal hypoperfusion (caused by small vessel insufficiency)
- Vasospasm
- Venous thrombosis
- Takayasu's arteritis

Risk Factors
- Atherosclerosis
- Age (> 50 years)
- Female > Male
- Young-female (should consider median arcuate ligament syndrome as a cause)
- Hypertension
- Diabetes
- Hypercholesteremia
- Smoking
- Gastrointestinal disease
- Coronary disease (e.g., arrhythmia, congestive heart failure, etc.)
- Mesenteric venous thrombosis
- Risk factors for mesenteric venous thrombosis: obesity, cancer, oral contraceptives
- History of abdominal surgery
- Hernia
- Genetic prothrombotic conditions (e.g., clotting disorders, such as Factor V Leiden)
- Aortic dissection
- Arteritis

Mechanism of Disease
Mesenteric blood flow is regulated by several mechanisms; intrinsic (metabolic) and extrinsic (neural and hormonal).[97]
- Atherosclerosis or vasospasm can significantly narrow the arterial vessels supplying the intestinal organs.[72] Emboli are a common cause of acute ischemia.[99]
- A lack of oxygen to the mesenteric organs causes cellular injury and mucosal ischemia within the intestines. Tissue necrosis and metabolic acidosis are significant consequences.
- Extracellular volume decreases. The renin-angiotensin system is activated, releasing renin which increases angiotensin II levels, causing vasoconstriction.[99]
- Plasma volume decreases and fluid concentrations increase abnormally resulting in the release of vasopressin (antidiuretic hormone) from the pituitary gland, causing mesenteric vasoconstriction and venorelaxation.[99]
- A low cardiac output state can cause a non-occlusive form of acute mesenteric ischemia.[101] This is commonly seen in ICU patients who are in heart failure or who are on multiple pressors (medication) to help support blood pressure.
- Compression of the celiac trunk by the median arcuate ligament of the diaphragm is another mechanism for mesenteric ischemia.[99] Lumenal stenosis is thought to be caused by intimal fibrosis resulting from the compression. Compression is increased during expiration.[100]

Mesenteric ischemia is categorized as chronic or acute:
- **Chronic Mesenteric Ischemia**
  » Most commonly caused by progression of atherosclerotic disease (stenosis or occlusion) in the aorta, celiac or proximal mesenteric arteries.
  » Less common causes include arteritis, aneurysm, mesenteric artery dissection and hypercoaguable conditions.

Acute mesenteric ischemia has a high mortality rate.[100]

Acute Mesenteric Ischemia [99,100,98]
- Can be caused by arterial occlusion, usually due to a cardiac embolism, occurring most frequently in the SMA due to its smaller size.[111]
- Can be caused by arterial occlusion due to thrombosis most commonly in the SMA
- Can be caused by small vessel insufficiency (e.g., poor collateral circulation)
- In acute ischemia, intestinal collaterals are able to partially compensate for the blocked mesenteric arteries, delaying substantial injury for approximately 12 hours.[98]

Location of Disease
- Superior mesenteric artery (most common site of embolic occlusion)
- Celiac artery (CA)
- Inferior mesenteric artery

The SMA is almost always one of the "two out of three" arteries involved in cases of chronic ischemia.[99,100]

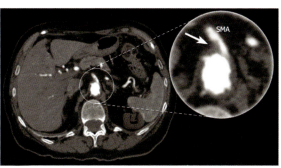

Fig. 12-34: *Mesenteric artery stenosis detected by CT angiography*

Usually, an isolated celiac or inferior mesenteric artery obstruction does not cause symptoms.[99]

Differential Diagnosis
- Cholecystitis
- Diverticulitis
- Appendicitis
- Intestinal obstruction
- Cancer

Correlation
- Duplex ultrasonography
- CT angiography
- MR angiography
- Endoscopy–upper/lower GI
- Colonoscopy/sigmoidoscopy
- Angiography
- Explorative surgery

Medical Treatment
- Serial imaging exams to monitor changes
- Risk factor management
- Systemic heparinization (acute cases)
- Treatment of contributing conditions (e.g., cardiac, hypovolemia or sepsis)

Surgical Treatment
- Mesenteric bypass (e.g., aorto-celiac-SMA, Ileo-SMA)
- Thromboendarterectomy
- Laparotomy
- Resection of dead bowel
- Decompression of the median arcuate ligament with bypass grafting

Emergent surgical/endovascular treatment is often required for acute mesenteric ischemia. [99]

Endovascular Treatment
- Angioplasty
- Stenting

Neointimal and Intimal Hyperplasia

Many use the terms intimal hyperplasia and neointimal hyperplasia interchangeably. This section discusses both.

The reader is cautioned to consider what they mean to convey when using the terms *intimal hyperplasia* and *neointimal hyperplasia* and to define their use of the terms when necessary for clarity.

Many exclude atherosclerosis and use intimal hyperplasia to mean an increase in intimal thickness due to an increase in smooth muscle cell number in the intima and their synthesis of extracellular matrix.

From the ancient Greek language, *neointimal hyperplasia* translates to "over-formation of a *young* intima." Neointimal hyperplasia is often used in connection with the growth of an existing intima. This is similar to the definition for intimal hyperplasia. It is used by many to mean either an increase in the thickness of the intima, as occurs in vein grafts, or the formation of a new intima due to an increase in smooth muscle cell number.

Intimal hyperplasia (IH) strictly means an increase in cell number in the intima. This would include atherosclerosis, where there is a large increase in the number of macrophages and a smaller increase in smooth muscle cell number.

Neointimal hyperplasia could also be defined as *pathologic* intimal hyperplasia that occurs in response to blood vessel injury.

Etiology
- Endovascular trauma
- Surgical intervention
- Other injury or trauma

Risk Factors
- Surgical or endovascular procedures including:
  - » Angioplasty
  - » Vein grafting
  - » Arteriovenous fistula creation
  - » Arteriovenous graft
  - » Stenting

Mechanism of Disease [123]
- Intimal hyperplasia (IH) occurs in arteries exposed to abnormal mechanical forces, low wall fluid shear stress and/or high mural tensile stress. [106]
- IH will reduce lumen diameter and/or increase wall thickness depending upon vessel remodeling. [13] A reduction in lumen diameter, which causes an increase blood flow velocity will increase wall shear stress.
- Wall shear stress is directly proportional to velocity and inversely proportional to the radius cubed.
- IH tends to be concentric in straight vessels as wall shear stress is constant around the circumference of the vessel.
- In vessels such as branches, bifurcations, and bends, the growth is asymmetric occurring in regions of low shear stress.

- There are slight differences in IH mechanisms, though it always involves a change in the regulation of the smooth muscle cells by the endothelial cells. The endothelial cells are either lost or become dysfunctional. In contrast to early hypotheses, inflammatory cells are being discovered to be a key component of IH.

Intimal hyperplasia (IH) is the principle cause for graft failure and occlusion of stented arteries. [114] Over distension of the lumen during graft preparation causes IH in vein grafts. [103] Mis-sizing of stents causes continual physical trauma resulting in IH.

- IH is characterized by the proliferation of smooth muscle cells in the media, followed by their migration to the intima where proliferation continues and then their synthesis of an abundance of extracellular matrix. [104,105,107] IH lesions that reach a steady state are approximately 80-90% extracellular matrix and 10-20% mainly smooth muscle cells. [108]
- Mechanical injury to vessel walls causes IH after procedures such as percutaneous transluminal angioplasty, stenting, etc.
- *Pathological intimal hyperplasia* occurs most often after a surgical or endovascular procedure that results in the loss or dysfunctionality of endothelial cells, which plays an important role in the development of intimal hyperplasia.
  - » Endothelial cell dysfunction also occurs with exposure to a dramatically different hemodynamic environment. Such a change occurs when veins are used as grafts.
    - This results in the endothelial cells being exposed to arterial level shear stresses, which are significantly greater than those in the venous circulation.
    - The creation of an arterio-venous fistula or graft for dialysis access also exposes venous endothelial cells to sudden increases in shear stress levels. In this case, the venous flow pattern also becomes nonlaminar, which is pathological for endothelial cells.
- Endothelial cells are primary regulators of smooth muscle cells.
  - » In a healthy vessel, smooth muscle cells contract and relax to maintain vascular tone. There is low proliferation, migration and extracellular matrix synthesis rates at this stage. Functional endothelial cells secrete factors such as nitric oxide and prostacyclin to control normal function.
  - » In pathological conditions, like intimal hyperplasia, the cells increase their rates of proliferation, migration and protein synthesis. Dysfunctional endothelial cells secrete nitric oxide and prostacyclin, as well as other factors at a significantly lower level.
- Endothelial cells also regulate the adherence of monocytes and platelets to the vessel wall. Monocytes and activated platelets secrete smooth muscle cell mitogens.
- Chemoattractants required for the migration of the smooth muscle cells from the media to the intima in intimal hyperplasia. Monocytes adhere directly to endothelial cells by binding specific proteins (receptors) on the endothelial cell surface.
  - » In a healthy vessel, these receptors are absent or present at a very low level.
  - » In intimal hyperplasia there is an increase in receptors, which increases the number of adhered monocytes.

» Endothelial cells prevent platelet adhesion and activation by maintaining a nonthrombogenic surface at the interface of the blood and vessel wall, and by secreting factors such as nitric oxide and prostacyclin, to inhibit platelet activation and adhesion. They cover thrombogenic factors in the subendothelial matrix such as collagen and platelet activating factor. [107] When the endothelial cells detach, these factors are exposed and platelet adhesion and activation ensue.

- The extracellular matrix must also be modified for the smooth muscle cells to be able to migrate through as they move from the media to the intima. This is done by *proteolysis* in which enzymes break down the proteins that comprise the extracellular matrix. [105,109]

Location of Disease
- The location of disease can be focal or diffuse throughout a vessel and affect any level or multiple levels.
- Most commonly occurs in vessels that have had surgical or endovascular intervention, especially procedures which remove or damage the endothelial cells.

IH occurs pathologically and during normal development, e.g. the closure of the ductus arteriosus shortly after birth.

Differential Diagnosis
- Atherosclerosis

Correlation
- Duplex ultrasonography
- CT angiography
- MR angiography
- Angiography

Medical Treatment
- Supervised exercise programs

Surgical Treatment
- Bypass grafting

Endovascular Treatment
- Angioplasty
- Drug coated stents
- Atherectomy
- Laser-assisted angioplasty
- Endovascular irradiation

Pseudoaneurysm

A pseudoaneurysm, (PA) or "false aneurysm" forms due to trauma to all three layers of the arterial wall. The "false aneurysm" is actually a hematoma, receiving its blood supply from the communication with an adjacent artery via a small channel or patent "neck." These "necks" vary in size and length.

Etiology
- Trauma
- Penetrating trauma (e.g., gunshot wound, blunt trauma, iatrogenic arterial puncture)
- Infection

Risk Factors
- Post-cardiac catheterization
- Post-angiography
- Post-operative arterial intervention (bypass graft)
- Post-endarterectomy
- Renal dialysis; PA commonly develop in synthetic grafts
- Intravascular drug abuse

Mechanism of Disease
- Insertion of a needle for diagnostic, therapeutic or recreational purposes is a trauma to the arterial wall and may cause a pseudoaneurysm.
- Reasons for pseudoaneurysm at an anastomotic site include; infection, tension at the anastomosis, thin-walled arteries, suture deterioration or improper suture technique. [38]
- Repeated puncture of hemodialysis grafts leads to formation of subcutaneous hematomas. [39]

In dialysis conduits, there are risks of graft thrombosis, infection and bleeding associated with pseudoaneurysms.[39] Difficulty with graft access during a hemodialysis session can also be an issue.

Pseudoaneurysm formation is less common in AV fistulas compared to prosthetic grafts.[39]

- A reduction in tensile strength post-endarterectomy may weaken the arterial wall, increasing the risk of a pseudoaneurysm. [31]

Location of Disease
- Common femoral artery
- Superficial femoral artery
- External iliac artery
- Deep femoral artery
- Brachial artery
- Axillary artery
- Radial artery
- Carotid artery
- Anastomotic sites
- Hemodialysis grafts or AV fistulas
- Thoracic aorta (due to trauma)

Correlation
- Duplex ultrasonography
- CT angiography
- Angiography

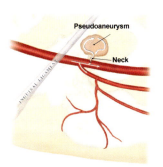
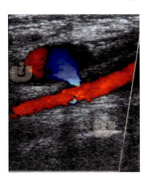

Fig. 12-35: *Arterial pseudoaneurysm off the superficial femoral artery*

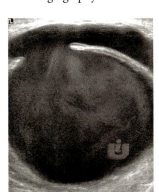

Fig. 12-36: *Duplex ultrasound image of a pseudoaneurysm off a dialysis graft*
Courtesy of Philips Healthcare

Medical Treatment

- Follow-up observation for pseudoaneurysms <2cm in diameter
- Thrombin injection under duplex ultrasound guidance
  - » Can be performed electively
  - » Performed if pseudoaneurysm:
    - Persists beyond 2 weeks
    - Causes significant compression and associated symptoms
    - Enlarges
- Duplex guided compression repair

Pseudoaneurysms may spontaneously thrombose. [115,41]

Surgical Treatment

- Open repair to evacuate the hematoma and repair the arterial wall.
- Resection of the pseudoaneurysm site and surrounding graft in hemodialysis conduits.
- Interposition graft placement or bypass around the affected section.

Endovascular Treatment

- Covered stent graft placed within existing dialysis access.

After a repair, observe the patient for distal symptoms (e.g., toe discoloration) which may result from a micro-thrombotic embolization that may have occurred as a result of the procedure. [40,41]

Popliteal Artery Entrapment Syndrome

Dynamic compression of the popliteal artery by surrounding muscles or tendons which may result in intermittent reduction of blood flow to the tibial arteries. If untreated, a thrombus may form in the artery. The resulting abnormal hemodynamics can also lead to atherosclerosis. Post-stenotic aneurysm or dilatations are not uncommon findings in popliteal entrapment cases. [32,83]

Etiology

- Anatomic variations in the popliteal fossa
- Popliteal entrapment can also occur due to muscle hypertrophy induced by exercise.

Risk Factors

- Middle-aged, sedentary males (anatomic entrapment)
- Young male (functional entrapment)

Males are twice as likely to suffer from popliteal entrapment than females. [82]

Mechanism of Disease

- The popliteal artery courses between the medial and lateral heads of the gastrocnemius muscles in the popliteal fossa. Variations during embryonic development result in an entrapment of the popliteal artery by neighboring muscles/tendons. [81,82]
- In one type of entrapment known as "functional," symptoms occur without evidence of an anatomic variant. [82]
- During plantar flexion, the gastrocnemius muscle compresses the popliteal artery which can result in the loss of distal pulses. [82]
- An acquired form of entrapment is possible after infragenicular bypass surgery.

Types of Entrapment [105,106]

- **Type I (classic):** occurs when the distal popliteal artery forms before the medial head of the gastrocnemius muscle is able to get into position. As a result, the popliteal artery will lay more medial than it normally does when the gastrocnemius muscle is already in place to properly position the artery.
- **Type II:** the popliteal artery displaces the medial head of the gastrocnemius muscle laterally.
- **Type III:** abnormal muscle bundles surround the popliteal artery due to the persistence of mesodermal tissue or embryonic cells in the popliteal fossa.
- **Type IV:** atypical development of the popliteal artery, deeper than usual within the popliteal fossa which leads to entrapment by the popliteal muscle or a fibrous band.
- **Type V:** both the popliteal artery and vein are compressed.
- **Type VI (type F):** the popliteal artery is compressed by certain maneuvers of the leg but the reason for the compression is unknown. This type is also referred to as *functional entrapment.*

Location of Disease

- Popliteal artery (often bilateral)

Differential Diagnosis

- Popliteal adventitial cystic disease (ACD)
- Synovial cyst
- Popliteal artery occlusive disease
- Extrinsic compression (from hematoma, cyst or tumor)

Correlation

- Duplex ultrasonography (while performing active plantarflexion)
- MRI
- MR angiography
- CT angiography
- Angiography

Duplex findings include obliteration of the popliteal artery waveform with plantarflexion of the knee. [82]

Medical Treatment

- None

Surgical Treatment

- Division of the muscle and replacement of the damaged artery with a bypass graft if needed.

Endovascular Treatment

- Balloon angioplasty (most successful if source of entrapment is also addressed)

Raynaud's Syndrome

The Raynaud's syndrome consists of **Raynaud's disease** and **Raynaud's phenomenon**. Digits display episodes of cyanosis or pallor due to vasoconstriction of the small, digital arteries or arterioles during times of cold or emotional stress.

Etiology

Patients exhibiting digital ischemia are divided into two categories: [75]

- **Raynaud's disease:** primary vasospastic disorder without an identifiable underlying cause
- **Raynaud's phenomenon:** vasospasm is secondary to some underlying condition (e.g., lupus, scleroderma, etc.)

Approximately 28 million (5-10%) of people in the U.S. suffer from Raynaud's phenomenon. [76]

Arterial Diseases

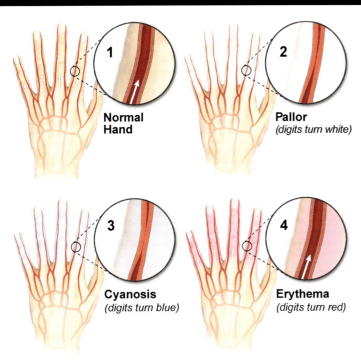

Fig. 12-37: Changes experienced in the digits with Raynaud's Syndrome

Risk Factors
- Young females
- Age (between 11-45 years)
- History of autoimmune disease
- Cooler climates (including England, Denmark, France)
- Diabetes
- Patients on hormone therapy
- Certain occupations at risk for "occupational arterial disease" (e.g., hammer syndrome, vibration white finger, thermal damage)
- Drug use
- Smoking
- Heart disease/myocardial infarction
- Family history of Raynaud's syndrome

Raynaud's affects women nine times more than men.[76]

Mechanism of Disease[98]
- The majority of blood flow to the digits is for thermoregulation of the body. The skin contains nerve fibers which sense temperature.
- The hypothalamus in the brain controls body temperature by varying the sympathetic outflow to the digital vessels using the medulla, spinal chord, sympathetic ganglion and local nerves. Sympathetic nerves stimulate smooth muscle cells in the digits to constrict the vessel. Vessel dilatation cools the body while constriction serves to warm/conserve body heat.
- Alpha-2 adrenoceptors are located in and on the smooth muscle cells in the thermoregulatory blood vessels, which help control body temperature. As the body is cooled additional alpha-2c adrenoceptors move from inside the cell to the surface. Here they are activated by the sympathetic nerves causing the smooth muscle cell to contract and thus the vessel to constrict. Constriction increases as the number of receptors on the cell surface increases. It has been suggested that in individuals with Raynaud's phenomenon, the receptors may abnormally accumulate on smooth muscle cell surfaces under certain circumstances, causing pathological vessel constriction.[112,113]

- Static blood in the capillaries becomes deoxygenated causing the digits to appear bluish in color.
- Post-ischemic vasodilatation causes hyperemia and rubor or *erythema* (redness) of the digit once the vasospastic episode is over.
- When there is an underlying cause for vasospasm, rewarming of the finger oftentimes results in pain, since the blood flow cannot return fast enough to meet the metabolic need of the digit.
- Individuals with low blood pressure have a decreased ability to dilate their arteries. Contraction of smooth muscle cells can result in vessel closure.
- An episode of vasospasm can be triggered by cold or emotionally stressful situations.

Holding an iced-drink or taking something out of a freezer can be enough to trigger a Raynaud's attack.

- Sympathetic nerves respond to stress by releasing neurotransmitters that cause smooth muscle cell contraction.
- Endothelial cells release vasoactive factors (e.g., nitric oxide, angiotensin II) which control smooth muscle cell contraction and relaxation causing vasodilation/vasoconstriction. Dysfunctional endothelial cells may not release these factors appropriately resulting in abnormal regulation of vessel constriction/relaxation.
- Endothelial damage caused by repetitive movements or use of vibrational tools (e.g., jack hammers) can lead to intralumenal thrombosis and embolism.
- Connective tissue disorders, such as scleroderma, cause fibrosis and disease of small arteries, arterioles and capillaries resulting in tissue ischemia from vasoconstriction.

In some Raynaud's patients, there may be underlying fixed digital occlusive disease that is complicated by digital vasospasm (both disease and phenomenon can exist simultaneously).

Location of Disease
- Fingers (most common)
- Toes
- Nose (rare)
- Ear (rare)
- Nipples (rare)

Only one or two digits may be affected by a Raynaud's attack. Attacks can last anywhere from a few minutes to several hours. Raynaud's attacks do not always affect the same digits.

Differential Diagnosis
- Atherosclerosis
- Buerger's disease (thromboangiitis obliterans)
- Giant cell arteritis
- Trauma
- Vasculitis (such as Wegener's granulomatosis)
- Scleroderma (or other connective tissue disorders such as lupus, rheumatoid arthritis, etc.)
- Myeloma
- Hematological cancers
- Malignancy
- Prinzmetal's angina
- Infection (hepatitis B and C, parovirus)
- Embolic (arterial or cardiac)
- Thoracic outlet syndrome
- Toxin induced vasospasm
- Hepatitis antigenemia
- Cryoglobulinemia
- Carpal tunnel syndrome
- Frostbite
- Neurological disorders

Correlation
- Non-invasive vascular testing:
  » Upper extremity arterial testing, including digital plethysmography
  » Cold immersion
  » Digital temperature recovery testing
  » Duplex ultrasonography
- Laser Doppler
- Laboratory blood tests (for Raynaud's phenomenon only)
- Platelet count, sedimentation rate, etc.

Medical Treatment
- Vasodilators (calcium channel blockers)
- Treatment of underlying condition
- Nerve block injection
- Risk factor management (smoking cessation, avoidance of cold)
- Thermal biofeedback

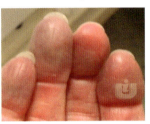
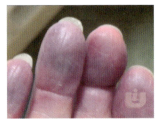

Fig. 12-38: *Typical presentation of Raynaud's (with cyanotic episode-right)*

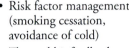

Surgical Treatment
- Open digital sympathectomy
- Amputation

Endovascular Treatment
- None

Renovascular Hypertension

Elevated blood pressure caused by decreased kidney perfusion due to stenosis or occlusion of the renal arteries.

Etiology
- Atherosclerosis
- Acute arterial thrombosis
- Embolism
- Fibromuscular dysplasia
- Renal artery trauma
- Aneurysm
- Aortic dissection
- Renal artery malformation
- Polyarteritis nodosa
- Neurofibromatosis
- Fibrosis, post-radiation
- Inadequate immune system or poor diet during pregnancy

Risk Factors
- Any risk factors for atherosclerosis
- Ethnicity
- Younger female (due to FMD, pregnancy)
- Elderly male (due to atherosclerosis)
- Younger than 20 years of age and older than 50 years of age

The most common cause of renal artery disease in children is FMD (fibromuscular dysplagia). [178]

- Smoking
- Malignant or accelerated hypertension
- Radiation therapy
- Renal artery intimal dysplasia in children

Mechanism of Disease [151,152]
- The kidney maintains blood pressure by regulating the balance of sodium and water retention.
- Renal arterial stenotic/occlusive disease results in decreased renal blood flow to the kidney.
- When *baroreceptors* (pressure sensors in the arterial wall) detect a decrease in renal blood flow, the enzyme renin is released.
- The renin-angiotensin system is activated which increases angiotensin II levels. Angiotensin II increases blood pressure and causes peripheral vasoconstriction.
- Angiotension II increases the synthesis of aldosterone by the adrenal gland. Aldosterone increases sodium and water retention, which increases blood pressure. If the contralateral kidney is healthy, increased renal perfusion causes a decrease in sodium reabsorption and increase sodium excretion. Blood pressure will decrease, which will decrease perfusion pressure of the stenotic kidney and increase the release of renin.
- When there is only a single functioning kidney with a renal artery is obstructed, the kidney cannot rely on increased urine output from the contralateral kidney to prevent sodium and water retention. The volume expansion which results causes elevated blood pressure and suppresses renin production by the stenotic kidney.
- In fibromuscular dysplasia, the lack of vasa vasorum in the long renal arterial segment may result in vessel wall ischemia and dysplasia. [94]

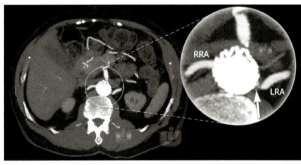

Fig. 12-39: *CT image illustrating left renal artery stenosis*

Location of Disease
- Renal ostia or proximal renal arterial segment (atherosclerosis as etiology)
- Middle-distal renal arterial segments (FMD as etiology)
- Stenosis of the renal artery may be unilateral, although bilateral renal stenosis is possible, especially when caused by atherosclerosis. [97]

Renovascular hypertension is the most common type of secondary hypertension (HTN). A "secondary condition" is a condition caused by another medical condition (e.g., HTN due to atherosclerosis or FMD).

Differential Diagnosis
- Other forms of hypertension
- Pheochromocytoma
- Primary hyperaldosteronism

Correlation
- Duplex ultrasonography
- Renal vein renin assay
- CT angiography
- MR angiography
- Renal arteriography

Medical Treatment
- Serial renal artery duplex exams to monitor for change
- Drug therapy
- Smoking cessation

Surgical Treatment
- Endarterectomy
- Bypass grafting (e.g., aorto-renal, splachno-renal)
- Renal artery reimplantation
- Ex-vivo reconstruction

Endovascular Treatment
- Angioplasty
- Stenting
- Endovascular neuro-ablation in trials

Subclavian Steal Syndrome

The vertebral artery flow reverses (flows away from the brain, in a retrograde direction) in an attempt to provide circulation to the upper extremity when the subclavian or right innominate artery is severely stenosed or occluded.

Bidirectional flow may occur in the vertebral artery if there is a hemodynamically significant stenosis in the ipsilateral subclavian artery at its ostia. The patient may complain of dizziness with use of the arm.

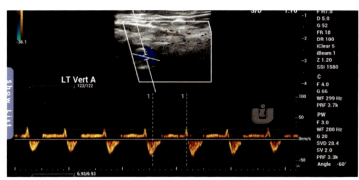

Fig. 12-40: *Bidirectional flow in the vertebral artery*

Subclavian steal phenomenon is diagnosed when there is retrograde vertebral flow without neurological symptoms related to cerebral ischemia.[93]

Etiology
- Atherosclerosis
- Takayasu's arteritis

Risk Factors
- Caucasian
- Males
- Females with Takayasu's arteritis
- Age
- Diabetes
- Smoking
- Hypercholesteremia
- Hypertension

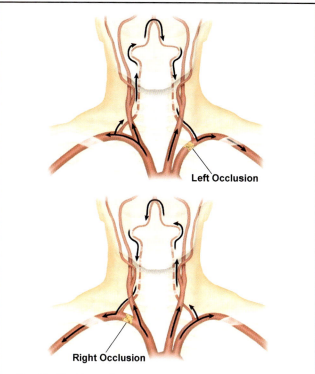

Fig. 12-41: *Hemodynamically significant disease in the subclavian creates subclavian steal syndrome. Flow reverses in the vertebral artery to supply the brachial artery and the upper extremity. Flow in the CCA is uneffected.*

Mechanism of Disease
- The vertebral artery is typically a low resistant pathway. Blood normally flows from the aorta to the subclavian (via the innominate on the right) to the vertebral artery, which is a branch of the subclavian.
- Hemodynamics change when there is an obstruction between the aorta and the vertebral artery. This path becomes high resistant, but fluids prefer to flow along the path of least resistance. The blood flows around the obstruction by going up the carotids and/or contralateral vertebral artery and then down the ipsilateral vertebral artery (retrograde direction) to the subclavian artery in order to supply the ipsilateral upper extremity.
- For some individuals, the flow rate down the vertebral artery is too great and blood is stolen from the cerebrum resulting in ischemia.
- Most cases of physiologic steal are neurologically asymptomatic.[93]

Location of Disease
- Origin of the left subclavian artery
- Subclavian artery (either side)
- Right innominate artery

The majority of subclavian steal cases occur on the left side (3x more than on the right side).[96]

Differential Diagnosis
- Arteritis
- Tumor
- Multiple sclerosis
- Cerebellar degeneration or neoplasm
- Neurologic

Correlation
- Duplex ultrasonography
- CT angiography
- MR angiography
- Angiography

Medical Treatment
None

Surgical Treatment
- Carotid-subclavian artery bypass
- Endarterectomy
- Subclavian transposition
- Vertebral transposition
- Subclavian endarterectomy
- Brachiocephalic endarterectomy
- Aorto-subclavian bypass

Endovascular Treatment
- Angioplasty
- Stenting

Thoracic Outlet Compression Syndrome (TOS)

Compression of the brachial plexus, subclavian artery or subclavian vein in the *thoracic outlet* or space between the collarbone and first rib of the upper extremity, resulting in symptoms of pain or neurologic deficit.

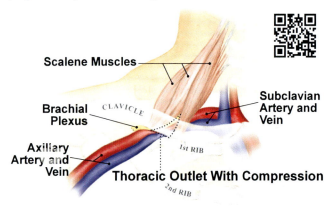

Fig. 12-42: *Arteries/veins can be compressed in the space known as the thoracic outlet*

Etiology
- Congenital (cervical rib, costoclavicular tendon)
- Trauma
- Occupational related injury
- Sports related injury
- Vasculitis
- Atherosclerosis
- Thrombus
- Embolization from the subclavian or axillary arteries
- Aneurysm
- Pseudoaneurysm
- Intimal hyperplasia
- Traumatic occlusion
- Extrinsic compression
- Radiation arteritis

"White-finger syndrome" resulting in small artery vasospasm can occur with the repetitive use of vibrating tools. [85]

Risk Factors
- Age (young)
- Males > females
- Athletic, active lifestyle
- Family history
- Obesity
- History of radiation

Weight training can result in muscle enlargement significant enough to cause compression in the thoracic outlet. [85]

Mechanism of Disease
- TOS results from mechanical compression of the subclavian vein, artery or brachial plexus in the thoracic outlet region. One cause may be an anatomical defect such as congenital abnormalities of the first rib or fracture of the clavicle, which would be a source of compression.

- Types of thoracic outlet syndrome: [84,85]
  » **Neurogenic** (most common): compression of the brachial plexus from the cervical ribs, first rib, anterior scalene muscles, congenital myofascial bands and ligaments.
  » **Venous:** also known as *effort thrombosis* or *Paget-Schroetter syndrome* results from repetitive trauma to the subclavian vein (SCV). Arm abduction causes the SCV to be compressed against the first rib and scalenus anticus muscle, resulting in this trauma.
    - Venous trauma may result in venous thrombosis. [86]
    - In cases of venous compression, the severity of symptoms relates to the length of the thrombosed segment and activity level of the patient.
  » **Arterial** (least common): The head of the humerus can cause arterial compression when the arm is abducted and externally rotated. Due to such repetitive extrinsic compression of the SCA, post-stenotic dilatation or frank aneurysm develops. The typical pathogenesis then is focal compression, dilation, ulceration, and thrombus formation. [1]
    - Most of these patients will present with thromboembolic symptoms.
    - Patients also present with ischemic complications secondary to repeated episodes of embolization.
- The cause of TOS is neurogenic in 93% of cases. A venous cause is present in 5%, while an arterial cause is present in only 1% of cases. [85]
- Venous or arterial compression results in:
  » **Stenosis:** Significant narrowing of the artery or vein decreasing the vessel lumen and possibly resulting in decreased blood flow.
  » **Occlusion:** Plaque, thrombus, or external compression of the artery completely blocking blood flow in that arterial segment.
  » **Embolization:** Contents of a plaque and/or fragments of an organized thrombus become lodged in a distant blood vessel.
  » **Swelling:** significant compression of the subclavian vein causes limb swelling.

Location of Disease
- Subclavian vein
- Subclavian or axillary artery
- Brachial plexus

Differential Diagnosis
- Spinal stenosis
- Carpal tunnel syndrome
- Nerve impingement (herniated disc)
- Raynaud's disease
- Venous thrombosis
- Neuropathy
- Muscle/tendon strains or tears
- Arthritis
- Tumors, including *Pancoast's tumors* (lung tumor which grows in the thoracic area)
- Degenerative spinal chord diseases (MS)
- Orthopedic shoulder problems
- Angina pectoris

Correlation
- Non-invasive arterial vascular testing
  » UE including volume pulse recording and digital testing
  » Duplex ultrasonography
- X-ray (chest, cervical spine)
- Electromyography
- Nerve conductivity testing
- CT angiography
- MRI
- MR angiography
- Arteriography
- Positional venography

Medical Treatment

- Modify risk factors
- Anti-inflammatory medication (e.g., aspirin)
- Muscle relaxants
- Physical therapy
- Nerve block treatments
- Anticoagulation (warfarin)
- Thrombolytic therapy (acute blockage)

Surgical Treatment

- Thoracic outlet decompression
- Removal of the first rib or cervical rib
- Dividing scalene muscle attachments and fibromuscular bands
- Cervical sympathectomy
- Resection of aneurysmal disease with bypass grafting
- Embolectomy
- Bypass grafting

Endovascular Treatment

- Thrombolysis
- Angioplasty
- Stent

Vasculitis

Inflammation of the vessel wall resulting in damage to the blood vessel. This can occur in all blood vessels and is classified based on vessel size: large, medium or small vessel vasculitis. Arteritis is a type of "vasculitis" or "angiitis."

Etiology

- Autoimmune
- Infection
- Radiation therapy
- Drug abuse

Risk Factors

- Age (young, for some types of arteritis)
- Female
- Arthritic conditions (e.g., polymyalgia rheumatica, which is often seen with temporal arteritis)
- Far Eastern, Asian or Middle Eastern descent
- Young, Japanese and Korean males (Kawasaki disease)
- HIV positive

Mechanism of Disease

- The causes of vasculitis are still under study. Genetics, infectious and toxic factors are suspected. Since there are wide variations in patient demographics and histopathological findings for vasculitis, they likely have significant differences as well as similarities in their pathogenic pathways.
- Giant cell arteritis, a large vessel vasculitis is the most common type of vasculitis and the most studied. The following is a brief description of the pathogenic mechanisms: [67,68,69,70]
  - » Giant cell arteritis, is a T-cell dependent disease. Next to the external elastic lamina are resident dendritic cells. *Dendritic cells* are antigen-presenting cells required for the activation of T-cells in vessel walls.
  - » In a healthy vessel, dendritic cells are characterized as immature and unactivated.
  - » Mature dendritic cells are required for the activation of T-cells. The maturation and activation of dendritic cells is considered to be the first step in the pathogenesis of giant cell arteritis. There is a significant increase in the number of dendritic cells in the adventitia during giant cell arteritis.

- » Circulating T-cells exit the blood only if endothelial cells have been activated. T-cells bind activated endothelial cells and then migrate into the vessel wall. In giant cell arteritis, this occurs in the vasa vasorum, not in the macrolumen.
- » The other requirement for the departure of T-cells is the synthesis of chemokines in the tissue. *Chemokines* are chemotactic cytokines, which induce directed chemotaxis. *Chemotaxis* is the migration of cells along a chemical concentration gradient. Activated dendritic cells synthesize chemokines, which attract T-cells.
- » *Granulomas* are small delineated collections of immune cells, primarily macrophages that are highly activated. The formation of granulomas in the media is dependent upon T-cells. The T-cells in the adventitia release interferon-gamma, which recruits and activates macrophages. These interferon-gamma stimulated macrophages are responsible for the granulomatous reaction.
- » Macrophages synthesize *matrix metalloproteinases (MMPs)* which are thought to be responsible for the fragmentation of the internal elastic lamina. Macrophages also mediate oxidative stress which causes smooth muscle cell injury and *apoptosis*, programmed cell death.
- » Macrophages join together to form giant cells, which may be present along the fragmented internal elastic lamina. In the adventitia, they optimize T-cell stimulation by the release of pro-inflammatory cytokines.
- » Giant cell arteritis can lead to ischemia if there is occlusion of the lumen. This is caused by rapid concentric intimal hyperplasia. Rarely does thrombotic occlusion contribute to the blockage of blood flow.
- » The critical growth factor for intimal hyperplasia is most likely *platelet derived growth factor* (PDGF), as it correlates with the degree of luminal stenosis. Smooth muscle cells synthesize PDGF, but the predominate sources are macrophages and giant cells.
- » In healthy vessels, the vasa vasorum is limited to the adventitia. In giant cell arteritis neovascularization of the media and hyperplastic intima occurs through the formation of microvessels. The number of neocapillaries correlates with the level of *vascular endothelial growth factor (VEGF)*, a stimulator of angiogenesis. Macrophages and giant cells are the primary producers of the VEGF.
- » In Takayasu's arteritis, another large vessel vasculitis, T-cells may contribute to the weakening of the wall by secreting *perforin*, a pore-forming protein.

- Radiation therapy causes injury to the vasa vasorum and necrosis of the vessel wall. Endothelial cells lining the arterial walls of vessels in the irradiated field are susceptible to damage. Lipid-containing plaques can then form in the intimal layer of the artery. [70]

Location of Disease

- Superficial temporal artery
- Aortic artery
- Renal artery
- External iliac artery
- Mesenteric artery
- Subclavian artery
- Axillary artery
- Innominate artery
- Carotid arteries

Aneurysms will form in the aorta but not in medium size arteries.

Common Types of Vasculitis [88,89,90]

A classification system for vasculitis developed in the early 1990s by the American College of Rheumatology and the Chapel Hill Consensus Conference was limited and controversial. This criterion was revised and published as the "Overview of the 2012 International Chapel Hill Consensus Conference Nomenclature of Vasculitides." [178]

Note: This is not a complete list. [178]

Large Vessel

- **Takayasu's arteritis**: predominately affects the aorta and its branches, usually causing a dilatation and an aneurysm, stenosis rarely occurs.
  - » Primarily affects females (80-90%) under the age of 50 years, especially those between 20-40 years of age. [71]
  - » Is more frequent in Asia and India than in Western Europe or North America. [72]
  - » Japanese with Takayasu's arteritis have a higher incidence of aortic arch involvement. The arteries most commonly involved in United States (US) patients suffering from Takayasu's arteritis are the left subclavian, superior mesenteric and abdominal aorta. [71]
- **Giant cell arteritis** (temporal arteritis): affects medium and large size vessels. The extracranial branches of the carotid, especially the temporal artery, are susceptible.
  - » Giant cell arteritis is typically seen in Caucasian women >50 years of age, especially those who are 75-85 years of age. The mean age is 72 years. [93]
  - » Women develop temporal arteritis 2-3x more than men. [93]

Medium Vessel

- **Polyarteritis nodosa**: Occurs in any organ, resulting in aneurysm, thrombosis, hemorrhage or tissue infarction.
- **Kawasaki disease**: Affects small and medium sized arteries (including coronary) in young children between the ages of 2-5 years of age.
  - » Most commonly affects the Japanese-American population. Outside of the US, the disease most frequently occurs in Japan. [73]
  - » Japanese children exhibit the disease at a younger age (6-12 months) than American children (18-24 months). [73]
  - » In the US, Kawasaki disease patients are most commonly middle and upper-middle class children. [73]
  - » Kawasaki's disease is 1.5x more common in males than females. [73]

Small Vessel

- **Wegener's granulomatosis**: Necrotizing vasculitis involving the kidney or upper/lower respiratory tracts.
- **Churg-Strauss angiitis**: Affects the nose, sinuses, lungs, nerves and intestines.
- **Cryoglobulinemia vasculitis:** Caused by abnormal proteins in the blood which affect the spleen, skin, nerves and kidneys
- **Henoch-Schonlein purpura (IgAV)**: Affects kidneys.
- **Microscopic polyangiitis**: Affects kidneys, lung, nerves, skin, and joints.

Variable Vessel Vasculitis

- **Cogan's syndrome:** Affects vision and hearing typically of young white adults in their 30s.

- **Behcet's disease**: results in mouth/genital sores, inflammation of the eyes.
  - » Uncommon in the US, but common in the Mediterranean, Middle and Far Eastern regions. [70,74]
  - » Men are affected more often than women by Behcet's disease (in some regions 24:1). The disease also seems to be more severe in men. [74]

Vasculitis Associated with Systemic Disease

- **Lupus**
- **Rheumatoid vasculitis**
- **Sarcoid vasculitis**

Differential Diagnosis

- Childhood diseases (e.g., scarlet fever)
- Juvenile rheumatoid arthritis
- Toxic shock syndrome
- Measles
- Epstein-Barr syndrome
- Crohn's disease
- Marfan's syndrome
- Ehlers-Danlos syndrome
- Sarcoidosis
- Aortic dissection
- Appendicitis
- Cholecystitis
- Intestinal perforation

Correlation

- Duplex ultrasonography
- MRI
- MR angiography
- CT angiography
- Angiography

Medical Treatment

- Aspirin therapy
- Corticosteroids

Surgical Treatment

- Biopsy of affected tissue (e.g., of temporal arteries to confirm diagnosis of giant cell arteritis)
- Bypass

Endovascular Treatment

- Angioplasty (percutaneous or coronary)
- Stenting

REFERENCES

1. Zarins CK, Xu C, Glagov S. (2005). Artery wall pathology in atherosclerosis. In Rutherford Vascular Surgery 6th edition. (123-148). Philadelphia. Elsevier Saunders.
2. Curci JA, Baxter TB, Thompson RW. (2005). Artery aneurysms. In Rutherford Vascular Surgery 6th edition. (475-492). Philadelphia. Elsevier Saunders.
3. López-Candales A, Holmes DR, Liao S, Scott MJ, Wickline SA, Thompson RW. Decreased vascular smooth muscle cell density in medial degeneration of human abdominal aortic aneurysms. (1997). Am J Pathol. March; 150(3): 993–1007.
4. Henderson, E. L., Y.-J. Geng, et al. (1999). "Death of Smooth Muscle Cells and Expression of Mediators of Apoptosis by T Lymphocytes in Human Abdominal Aortic Aneurysms." Circulation 99(1): 96-104.
5. Krettek, A., G. K. Sukhova, et al. (2003). "Elastogenesis in human arterial disease: a role for macrophages in disordered elastin synthesis." Arteriosclerosis, thrombosis, and vascular biology 23(4): 582-587.
6. Szilagyi, D. E., R. F. Smith, et al. (1966). "Contribution of abdominal aortic aneurysmectomy to prolongation of life." Annals of Surgery 164(4): 678-699.
7. Sterpetti, A. V., A. Cavallaro, et al. (1991). "Factors influencing the rupture of abdominal aortic aneurysms." Surgery, Gynecology & Obstetrics 173(3): 1750178.
8. Darling, R. C., C. R. Messina, et al. (1977). "Autopsy study of unoperated abdominal aortic aneurysms. The case for early resection." Circulation 56(3 Suppl): II161-164.
9. Walker, D. I., K. Bloor, et al. (1972). "Inflammatory aneurysms of the abdominal aorta." British Journal of Surgery 59(8): 609-614.
10. Ritman, E. L. and A. Lerman (2007). "The dynamic vasa vasorum." Cardiovascular research 75(4): 649-658.
11. Halka AT, Turner NJ, Carter A, Ghosh J, Murphy MO, Kirton JP, Kielty CM, Walker MG. (2008). The effects of stretch on vascular smooth muscle cell phenotype in vitro. Cardiovascular Pathology. (98-102). March-April;17(3).
12. Stary HC, Chandler AB, Glagov S, Guyton JR, Insull W, Rosenfeld ME, Schaffer SA, Schwartz CJ, Wagner WD, Wissler RW. A definition of intimal, fatty streak and intermediate lesions of atherosclerosis. (2462-2478). Circulation 1994; 89.
13. Glagov S, Weisenberg E, Zarins C, et al. (1987). Compensatory enlargement of human atherosclerotic coronary arteries. (1371-5). N Engl J Med; 316.
14. Stary HC, Chandler AB, Dinsmore RE, Fuster V, Glagov S, Insull W, Rosenfeld ME, Schwartz CJ, Wagner WD, Wissler RW. A definition of advanced types of atherosclerotic lesions and histological classification of atherosclerosis. Atherosclerosis, Thrombosis and Vascular Biology. 1995; 15; 1521-1531.
15. Easton JD, Saver JL., et al. (2009). "Definition and Evaluation of Transient Ischemic Attack." Stroke 40(6): 2276-2293.
16. Bamford J, Sandercock P., et al. (1987). "The natural history of lacunar infarction: the Oxfordshire Community Stroke Project." Stroke 18(3): 545-551.

17. Petty GW, Brown RD, et al. (2000). "Ischemic Stroke Subtypes: A Population-Based Study of Functional Outcome, Survival, and Recurrence." Stroke 31(5): 1062-1068.
18. Torvik, A. (1984). "The pathogenesis of watershed infarcts in the brain." Stroke 15(2): 221-223.
19. Mangla R, Kolar B., et al. (2011). "Border Zone Infarcts: Pathophysiologic and Imaging Characteristics." Radiographics 31(5): 1201-1214.
20. Momjian-Mayor I, and Baron JC., (2005). "The Pathophysiology of Watershed Infarction in Internal Carotid Artery Disease." Stroke 36(3): 567-577.
21. Vermeer SE, Longstreth Jr WT., et al. (2007). "Silent brain infarcts: a systematic review." The Lancet Neurology 6(7): 611-619.
22. Morgenstern LB, Hemphill JC, et al. (2010). "Guidelines for the Management of Spontaneous Intracerebral Hemorrhage." Stroke 41(9): 2108-2129.
23. Adams HP, del Zoppo G, et al. (2007). "Guidelines for the Early Management of Adults With Ischemic Stroke." Stroke 38(5): 1655-1711.
24. Mitchell ME, Sidaway AN. (2005). Basic considerations of the arterial wall in health and disease. In Rutherford Vascular Surgery 6th edition. (62-75). Philadelphia. Elsevier Saunders.
25. Schermerhorn ML, Cronenwett JL. (2005). Abdominal aortic and iliac aneurysms. In Rutherford Vascular Surgery 6th edition. (1408-1452). Philadelphia. Elsevier Saunders.
26. Shepard RJ, Rooke T. (2005). Uncommon arteriopathies. In Rutherford Vascular Surgery 6th edition. (453-474). Philadelphia. Elsevier Saunders.
27. Reddy DJ, Weaver MR. (2005). Infected aneurysms. In Rutherford Vascular Surgery 6th edition. (1581-1596). Philadelphia. Elsevier Saunders.
28. Gerhard-Herman M, Gardin JM, Jaff M, Mohler E, Roman M, Naqvi TZ. (2006). Guidelines for non-invasive vascular laboratory testing: a report from the American society of echocardiography and the society of vascular medicine and biology. J Am Soc Echocardiogr 19:955-972.
29. Nordon IM, Hinchliffe RJ, Loftus IM, Thompson MM. (2010). Pathophysiology and epidemiology of abdominal aortic aneurysms Nat Rev Cardiol. Nov 16.
30. Lawrence PF, Rigberg D. (2010). Arterial aneurysms: general considerations. In Rutherford Vascular Surgery 7th edition. (Chapter 126). Philadelphia. Elsevier Saunders.
31. Sumner DS, Zierler RE. (2005). Vascular physiology: essential hemodynamic principles. In Rutherford Vascular Surgery 6th edition. (75-123). Philadelphia. Elsevier Saunders.
32. Van Bockel JH, Hamming JF. (2005). Lower extremity aneurysm. In Rutherford Vascular Surgery 6th edition. (1534-1551). Philadelphia. Elsevier Saunders.
33. Upchurch GR, Zelenock GB, Stanley JC. (2005). Splanchnic artery aneurysms. In Rutherford Vascular Surgery 6th edition. (1565-1581). Philadelphia. Elsevier Saunders.
34. Isselbacher EM, 2005, "Thoracic and Abdominal Aortic Aneurysms," Circulation, 111(6), pp. 816-828.
35. Clouse WD, Hallett JW Jr., Schaff HV, Spittell PC, Rowland CM, Ilstrup DM, and Melton LJ 3rd, 2004, "Acute Aortic Dissection: Population-Based Incidence Compared with Degenerative Aortic Aneurysm Rupture," Mayo Clinic proceedings. Mayo Clinic, 79(2), pp. 176-80.
36. Centers for medicare and medicaid services. (09/20/2010 1:09:09 PM). Retrieved from https://www.cms.gov/deficitreductionact.
37. Beridze N, Frishman WH. 2012, "Vascular Ehlers-Danlos syndrome: pathophysiology, diagnosis, and prevention and treatment of its complications." Cardiol Rev. Jan-Feb; 20(1):4-7.
38. Casey PJ, LaMuraglia GM. (2005). Anastomotic aneurysms. In Rutherford Vascular Surgery 6th edition. (894-902). Philadelphia. Elsevier Saunders.
39. Adams ED, Sidway AN. (2005). Nonthrombotic complications of arteriovenous access for hemodialysis. In Rutherford Vascular Surgery 6th edition. (1692-1706). Philadelphia. Elsevier Saunders.
40. Kang, SS, (2005). Pseudoaneurysm: diagnosis and treatment. In Mansour MA, Labropoulos N. (Eds.), Vascular Diagnosis, (319-323). Philadelphia: Elsevier Saunders.
41. Rowe VL, Yellin AE, Weaver FA. (2005). Vascular injuries of the extremities. In Rutherford Vascular Surgery 6th edition. (1044-1058). Philadelphia. Elsevier Saunders.
42. Black JH, Cambria RP. (2005). Aortic dissection: perspectives for the vascular/endovascular surgeon. In Rutherford Vascular Surgery 6th edition. (1512-1533). Philadelphia. Elsevier Saunders.
43. Zwiebel, WJ. Pellerito JS. (2005). Carotid occlusion, unusual carotid pathology, and tricky carotid cases. In Zwiebel WJ, Pellerito JS (Eds.), In Introduction to Vascular Ultrasonography 5th ed, (192-210). Philadelphia: Elsevier Saunders.
44. Krupski WC. (2005). Uncommon disorders affecting the carotid arteries. In Rutherford Vascular Surgery 6th edition. (2064-2092). Philadelphia. Elsevier Saunders.
45. Saldana, M. J., L. E. Salem, et al. (197). "High altitude hypoxia and chemodectomas." Human Pathology 4(2): 251-263.
46. Jech M, Alvarado-Cabrero L, et al. (2006). "Genetic analysis of high altitude paragangliomas." Endocrine Pathology 17(2): 201-202.
47. McNicol A.M. (2010). Adrenal Medulla and Paraganglia in Endocrine Pathology: Differential Diagnosis and Molecular Advances. R.V. Lloyd (Ed). Springer Science + Business Media LLC.
48. Baysal, BE, Ferrell RE, et al. (2000). "Mutations in SDHD, a mitochondrial complex II gene, in hereditary paraganglioma." Science 287(5454): 848-851.
49. Niemann S. and Muller U. (2000). "Mutations in SDHC cause autosomal dominant paraganglioma, type 3." Nature genetics 26(3): 268-270.
50. Astuti, D, Latif F, et al. (2001). "Gene mutations in the succinate dehydrogenase subunit SDHB cause susceptibility to familial pheochromocytoma and to familial paraganglioma." American journal of human genetics 69(1): 49-54.
51. Hao,HX, Khalimonchuk O, et al. (2009). "SDH5, a Gene Required for Flavination of Succinate Dehydrogenase, Is Mutated in Paraganglioma." Science 325(5944): 1139-1142.
52. Baysal B E, McKay SE, et al. (2011). "Genomic imprinting at a boundary element flanking the SDHD locus." Human molecular genetics 20(22): 4452-4461.
53. Neumann, H. P. and Z. Erlic (2008). "Maternal transmission of symptomatic disease with SDHD mutation: fact or fiction?" The Journal of clinical endocrinology and metabolism 93(5): 1573-1575.
54. Mariman EC, van Beersum, SE. et al. (1995). "Fine mapping of a putatively imprinted genefor familial non-chromaffin paragangliomas to chromosome 11q13.1: evidence for genetic heterogeneity." Human Genetics 95(1): 56-62.
55. Van Schothorst, EM, Beekman M, et al. (1998). "Paragangliomas of the head and neck region show complete loss of heterozygosity at 11 q22-q23 in chief cells and the flow-sorted dna aneuploid fraction." Human Pathology. 29(10): 1045-1049.
56. Baysal BE. (2008). "Clinical and molecular progress in hereditary paraganglioma." Journal of Medical Genetics 45(11): 689-694.
57. Arias-Stella J, Human carotid bodies at high altitudes. (Abstract) American Journal of Pathology 1969; 55: 82a. (not in endnotes library)
58. Arias-Stella, J. and J. Valcarcel (1973). "The human carotid body at high altitudes." Pathologia et microbiologia 39(3): 292-297.
59. Lack, E. E. (1977). "Carotid body hypertrophy in patients with cystic fibrosis and cyanotic congenital heart disease." Human Pathology 8(1): 39-51.
60. Heath, D., C. Edwards, et al. (1970). "Post-mortem size and structure of the human carotid body." Thorax 25(2): 129-140.
61. Rush BF. Jr. (1963). "Familial bilateral carotid body tumors." Annals of Surgery 157: 633-636.
62. Pratt, LW. (1973). "Familial Carotid Body Tumors." Arch Otolaryngol 97(4): 334-336.
63. Grufferman S, Gillman MW et al. (1980). "Familial carotid body tumors: Case report and epidemiologic review." Cancer 46(9): 2116-2122.
64. Koenigsberg RA, Dastur BS. (1-29-2008). "Imaging of Head and Neck Glomus Tumors" Emedicine. medscape.com Retrieved from http://www.emedicine.medscape.com/article/382908 (12-4-2010).
65. Sevilla, MA, Hermsen MA, et al. (2009). "Chromosomal changes in sporadic and familial head and neck paragangliomas." Otolaryngology--head and neck surgery: official journal of American Academy of Otolaryngology-Head and Neck Surgery 140(5): 724-729.
66. Weyand, CM and Goronzy, JJ. (2003). "Medium- and Large-Vessel Vasculitis." New England Journal of Medicine 349(2): 160-169.
67. Michael B Gravanis. (2000). "Giant cell arteritis and Takayasu aortitis: morphologic, pathogenetic and etiologic factors." International Journal of Cardiology 75, Supplement 1(0): S21-S33.
68. Yilmaz, A and Arditi M. (2009). "Giant Cell Arteritis." Circulation Research 104(4): 425-427.
69. Weyand, CM, Ma-Krupa W., et al. (2004). "Immunopathways in giant cell arteritis and polymyalgia rheumatica." Autoimmunity Reviews 3(1): 46-53.
70. Shepard RJ, Rooke T. (2005). Uncommon arteriopathies. In Rutherford Vascular Surgery 6th edition. (453-474). Philadelphia. Elsevier Saunders.
71. Hajj-Ali RA, Mandell B. (2005). Approach to and management of inflammatory vasculitis. In Rajagopalan S, Mukherjee D, Mohler E. (Eds). Manual of Vascular Diseases. (353-375). Philadelphia. Lippinott Williams & Wilkins.
72. Parrillo SJ, Parrillo CV. (3-18-2010). "Pediatrics, Kawasaki disease" Emedicine.medscape.com. http://emedicine.medscape.com/article/804960-overview (12-4-2010).
73. Yousefi M, Ferringer T, Lee S, Bang, D. (6-19-2009). "Bechet disease" Emedicine.medscape.com. http://emedicine.medscape.com/article/1122381-overview (12-4-2010).
74. Shepherd RFJ. (2005). Raynaud's syndrome: vasospastic and occlusive arterial disease involving the distal upper extremity. In Rutherford Vascular Surgery 6th edition. (1319-1346). Philadelphia. Elsevier Saunders.
75. "What is Raynaud's" (2010). Raynaud's Association. www.raynauds.org (12-4-2010).
76. Shah SN. (10-2-2008). Aortic Coarctation. Emedicine.medscape.com. Retrieved from http://www.emedicine.medscape.com/article/150369 (12-4-2010).
77. "Coarctation of the aorta" (3-2-2010). Mayo Clinic. Retrieved from http://www.mayoclinic.com/health/coarctation-of-the-aorta/DS00616. (12-4-2010).
78. Narvencar K PS, Jaques e Costa AK, Patil VR. "Shones complex" May 2009 Journal of Association of Physicians of India, 57: 415-416. http://www.japi.org/may_2009/article_12.pdf. (12-4-2010).
79. Giordano JM. (2005). Embryology of the vascular system. In Rutherford Vascular Surgery 6th edition. (53-62). Philadelphia. Elsevier Saunders.
80. Levien LJ. (2005). Nonatheromatous causes of popliteal artery disease. In Rutherford Vascular Surgery 6th edition. (1236-1255). Philadelphia. Elsevier Saunders.
81. Myers K, Clogh A, (2004). Disease of arteries to the lower limbs. In Making Sense of Vascular Ultrasound, (141-180). London: Hodder Arnold.
82. Kreienberg PB, Shah, DM, Darling III, RC, Change BB, Paty SK, Roddy SP, Ozsvath KJ, Manish,, (2005). Thoracic Outlet Syndrome: In Mansour MA, Labropoulos N. (Eds.), Vascular Diagnosis, (517-522). Philadelphia,: Elsevier Saunders.
83. Thompson RW, Bartoli MA. (2005). Neurogenic thoracic outlet syndrome. In Rutherford Vascular Surgery 6th edition. (1347-1365). Philadelphia. Elsevier Saunders.
84. Green RM. (2005). Subclavian-axillary vein thrombosis. In Rutherford Vascular Surgery 6th edition. (1371-1392). Philadelphia. Elsevier Saunders.
85. Eskandari MK, Yao JST. (2005). Occupational vascular problems. In Rutherford Vascular Surgery 6th edition. (1393-1401). Philadelphia. Elsevier Saunders.
86. Flanigan DP, Burnham SJ, Goodreau JJ, Bergan JJ. Summary of cases of adventitial cystic disease of the popliteal artery. Ann Surgery 1979 Feb: 189 (2): 165-75.
87. Stanley JC, Wakefield TW. (2005). Arterial fibrodysplagia. In Rutherford Vascular Surgery 6th edition. (431-452). Philadelphia. Elsevier Saunders.
88. Paciaroni M, Eliasziw M, Kappelle LJ, Finan JW, Ferguson GG, Barnett HJ. Medical complications associated with carotid endarterectomy. North American Symptomatic Carotid Endarterectomy Trial (NASCET). Stroke. 1999 Sep;30(9):1759-63.
89. Walker, MD, Marler JR, Goldstein M, Grady PA, Toole JF, Baker WH, Castaldo JE, Chambless LE, Moore WS, Robertson JT, Young B, Howard VJ, Marler JR, Ourvis S, Vernon D, Needham K, Beck P, Celani VJ, Sauebeck L, von Rajcs JA, Atkins D. Endarterectomy for Asymptomatic Carotid Artery Stenosis JAMA 1995; 273: 1421-1428.
90. Labropoulos N, Erzurum V, Sheehan MK, Maker WH. (2005). Cerebral vascular color-flow scanning techniques and applications. In Mansour MA, Labropoulos N. (Eds.), Vascular Diagnosis, (91-104). Philadelphia: Elsevier Saunders.
91. Chaaban M, Stenson KM. (5-5-2009). "carotid body tumors. Emedicine.medscape.com. Retrieved from http://www.emedicine.medscape.com/article/1575155. (12-4-2010).
92. Schneider DB, Stanley JC, Messina LM. (2005). Renal artery fibrodysplagia and renovascular hypertension. In Rutherford Vascular Surgery 6th edition. (1789-2371). Philadelphia. El sevier Saunders.
93. Schneider PA. (2005). Endovascular and surgical management of extracranial carotid fibromuscular arterial dysplagia. In Rutherford Vascular Surgery 6th edition. (2044-2051). Philadelphia. El sevier Saunders.
94. Schneider DB, Stanley JC, Messina LM. (2005). Renal artery fibrodysplagia and renovascular hypertension. In Rutherford Vascular Surgery 6th edition. (1789-2371). Philadelphia. El sevier Saunders.
95. Hallett JW, Brewster DC, Rasmussen TE. (2001). Cerebrovascular diseases. In: Handbook of Patient Care in Vascular Diseases. (131-149), Philadelphia Lippincott Williams & Wilkins.
96. Davies MG. (2005). Intimal hyperplasia: basic response to arterial and vein graft injury and reconstruction. In Rutherford Vascular Surgery 6th edition. (149-172). Philadelphia. Elsevier Saunders.
97. Wyers MC, Zwolak RM. (2005). Physiology and diagnosis of splachnic arterial occlusion. In Rutherford Vascular Surgery 6th edition. (1707-1717). Philadelphia. Elsevier Saunders.
98. Stamatakos M, Stefanaki C, Mastrokalos D, Arampatzi H, Safioleas P, Chatziconstantinou C, Xiromeritis C, Safioleas M. (2008). Mesenteric ischemia: still a deadly puzzle for the medical community. Tohoku J Exp Med. 216: 197-204.
99. Hallett, JW, Brewster DC, Rasmussen TE, (2001) Intestinal ischemia. In Handbook of Patient Care in Vascular Diseases, (231-237), Philadelphia: Lippincott Williams & Wilkins.
100. Aziz F, Comerota AJ. (12-3-2009). Abdominal Angina. eMedicine. Retrieved from http://emedicine.medscape.com/article/188618-overview. (12-11-2010).
101. Johansen K. (2005). Portal hypertension. In Rutherford Vascular Surgery 6th edition. (1752-1761). Philadelphia. Elsevier Saunders.
102. Carale J, Murherjee S. (9-24-2010). Portal Hypertension. eMedicine. Retrieved from http://emedicine.medscape.com/article/182098-overview. (12-10-2010).
103. Raja SG, Haider Z, Ahmad M, Zaman H. Saphenous vein grafts: Heart Lung Circ. 2004;13:403-409.
104. Bauters, C., Meurice, T., Hamon, M., Mcfadden, E., Lablanche, J. M., and Bertrand, M. E., 1996, "Mechanisms and Prevention of Restenosis: From Experimental Models to Clinical Practice," Cardiovascular research, 31(6), pp. 835-46.
105. Newby, A. C., and Zaltsman, A. B., 2000, "Molecular Mechanisms in Intimal Hyperplasia," The Journal of pathology, 190(3), pp. 300-9.
106. Glagov, S., Zarins, C. K., Masawa, N., Xu, C. P., Bassiouny, H., and Giddens, D. P., 1993, "Mechanical Functional Role of Non-Atherosclerotic Intimal Thickening," Frontiers of medical and biological engineering: the international journal of the Japan Society of Medical Electronics and Biological Engineering, 5(1), pp. 37-43.
107. Zargham, R., 2008, "Preventing Restenosis after Angioplasty: A Multistage Approach," Clinical science, 114(4), pp. 257-64.
108. Allaire, E., and Clowes, A. W., 1997, "Endothelial Cell Injury in Cardiovascular Surgery: The Intimal Hyperplastic Response," The Annals of thoracic surgery, 63(2), pp. 582-91.
109. Fay, W. P., Garg, N., and Sunkar, M., 2007, "Vascular Functions of the Plasminogen Activation System," Arteriosclerosis, thrombosis, and vascular biology, 27(6), pp. 1231-7.
110. Zwiebel, WJ (2005). Ultrasound assessment of the hepatic vasculature. In Zwiebel WJ, Pellerito JS (Eds.), Introduction to Vascular Ultrasonography 5th ed, (586-609). Philadelphia: Elsevier Saunders.
111. McKinsey JF, Gewertz BL. (1077) Acute mesenteric ischemia. Clin North Am; 77:301-318.
112. Jeyaraj SC, Chotani MA, Mitra S, Gregg HE, Flavahan NA, Morrison KJ. Cooling evokes redistribution of ⊠2C-adrenoceptors from golgi to plasma membrane in transfected HEK293 cells. Mol Pharmacol. 2001;60:1195–1200. [HYPERLINK "/pubmed/11723226"PubMed]
113. Nicholas A. Flavahan, PhD Rheumatic Disease Clinics of North America; "Regulation of Vascular Reactivity in Scleroderma: New Insights into Raynaud's Phenomenon" Volume 34, Issue 1, February 2008, Pages 81–87
114. Davies MG. (2005). Intimal hyperplasia: basic response to arterial and vein graft injury and reconstruction. In *Rutherford Vascular Surgery 6th edition.* (149-172). Philadelphia. Elsevier Saunders.
115. Lumsden AB, Peden E, Bush RL, Lin PH. (2005). Complications of endovascular procedures. In Rutherford Vascular Surgery 6th edition. (809-820). Philadelphia. Elsevier Saunders.

CEREBROVASCULAR TESTING
13. Carotid Artery Duplex Ultrasound

Definition
The combination of real-time B-mode imaging with spectral and color Doppler to evaluate the extracranial vessels.

Etiology
- Atherosclerosis (90%)
- Intimal hyperplasia
- Dissection
- Traumatic occlusion
- Extrinsic compression
- External radiation
- Carotid body tumor
- Fibromuscular dysplasia
- Post-traumatic pseudoaneurysm

Risk Factors
- Age
- Hypertension
- Diabetes
- Hypercholesterolemia
- Smoking
- Obesity
- Physical inactivity
- Genetic predisposition
- Homocysteinemia
- Cardiac disease
- Previous TIA or stroke
- Patent foramen ovale

Indications for Exam
- Carotid bruit
- Follow-up of known carotid stenosis
- Syncope
- Abnormality of gait
- Hemiparesis/hemiplegia
- Paresthesia
- Aphasia
- Positional vertigo
- Visual symptoms (e.g., amaurosis fugax, retinal ischemia, transient visual loss, etc.)
- Transient ischemic attack (TIA)
- Stroke: Cerebrovascular Accident (CVA)
- Follow-up (carotid endarterectomy, stent, bypass)
- Infarction (previously known as RIND: reversible ischemic neurologic deficit)
- Neck trauma
- Pulsatile mass in the neck
- Fibromuscular dysplasia
- Moyamoya disease
- Carotid artery dissection
- Seizure

Contraindications/Limitations
- Patients with extensive bandages or cervical collars
- Patients with neck IV
- Poor visualization due to vessel depth

Location of Disease
- First 1-2cm of the internal carotid artery (most common)
- Common carotid artery
- Diffuse arterial wall calcification may interfere with acquisition of duplex information
- Patients who cannot be adequately positioned.
- Subclavian artery
- Origin of the vertebral artery
- External carotid artery

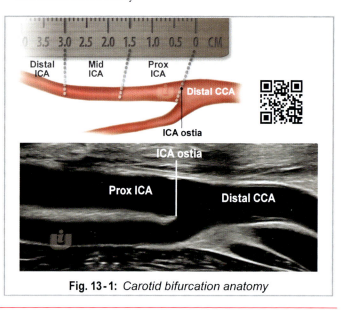

Fig. 13-1: Carotid bifurcation anatomy

Labs may use different terminology when sampling the carotid arteries. The "bulb" is a dilated segment usually of the ICA which sometimes includes part of the distal common carotid artery. The "ostia" (e.g., ICA ostia, ECA ostia) refers to the opening into a vessel.

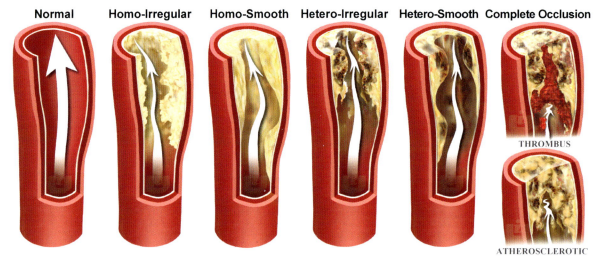

Fig. 13-2: Presentations of atherosclerosis within an artery

Table 13-1: **B-mode and Plaque Morphology**

Echogenicity	Composition	Texture	Surface
Reflections determined by plaque's composition of lipids, collagen, hemorrhage and calcification	Determined by levels of lipid, hemorrhage, collagen and calcification		

Echogenicity

Anechoic
- No echogenicity (lipids, intraplaque hemorrhage)

Hypoechoic
- Low echogenicity (fibrofatty plaque)

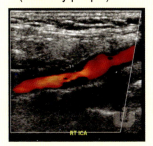

Hyperechoic
- Moderate echogenicity (fibrous plaque) acoustic shadowing may or may not be present

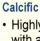

Calcific
- Highly reflective plaque(s) with acoustic shadowing

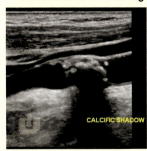

Composition

Fibrofatty plaque
- Contains lipid material
- Lightly echogenic
- Acoustics similar to blood: uniform echo distribution

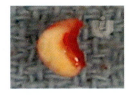

Fibrous plaque
- Moderate to strong echogenicity
- Lipid or thrombus may create hypoechoic regions

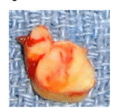

Complex plaque
- Multiple levels of echogenicity
- Acoustic calcific shadowing may or may not be present.

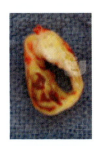

Texture

Homogeneous
- Uniform echo pattern and composition
- May be echogenic or echolucent

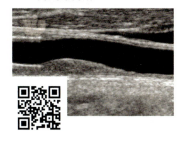

Heterogeneous
- Non-uniform echo pattern, multiple echo densities of anechoic and hyperechoic areas.
- May be classified as primarily echolucent if greater than 50% of the plaque is dark.

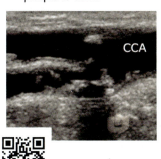

- May be classified as primarily echogenic if greater than 50% of the plaque demonstrates brighter echoes

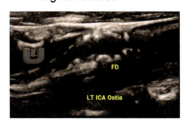

Surface

Smooth
- Surface plaque appears continuous with no irregularities

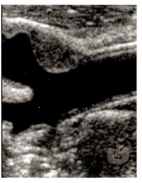

Irregular
- Plaque surface is discontinuous, may have multiple echoes present
- Possibility of ulceration on such surfaces. However, presence of ulcer cannot always be determined by duplex ultrasound

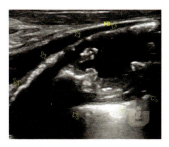

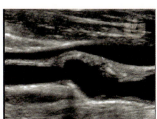

Images courtesy of Philips Healthcare

Mechanism of Disease for Carotid Artery Stenosis
Atherosclerosis
- Atherosclerosis is the most common arterial disease.
- Atherosclerotic plaque forms in the arterial wall and decreases or stops blood flow by either narrowing the lumen (stenosis) or completely blocking the artery (occlusion).
- Hemodynamically significant obstruction refers to a stenosis or an occlusion. This term typically describes an obstruction >50% diameter reduction. [1]
- Typically, a stenosis must narrow the diameter of the artery by at least 50% to increase the peak systolic velocity significantly.

Emboli
- An *embolus* is a piece of plaque or thrombus that moves from a proximal point, stopping in the artery too narrow for it to pass. This causes an *infarction*, a sudden reduction of flow to a part.
- A cerebral embolus is frequently a piece of carotid plaque or thrombus from a plaque in the heart, but it may originate elsewhere.
- If the embolus originates from the heart, it is classified as a *cardioembolic infarction*.
- *Territorial infarcts* are restricted to territories supplied by major intracerebral arteries, their branches or the *pial arteries* that surround the brain and spinal cord.

Additional Mechanisms of Disease
Dissection
- A tear in the intimal lining of an artery, with or without outer medial wall involvement. Blood enters the media of the vessel through this tear creating a "false lumen." Simultaneously, blood is also flowing through the original or "true lumen."
- Blood flows through the tear in the intimal layer and sometimes clots.
- Can be spontaneous or result from trauma or an iatrogenic complication.
- ICA dissection typically starts in the first 2-4cm of the ICA
- Expansion of the false lumen that develops during dissection can narrow the true carotid lumen. [5,7]
- CCA dissection may be an extension of an aortic dissection or blunt trauma.
- The false lumen can progressively dilate into a pseudoaneurysm. [2]

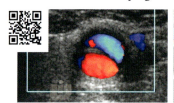
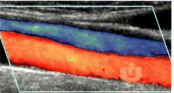

Fig. 13-3: Arterial dissection showing 2 distinct flow channels by color

Kinking and Tortuosity
- Kinking or tortuosity refers to a sharp angle of 90° or less usually located 2-4cm above the bifurcation.
- Blood flow is compromised in kinked arteries and is often associated with plaque and arterial stenosis.
- The most important difference between a tortuous, coiled and kinked vessel is that the kinked vessel is most often associated with symptoms of cerebral ischemia.
- Congenital kinks are a result of faulty descent of the vessels during embryonic development.
- Kinks can be acquired with age; arteries can elongate and at the same time, the medial layer degenerates. [3]
- Approximately 25% of the population are affected by this condition which is often bilateral. [4]

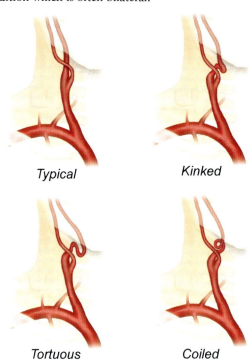

Fig. 13-4: Common shape distortions found at the extracranial internal carotid artery

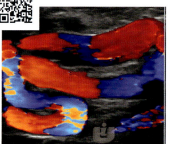
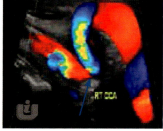

Fig. 13-5: Duplex image of a tortuous artery-ICA

Fig. 13-6: Duplex image of a kinked-CCA

Images courtesy of Patrick Washko, BS RT RDMS RVT

The ICA may be coiled or tortuous typically located in the first 2-3cm of the artery; creating an "S" curve or "C" shape which may produce a bruit. The patient is usually asymptomatic. [11] Carotid artery kinks occur four times more often in women than men. [7,11]

Fibromuscular Dysplasia (FMD) [1,7,8,9]
- Non-atherosclerotic arterial disease resulting in either a focal stenosis or multifocal stenoses. Multifocal FMD accounts for 90% of cases while the less common focal type occurs more in pediatric cases.
- On duplex ultrasound especially when there is multifocal stenoses, there will be a series of tandem stenoses or significant increases in peak systolic velocity with extensive turbulence followed by dilated arterial segments which resemble a "string of beads."

- FMD affects medium and large sized vessels, especially the renal and internal carotid arteries. Coexisting FMD in the renal and carotid arteries is not an uncommon occurrence. [10]
- Usually occurs in females in the mid-section of the internal carotid artery. [5,6]
- The carotid bulb/proximal ICA segment typically is not affected by FMD. [10]

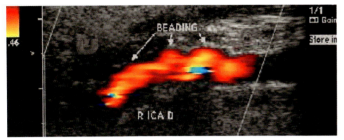

Fig. 13-7: *Detection of FMD in the distal ICA at the level of the mandible by color duplex*

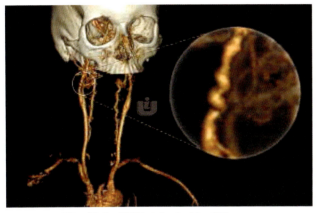

Fig. 13-8: *FMD detected by CT scan*

Carotid Body Tumor

- The carotid body is a small cluster of primarily chemoreceptor cells located at the split of the carotid bifurcation.
- Chemoreceptors are part of the autonomic nervous system and regulate the levels of oxygen, carbon dioxide and hydrogen ions in the arteries. They can signal vasoconstriction when necessary.
- A carotid body tumor (CBT) is a *paraganglioma* (tumor or ganglioma comprised of chromaffin). They arise off the ganglion of the glossopharyngeal nerve.
- In most cases, the external carotid artery supplies blood to the tumor. [3, 10] Flow will be low resistant. As the tumor grows, blood flow can also be supplied by the internal carotid, vertebral artery or thyrocervical trunk. [54]
- CBT are unilateral in 95% of reported cases [3] and females suffer from carotid body tumors 3-5 more times than men. [54] The tumors are benign in 90-95% of all cases. [28] CBTs are more frequent in people living at higher altitudes. [29, 30]

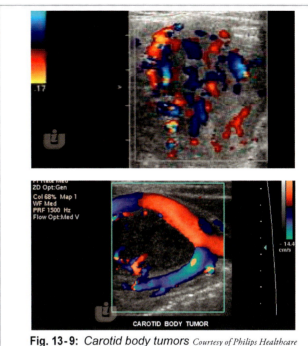

Fig. 13-9: *Carotid body tumors* Courtesy of Philips Healthcare

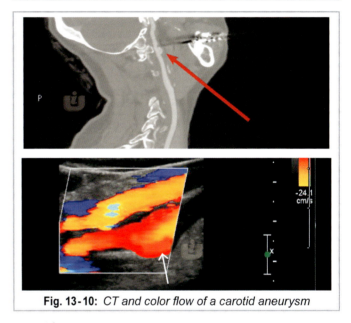

Fig. 13-10: *CT and color flow of a carotid aneurysm*

Carotid Aneurysm

- Carotid aneurysms and pseudoaneurysms are very rare.
- A reduction in tensile strength of the wall post-endarterectomy may weaken the arterial wall, increasing the risk of a pseudoaneurysm. [13]
- Reasons for pseudoaneurysm at a carotid bypass anastomotic site include; infection, tension at the anastomosis, thin-walled arteries, suture deterioration or improper suture technique. [14]

Radiation Injury

- Radiation therapy causes injury to the vasa vasorum and necrosis of the vessel wall. Endothelial cells lining the arterial walls of vessels in the irradiated field are susceptible to damage. Lipid-containing plaques can then form in the intimal layer of the artery. [15]

Vasculitis
- Inflammation of the vessel wall results in damage to the blood vessel.
- The causes of vasculitis are still under study. Genetics, infectious and toxic factors are suspected.
- Giant cell or temporal arteritis affects the extracranial branches of the carotid. The temporal artery is especially susceptible.

Patient History

Anterior Circulation Symptoms (Internal Carotid Artery) Disease Suspected
- Transient ischemic attack (resolves within 24 hours)
- Cerebral vascular accident (permanent deficit)
- Amaurosis fugax: partial or complete loss of vision (often described as a "window shade being pulled down")
- Hemiparesis/hemiplegia: weakness or complete loss of function to one limb or one side of the body
- Paresthesia (tingling, numb or burning sensation)
- Aphasia: inability to speak or comprehend language
- Homonomous hemianopia (blindness or visual defect in half of the field of vision)

Posterior Circulation Symptoms (Vertebrobasilar Artery) Disease Suspected
- Ataxia (lack of muscle coordination which can affect walking, swallowing, eye movements, speech, etc.)
- Confusion
- Diplopia (double vision)
- Dizziness
- Dysarthria (abnormal speech or difficulty with speech)
- Drop attacks (sudden fall while walking or standing that is recovered from quickly)
- Dysphagia (difficulty swallowing)
- Headache
- Motor/sensory disturbances (unilateral, bilateral, alternating)
- Syncope (fainting)
- Vertigo ("spinning" or sensation that your surroundings are moving around you)
- Subclavian steal syndrome

Physical Examination
- Carotid auscultation for bruits
- Bilateral blood pressure (>20mmHg difference between right and left arm may indicate significant pathology, e.g., subclavian obstruction on the side with the lower pressure resulting in a subclavian steal)

Table 13-2: Identification of ICA vs ECA Vessels

Characteristic	Internal Carotid Artery	External Carotid Artery
Anatomical location	Posterolateral	Anteromedial
Branch vessels in neck	Extremely rare	Yes
Luminal size	Larger diameter	Smaller diameter
Responds to temporal tap*	No	Yes
Doppler flow pattern	Low resistance	High resistance
Normal PSV	Varies, <180cm/s	Varies, <200cm/s

*Tapping too hard can cause reverberation in the ICA. Best to tap the STA while listening to each vessel and compare the waveforms for the strongest response.

Carotid Artery Examination Protocol
- Obtain a patient history to include symptoms and risk factors, past vascular interventions and general dates of surgery.
- Obtain bilateral brachial blood pressures.
- Patient is examined in the supine position with the head supported by a small pillow or towel, turning the head approximately 45° toward the opposite side.
- Some patients may require the use of a range of transducers, including high-frequency (5-7 MHz), (8-15 MHz) transducers and a lower frequency (1-4 MHz) transducer to assist with large, short necks.

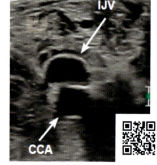

- Locate the common carotid artery (CCA) at the base of the neck in the transverse (short axis) plane.
- Obtain and record B-mode images in transverse view of the following:
  » Common carotid artery
  » Carotid bifurcation; distal CCA before the complete split of the proximal internal and external carotid arteries.
  » Internal carotid artery (ICA); can be in same view with ECA.
  » These images can be repeated with color flow Doppler.

Fig. 13-11: B-mode imaging of the carotid artery system

- Obtain and record B-mode images in the longitudinal (sagittal) view of the following:
  » Common carotid artery
  » Carotid bifurcation, distal CCA into the ICA, this is the most diagnostic image.
  » Carotid bifurcation; distal CCA into the ECA
  » Proximal, mid and distal ICA
  » ECA

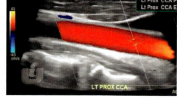

Fig. 13-12: Long view of the CCA with color

- These images can be repeated with color flow Doppler.
- Use a 60° spectral Doppler angle or less with the angle cursor set parallel to the vessel wall or to flow and the sample volume placed center stream. It is VITAL to velocity measurements that the angle be accurate. Document the peak systolic (PSV) and end diastolic velocity (EDV) for the following:
  » Proximal, mid and distal CCA
  » Proximal ECA
  » Proximal, mid and distal ICA
  » Vertebral artery
- Subclavian artery when clinically indicated (PSV only). Although the subclavian artery is not considered a part of the intra or extracranial system, many testing centers include the subclavian artery in the carotid duplex exam.
- It is extremely important to "walk" the spectral Doppler sample volume through an area of stenosis to obtain the maximum peak systolic velocity and end-diastolic velocities.
- Take additional spectral Doppler measurements as appropriate. Areas of stenosis should include pre, at and post stenosis waveform measurements. Use color Doppler as needed to define anatomy and areas of stenosis.

Carotid Artery Duplex Ultrasound 103

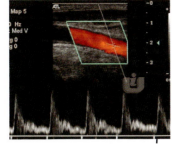
Fig. 13-13: Normal ICA

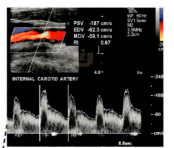
Fig. 13-19: Abnormal ICA with elevated PSV and spectral broadening

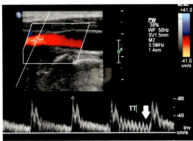
Fig. 13-14: Normal ECA

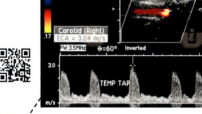
Fig. 13-20: Abnormal ECA with elevated PSV and spectral broadening

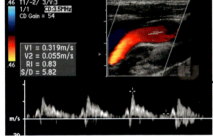
Fig. 13-15: Normal waveform in the bulb

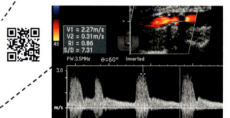
Fig. 13-21: Abnormal waveform in the bulb with elevated PSV and spectral broadening

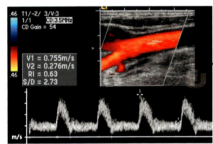
Fig. 13-16: Normal CCA

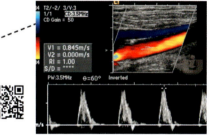
Fig. 13-22: Abnormal CCA (no diastolic flow)

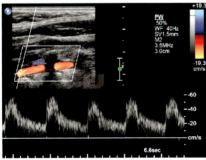
Fig. 13-17: Normal vertebral

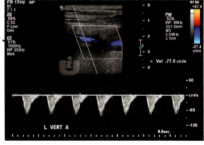
Fig. 13-23: Abnormal (retrograde) vertebral

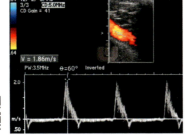
Fig. 13-18: Normal subclavian

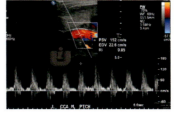
Fig. 13-24: Abnormal subclavian with elevated PSV and spectral broadening

- Document additional B-mode and color images in areas of suspected stenosis. Measure lumenal reduction, especially when lesions cause a hemodynamically significant velocity increase. This provides backup information for the velocity data.

Duplex % diameter stenosis = $(1 - \frac{\text{residual lumen}}{\text{true lumen}}) \times 100$

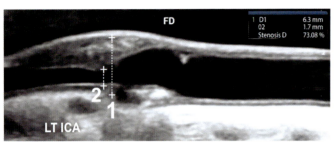

Fig. 13-25: *The true/residual lumen can be measured at the point of stenosis on B-mode. 1 = true lumen; 2 = residual lumen*

» Measure in multiple planes to get full effect of plaque: transverse, longitudinal-anterior/posterior, longitudinal-lateral. Use the oblique plane as needed to follow tortuous vessels.
  - Use color only if needed to clearly define the edges of plaque, and update with B-mode frequently to avoid color overgain.
  - Most difficult point to define is the true lumen. Look for the black line separating wall from plaque.
» Calculate and report the average of 2-3 measurements from these different planes.

- Document any additional abnormal findings with B-mode and color imaging (e.g., aneurysmal formation, thrombus, wall irregularity, aneurysm, etc).
- When arterial occlusion is suspected, document the lack of flow with spectral Doppler. Decrease the color and velocity scales to detect low flow and confirm occlusion.
- A suspected occlusion must be examined and documented in both longitudinal and transverse planes.
- Optimize exam; sample volume, gain and scales may all need to be adjusted.
- Determine classification of stenosis according to laboratory diagnostic criteria. *(See diagnostic criteria tables).*
- Repeat on the opposite side.

Duplex Exam Considerations After Carotid Endarterectomy or Carotid Bypass Graft
- First exam is usually within 30 days of the procedure. Most labs use the patient's first duplex exam post CAS values as their baseline for subsequent duplex exams.
- Exams performed within the first few days may encounter shadowing from air entrapment associated with a synthetic patch or graft, multiple views may be required to view the vessel.
- In addition to standard duplex, the following conditions should be noted: [3]
  - » Restenosis
  - » Residual plaque
  - » Tissue flaps
  - » Vessel narrowing
  - » Neointimal hyperplasia
  - » Hematoma
  - » Extravascular leak
  - » Pseudoaneurysm (associated with a synthetic patch)
- The length of the surgical area is dependent on the extent and level of disease.

- With patch angioplasty closure, a wider vessel will be noted and sutures may be visible as small echoes regularly spaced on the wall of the vessel.

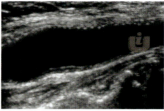
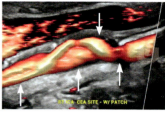

Fig. 13-26: *B-mode image of a carotid patch*
Courtesy of Philips Healthcare

Fig. 13-27: *Flow through the patch by power Doppler*

Table 13-3: Carotid Artery Examination Protocol Summary

Scan transverse (short-axis) with B-mode and color flow Doppler	Scan longitudinal (sagittal) with B-mode, color flow and spectral Doppler
• CCA (Proximal, mid, distal)	• CCA (Proximal, mid, distal)
• Carotid bifurcation	• Proximal ECA*
• Proximal ECA	• ICA (Proximal, mid, distal)
• ICA (Proximal, mid, distal)	• Vertebral
* Measure only the PSV	• Subclavian*

- Determine plaque location, plaque surface characteristics, plaque texture and vertebral flow direction
- Measure highest peak systolic velocity (PSV) and end-diastolic velocity (EDV)
- At areas of stenosis measure PSV and EDV proximal, within and distal to the stenosis
- Calculate systolic ICA/CCA ratio bilaterally using the highest PSV of the ICA and the mid/distal CCA just proximal to the bulb where the CCA walls are parallel

ICA/CCA ratio = $\frac{\text{Maximum PSV from the proximal ICA}}{\text{PSV from the mid/distal CCA}}$

- Determine classification of disease using the velocity criteria chosen by the laboratory

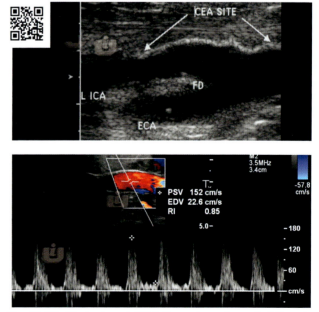

Fig. 13-28: *Typical post-CEA B-mode and spectral Doppler*

Duplex Evaluation Considerations for Carotid Stents

- First exam is usually within 30 days of the procedure.
- In addition to standard duplex, the following additional views are to be documented:
  » Proximal native artery
  » Distal attachment site
  » Proximal stent attachment
  » Native artery beyond the stent
  » Proximal, mid and distal stent
- In-stent restenosis is infrequent,[16] stent borders are the most common site of restenosis. Stents can overlap.
- Walk the Doppler through areas of hyperplasia for stent fractures which can cause elevated velocities.
- Follow flow changes over time.

Color Doppler may be helpful to evaluate residual lumens.

- When scanning post-stent placement, the proximal and distal ends of the stent should not reveal any major flow abnormalities. Make comparisons over serial studies and observe for any flow changes over time.

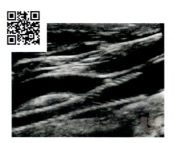
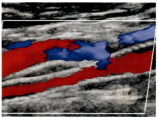

Fig. 13-29: *The proximal end of this stent is in the distal CCA with the distal end in the ICA*

Color flow can obscure the true lumenal reduction if the color gain is set too high. Measure luminal reduction in B-mode whenever possible.

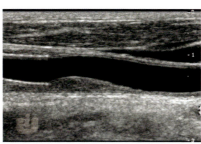
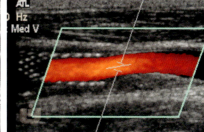

Fig. 13-30: *Intimal hyperplasia proximal to the stent*
Courtesy of Philips Healthcare

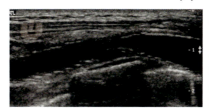
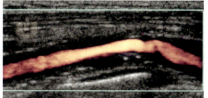

Fig. 13-31: *B-mode image and power Doppler of the residual lumen within a stent* Courtesy of Philips Healthcare

Table 13-4: Extracranial Vessels Characteristics

Vessel	Normal PSV	Normal EDV	Flow Pattern	Abnormal Flow	Area Supplied
Subclavian	Varies	Reversal of flow with high diastolic component	High resistance triphasic flow	High PSV may indicate stenosis; biphasic or monophasic waveform associated with obstruction	Vertebral artery and arm
Common Carotid	Varies	Between ECA and ICA EDV	Low resistance	Low or zero EDV may indicate distal CCA, and/or proximal ICA high-grade stenosis or occlusion	ICA and ECA
External Carotid	Typically higher than normal ICA	Low diastolic flow; may have reversal of flow	High resistance	>200cm/s with post-stenotic turbulence and plaque in the image	Face and scalp
Internal Carotid	<180cm/s with no or minimal spectral broadening PSV varies widely across labs	Diastolic flow beyond the bulb with velocities usually <40cm/s	Low resistance	Increased PSV and EDV with post-stenotic turbulence and plaque in the image	Middle cerebral and ophthalmic arteries
Vertebral	20-60cm/s but can vary from side to side	Flow above the baseline; less diastolic flow than the ICA	Low resistance	Reversed flow pattern may indicate subclavian steal syndrome	Intracranial vessels

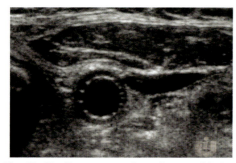

Fig. 13-32: *Transverse view of a carotid stent*
Courtesy of Philips Healthcare

Duplex Evaluation for Temporal Arteritis
- Use a high-frequency transducer (5-7 MHz, 8-15 MHz, etc).
- Image the superficial temporal, frontal and parietal arteries bilaterally in the transverse and longitudinal planes.
- Observe the lumen of these small arteries using B-mode image to:
  » Measure the anterior and posterior diameters (mm) of the arteries. Some laboratories will measure the diameter of the "halo's thickness" (similar to measuring CIMT).
  » Assess the arterial walls for a hyperechoic area or "halo" effect on B-mode image.
- Use color Doppler to assess and document patency.
- Use spectral Doppler to document the PSV and EDV using a ≤60° spectral Doppler angle with the cursor set parallel to the vessel wall or to flow and the sample volume placed center stream.

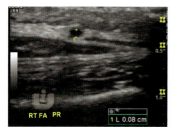

Fig. 13-33: *Transverse arterial diameter of the frontal artery*

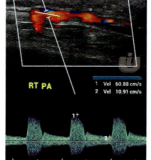

Fig. 13-34: *Spectral Doppler of the parietal artery*

PRINCIPLES OF INTERPRETATION

B-mode Imaging and Color Doppler
- Assess all arteries for intraluminal echoes. Determine plaque location and plaque characteristics:
  » **Diffuse plaque:** long segment of the artery lined with plaque, but <50% diameter reduction at any point.
  » **Stenotic:** lumen is narrowed and velocity increases. A hemodynamically significant stenosis typically occurs when narrowing results in a >50% diameter reduction (75% area reduction). A stenosis can be focal or involve a long segment.
  » **Calcific:** highly reflective plaque(s) with acoustic shadowing
  » **Occluded:** complete occlusion of the vessel
- Assess color filling and flow direction for each artery.

Spectral Doppler Waveforms and Flow Velocities
- Assess PSV/EDV and waveforms of the CCA and ECA and compare right and left sides.
- Assess the PSV and waveforms of the VA and SCA and compare right and left sides.
- Categorize ICA disease by PSV, EDV ratio and image according to the diagnostic criteria. Make sure these measurements support each other and give a possible explanation if they do not correlate (e.g., compensatory flow, inflow obstruction).

Interpretation/Diagnostic Criteria

Normal

(Absence of a hemodynamically significant stenosis, <50%)

B-mode Imaging and Color Doppler
- The arteries are free of significant intraluminal echoes (>50%).
- When utilized, color Doppler fills the entire arterial lumen.

Spectral Doppler Waveforms and Flow Velocities
- Normal carotid artery waveforms demonstrate antegrade, low-resistance in the CCA, ICA and vertebral. Waveforms demonstrate high-resistance in the ECA.
- PSV should be relatively uniform throughout the carotid arteries. Specific normal PSV values vary across labs with normal velocity ratios <2.0. Peak velocities <200 cm/s are generally expected in the ECA and <125-180 cm/s is expected in the ICA.

Always compare flow velocities from side-to-side.

- Velocities are higher in younger people
- Vertebral flow velocities can vary from side to side due to one vertebral artery being dominant. The left side is commonly dominant.
- Subclavian artery waveform configuration is normally triphasic.
- The EDV is generally above the zero baseline with these possible exceptions:
  » CCA or ECA may have a short duration of reversed flow at end systole
  » Areas of the bulb (wider area usually found between the distal CCA-proximal ICA) may have reversed flow

Abnormal

B-mode Imaging and Color Doppler
- There are intraluminal echoes observed in the arteries.
- Exact location and plaque characteristics should be described:
  » Homogeneous, echolucent
  » Homogeneous, echodense
  » Heterogeneous, primarily echolucent
  » Heterogeneous, primarily echodense
  » Smooth vs. irregular
- When utilized, color Doppler does not fill the entire arterial lumen and should correlate with echoes noted on B-mode imaging.
- Measure a diameter reduction when indicated in the longitudinal and transverse planes with and without color flow and report the average diameter calculated.
- Modest flow disturbances seen early after CEA may disappear on subsequent studies due to natural vessel remodeling.

Spectral Doppler Waveforms and Flow Velocities
- Check that the ICA/CCA ratio and image measurement agree with the category of disease suspected.

Common Carotid Artery (CCA)
- Low or zero end-diastolic velocity may indicate distal common carotid artery, carotid bifurcation and/or proximal internal carotid artery high grade stenosis or occlusion.
- No particular velocity value is considered abnormal. A hemodynamically significant lesion (>50%) will result in a focal velocity increase (at least double the velocity in the proximal arterial segment) and post-stenotic turbulence.
- Compare right and left CCA velocities, if there is approximately 30cm/s or more difference between CCAs at multiple levels, consider the following:
  » Proximal CCA with slow upstroke and lower velocity waveform indicates proximal obstruction.
  » Higher proximal CCA velocities can result from vessel tortuosity.
  » Proximal CCA waveforms with a quick upstroke but low velocities may indicate a tight distal CCA stenosis. A tight distal CCA stenosis is sometimes labeled mistakenly for a stenosis at the origin of the ICA, so watching for the low proximal and mid CCA velocities will may help recognize the difference.
  » CCA velocities which are much higher compared to the other side may be a sign of compensatory flow due to a contralateral occlusion.
- Long duration reversed flow may be due to aortic regurgitation if noted bilaterally in the CCA

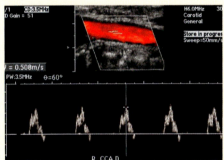

Fig. 13-35: *Loss of diastolic flow in the CCA due to ICA occlusion*

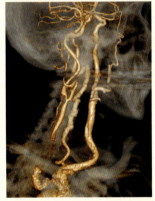
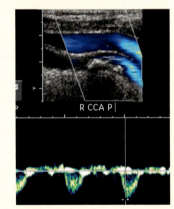

Fig. 13-36: *Reversal of flow in the CCA due to occlusion of the brachiocephalic artery*

Internal Carotid Artery (ICA)
- Depending on which criterion is used, peak systolic velocities >125cm/s may be considered abnormal. Spectral broadening will increase as the higher velocities are reached.
- End-diastolic velocity >40cm/s

The criterion for abnormal carotid artery duplex varies across institutions.

- Use the highest PSV and EDV from the pre-bulb CCA and first 3cm of the ICA to calculate the ICA/CCA ratio. Refer to criteria options in this chapter.

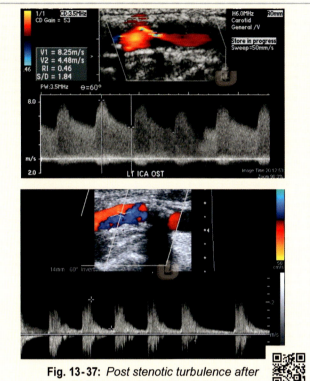

Fig. 13-37: *Post stenotic turbulence after a high-grade obstruction in the ICA*

External Carotid Artery (ECA)
- Peak systolic velocity >150-200cm/s with evidence of plaque and post stenotic turbulence indicates >50% stenosis [16]
- Some labs define a hemodynamically significant ECA lesion (>50%) by a focal velocity increase (at least double the velocity in the proximal ECA segment), with post-stenotic turbulence and a possible color bruit.
- Low resistance flow patterns may occur due to severe ICA stenosis/occlusion resulting in the ECA acting as a collateral to feed the low resistance vessels of the brain. In this case it is important to look for branches to identify this vessel as the ECA.
- In cases of CCA occlusion, ECA flow direction will often reverse in order to perfuse the ICA and the brain ECA flow will be retrograde to the bifurcation to give antegrade flow to the ICA.
- Performing a temporal tap helps identify the ECA. The spectral trace should "oscillate" when you tap on the superficial temporal artery (STA).

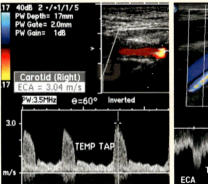
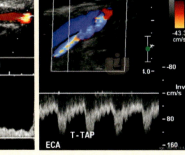

Fig. 13-38: *Internalized ECA signal*

Fig. 13-39: *Reversal of flow in the ECA supplying the ICA due to CCA occlusion*

Vertebral Artery (VA)

- Vertebral artery stenoses occur most frequently in the proximal VA which is often not directly assessed. Some labs define a hemodynamically significant VA lesion (>50%) by a focal velocity increase (at least double the velocity in the proximal VA segment), with post-stenotic turbulence and a possible color bruit.
- Since flow direction is usually antegrade, reversed flow pattern may indicate subclavian steal syndrome and should be confirmed with abnormal subclavian artery waveform documentation or brachial pressure decrease of >20mmHg on the same side.
- Loss of EDV may indicate a distal occlusion
- No flow despite low scales and higher gains in spectral and color analysis along with a well visualized artery below the vein indicates vertebral occlusion.
- Pendulum waveforms (a.k.a. bunny ears) suggests subacute subclavian steal syndrome.

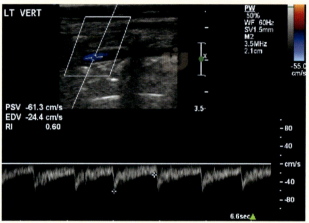

Fig. 13-40: *Reversed flow in the vertebral artery suggesting subclavian steal syndrome.*

Subclavian Artery (SA)

- There is no absolute abnormal velocity, but velocities are typically higher than the carotid arteries.
- A hemodynamically significant SA lesion (>50%) is indicated by a focal velocity increase (at least double the velocity in the proximal SA segment), with post-stenotic turbulence and a possible color bruit.
- Biphasic or monophasic signals may be observed when significant stenosis or occlusion is present in the SA.
  » Biphasic arterial signals (or alternative terms used including multiphasic or high-resistive) are characterized by strong forward flow in arterial systole (sharp upstroke) with a loss of flow reversal in early diastole (no flow below the baseline) and either forward flow or no flow in the late diastolic component.
  » Monophasic arterial signals (or alternative terms used including intermediate and low-resistive) are characterized by reduced pulsatility or forward flow in late systole (blunted upstroke). A diastolic flow component may or may not be apparent. Continuous forward flow and a slow, blunted systolic component is another way to describe monophasic flow.

Occlusion

- An occlusion of the artery is present when no flow is detected by color or spectral Doppler. Determine the extent of the occlusion when possible.
- To confirm occlusions:

» Decrease scales
» Increase color and spectral gain
» Decrease filter
» Increase sample volume but avoid ECA branches and veins

- Use spectral and color Doppler to investigate distal to the bulb in the transverse and longitudinal views. Never measure the velocity in transverse since the angle to flow direction cannot be measured accurately.
- ICA occlusions may result in the loss of diastolic flow in the CCA.
- ICA may be filled in with plaque or thrombus and horizontal motion with each pulse may be noted in B-mode.
- A "staccato" waveform often indicates that there is downstream occlusion.
- Intracranial ICA occlusion can cause a loss in EDV in the distal ICA

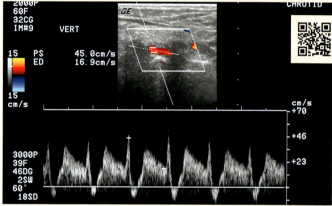

Fig. 13-41: *Early systolic deceleration in the vertebral waveform suggestive of subclavian artery stenosis.*
Image courtesy of Robert Scissions, RVT

It is important to clearly demonstrate that the ICA is occluded and that there is no "trickle" flow present during the duplex scan since carotid endarterectomy is not usually performed on completely occluded ICAs.

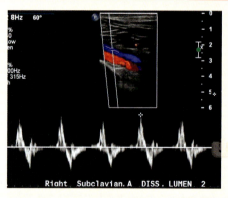

Fig. 13-42: *Dissection of the subclavian artery. Note the flow above and below the baseline in the spectral Doppler waveform*

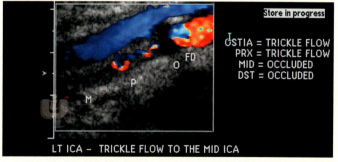

Fig. 13-43: *Trickle flow noted in the ICA. These images represent a functionally occluded ICA or a "string sign."*

Compensatory Flow

- With occlusion or very high grade stenosis on one side, the opposite carotid artery may be feeding both sides of the brain which increases flow, including velocities throughout the CCA, ECA and ICA.
- Sometimes there is no compensatory flow due to other contributions from other collateral systems.
- When compensatory flow is present contralateral to an occlusion, a stenosis may be placed in a higher category based on the absolute velocities alone, e.g., although the stenosis would normally fall into the 50-79% category, the velocities in the stenosis may reach the 80-99% range because the incoming velocities are higher from the compensatory flow state.
- Multiple pieces of evidence identify when a stenosis appears higher due to compensatory flow and should be used in the interpretation:
  » ICA/CCA ratio is in a lower category than the absolute velocity criteria
  » Image measurement is in a lower category than the absolute velocity criteria
  » PSV throughout the CCA is generally higher than normal and higher than the contralateral side
  » The interpretation should indicate which velocities are suspected to be falsely elevated and it should be explained that compensatory flow is the likely cause.

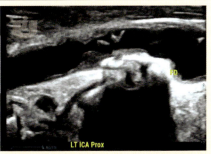
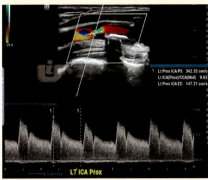
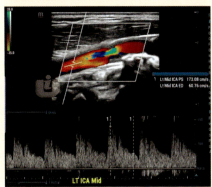

Fig. 13-44: *This series of images represent a high grade stenosis*
Image courtesy of Steve Knight, BSc, RVT, RDMS

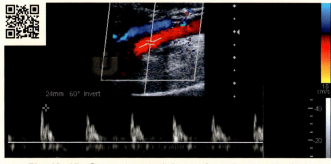

Fig. 13-45: *Staccato arterial waveform (pre-occlusive)*

Use color flow as a guide to identify an occluded artery. But always confirm flow by placing the Doppler sample volume in the vessel lumen.

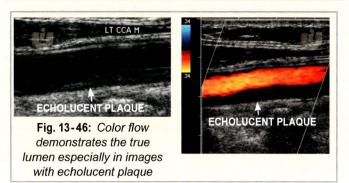

Fig. 13-46: *Color flow demonstrates the true lumen especially in images with echolucent plaque*

The following tables represent popular criteria that may still be used by some labs.

Table 13-5: IAC Updated Recommendations for Carotid Stenosis Interpretation Criteria

	Primary Parameters		Additional Parameters	
Degree of Stenosis (%)	ICA PSV (cm/s)	Plaque Estimate*	ICA/CCA PSV Ratio	ICA EDV (cm/s)
Normal	<180	None	<2.0	<2.0
<50	<180	<50%	<2.0	<2.0
50-69%**	180-230	>50	2.0-4.0	2.0-4.0
>70 but less than near occlusion	>230	>50	>4.0	>100
Near occlusion	High, low or undetectable	Visible	Variable	Variable
Total Occlusion	Undetectable	Visible, No detectable Lumen	Not applicable	Not applicable

*Plaque estimate (diameter reduction) with B-mode and color Doppler US
**PSV 125-180cm/s and ICA/CCA PSV ration ≥2.0 is also consistent with 50-69% stenosis

Modified from diagnostics criteria proposed by Society of Radiologists in Ultrasound (SRU) Consensus Conference IAC. (2023 November). Updated Recommendations for Carotid Stenosis Interpretation Criteria. Intersocietal.org. https://intersocietal.org/wp-content/uploads/2023/11/IAC-Updated-Recommendations-for-Carotid-Stenosis-Interpretation-Criteria_11.1.23.pdf

Table 13-6: University of Washington Diagnostic Criteria for Classification of Internal Carotid Artery Disease

Category	Peak Systolic Velocity	End Diastolic Velocity	Spectral Waveform Characteristics
Normal (0%)	<125cm/s	–	Minimal or no spectral broadening; boundary layer separation present in the carotid bulb
Mild (1-15%)	<125cm/s	–	Spectral broadening during deceleration phase of systole only
Moderate (16-49%)	<125cm/s	–	Spectral broadening throughout systole
Severe (50-79%)	>125cm/s	<140cm/s	Marked spectral broadening
Critical (80-99%)		≥140cm/s	Marked spectral broadening
Occlusion	No Flow	No Flow	No flow signal in the internal carotid artery; decreased diastolic flow in the ipsilateral common carotid artery

ICA/CCA Ratio: >60% >3.2
>70% = >4.0

Moneta GH, Edwards JM, Chitwood RW, et al. Correlation of North American Symptomatic Carotid Endarterectomy Trial (NASCET) angiographic definition of 70-99% internal carotid artery stenosis with duplex scanning. J Vasc Surg. 17:152-159, 1995

Moneta GH, Edwards JM, Papanicolaou G, et al. Screening for asymptomatic internal carotid artery stenosis; duplex criteria for discriminating 60-99% stenosis, J Vasc Surg, 21(6): 989-994, 1995

Table 13-7: University of Chicago Diagnostic Criteria for Classification of Internal Carotid Artery Disease

Category of Disease	Peak Systolic Velocity	End Diastolic Velocity	ICA/CCA Ratio
0-49 %	<155cm/s		<2.0
50-79%	>155cm/s	<140cm/s	>2.0
80-99%	>370cm/s	>140cm/s	>6.0
Occluded	N/A	N/A	N/A

ICA/CCA Ratio: >70% >4.2

Source: Internally validated at the University of Chicago Medical Center Vascular Laboratory.

Table 13-8: Bluth Diagnostic Criteria for Classification of Internal Carotid Artery Disease

Category	PSV	EDV	Systolic Velocity Ratio ICA/CCA	Diastolic Velocity Ratio ICA/CCA	Spectral Broadening (cm/s)
Normal 0%				<2.4	<30
Mild 1-39%	<110	<40	<1.8	<2.4	<40
Moderate 40-59%	<130	<40	<1.8	<2.4	<40
Severe 60-79%	>130	>40	>1.8	>2.4	>40
Critical 80-99%	>250	>100	>3.7	>5.5	>80
Occluded	N/A	N/A	N/A	N/A	N/A

Bluth, EI, Wetzner, SM, Baker, JD, et al: Carotid duplex sonography: a multicenter recommendation for standardized imaging and Doppler criteria. Radiographics 8:487-506, 1988. [19]

Table 13-9: Velocity Criteria Defining Stenoses in the Stented Carotid Artery Compared to Criteria for the Native Carotid Artery

Stenosis %	Stented Carotid Artery	Native Carotid Artery
0-19%	PSV* <150cm/s and ICA/CCA ratio <2.15	PSV <130cm/s
20-49%	PSV 150-219cm/s	PSV 130-189cm/s
50-79%	PSV 220-339cm/s and ICA/CCA ratio ≥2.7	PSV 190-249cm/s and EDV <120cm/s
80-99%	PSV ≥340cm/s and ICA/CCA ratio ≥4.15	PSV ≥250cm/s and EDV <120cm/s, or ICA/CCA ratio ≥3.2

PSV: Peak systolic velocity; EDV: end diastolic velocity; ICA: Internal carotid artery; CCA: common carotid artery. *PSV and EDV measurements for stented carotid arteries are performed within the stented segments.

Lal BK, Hobson II RW, Tofighi B, Kapadia I, Cuadra S, and Jamil Z. Duplex ultrasound velocity criteria for the stented carotid artery. 2007. Journal of Vascular Surgery Volume 47, Number 1. pp 63-73. [17]

Other Pathology

- **Aneurysm:** An aneurysm is defined as a focal enlargement of an artery at least twice the diameter of the proximal segment. Intraluminal thrombus may be observed and is a possible source of distal emboli.[12] PSV are typically reduced with abnormal flow patterns within an aneurysm.[22]

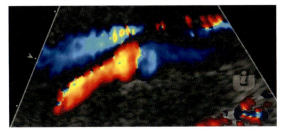

Fig. 13-47: *Mid ICA aneurysm*

- **Arterial dissection:** A dissection of the arterial lumen is recognized by two distinct flow channels by B-mode and/or color Doppler separated by the dissected intima seen as a white line within the lumen. One lumen is known as the "true lumen" while the other is referred to as the "false lumen. Each lumen has a distinctly different flow pattern or one lumen may be occluded.[23]

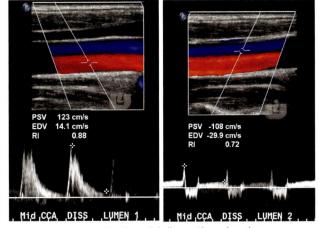

Fig. 13-48: *Arterial dissection showing flow in the true/false lumens.*

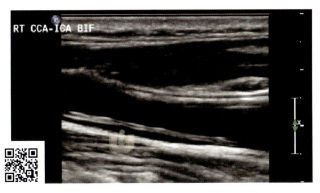

Fig. 13-49: *The double white line in the arterial lumen indicates there is a carotid artery dissection.*

- **Fibromuscular dysplasia:** When a focal or series of hemodynamically significant velocity increases are noted in the mid/distal segment of the ICA accompanied by significant turbulence, FMD is suspected.[20] A "string of beads" is the classic appearance on B-mode and color Doppler images (where segments of the artery can be seen narrowing and then widening in series).[24, 25]

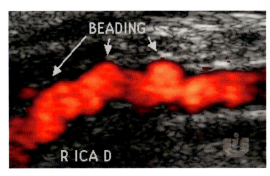

Fig. 13-50: *Typical "string of pearls" sign noted in the ICA*

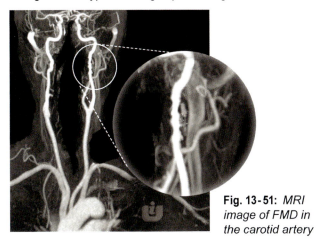

Fig. 13-51: *MRI image of FMD in the carotid artery*

Temporal Arteritis

Normal: Reported diameters for the superficial temporal artery (STA) are about 1.4-2mm normally.

- In one study, the average arterial diameters reported were: common STA 2.03mm; frontal branch, 1.74mm; and parietal branch, 1.83mm.[31]
- Some labs measure the thickness of the "halo" instead. Studies suggest using 0.3-0.6mm as the cut-off measurement for normal halo-thickness.[32, 33]
- Uniform PSV and average arterial diameters do not support the presence of temporal arteritis.

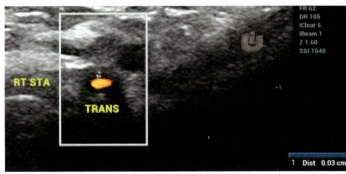

Fig. 13-52: *The "halo" measures 0.3mm in the STA.*

Abnormal: spectral Doppler and increased diameters support the presence of temporal arteritis.

- Arterial diameters are reported to be larger in patients with temporal arteritis.
  - » In one study, the mean (±SD) abnormal diameters were as follows: common superficial temporal artery, 1.7±0.43mm; frontal (1cm distal to the bifurcation), 2.2±0.38mm; and parietal (1.5cm distal to the bifurcation), 2.3±0.38mm.[31]
- A hemodynamically significant lesion (>50%) will result in a focal velocity increase (at least double the velocity in the proximal arterial segment) and post-stenotic turbulence or occlusion.

- Research has suggested abnormal halo thickness >0.3mm.[33] Other studies have suggested using >0.6mm as abnormal.[32]

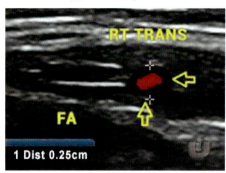

Fig. 13-53: *The hyperechoic area surrounding the artery and increased diameters are suggestive of arteritis.*

Differential Diagnosis for CVA/TIA

- Vasculitis (e.g. arteritis)
- Fibromuscular dysplagia
- Moyamoya disease
- Cerebral hemorrhage
- Carotid artery dissection
- Seizure
- Lupus
- Metabolic problems (e.g., glucose derangement)
- Migraines
- Cardiac embolization
- Nonatherosclerotic vasculopathy
- Systemic infections
- Mass lesions
- Intracranial tumor
  » Primary central nervous system (CNS)
  » Metastatic subdural hematoma
- Cerebral abscess
- Multiple sclerosis
- Alcohol or drug abuse
- Cardiac failure
- Syncope
- Positional vertigo

Correlation

- Spiral CT scan
- MRA
- MRI
- Cerebral arteriography

Medical Treatment

- Modify risk factors (e.g., Smoking cessation, lower cholesterol, etc.)
- Statin therapy
- Antithrombotics
- Tissue plasminogen activator (TPA) therapy: to treat ischemic stroke, within three hours of onset of symptoms
- Anticoagulation (e.g., Warfarin)

Surgical Treatment

- Carotid endarterectomy
- ICA resection and reanastomosis (for kinking)
- Carotid thrombectomy
- Bypass (subclavian-carotid or carotid-carotid)
- Vertebral artery transposition to CCA
- Vertebral artery reconstruction
- Direct focal repairs (e.g., subclavian artery, vertebral)

NASCET (North American Symptomatic Carotid Endarterectomy Trial) demonstrated that the long-term benefit of CEA was significantly greater than medical treatment in symptomatic patients with >70% stenosis.[26]

ACAS (Asymptomatic Carotid Atherosclerosis Study) demonstrated marginal benefit of carotid endarterectomy in asymptomatic male patients with >60% stenosis.[27]

Endovascular Treatment

- Carotid angioplasty
- Carotid stent

CREST was the largest randomized clinical trial for patients at risk for stroke from carotid artery disease due to either CEA or carotid stent placement with embolic protection.

REFERENCES

1. Zarins CK, Xu C, Glagov, S. (2005). Artery wall pathology in atherosclerosis. In Rutherford Vascular Surgery 6th edition. (123-148). Philadelphia. Elsevier Saunders.
2. Henderson, E. L., Y.-J. Geng, et al. (1999). "Death of Smooth Muscle Cells and Expression of Mediators of Apoptosis by T Lymphocytes in Human Abdominal Aortic Aneurysms." Circulation 99(1): 96-104.
3. Black JH, Cambria RP. (2005). Aortic dissection: perspectives for the vascular/endovascular surgeon. In Rutherford Vascular Surgery 6th edition. (1512-1533). Philadelphia. Elsevier Saunders.
4. Kupinski, Anne Marie (2013) In The Vascular System 1st edition (p 66, 81), Philadelphia. Wolters Kluwer.
5. Shepard RJ, Rooke T. (2005). Uncommon arteriopathies. In Rutherford Vascular Surgery 6th edition. (453-474). Philadelphia. Elsevier Saunders.
6. Young JR, Graor RA, Olin JW, Bartholomew JR. (1991). "Vasospastic disease" in Peripheral Vascular Diseases. (361-378). St Louis : Mosby Elsevier Health Science.
7. Rowe VL, Yellin AE, Weaver FA. (2005). Vascular injuries of the extremities. In Rutherford Vascular Surgery 6th edition. (1044-1058). Philadelphia. Elsevier Saunders.
8. Hom C. (8-25-2010). "Takayasu's arteritis" Emedicine.medscape.com. http://emedicine.medscape.com/article/1007566-overview (12-4-2010).
9. Hajj-Ali RA, Mandell B. (2005). Approach to and management of inflammatory vasculitis. In Rajagopalan S, Mukherjee D, Mohler E. (Eds). Manual of Vascular Diseases. (353-375). Philadelphia. Lippinott Williams & Wilkins.
10. Basu N, Watts R., et al. (2010). "EULAR points to consider in the development of classification and diagnostic criteria in systemic vasculitis." Annals of the Rheumatic Diseases 69(10): 1744-1750.
11. Krupski WC. (2005). Uncommon disorders affecting the carotid arteries. In Rutherford Vascular Surgery 6th edition. (2064-2092). Philadelphia. Elsevier Saunders.
12. Saldana, M. J., L. E. Salem, et al. (1973). "High altitude hypoxia and chemodectomas." Human Pathology 4(2): 251-263.
13. Sumner DS, Zierler RE. (2005). Vascular physiology: essential hemodynamic principles. In Rutherford Vascular Surgery 6th edition. (75-123). Philadelphia. Elsevier Saunders.
14. Casey PJ, LaMuraglia GM. (2005). Anastomotic aneurysms. In Rutherford Vascular Surgery 6th edition. (894-902). Philadelphia. Elsevier Saunders.
15. Shepard RJ, Rooke T. (2005). Uncommon arteriopathies. In Rutherford Vascular Surgery 6th edition. (453-474). Philadelphia. Elsevier Saunders.
16. Zieler, R. Eugene (2010) In Strandness's Duplex Scanning in Vascular Disorders. 4th edition (93, 100, 117-121), Philadelphia. Wolters Kluwer.
17. Lal BK, Hobson II RW, Tofighi B, Kapadia I, Cuadra S, and Jamil Z. Duplex ultrasound velocity criteria for the stented carotid artery. 2007. Journal of vascular surgery Volume 47, Number 1. pp 63-73.
18. Grant, E., Benson, C., et al, Carotid Artery Stenosis: Gray-Scale and Doppler US Diagnosis—Society of Radiologists in Ultrasound Consensus Conference, Radiology 229 (2): 340-346, 2003.
19. Bluth, EI, Wetzner, SM, Baker, JD, et al: Carotid duplex sonography: a multicenter recommendation for standardized imaging and Doppler criteria. Radiographics 8:487-506, 1988.
20. Karnik, S. K., B. S. Brooke, et al. (2003). "A critical role for elastin signaling in vascular morphogenesis and disease." Development 130(2): 411-423.
21. Krettek, A., G. K. Sukhova, et al. (2003). "Elastogenesis in human arterial disease: a role for macrophages in disordered elastin synthesis." Arteriosclerosis, thrombosis, and vascular biology 23(4):582-587.
22. Patel, M. I., J. Melrose, et al. (1996). "Increased synthesis of matrix metalloproteinases by aortic smooth muscle cells is implicated in the etiopathogenesis of abdominal aortic aneurysms." Journal of Vascular Surgery 24(1): 82-92.
23. Henderson, E. L., Y.-J. Geng, et al. (1999). "Death of Smooth Muscle Cells and Expression of Mediators of Apoptosis by T Lymphocytes in Human Abdominal Aortic Aneurysms." Circulation 99(1): 96-104.
24. López-Candales A, Holmes DR, Liao S, Scott MJ, Wickline SA, Thompson RW. Decreased vascular smooth muscle cell density in medial degeneration of human abdominal aortic aneurysms. (1997). Am J Pathol. March; 150(3): 993–1007.
25. Hellmann, D. B., D. J. Grand, et al. (2007). "Inflammatory Abdominal Aortic Aneurysm." JAMA: The Journal of the American Medical Association 297(4): 395-400.
26. Young JR, Graor RA, Olin JW, Bartholomew JR. (1991). Miscellaneous arterial disease" in Peripheral Vascular Diseases. (379-394). St Louis :Mosby Elsevier Health Science.
27. Walker, MD, Marler JR, Goldstein M, Grady PA, Toole JF, Baker WH, Castaldo JE, Chambless LE, Moore WS, Robertson JT, Young B, Howard VJ, Marler JR, Ourvis S, Vernon D, Needham K, Beck P, Celani VJ, Sauebeck L, von Rajcs JA, Atkins D. Endarterectomy for Asymptomatic Carotid Artery Stenosis JAMA 1995; 273: 1421-1428.
28. Watts RA, and Scott DGL, (2010). Classification and Epidemiology of Vasculitis in Clinical Practice. R. A. Watts and D. G. I. Scott, Springer London: 7-11.
29. Basu N, Watts R., et al. (2010). "EULAR points to consider in the development of classification and diagnostic criteria in systemic vasculitis." Annals of the Rheumatic Diseases 69(10): 1744-1750.
30. Johns Hopkins Vasculitis Clinic "Giant cell arteritis" Johns Hopkins Medicine (2009).http://vasculitis.med.jhu.edu/types of/giantcell.html (12-4-2010).
31. Schmidt, W. A., Kraft, H. E., Vorpahl, K., Völker, L., & Gromnica-Ihle, E. J. (1997). Color duplex ultrasonography in the diagnosis of temporal arteritis. The New England journal of medicine, 337(19), 1336–1342. https://doi.org/10.1056/NEJM199711063371902
32. Kaandorp, B. I., Raterman, H. G., Stam, F., Gamala, M., Meijer-Jorna, L. B., Kalb, F. B., & Wallis, J. W. (2024). Determination of the Value of Color Doppler Ultrasound in Patients With a Clinical Suspicion of Giant Cell Arteritis. ACR open rheumatology, 6(2), 56–63.
33. Pouncey, A. L., Yeldham, G., Magan, T., Lucenteforte, E., Jaffer, U., & Virgili, G. (2024). Halo sign on temporal artery ultrasound versus temporal artery biopsy for giant cell arteritis. The Cochrane database of systematic reviews, 2(2), CD013199.

CEREBROVASCULAR TESTING
14. Carotid Intima-Media Thickness

Definition
The use of real time B-mode ultrasonography to identify areas of increased thickness along the lumen-intima and media-adventitia interfaces of an extracranial carotid artery in order to predict early atherosclerosis or classify patients with cardiovascular disease (CVD). CIMT testing is sometimes used in clinical trials to help determine if there is any benefit to certain drugs or treatment for cardiovascular disease.

Carotid intima-media thickness (CIMT) has been shown to be associated with increased risk of myocardial infarction (MI), stroke and/or death from heart disease. [1,5,6] There is a link between greater CIMT and more extensive/severe cases of coronary heart disease. CIMT testing is used to predict major critical CVD events in symptomatic and asymptomatic patients, with and without prevalent CVD. [1,7] CMIT varies across race, region, age and sex. Values are typically higher in African and Americans than in Asians and Eastern Mediterranean populations. Normal values are higher in males than females. [9]

The common carotid artery is typically used for this evaluation since it is often free of plaque. The clear interface between the anechoic arterial lumen and the echoic intima makes definition of these interfaces and opportunity for measurement possible.

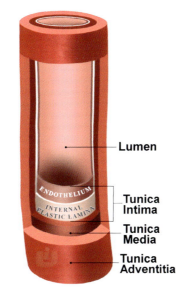

Fig. 14-1: *Arterial wall anatomy*

Etiology (of carotid atherosclerosis)
- Endothelial dysfunction
- Hemodynamic forces

CIMT testing is a cardiovascular risk assessment tool and should not be used as a substitute for a clinically indicated carotid ultrasound duplex exam. [1]

Risk Factors (to predict cardiovascular risk)
- Genetic predisposition
- Gender (Males >Females)
- Race
- Obesity
- Smoking
- Diabetes
- Radiation therapy

Indications for Exam
- History of early cardiovascular disease in an immediate family member (men <55 years and women <65 years of age). [1,2]
- Patients younger than 60 years of age who are not candidates for drug therapy but have severe abnormalities involving a single risk factor. [1]
- Women, younger than 60 years of age with >2 CVD risk factors. [1]

Imaging should not be performed in patients with known significant atherosclerotic disease or if results would not alter patient management. [1]

Contraindications/Limitations
- Suboptimal visualization by B-mode image (including, but not limited to the lack of visible "double line" along the far arterial wall, motion artifact from the jugular vein or deep vessels).
- Tortuous carotid arteries
- Intraobserver variability of CIMT measurements range between 3.7-7.8% according to published data. [2]

Location (of arteries for testing)
- Distal common carotid artery (most common)
- Carotid bifurcation
- Proximal internal carotid artery

Patient History

Increased CIMT has been associated with higher risks for peripheral vascular disease and stroke. [2]

- CVD
- Risk factors for CVD [3]
  » Hypertension
  » Hyperlipidemia
  » Diabetes
  » Obesity
  » Sedentary lifestyle
  » Smoking
  » Stress
  » Poor diet

Physical Examination
- Carotid bruit (abnormal sound heard through auscultation caused by vibration of tissue from turbulent flow).

Carotid Intima-Media Thickness (CIMT) Protocol

CIMT evaluation using B-mode imaging is preferred over M-mode imaging since B-mode provides better perpendicular images and is capable of providing thickness values for longer segments of the artery, rather than just a single point. [1]

- The patient is examined in the supine position with the head elevated.
- Some patients may require the use of a range of transducers for superficial vessels including high frequency, linear-array (5-7 MHz) (8-15 MHz) transducers.
- The typical depth used for scanning is 4cm, although increased depths may be necessary in patients with deeper arteries or larger necks.
- Optimize the B-mode image by making adjustments to the TGC to obtain a clear image of the anterior-posterior intimal interfaces between the lumen and vessel walls. Manually adjust additional settings such as the overall gain, focal zone (single is preferred), dynamic range (high), persistence and harmonics so near and far walls of the endothelium are clearly defined.
- Evaluate the common carotid artery (CCA), carotid bifurcation and internal carotid artery (ICA) for any carotid plaque with B-mode and color imaging in both the transverse (short-axis) and longitudinal (sagittal) planes. Adjust the color scale to accurately fill the arterial lumen around any observed plaque without resulting in color-bleeding.

> CIMT measurements should be performed using the far wall of the carotid artery. Near-wall CIMT is less accurate since the US beam has to travel from a more echogenic to a less echogenic interface. An ultrasound phantom is suggested to ensure accurate resolution of the transducer. [1]

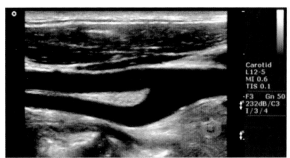

Fig. 14-2: B-mode image of the carotid bifurcation
Courtesy of Philips Healthcare

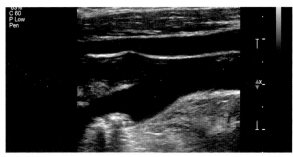

Fig. 14-3: Plaque noted by B-mode imaging
Courtesy of Philips Healthcare

- Document and report the location of carotid plaque (e.g., near/far wall, proximal/mid or distal CCA segment). Report the presence of any calcific arterial shadowing which may result in technically suboptimal images.

> A carotid plaque has been defined as CIMT ≥1.5mm or ≥50% of the surrounding IMT by the Manheim Intima Media Thickness Consensus Panel. Some physicians consider CIMT >1.0mm as a significant plaque. [6]

- Measure and record the peak systolic velocity (PSV) of the CCA and ICA in longitudinal view using spectral Doppler (60° Doppler angle or less, with the angle cursor parallel to the vessel walls in the center of the flow stream).
- Identify a straight segment of the distal CCA in the longitudinal plane, approximately 1cm from the flow divider. Using the heel-toe transducer method, align the CCA so that the artery is perfectly horizontal on the ultrasound screen. Optimize the B-mode image to see the characteristic "double line" representing the lumen-intima-and media-adventitia interfaces. In cases where the wall interfaces are suboptimal, you can trace a segment <1cm in length. Do not trace any interfaces that are not clearly visualized.

> (ASE consensus) Histologic studies have confirmed that the two echogenic lines produced by B-mode imaging correspond to the lumina-intima and media-adventitia interfaces.

> Repeat measurements should be within 0.05mm of each other.

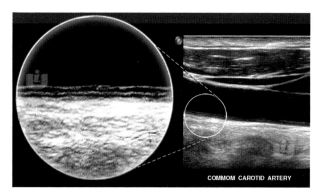

Fig. 14-4: Characteristic "double line" between the lumen-intima and media-adventitia interfaces
Courtesy of Philips Healthcare

- Record loops or still frames of this distal CCA segment using each of the carotid scan windows: anterior, anterio-lateral and posterior-lateral. Loops should consist of 3-5 cardiac cycles.

> To prevent image degradation, digital images (e.g., DICOM) are preferred for analysis over digitized video capture. [1]

- Capture an image of the arterial wall when systolic-diastolic differences are at a minimum (during end-diastole). Capture multiple images of the distal CCA, concentrating on image optimization of the far-wall.
- Repeat the protocol for the contralateral carotid arteries.
- Use a manual or semiautomated border detection measuring technique to determine the CIMT value. It may be necessary to edit suboptimal borders generated by the automated programs.

> Semiautomated border detection software is thought to improve reproducibility and shorten reading time. Some critics of automated programs believe CIMT are thicker than those measured manually with or without electronic calipers. [1]

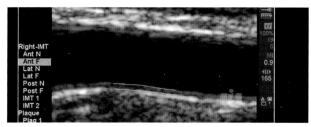

Fig. 14-5: Manual CIMT trace method

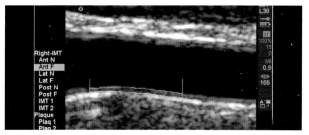

Fig. 14-6: Auto CIMT trace method *Image courtesy of SonoSite FUJIFILM*

- Using the best images recorded, trace the intima and media adventitia interfaces of the far-wall. Using 1cm length segments, repeat these measurements multiple times to ensure accuracy.
- Report the CIMT as an average of all of the recorded values. Mean CIMT values should also be reported using both right and left carotid data.

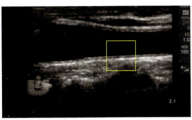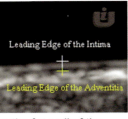

Fig. 14-7: *"Double-line" noted on the far wall of the carotid artery by B-mode imaging.* Image courtesy of SonoSite FUJIFILM

Table 14-1: Carotid Intima-Media Thickness Protocol at a Glance

1. Evaluate the CCA, bifurcation and ICA for disease in the transverse and longitudinal planes using B-mode and color imaging. Record representative images.
   - Record B-mode and color images. Document and describe the location of any carotid plaque.
   - Record representative spectral Doppler waveforms of the CCA and ICA.
2. Identify a relatively straight segment of the distal CCA in the longitudinal plane, approximately 1cm proximal to the flow divider and optimize visualization of the "double lined" far-arterial wall.
3. Record loops/stills of the distal CCA segment from three scan windows; anterior, anteriolateral and posteriolateral.
4. Repeat the protocol for the contralateral carotid artery.
5. Measure CIMT using manual or semiautomated detection software.
6. Report the average CIMT values for each side.

PRINCIPLES OF INTERPRETATION

- CIMT increases nearly 3-fold between the ages of 20 and 90 years of age.[1]
- Research shows that CIMT increases linearly with age from a mean value of 0.48 at age 40 to 1.02 by age 100.[4]

$$(0.009 \times age) + 0.116 = mean\ CIMT$$

"CIMT measurements have not been proven to be particularly precise and are best reported as a range in order to account for technical differences (e.g., instrumentation and techniques) since the US beam has to travel from a more echogenic to a less echogenic interface."
American Society of Echocardiography (ASE)

Interpretation/Diagnostic Criteria

- CIMT values less than or equal to the 25th percentile are considered at low-risk for cardiovascular disease (CVD).[1,5]
- CIMT values in the 25th-75th percentile are considered average and suggest no change in CVD risk.[1,5]
- CIMT values greater than the 75th percentile are considered elevated and suggest increased risk of CVD.[1,5]

A mean CMIT of 0.65mm was reported in one study for men in the 25th percentile with a mean CMIT of 0.84mm for men in the 75th percentile. In the same study, the value for women in the 25th percentile was 0.58mm and 0.74mm in the 75th percentile.[10]

Table 14-2: CIMT Diagnostic Criteria

Description	IMT
Normal	<0.8
Abnormal	>0.8

Age, gender and race should be documented for risk assessment.

Source: Stein JH, Fraizer MC, et al. (2004). Vascular age: Integrating carotid intima-media thickness measurements with global coronary risk assessment. *Clin Cardiol.* (388-392) 27.

Table 14-3: Risk for CVD Based on CIMT Values

Risk of CVD	CIMT value (in percentile)
Low	≤25th
Average	25-75th
High	>75th

Source: Stein JH MD FASE, Korcarz CE DVM RDCS FASE, Hurst RT MD, Lonn E MD MSc FASE, Kendall CB BS RDCS, Mohler ER MD, Najjar SS MD, Remboldcm MD, Post WS MD MS. (2008). Use of carotid ultrasound to identify subclinical vascular disease and evaluate cardiovascular risk: A consensus statement from the American society of echocardiography carotid intima-media thickness task force endorsed by the society for vascular medicine. *Journal of the American Society of Echocardiography* Feb; 21(2):93-106.

Correlation

- CT scan to measure coronary artery calcification score. CAC scoring (coronary artery calcium).
- Transesophageal echocardiography (TEE)
- Intravascular ultrasound (IVUS) during arteriography
- MRI yield similar results to DUS and is said to be highly reproducible.[11]

Medical Treatment

- Statin therapy
- Modify risk factors (e.g., reduce cholesterol/HTN, manage DM, smoking cessation)
- Exercise regimen
- Antihypertensive medication

REFERENCES

1. Stein JH MD FASE, Korcarz CE DVM RDCS FASE, Hurst RT MD, Lonn E MD MSc FASE, Kendall CB BS RDCS, Mohler ER MD, Najjar SS MD, Remboldcm MD, Post WS MD MS. (2008). Use of carotid ultrasound to identify subclinical vascular disease and evaluate cardiovascular risk: A consensus statement from the American society of echocardiography carotid intima-media thickness task force endorsed by the society for vascular medicine. Journal of the American Society of Echocardiography. Feb; 21(2):93-106.
2. Leon Jr, LR, Brewster LP, Labropoulos N. (2005). Non-invasive screening and utility of carotid intima-media thickness. In Mansour MA, Labropoulos N. (Eds.), Vascular Diagnosis. (157-173). Philadelphia: Elsevier Saunders.
3. National Heart Lung and Blood Institute. (12/3/2011 10:58 PM). Retrieved from http://www.nhlbi.nih.gov/.
4. Zwiebel, WJ. Pellerito JS. (2005). Ultrasound assessment of carotid plaque. In Zwiebel WJ, Pellerito JS (Eds.), In Introduction to Vascular Ultrasonography 5th ed, (155-169). Philadelphia: Elsevier Saunders.
5. Nambi J MD, Chambless L PhD, Folsom AR MD, He M, Hu Y, Mosley T PhD, Volcik V PhD, Boerwinkle F PhD, Ballantynecm MD. Carotid intima-media thickness and presence or absence of plaque improves prediction of coronary heart disease risk in the Atherosclerosis Risk in Communities (ARIC) study. (2010). J Am Coll Cardiol. 2010 April 13; 55(15): 1600–1607.
6. Cobble M, Bale B (2010). Carotid intima-media thickness: knowledge and application to everyday practice. Postgrad Med. Jan; 122 (1): 10-8.
7. Tabor A RVT, Size GP RVT RVS RPhS FSVU (2007). What is IMT? Sonosite. PowerPoint slides].
8. Carotid intima-media thickness and presence or absence of plaque improves prediction of coronary heart disease risk in the Atherosclerosis Risk in Communities (ARIC) study. Nambi V, Chambless L, Folsom AR, He M, Hu Y, Mosley T, Volcik K, Boerwinkle E, and Ballantynecm, Am Coll Cardiol. 2010 April 13; 55(15): 1600–1607. doi:10.1016/j.jacc.2009.11.075.
9. Abeysuriya V, Perera BPR, Wickremasinghe AR (2022) Regional and demographic variations of Carotid artery Intima and Media Thickness (CIMT): A Systematic review and meta-analysis. PLOS ONE 17(7): e0268716. https://doi.org/10.1371/journal.pone.0268716
10. Nambi, V., Chambless, L., Folsom, A. R., He, M., Hu, Y., Mosley, T., Volcik, K., Boerwinkle, E., & Ballantyne, C. M. (2010). Carotid intima-media thickness and presence or absence of plaque improves prediction of coronary heart disease risk: the ARIC (Atherosclerosis Risk In Communities) study. Journal of the American College of Cardiology, 55(15), 1600–1607.
11. Doneen, A. L., & Bale, B. F. (2013). Carotid intima-media thickness testing as an asymptomatic cardiovascular disease identifier and method for making therapeutic decisions. Postgraduate medicine, 125(2), 108–123. https://doi.org/10.3810/pgm.2013.03.2645
12. Doneen, A. L., & Bale, B. F. (2013). Carotid intima-media thickness testing as an asymptomatic cardiovascular disease identifier and method for making therapeutic decisions. Postgraduate medicine, 125(2), 108–123. https://doi.org/10.3810/pgm.2013.03.2645

Fig. 15-1: *Circle of Willis Posterior View*

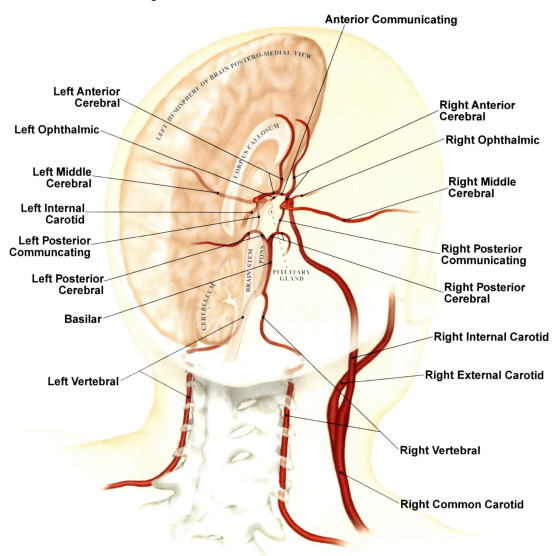

Definition

Intracranial cerebrovascular testing is performed to assess arterial patency and measure flow velocities within the Circle of Willis using transcranial Doppler (TCD) or transcranial imaging (TCI). The hemodynamic effects of stenosis or occlusion can be studied in real-time.

TCD and TCI are able to determine the extent and patterns of collateral circulation in patients with known cerebrovascular disease and can be used to monitor patients with vasospasm after subarachnoid hemorrhage and detect embolic events (e.g., during surgery).

Transcranial testing can help surgeons detect hyperperfusion syndrome post-CEA; symptoms include headache, seizure and intracranial hemorrhage.[1,18] Preoperative screening (e.g., CO_2 challenge) and post-operative monitoring can be useful tools to identify patients at-risk.[22]

Rationale

TCD uses range-gated spectral Doppler to penetrate "windows" or openings through the cranium and assess intracranial cerebrovascular blood flow. TCI adds imaging and utilizes color flow as a guide during the examination.

Etiology of Intracranial Disease

- Atherosclerosis, resulting in stenosis or occlusion
- Embolus
- Thrombosis
- Vasculitis
- Carotid aneurysm
- Carotid dissection (spontaneous or post-traumatic)
- Arteriovenous malformations (AVM)
- Non-atherosclerotic causes; e.g., carotid coiling or kinking
- Fibromuscular dysplasia (FMD)

Fig. 15-2: *Most Common Variations of the Circle of Willis*

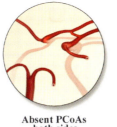
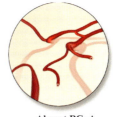
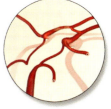

| Absent ACA (A1) 25% | Absent ACoA 1% | Absent PCoA one side 9% | Absent PCoAs both sides 9% | Absent PCoA and contralateral PCA (P1) | Absent PCA (P1) fetal origin 9% |

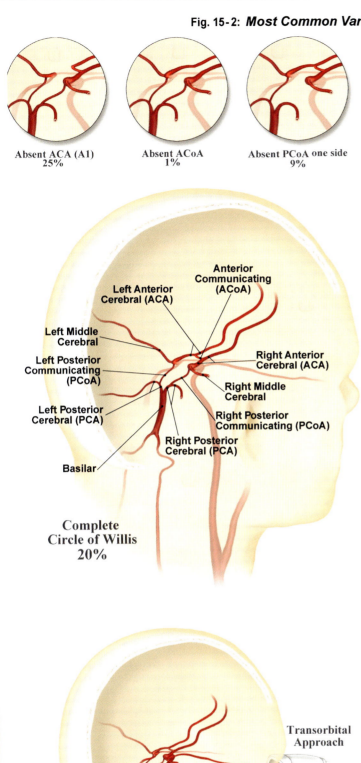

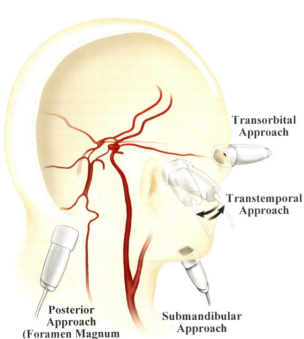

Fig. 15-3: *Acoustical windows used in transcranial testing*

Risk Factors
- Hypertension
- Hypercholesteremia
- Diabetes
- Smoking
- Age
- Gender (Male >Female)
- History of peripheral vascular disease (PVD)
- History of coronary artery disease (CAD) or atrial fibrillation (A-fib)
- History of cerebrovascular disease (CVA, TIA, subarachnoid hemorrhage or intracranial aneurysm)
- Vasculitis
- Family history
- Trauma, especially to the cranium

Indications for Exam
- Detect hemodynamically significant stenosis (>65%) of the intracranial cerebral arteries
- Assess collateral circulation in patients with regions of known severe disease
- Determine the effects of hemodynamically significant stenosis/occlusion of the extracranial arteries on intracranial circulation
- Evaluate patients with cerebral vasospasm (e.g., subarachnoid hemorrhage patients)
- Detect AVM and determine flow patterns and supplying arterial flow
- Suspected intracranial aneurysm
- Embolism detection during operative procedures. Middle cerebral arterial (MCA) flow is monitored during carotid endarterectomy (CEA) and other revascularization procedures, such as cardiac surgery.
- Detection of cerebral ischemia during surgery (e.g., when cross-clamping)
- Detection and management of post-operative hyperemia
- Suspected carotid dissection, post-angiography
- Evaluation of pediatric patients with various blood vessel disease such as sickle cell disease, Moyamoya disease, etc. to assess the risk of stroke (CVA)
- Evaluate vasomotor reserve (VMR) with the use of CO_2 challenge testing
- Detection of right to left cardiac or pulmonary shunts using bubble studies (e.g., patent foramen ovale (PFO))

Although transesophageal echo (TEE) is the current gold-standard for detecting PFO, but a study by Palazzo from 2019 suggests a TCD bubble study may be more sensitive for detecting some PFO. [34]

- Evaluate intracranial flow, post-cranial injury
- Evaluate patients for suspected brain death

Contraindications/Limitations

- Inadequate cranial windows preventing insonation of the Circle of Willis
  » Thicker (skull) bone may inhibit visualization through the transtemporal window in older, especially female and/or African American patients. This condition is referred to as *hyperkeratosis* and is caused by increased density and thickness of the skull. [1,18]

Visualization through the transtemporal window may be technically difficult in 10-15% of cases. [23]

- Uncooperative or agitated patients (e.g., post-operative, patients with cranial injury or some pediatric patients, etc.)
- Exams can be time consuming.
- Exams can be limited due to severity of the patient's condition or poor patient positioning.
- Since the Circle of Willis anatomy can vary and TCD does not involve direct imaging, incorrect identification of vessels is possible.
- TCI is dependent on color flow. Vessel walls are not well visualized.
- Spectral Doppler can produce aliasing in very high-grade intracranial stenoses.
- Collaterals or vasospasms can be misinterpreted as a stenosis.
- Transcranial testing is not sensitive for smaller intracranial aneurysms.
- Recent eye surgery may be a contraindication for imaging through the transorbital window.
- Patients with SAH and craniotomies will usually have bandaging covering their transtemporal windows which will need to be loosened in order to gain access for transcranial testing.

Circle of Willis

The Circle of Willis refers to the intracranial arteries. The polygonal shape of this "circle" allows blood to flow between the right and left hemispheres of the brain. There is an anterior (carotid) and posterior (vertebrobasilar) supply to the Circle of Willis.

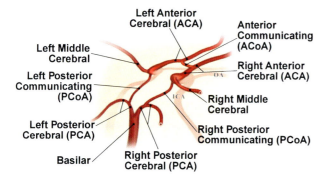

Location of the intracranial windows and their accessible arteries

There are several acoustic windows used to access the intracranial vessels. These are thinner areas or openings (*foramina*) of the cranium that transcranial testing uses to visualize the following arteries:

- Transorbital
  » OA (Orbital Artery)
  » Carotid siphon
- Transtemporal
  » MCA (Middle Cerebral Artery)
  » ACA (Anterior Cerebral Artery)
  » MCA-ACA bifurcation
  » PCA (Posterior Cerebral Artery)
  » tICA (Terminal Internal Carotid Artery (ICA))
  » ACoA and/or PCoA when functioning as collateral pathways (Anterior and Posterior Communicating Arteries)
- Submandibular (retromandibular)
  » Distal cervical portion of the ICA
- Transforaminal (suboccipital)
  » VA (Vertebral Arteries)
  » BA (Basilar Artery)

Staples, bandaging, scar tissue, etc. may limit scan windows.

Mechanism of Disease

Examples of cerebrovascular disease include aneurysm and stroke. An aneurysm of the intracranial arteries occurs due to weakening of the arterial wall. Stroke is defined as a temporary or permanent loss of function or consciousness caused by an interruption in blood flow. Atherosclerosis causes stenosis or occlusion which can lead to such a disruption in blood flow, damaging brain tissue. (*See the Arterial Vascular Diseases chapter for a detailed description of atherosclerosis and plaque evolution.*) Arterial rupture or venous malformation results in another type of stroke (hemorrhagic). When the patient experiences a permanent neurological deficit (motor, sensory, speech deficit, etc.) it is known as a completed stroke or CVA (cerebrovascular accident). A TIA (transient ischemic attack) is any deficit lasting less than 24 hours.

Common types of stroke are ischemic and hemorrhagic. Symptoms or deficits can be permanent (CVA) or temporary (transient ischemic attack). [5,6]

Ischemic Stroke

- Most common (approximately 87% of all strokes). This stroke is due to a decrease in blood flow to the brain caused by an arterial narrowing or blockage. Sub classification of ischemic stroke include:
  » **Cardioembolic (embolic):** an embolus from a cardiac or pericardiac source causes a territorial infarction. The most common cause is atrial fibrillation, where there is pooling of the blood in the heart which can lead to the formation of blood clots. Plaque or fragments of an organized thrombus loosen and flow upstream. Emboli become lodged in a distant blood vessel, causing arterial occlusion and reduction of flow.
  » **Large Vessel Atherosclerosis:** (atherothrombotic), Occlusion or stenosis >50% of the major intra- and extracranial arteries (internal carotid, common carotid, vertebral, basilar, middle cerebral, anterior cerebral or posterior cerebral) supplying the vascular territory of the stroke. Decrease in lumenal area due to atherosclerosis and/or thrombosis.
  » **Lacunar:** (Small vessel disease) account for approximately 25% of all acute ischemic strokes. [6,7] Lacunar infarcts are small infarcts (3-20mm in diameter) in the deeper noncortical parts of the cerebrum and brainstem. They result from occlusion or stenosis of penetrating branches of the large cerebral arteries.

- » **Stroke of other determined etiology:** these rare cases normally occur in the young who have no stroke risk factors. They include coagulopathies, vasculopathies, genetic disorders and metabolic disorders.
- » **Stroke of undetermined etiology:** In a significant number of cases (≤40%), no clear explanation can be found for an ischemic stroke despite an extensive diagnostic evaluation.

Hemorrhagic Stroke *(approximately 15% of all strokes)*

- Occurs due to arterial rupture or venous malformation in the brain. Blood accumulates and compresses the surrounding brain tissue. In addition, there is no or little blood flow distal to the rupture site. Hemorrhagic strokes are classified as either subarachnoid hemorrhage or intracerebral hemorrhage:
  - » **Subarachnoid Hemorrhage (SAH):** most commonly due to trauma but also occur due to rupture of a cerebral aneurysm. In 10-20% of spontaneous, nontraumatic cases no cause is found.
  - » **Intracerebral Hemorrhage:** (parenchymatous) Rupture of a blood vessel within the parenchyma often the result of chronic hypertension or an intrinsic vessel problem such as amyloid angiopathy or other vascular malformation. May also be caused by a brain tumor.

The incidence of SAH in the United States is approximately 25,000 to 30,000 cases yearly. There is an 1.5-3 fold increased risk of death during the first 2 weeks after SAH. TCD has been shown to identify this condition 1-2 days before the patient becomes symptomatic, which can expedite treatment. [19,20]

Transient Ischemic Attack

- The cerebral blood supply is blocked for a limited amount of time and the patient's symptoms last less than 24 hours. A TIA is often thought to be a warning for future stroke.

The mechanism of disease for other cerebrovascular events include:

- **Vasospasm:** decreased perfusion caused by a gradual constriction of cerebral arterial flow in the subarachnoid space following subarachnoid hemorrhage (SAH). Narrowing of the cerebral arteries usually begins 2-4 days after the SAH and can last for up to 3 weeks. Normal arterial wall vasodilatation/ vasoconstriction is disrupted due to the changes in metabolism and arterial wall structure. A higher risk of cerebral infarction exists due to the constricted arterial flow caused by the surrounding blood clot. [8] Vasospasm increases vascular resistance along with the decrease in blood flow. [25]
- **Vasculitis:** hyperactivity of the immune system causing inflammation of the vessel walls. Inflammation can lead to arterial narrowing and a subsequent decrease in cerebral perfusion.
- **Intracerebral Aneurysm:** Aneurysmal disease results from weakening of the structural proteins (elastin and collagen) within the medial layer of the arterial wall. Large aneurysms can constrict surrounding arterial flow and also carry the risk of rupture, subsequent SAH and cerebral infarct. The basilar artery bifurcation, vertebral artery junction and ACoA are areas prone to aneurysmal formation because of the high wall sheer stress, hydrostatic and translumenal pressures through these segments. Also, individuals with an incomplete Circle of Willis may also have a higher risk for aneurysmal formation since there is greater flow resistance through their arterial pathways. [9]

Transcranial imaging can be used to study the effects of temporary vessel occlusion when treating patients with tumors, fistulas or aneurysms.

- **Carotid Dissection:** tears in the intimal layer of the arterial wall allowing blood flow to access the carotid media. Trauma can cause a dissection, though it also occurs due to aging or connective tissue disorders when the breakdown of collagen and elastin fibers, render the arterial wall weak and at risk for tears. [10,13] Blood flows through the tear in the intimal layer and sometimes clots. Pulsatile flow and high blood pressure cause propagation of the dissection. [10] Dissection between the medial and adventitial layers may result in a false lumen, which can narrow the true carotid lumen. [10]
- **Arteriovenous Malformations:** abnormal connection between an artery and vein where blood flows directly from the artery into the venous system without passing through the tissues and capillary bed. The exact cause of AVM is unknown. AVM can be a congenital condition, with the onset of symptoms occurring at any age.
- **Carotid Coiling/Kinking:** Coils and kinks are thought to normally be present during the embryonic stage of development. The arteries typically straighten once the fetal heart and larger vessels descend into the thoracic cavity. In some patients, these coils/kinks linger. [11] Intralumenal folds involving all three arterial layers have been observed on histological study along with increased fibrous tissue, and a loss of elastic tissue and smooth muscle cell within the medial layer. Some believe that atherosclerotic occlusive disease must be present before patients with coils/kinks become symptomatic. [12]
- **Sickle Cell Disease (SCD)** is a hereditary condition primarily affecting pediatric patients. Sickle cell anemia carries a significant risk of stroke in children before the age of 20 years. [26]
- **Fibromuscular Dysplasia:** non-atherosclerotic arterial disease which affects medium and large-sized vessels, including the internal carotid artery (ICA). A significant decrease in blood flow through the ICA can result in decreased cerebral perfusion.
- **Patent Foramen Ovale (PFO):** During fetal development, there is normally an opening in the atrial septum known as the "foramen ovale." Through the foramen ovale, oxygenated blood can easily pass from the mother to the fetus without having to pass through the lung. This opening, which normally closes within a year after birth, remains open in approximately 20-25% of the population.
  - » The patent foramen ovale is a flap-like opening within the heart which can grow and stretch as the individual ages. The high pressure of the left atrium usually keeps the flap closed, though certain straining actions like lifting, sneezing or coughing can result in a pressure gradient between the right and left atria.
  - » It is possible for an emboli to cross directly through this opening and travel to the brain, bypassing the lung filter. For this reason, patients with PFO are at risk for a cerebrovascular event. There is also the theory that maybe the PFO tunnel itself may develop thrombus and be a source of emboli. [15]

Location of Disease

- For stenosis: MCA, carotid siphon and terminal ICA
- For aneurysm: ACoA, MCA, PCA
  - » The ACoA is the most common site for an intracranial aneurysm, especially those associated with subarachnoid hemorrhage.
  - » The PCoA and MCA bifurcation are also common sites for aneurysm development. [1]

Patient History

- Aphasia (difficulty expressing or understanding language)
- Dysphagia (difficulty swallowing)
- Dysarthria (language issues (ranging from slurred speech to mumbling)
- Visual disturbances
- Numbness/tingling
- Paresthesia (hemiparesis or monoparesis)
- Syncope
- Ataxia (gait disturbance)

Physical Examination

- Assess responsiveness (ranging from awake and responsive to unresponsive)
- Ability to follow commands (grip objects, open and close eyes, etc.)
- Facial paralysis
- Ability to move arms/legs independently
- Sensory loss
- Language difficulties (e.g., aphasia, dysarthria)
- Visual loss (monocular or binocular)

Intracranial Testing Consideration

- Obtain a patient history to include symptoms and risk factors whenever possible.

Transcranial protocols may vary at different institutions.

- A quiet room is helpful when performing TCD examinations, otherwise headphones can also be used. Some technologists prefer using headphones to block out any background noise during transcranial exams.

Equipment and Supplies

- A non-imaging TCD system or color duplex ultrasound for TCI exams with spectral Doppler and bidirectional spectral analysis capabilities.
  - » Real-time spectral Doppler waveforms will produce a bidirectional signal which will display flow toward the transducer, above the baseline and flow away from the transducer, below the baseline.
  - » Both non-imaging and imaging systems should allow for adjustment of sample gate, audiovisual output, permanent recording and measurement of velocities using manual calipers.
  - » Improper gain adjustments can result in invalid automatic calculations by machines. Manual calculations for TAMV should be performed by placing the cursor at the point where the peak velocity area in systole and peak velocity area in diastole are equal. Manual calculation can also be performed for pulsatility index when necessary. [4]
- A low frequency (1.0 to 2.0 MHz) spectral Doppler transducer should be used for TCD imaging. A low frequency transducer (1.8 to 2.5 MHz) is used for TCI examinations.
- A small amount of ultrasound gel is needed to start. Additional gel may be necessary to maintain contact with the skin when having to tilt the transducer in order to obtain the best angle.
- Output power should be reduced when scanning patients with "burr holes" or removed and replaced pieces of the skull bone.

Patient Positioning

- The patient is examined in the supine position with the head supported and neck straight for evaluations through the transtemporal, transorbital and submandibular windows.
- Have the patient lie on their side or ask the patient to sit and lower their head towards their chest in order to access the transforaminal window.
- The technologist should try to be seated at the head of the bed whenever possible with their arms supported.

- When imaging through the transorbital window, ask the patient to gently close their eyelids during the examination and focus their eye to the opposite side that is being studied.

Table 15-1: **Windows Used for Visualization of the Intracranial Arteries**	
Window	**Arteries Visualized**
Transtemporal	MCA
	ACA
	ACoA
	PCA
	PCoA
	Terminal ICA
Transorbital	OA
	Carotid siphon
Transforaminal	VA
	Basilar
Submandibular	ICA

Transcranial Doppler and Imaging Techniques

Flow direction is relative to the transducer; toward, or away from the transducer or in both directions (bidirectional).

- Search for the highest pitched signal (strongest signal with the highest velocity and amplitude) through the various acoustical windows (transtemporal, transorbital, transforaminal and submandibular) while adjusting the depth, angle and location of the transducer. Usually, small maneuvers and minimal transducer pressure are all that is necessary.
- The diameter of a child's head should be considered before TCD testing. Determining where the child's midline to assist in selection of proper depths f or analysis. Children have larger transtemporal windows than adults, so the overall power can be reduced before study. Note the child's demeanor during testing, since crying and sleeping can affect intracranial velocities. [1]

If no audible signal is located, try changing windows.

- Use a large sample volume between 10-15mm. When studying a child, a smaller sample volume (6mm) may be used.
- Adjust the Doppler gain as needed throughout the examination to fill the peak velocity outline of the spectral waveform found on many types of transcranial equipment.
- Increase output power while searching for intracranial signals if necessary. Once the signal has been located, consider lowering the output power to a level where signals can still be assessed.
- Record the PSV, EDV and MV in each vessel.

MV is more accurate than PSV since MV is unaffected by systemic factors (e.g., heart rate).

- Use a zero-degree Doppler angle for TCI examinations. The exact angle is unknown between the ultrasound beam and the intracranial vessel, especially in TCD.
- During a TCI exam, the PRF, filters and color scales should be adjusted appropriately (e.g., decreased PRF and increased color scale for low-flow). Using both color and power Doppler may be helpful.
- The examination should be performed bilaterally.

Transtemporal Window

- Place the transducer superior to the zygomatic arch, over the temporal bone. Set the sample volume depth for 50-60mm and the output power to 100%. Locate the best sample area within this window. Once the signal is located, decrease the output power as much as possible without losing the arterial signal.
- Some TCD machines use multigate or M-mode (power motion) Doppler to display multiple gates and depths of information (6.5cm path). This enables capture of hemodynamic data from multiple depths simultaneously. This method may increase accuracy when detecting emboli.[1]

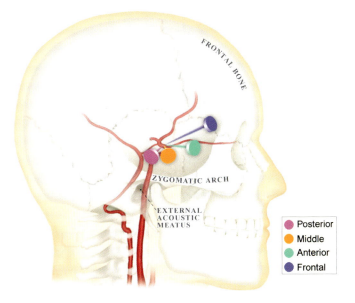

Fig. 15-4: Transtemporal Probe Positioning

- There are three main areas of the transtemporal window: anterior, middle and posterior. A fourth area known as the frontal is also considered by some technologists. Explore these areas, rotating the angle of the transducer while searching for the best signal.

The size and location of the transtemporal window may vary from side to side on the same patient. Visualization through the transtemporal window may be technically difficult in 10-15% of cases.[23]

- » **Anterior:** move the transducer 1.5cm in front of the middle window, slightly superior to the zygomatic arch and angle posteriorly.
- » **Middle:** move the transducer forward from the upper edge of the zygomatic arch, about 1.5cm in front of the posterior window.
- » **Posterior:** point the transducer anteriorly and superiorly, above the zygomatic arch and in front of the external auditory meatus. This area often provides the best access of the three.[4]
- » **Frontal:** place the transducer over the frontal bone, superior and in front of the anterior window, angling posteriorly.

Increase the sample volume depth to 60-70mm if no signals are obtained at 50-60mm in order to rule out MCA occlusion.

- **MCA:** Analyze the length of the MCA using a depth between 30-60mm. Angle anteriorly and superiorly. Flow direction should be toward the transducer. Starting at the shallowest depth, adjust the sample volume deeper using small increments (2-5mm) and small angle changes. Obtain and record the highest velocities in the proximal, mid and distal segments.

The M2 segment can usually be found between 30-40mm.

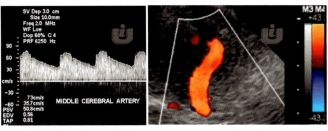

Fig. 15-5: MCA spectral and color Doppler

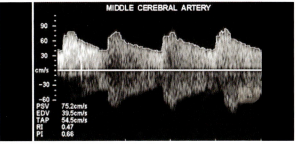

Fig. 15-6: Spectral Doppler signal at the MCA-ACA bifurcation

You may need to angle differently for each artery if the MCA and ACA are not directly in line with each other.

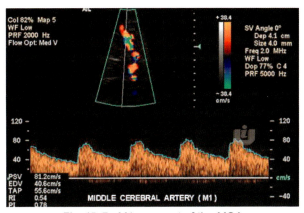

Fig. 15-7: M1 segment of the MCA
Courtesy of Philips Healthcare

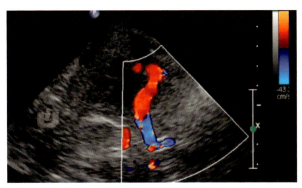

Fig. 15-8: Color flow image of the MCA-ACA bifurcation with antegrade flow towards the transducer in the MCA (red) and retrograde flow away from the transducer in the ACA (blue).

- **Terminal ICA (tICA):** Identify the terminal ICA (segment bifurcating into the MCA and ACA) for use as a reference point at a depth between 55-65mm. Angle anteriorly and superiorly. Start at the MCA and increase the depth until bidirectional flow is noted. Blood flow toward and away from the transducer represents simultaneous MCA and ACA flow. Obtain and record the highest velocity.

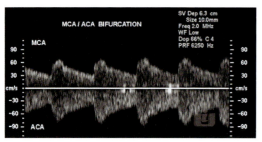

Fig. 15-9: *Doppler signal at the MCA/ACA bifurcation*

- **ACA:** Increase the depth to about 60-80mm from the terminal ICA to access the ACA. Angle anteriorly and superiorly. The A1 segment typically can be sampled between 70-80mm depth. Flow direction should be away from the transducer. Obtain and record the highest velocity.

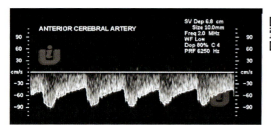

Fig. 15-10: *ACA Doppler signal*
Courtesy of Philips Healthcare

- A "false bifurcation" may be encountered near 50mm depths in larger diameter ACA that course medially. Although the spectral trace will appear similar to the ACA/MCA, the "true" bifurcation will be deeper. [4]

The A2 segment is easier to access in patients that have a "burr hole" (hole in the skull, made in the frontal bone).

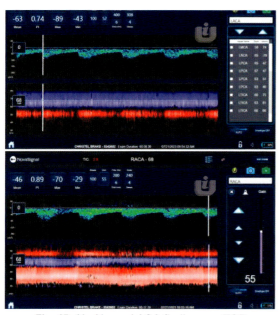

Fig. 15-11: *Normal ACA findings on TCD*

- **PCA:** Returning to the bifurcation for reference, rotate the transducer posteriorly and inferiorly using a depth between 60-70mm. Flow direction should be toward the transducer. Adjust the sample volume using small increments and small angle changes. Obtain the strongest signal and record the highest velocities.
  » Flow should be toward the transducer in the P1 segment of the PCA.
  » The PCA signal should drop out at a depth of 55-60mm.
  » Increase the depth to 70-80mm in order to access the contralateral P1 segment of the PCA. Flow should be away from the transducer.
  » The ipsilateral P2 segment of the PCA can be analyzed by returning to a depth of 60-70mm and angling more posteriorly. Flow should be away from the transducer.

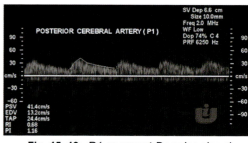

Fig. 15-12: *P1 segment Doppler signal*
Courtesy of Philips Healthcare

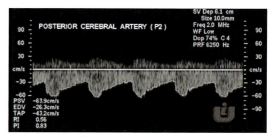

Fig. 15-13: *P2 segment Doppler signal*
Courtesy of Philips Healthcare

Table 15-2: Intracranial Artery Mean Diameter and Length

Artery	Mean Diameter	Mean Length of Artery
TICA	3.6-4.6mm	–
PCoA	–	1.5mm
MCA	2.5-3.8mm	16.2mm
ACA	1.8-3.0mm	
PCA		
P1 segment	–	6.3mm
P2 segment	1.96mm	6.3mm
BA	4.1mm (distally)	–

Source: Modified from Byrd-Raynor SA, Smith WB. (2010). Transcranial duplex imaging. In Zierler RE (Ed.), Strandess's duplex scanning disorders in vascular diagnosis 4th ed. (101-113). Philadelphia Wolters Kluwer Lippincott Williams & Wilkins

Collateral Vessels

- **ACoA:** When patent, the ACoA signal can be identified at a depth between 70-80mm. Flow is usually toward the hemisphere being supported by this collateral. The ACoA also becomes active when one A1 segment of the ACA is congenitally absent.
- **PCoA:** When patent, the PCoA may be identified by angling the transducer posteriorly and slightly inferior from the terminal ICA. Expect turbulence and increased velocities.

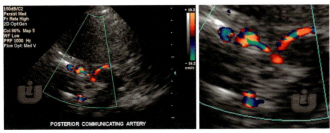

Fig. 15-14: *PCoA imaged using TCI*

Transorbital Window

- **OA:** Place the transducer on the orbital window, position laterally and point the transducer medially. Adjust the depth to 40-60mm and make small movements of the transducer to access the OA. Flow should be toward the transducer. Obtain and record the highest velocity.

The FDA recommends lowering the overall power to 10% and minimizing scan time to 10 second intervals or 3 spectral tracings to avoid retinal damage.

- **Carotid Siphon:** Increase the depth to 60-80mm in order to insonate the carotid siphon. Flow direction may vary due to tortuosity of this vessel in many individuals. Obtain and record the highest velocity.

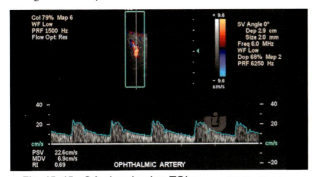

Fig. 15-15: *OA signal using TCI* Courtesy of Philips Healthcare

Transforaminal Window

- **VA:** Place the transducer at the midline of the nape of the neck (the spot where your hair begins in the back of the neck). Make sure there is enough gel to ensure transducer contact and aim the transducer towards the patient's nose. Using a depth between 40-85mm, move the transducer slightly to either side of midline. Flow direction should be away from the transducer.
- **BA:** Increase the depth from the vertebral arteries >80mm (90-100mm in some cases) to insonate the basilar segment. Flow direction should be away from the transducer.

The transforaminal window may also be studied with the patient in the prone position.

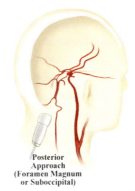
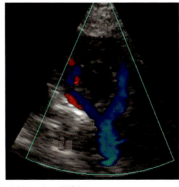

Fig. 15-16: *VA using TCI*

Limit the amount of time spent imaging through the transorbital window and use the lowest output power possible in order to obtain the spectral tracing (10% or 17mW/cm^2).

Visualization may be difficult through the Transforaminal window if the muscles are too tense from extending the patient's neck too far forward. [4]

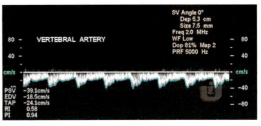

Fig. 15-17: *VA Doppler signal* Courtesy of Philips Healthcare

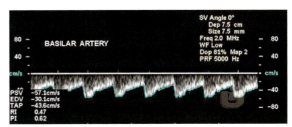

Fig. 15-18: *BA Doppler signal* Courtesy of Philips Healthcare

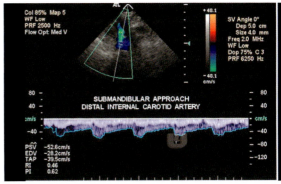

Fig. 15-19: *Distal ICA signal using TCI* Courtesy of Philips Healthcare

Submandibular Window

- **Distal ICA (proximal intracranial portion):** Place the transducer at the angle of the mandible and aim both slightly medial and toward the head. The ICA is usually found at a depth between 35-70mm. Flow direction should be away from the transducer. Expect a low-resistant signal. *Note: You may be listening to the ECA if the signal obtained with this approach demonstrates high-resistance.*
- Examination of the proximal intracranial portion of the ICA through the submandibular window can be used for patients with subarachnoid hemorrhage (SAH). [1,4]

- Other uses for this window include detection of spontaneous ICA dissection and FMD which often occur above the level of the jaw.
- Flow velocity ratios between the extracranial ICA and MCA can help distinguish vasospasm versus hyperemia in trauma patients.[4]

Intraoperative Monitoring for Embolism
(e.g., during CEA)

- Assess baseline intracranial velocities. Mark the transtemporal window on the skin for easier access peri-operatively.
- Head gear may be used to keep the transcranial equipment in place during the continuous MCA monitoring necessary during the procedure.
- Monitor the main trunk of the MCA with a 2MHz transducer at a depth of 45-55mm. Adjust the sample volume to exclude any ACA or tICA flow signals.
- Record the velocities in the MCA pre-clamp and at the time the artery is clamped. Determine an ischemic index by comparing velocities, pre and at-clamping. Other protocols suggest monitoring 10 minutes before CEA, as well as 10-15 minutes after CEA.[14]
- Document any signs of emboli (e.g., visible straight, bright lines through the spectral tracing) or changes in perfusion (e.g., mean velocities) during administration of anesthesia or during cross clamping procedures.
- Monitor for any of these changes during the different parts of the procedure (e.g., when the line is passed through the plaque to deploy the filter, balloon angioplasty, stent deployment, etc.).

Evaluation of Arteriovenous Malformation (AVM)

- Attempt to identify the artery feeding the AVM. Record flow velocities in the arterial branch.
- Record flow in the venous drainage vessel.
- Measure the diameter of the AVM when possible.

Evaluations for Subclavian Steal

- Evaluate the vertebral and basilar arteries, looking for reversed flow direction.
- If vertebrobasilar flow appears normal (no flow reversal or flow oscillates), there may be a "latent steal." The arm can be stressed if suspicion for steal is high:
  » Apply a blood pressure cuff to the ipsilateral arm with the suspected obstruction.
  » Monitor the ipsilateral VA flow. Inflate the cuff >20mmHg above the systolic pressure for approximately 3 minutes. Rapidly release the pressure in the cuff.
  » Record any changes in the vertebral Doppler signal or flow direction throughout the process.
  » Repeat on the contralateral side.

Evaluations for Vasospasm

SAH can last 12-16 days.[19] The onset of vasospasm is typically 3-5 days after the initial SAH and is usually at its worst between the 6-8th day.

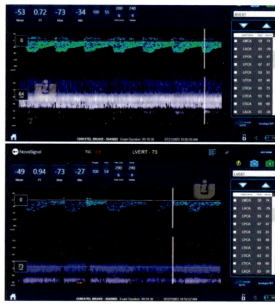

Fig. 15-20: Bilateral MCA waveforms recorded using TCD during eval for vasaospasm

Table 15-3: **Collateral Pathways of Intracranial Flow** *(Direction and Mean Velocity)*					
	Collateral path	MCA	ACA	PCA	BA
ACA	(Normal side)	Toward, normal	Away, elevated	P1: Toward, normal P2: Away, normal	Away, normal
	(Diseased side)	Toward, normal/increased	Toward, turbulent	P1: Toward, normal P2: Away, normal	Away, normal
PCoA	(Normal side)	Toward, normal	Away, elevated	P1: Toward, normal P2: Away, normal	Away, elevated also expect elevated VA(s)
	(Diseased side)	Toward, normal/increased	Toward, turbulent	P1: Toward, elevated P2: Away, normal	Away, normal
OA	(Normal side)	Toward, normal	Away, normal	P1: Toward, normal P2: Away, normal	Away, normal
	(Diseased side) OA flow will be away, increased	Toward, velocity dependent on capability of OA flow	Toward, velocity dependent on capability of OA flow	P1: Toward, normal P2: Away, normal	Away, normal

- Multiple exams are typically performed daily or every other day depending on the patient's symptoms and the level of clinical suspicion.
- Record the highest mean velocity from each artery.
- Record a cervical ICA velocity at a depth of 45-55mm without adjusting the angle in order to calculate a hemispheric ratio.
- Add approximately 2cm/depth for vessel depth post-craniotomy when patients are experiencing swelling.[4]

Evaluations During tPA Infusion
- Perform a baseline transcranial evaluation. Document any occlusion or other abnormality.
- Head-gear may be used to keep the transcranial transducer in place during the continuous intracranial monitoring necessary during the infusion of tPA.

TCD monitoring has been used to support physicians during infusion of tPA (tissue plasminogen activator) in acute stroke cases.

- Note the time and record any changes to the Doppler signal (e.g., reappearance of the signal, increase in velocity, change in waveform shape or evidence of embolization).
- Adjust sample volume depth according to the location of the obstruction. For example, use 55-60mm when the M1 segment is occluded and 80-100mm for the basilar artery.

Evaluation for Right-to-Left Cardiac Shunts (RLS)
- Examine the patient in the supine position with their head slightly elevated. Perform what is referred to as a "PFO bubble study" or "transcranial Doppler for microemboli detection" using an agitated saline solution injected into a peripheral vein, while TCD is continuously being monitored during normal respiration and while "straining" (Valsalva maneuver, for example).
- Perform a baseline transcranial evaluation of the MCA using a low frequency transducer at a depth between 50-60mm. Document any occlusion or other abnormality.
- A multigated TCD system is best for observation since screening multiple vessels and depths at the same time is possible and makes detection of HITS (*hyperintense transient signal*) often resembling a "chirp" or a "click" more reliable. Although a transtemporal window is preferred, observation of the distal ICA through the submandibular window is acceptable.[15]
- Head-gear may be used to keep the transcranial equipment in place during the continuous MCA monitoring necessary for the procedure. Monitoring should be performed bilaterally. The gain should be set low and sweep speed should be slow.
- A valsalvometer can be used during a RLS evaluation to performed a "calibrated Valsalva" which standardizes the Valsalva strain. The patient releases their breath into a tube for 10 seconds, trying to achieve 40mmHg of pressure on the valsalvometer gauge.[15]
  » Adequate strain will likely increase the pressure gradient between the right and left atria and open the PFO.[15,17]
  » Asking the patient to vigorously cough for 5 seconds is an alternative method used for a non-calibrated Valsalva technique.[17]
- Obtain and record the highest velocities. Make sure the TCD transducers will not move from their position.

- Qualified personnel insert an IV. A three-way stopcock device is attached to the inserted needle, along with two syringes. One syringe will remain empty while the other syringe will contain a mixture of 9mL saline and 1 mL air.[15,16] A small amount of blood (0.5mL) may be introduced into one of the syringes to optimize the procedure.[15,17] Once the stopcock is locked so no fluid can enter the vein, the saline-air mixture is agitated between the two syringes about 10 times in order to create microbubbles.[15] The saline is then introduced into the vein.

The pulmonary artery (PA) may also be monitored to determine how long it takes (number of cardiac cycles) for the microbubbles to reach the heart. Using a low frequency continuous-wave Doppler transducer, listen for an audible signal similar to a "washing machine."[15]

Knowing the number of cardiac cycles that will occur before the microbubbles reach the heart can be helpful. If the patient performs Valsalva AFTER the microbubbles have left the heart, there is a greater chance for false-positive or non-diagnostic results.[15]

- Begin monitoring the intracranial vessels after injection of the agitated saline solution while the patient is "at rest."
- Observe for visual and audible "HITS." Count and document the number of HITS bilaterally.

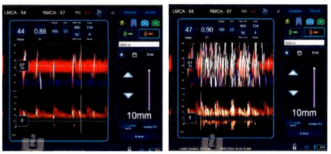

Fig. 15-21: *HITS visualized at rest in the MCA and with Valsalva*

- Repeat the observation while the patient performs the Valsalva maneuver. Ask the patient to inhale deeply and hold their breath. While holding this breath, the patient will need to contract the abdomen (or bear down). Instruct the patient to release the breath and relax the abdomen after 10 seconds.
- Observe for visual and audible "HITS" once again. Count and document the number of HITS bilaterally.
- A third observation for HITS may be performed, this time without a calibrated Valsalva.
- When only unilateral monitoring is possible, the number of HITS reported should be doubled.[15]

Evaluation for Brain Death
- Use multiple windows and obtain recordings from several intracranial arteries.

It may be helpful to mark the transtemporal window for serial study on patients suspected of brain death.

- Repeat examinations can prevent false positive results.

Common Carotid Artery Compressions/Oscillation Maneuvers
- A drop in pressure results when the common carotid artery (CCA) is compressed low in the neck or vibrated with brisk finger compressions (similar to a "temporal tap"). Effects on flow velocities, direction of flow and pulsatility of the intracranial vessels may be observed.

- Compression maneuvers should not be performed when there is evidence of high-grade stenosis/occlusion, low carotid bifurcations, calcification or complicated lesions in the CCA.
  » Palpate the CCA in the lower neck using the thumb, or first and second digits, above the clavicle and between the trachea and sternocleidomastoid muscle.
  » While insonating the intracranial vessel, apply downward pressure away from the trachea. Compress for 2-4 cardiac cycles and release.
  » Observe for any changes to intracranial flow.
  » Responses to CCA compression would include obliteration, diminished flow, alternating flow or change in flow direction.

PRINCIPLES OF INTERPRETATION

- Changes in heart rate, hematocrit levels, blood pressure, etc., can affect transcranial velocities and should be considered during the exam.
- Expect a low-resistant signal similar to the extracranial ICA with diastolic flow throughout systole, since the Circle of Willis feeds the brain, a low-resistance vascular bed.
- Significant extracranial disease can result in decreased ipsilateral intracranial artery velocities, a delay in systole, reduced PI and collateralization. In other cases of significant extracranial disease, there will be no effect on the Circle of Willis. [1]
- Doppler waveforms, spectral analysis and direction of flow are utilized to pinpoint the location of lesions and resulting collateralization. Comparisons should be made regarding the anterior and posterior circulation, as well as right/left sides. [1,3]
- **Mean velocity (MV):** mean of the peak velocity "envelope" over time. The "envelope" refers to a trace of the PSV as a function of time. MV or TAMV is a.k.a TAP (time average peak):

$$MV = \frac{PSV + (EDV \times 2)}{3} \quad \text{or} \quad MV = \frac{(PSV - EDV)}{3} + EDV$$

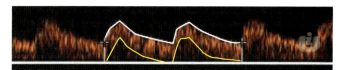

Fig. 15-22: Duplex scanners record the mean velocities or time-averaged maximum velocity (TAMAX or TAP). Note the average maximum velocities (white line) illustrated versus the average mean velocities (yellow line).

- **Pulsatility index (PI):** distal vascular resistance is measured through waveform analysis. Decreased diastolic flow caused by a decrease in cerebral perfusion pressure increases the pulsatility index. PI is calculated using the *Gosling equation* to calculate the difference between the maximum and minimum velocities divided by the mean velocity:

$$PI = \frac{PSV - EDV}{MV}$$

  » Elevated PI suggests increased vascular resistance.
  » Decreased PI suggests lower vascular resistance.

PI alone is not the most useful criteria for interpretation. The PI can be affected by the typical decrease in elasticity of vessel walls that accompanies certain conditions such as advanced age or diabetes.

- **Lindegaard ratio (LR):** is the ratio of MCA mean flow velocity divided by the extracranial internal carotid artery mean flow velocity.
  » When increased flow velocities are noted, this ratio may help differentiate focal vasospasm involving the MCA from systemic reasons for hyperdynamic blood flow like anemia or sepsis.

LR = MV of the MCA ÷ MV in the ipsilateral extracranial ICA

Normal [1,4]

Spectral Doppler Waveforms and Flow Velocities

Table 15-4: Transcranial Waveforms and Velocities

Vessel	Flow Direction *	Time Average Mean Velocity (TAMV) cm/s
MCA	Toward	55 + 12
MCA/ACA Bifurcation (terminal ICA)	Bidirectional	55 + 12
ACA	Away	50 + 11
PCA (P1 Segment)	Toward	39 + 10
PCA (P2 Segment)	Away	40 + 10
OA	Toward	21 + 5
VA	Away	38 + 10
BA	Away	41 + 10
Siphon	Either direction (due to tortuosity of the carotid siphon)	47 + 14

Flow should be toward or away from the transducer with the exception of normal bidirectional in some segments.

- There should be little difference between the right and left sides in asymptomatic patients.
- A normal PI value is usually between 0.5-1.2. [27, 28]

The PI should be higher in the OA since it supplies structures such as the ocular muscles and has anastomoses with ECA territories. [1]

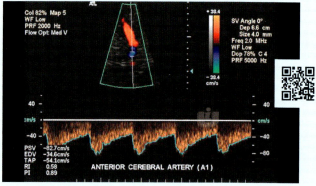

Fig. 15-23: ACA signal using TCI *Courtesy of Philips Healthcare*

- Expect higher velocities in the anterior versus the posterior circulation. MCA >ACA >PCA is often used to describe the normal velocity relationship between the three major intracranial arteries. When the PCA >MCA and ACA for example, this finding would suggest that the PCA is acting as a collateral pathway.[18]

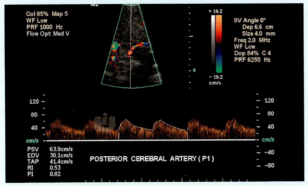

Fig. 15-24: *P1 segment using TCI* Courtesy of Philips Healthcare

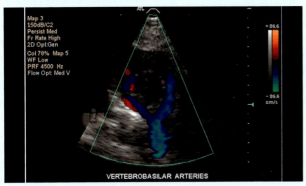

Fig. 15-25: *VA flow using TCI*

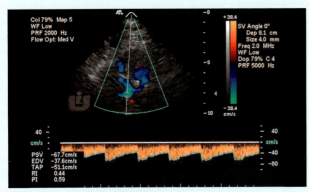

Fig. 15-26: *BA using TCI*

- A normal value for the Lindegaard ratio is < 3.0.[31]
- Distal ICA TAMV obtained from the submandibular approach are normally 37 ± 9cm/s.

Abnormal

Spectral Doppler Waveforms and Flow Velocities

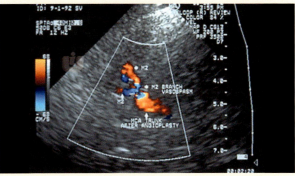

Fig. 15-27: *Mosaic color flow noted on TCI image of vasospasm*

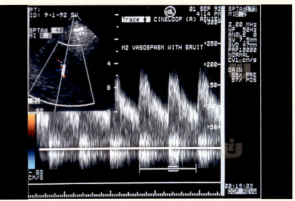

Fig. 15-28: *Increased velocities indicative of vasospasm*

Stenosis versus Vasospasm: A stenosis is characterized by a focal increase in velocity ≥30cm/s at 1-2 sample depths, while a vasospasm is characterized by a long segment velocity increase over several sample depths.

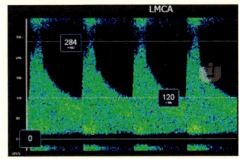

Fig. 15-29: *MCA waveform taken at 52mm depth with a peak velocity of 284cm/s and MV of 120cm/s.*

Stenosis

- Additional findings that support intracranial stenosis include: turbulence, post-stenotic drop in velocity, bruit/musical murmurs and compensatory flow in branching vessels.[1]
- A hemodynamically significant focal stenosis (≥50%) is characterized by a **minimum** two-fold increase in velocity compared to the proximal segment.[1]
  » A velocity ratio >3 suggests a MCA stenosis >70%.[29]
    - Significant extracranial disease can result in decreased ipsilateral intracranial artery velocities, a delay in systole, reduced PI and collateralization. In other cases of significant extracranial disease, there will be no effect on the Circle of Willis.[1] A mean velocity of 80cm/s suggests a significant stenosis in the MCA, ACA, PCA and terminal ICA.

- When the mean velocity is 120cm/s in the MCA, a ≥70 stenosis is highly suspected.[29]
- A mean velocity of 110cm/s is used to predict a stenosis in the BA and VA.[29] Other studies suggest >80cm/s as the threshold for VA vasospasm.[20]
- A velocity ratio >3 plus significantly increased mean velocities in the MCA, BA or VA increases TCD sensitivity for predicting a >70% stenosis.[29]

An isolated stenosis of the PCA or ACA is rare.[1]

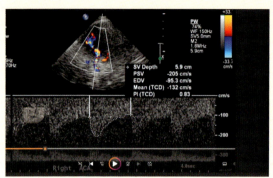

Fig. 15-30: *ACA waveform taken at 59mm depth with a peak velocity of 205cm/s and MV of 132cm/s.*

- **Pulsatility index:** PI >1.2 represents high resistance blood flow[28]
- Cardiac patients on an ECMO or an intra-aortic balloon pump may have reduced PI. Increased PI has also been described in patients with aortic regurgitation, severe carotid plaque, small vessel disease and dementia.[24] Combining PI with flow velocities for a more accurate interpretation.
- **Lindegaard ratio:** The LR is used in conjunction with flow velocity to differentiate between vasospasm versus another reason for increased velocities such as anemia or fever. Abnormal LR ratios >2.9 and elevated flow velocities suggest:[31]
  » LR 3-4.5: mild vasospasm
  » LR 4.5-6: moderate vasospasm
  » LR >6: severe vasospasm

Vasospasm
The criterion for vasospasm varies across institutions. This chapter includes a sample of criteria used to diagnosis vasospasms of the anterior (MCA) and posterior (BA) circulations.

Table 15-5: MCA Vasospasm Criteria

Category of Disease	Lindegaard Ratio	MV of MCA
Hyperemic	<3	<120cm/s
Mild	3-6	120-149cm/s
Moderate	3-6	150-200cm/s
Severe	>6	>200cm/s

Park SH, Kim TJ, et. al. (2022). Transcranial Doppler Monitoring in Subarachnoid Hemorrhage. J Neurosonol Neuroimag. 14, (1):1-9. DOI: https://doi.org/10.31728/jnn.2022.00115

- An increase of 50cm/s within a 24-hr period suggests vasospasm.[30]

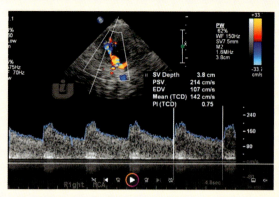

Fig. 15-31: *Mild vasospasm of the MCA with a MV of 142 cm/s*

Table 15-6: BA Vasospasm Criteria

Category of Disease	Lindegaard Ratio	MV of BA
Hyperemic	<2	<70
Mild	≥2	70-85cm/s
Moderate	>2.5	>85cm/s
Severe	>3	>85cm/s

A modified LR is used to calculate BA vasospasm. Instead of using the extracranial ICA, use the averaged MFV of the vertebral arteries.

Park SH, Kim TJ, et. al. (2022). Transcranial Doppler Monitoring in Subarachnoid Hemorrhage. J Neurosonol Neuroimag. 14, (1):1-9. DOI: https://doi.org/10.31728/jnn.2022.00115

Mean velocity increases >25cm/s each day suggest a poor prognosis.

- **Occlusion:** An MCA occlusion is suspected when there is absence of the MCA signal, but there is good window and recordable signals in the ipsilateral ACA, PCA and tICA. Increased ipsilateral ACA flow in such cases also supports MCA occlusion.[1]

The MCA can recanalize on serial TCD in cases of acute cerebral infarct.

Collateralization
- Increased velocities are not uncommon in a vessel acting as a collateral. For example, a patent ACoA signal with turbulence and increased velocities is often a signal of ICA obstruction.

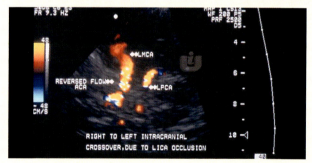

Fig. 15-32: *Collateralization observed using TCI (Note: antegrade ACA)* Courtesy of Philips Healthcare

Multiple collateral paths can occur at the same time in individuals.

- The most common collateral pathways include:[1,18]
  » **ACA (most common):** carrying flow from hemisphere to hemisphere. Expect increased velocities in the contralateral ACA (above those recorded in the MCA) while flow in the ipsilateral ACA is reversed.

» **PCoA:** carrying flow between the posterior and anterior circulation.
- This collateral pathway can be activated when there is bilateral extracranial obstruction, or when either the ACA/ACoA is absent.[18]
- The ipsilateral PCA will demonstrate increased velocities proximal to the PCoA origin, the PCA velocities will be decreased distally.

» **OA:** Flow will be reversed in the OA in cases of severe ICA obstruction. The OA acts as a collateral from ECA branches and its waveform patterns will be low resistant, since the OA will now have to supply the brain.

- **Subclavian steal:** Flow will be reversed in the vertebral or basilar arteries (toward the transducer, instead of away) in cases of subclavian steal. A vertebral-to-vertebral steal may also be observed.[1]

The BA is usually not affected unless the supplying VA is disease.

Other Pathologies
Aneurysms
- When a larger intracranial aneurysm is present (>1cm), decreased velocities, multiple systolic peaks, increased resistance, areas of turbulence and bruits may all be present.[1]

Since there will be a lack of color flow, TCI is not an appropriate study to assess a thrombosed intracranial aneurysm. Plus, vessel tortuosity and branching can be misdiagnosed as an aneurysm.[1]

» The neck of an aneurysm may project increased velocities.[1]
» Compression by the aneurysm is reflected by focal increases in velocity in any adjacent arteries.[1]

Arteriovenous malformations (AVM)
- In this condition, there is an abnormal tangle of blood vessels in the brain. The blood flows directly from an artery to a vein, without going through the capillaries. Surrounding tissue is at risk since blood is automatically shunted away from the tissue into the vein.
- Flow should be low resistant and the PI will be decreased.
- The "feeder artery" that supplies the AVM is usually larger in diameter. Blood flow will typically demonstrate increased velocities and reduced pulsatility.
- The veins involved will also be larger in diameter and flow will be pulsatile.

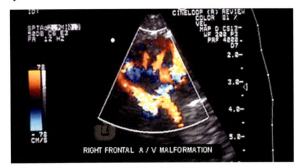

Fig. 15-33: *Image of an AVM using TCI Courtesy of Philips Healthcare*

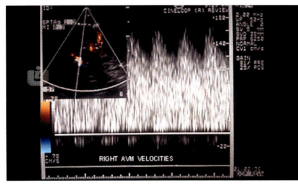

Fig. 15-34: *Doppler signal representing an AVM Courtesy of Philips Healthcare*

Stroke prediction in sickle cell patients
- MV is used for diagnosis rather than PSV in sickle cell cases to decrease the risk of false positive results. MV <170cm/s are considered normal.[19]
- MV between 171-199cm/s are considered "conditional."[19] Some labs will repeat the exam within 3-6 months to monitor for disease progression.
- Studies suggests that MCA velocities ≥200cm/s on two separate exams indicate a higher stroke risk for the child.[1,20]

For sickle cell patients with mean velocities ≥200cm/s, there is an estimated 40% stroke risk within 3 years.[19]

The Stroke Prevention Trial in Sickle Cell Anemia (STOP) study revealed elevated MCA velocities by TCD followed by blood transfusion reduced the rate of the first stroke in children.

Intraoperative monitoring during CEA
- Intraoperative TCD monitoring can help surgeons decide between clamping or shunting. If there is a significant velocity decrease after clamping, shunting is suggested.
- Microemboli are described as a change in the TCD signal, which is unilateral lasting <300 microseconds, with an amplitude that is at minimum 3dB higher than the background flow signal.
- The audible signal or HIT often resembles a "chirp" or a "click."[1] HITS appear as straight, bright lines through the spectral tracing.
- A decrease in MV of >75-90% in the ipsilateral MCA is considered significant.[14,33]
- **Post-operative hyperperfusion:** Elevated MCA velocities >175% has been associated with hyperperfusion.[22]
- **RLS shunts (e.g., PFO):** Observe for the appearance of microemboli after injection of the saline-contrast during the first 3-5 cardiac cycles. The criterion that exists in the literature predicts either the size of the opening or the amount of microemboli which may pass.
  » Contrast bubbles after 3-5 cardiac cycles often result from intrapulmonary AVM.

The absence of "HITS" during a RLS bubble study does not definitively rule out PFO.[15]

An initial decrease in velocities during the Valsalva maneuver indicates a good strain was performed.[15]

Table 15-7: SLS Grading System (Spencer Logarithmic Scale) [15,21]

Grade 0	No microemboli detected
Grade 1	1-10 embolic tracks
Grade 2	11-30 embolic tracks
Grade 3	31-100 embolic tracks
Grade 4	101-300 embolic tracks
Grade 5	>300 embolic tracks or "curtain effect"

Source: Spencer Logarithmic Scale. Modified from Sarkar, S., S. Ghosh, et al. (2007). "Role of Transcranial Doppler ultrasonography in stroke." Postgrad Med J 83(985): 683-689.

Table 15-8: International Consensus Criteria

Category	High-Intensity Transient Signal Appearance
1	No occurrence
2	1-10
3	11-25 but no curtain
4	>25 or curtain

Hutayanon P, Muengtaweepongsa S. The Role of Transcranial Doppler in Detecting Patent Foramen Ovale. Journal for Vascular Ultrasound. 2023;47(1):33-39. doi:10.1177/15443167221108512

Table 15-9: Quantification of RLS Shunts

Low-grade shunt	1-10 microbubbles
Mid-grade shunt	>10 microbubbles
High-grade shunt	numerous microbubbles which can no longer be identified separately ("curtain effect")

Source: Modified from Sarkar, S., S. Ghosh, et al. (2007). "Role of Transcranial Doppler ultrasonography in stroke." Postgrad Med J 83(985): 683-689.

- **Brain death:** Three different signals that are suggestive of brain death have been described:
  » The loss of EDV (to about 50% of the PSV) or loss of forward, antegrade flow through diastole. [1]
  » To and fro waveform, since blood flow oscillates within the blood column and does not perfuse the parenchyma of the brain. There will be an absence of net flow over time. [1,19]
  » Staccato signal- short systolic peak only. [1]
- Net flow velocities in the MCA <10cm/s also suggest brain death. [1]

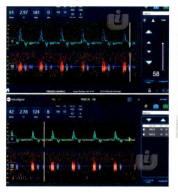

Fig. 15-35: TCD in patient with suspected brain death.

Fig. 15-36: No intracranial blood flow or parenchymal perfusion confirmed by NM brain scan with SPECT. Findings compatible with clinical diagnosis of brain death.

Confirmation of brain death is most commonly performed with a CT or spectamine scan.

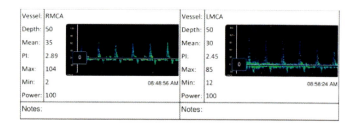

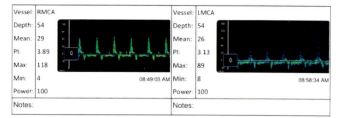

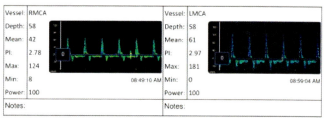

Fig. 15-37: Loss of EDV on TCD waveform suggestive of brain death

Differential Diagnosis
- Atherosclerosis
- Arterial dissection
- Vasculitis (giant cell arteritis, PAN, Wegener's, lupus, primary angiitis of CNS)
- Reversible cerebral vasoconstrictive syndrome
- Moyamoya disease
- CADASIL (cerebral autosomal dominant arteriopathy with subcortical infarcts and leukoencephalopathy)
- Syphilis
- Sarcoidosis
- Migraines
- Brain tumor
- Seizure
- Dementia, caused by Alzheimer's
- Stokes-Adams syndrome
- Bell's palsy
- Demyelinative diseases (multiple sclerosis, etc.)

Correlation
- CT scan
- MRI/MRA
- Digital subtraction cerebral angiography
- **Spectamine scan (SPECT):** nuclear medicine exam using radioisotope uptake to create images for assessment of cerebral blood flow.

The Glasgow coma scale is used for patients with brain injury to assess their level of consciousness. Eye movements and motor responses are considered. A normal score is 15. Noting changes in this score and correlating it to changes in serial transcranial exams may be a useful tool.

Medical Treatment

- Modify risk factors (e.g., reduce cholesterol, manage HTN and DM, smoking cessation)
- Anticoagulation (e.g., coumadin) or aspirin and statin therapy
- Heparin therapy, with monitoring for hemorrhage
- Drug therapy (e.g., calcium channel blockers) is used in conjunction with serial TCD monitoring in cases of vasospasm
- Blood transfusions to reduce the risk of stroke in sickle cell patients

Surgical Treatment

- EC-IC bypass (extracranial-intracranial bypass joining the superficial temporal to MCA)
- Aneurysm repair (e.g., clipping)
- Coil embolization

Endovascular Treatment

- Balloon angioplasty (vasospasm)
- Stenting

Table 15-10: Protocol and Diagnostic Criteria Summary for Intracranial Cerebrovascular Techniques

Artery	Transducer Position	Depth of Sample Volume	Flow Direction	Spatial Relationship of ACA/CA Bifurcation	Mean Velocity (cm/s)	Response of Ipsilateral Compression
MCA [M1]	Transtemporal	30-60	Toward	Same	55 ± 12	Obliteration Diminishment
ACA/MCA Bifurcation	Transtemporal	55-65	Bidirectional	–	–	Identical to ACA/MCA
ACA [A1]	Transtemporal	60-80	Away	Anterior and Superior	50 ± 11	Obliteration Diminishment Reversal
PCA [P1] *Fetal Origin	Transtemporal	60-70	Toward	Posterior and Inferior	39 ± 10	No Change Augmentation Diminishment* Obliteration*
PCA [P2] *Fetal Origin	Transtemporal	60-70	Away	Posterior and Inferior	40 + 10	No Change Diminishment* Obliteration*
TICA	Transtemporal	55-65	Toward	Inferior	39 ± 9	Obliteration Reversal
OA	Transorbital	40-60	Toward	–	21 ± 5	Obliteration
Carotid Siphon [Supraclinoid] [Genu] [Parasellar]	Transorbital	60-80	Away Bidirectional Toward	–	41 ± 11 – 47 + 14	Obliteration Reversal
VA	Transforaminal	60-90	Away	–	38 ± 10	–
BA	Transforaminal	80-120	Away	–	41 ± 10	–

Source– Fujioka KA, Douville CM. 1992. "Anatomy and Freehand Examination Techniques." Transcranial Doppler. Raven Press, Ltd. New York.

REFERENCES

1. Katz ML, Alexandrov AV. (2003). A Practical Guide to Transcranial Doppler Examinations. Littleton: Sumner Publishing.
2. McCartney JP, Lukes-Thomas KM, Gomez CR. (1997). Handbook of Transcranial Doppler. New York. Springer-Verlag
3. Naylor AR, Markose G. (2010) Cerebrovascular disease: diagnostic evaluation, In Cronenwett JL., Johnston KW. (Eds.) Rutherford's Vascular Surgery (7th ed.) (Chapter 93). Philadelphia. Saunders Elsevier.
4. Fujioka KA, Douville CM. 1992. "Anatomy and Freehand Examination Techniques." Transcranial Doppler. Raven Press, Ltd. New York.
5. Easton JD, Saver JL., et al. (2009). "Definition and Evaluation of Transient Ischemic Attack." Stroke 40(6): 2276-2293.
6. Bamford J, Sandercock P., et al. (1987). "The natural history of lacunar infarction: the Oxfordshire Community Stroke Project." Stroke 18(3): 545-551.
7. Petty GW, Brown RD, et al. (2000). "Ischemic Stroke Subtypes: A Population-Based Study of Functional Outcome, Survival, and Recurrence." Stroke 31(5): 1062-1068.
8. Weir, B., R. L. Macdonald, et al. (1999). "Etiology of cerebral vasospasm." Acta Neurochir Suppl 72: 27-46.
9. Penn DL, Komotar RJ, et al. (2011). "Hemodynamic mechanisms underlying cerebral aneurysm pathogenesis." J Clin Neurosci 18(11): 1435-1438.
10. Rowe VL, Yellin AE, Weaver FA. (2005). Vascular injuries of the extremities. In Rutherford Vascular Surgery 6th edition. (1044-1058). Philadelphia. Elsevier Saunders.
11. Desai, B. and J. F. Toole (1975). "Kinks, coils, and carotids: a review." Stroke 6(6): 649-653.
12. Trackler, RT, Mikulicich AG. (1974). "Diminished cerebral perfusion resulting from kinking of the internal carotid artery." J Nucl Med 15(7): 634-635.
13. Bickerstaff LK, Pairolero PC, et al. (1982). "Thoracic aortic aneurysms: a population-based study." Surgery 92(6): 1103-1108.
14. Rowed, D. W., D. A. Houlden, et al. (2004). "Comparison of monitoring techniques for intraoperative cerebral ischemia." Can J Neurol Sci 31(3): 347-356.
15. Hughes JP, Dubin R, Harley M, Renz J. (2007). "Transcranial Doppler in the Detection of Patent Foramen Ovale. Vascular US Today 12(5):77-96.
16. Rubiera, M., L. Cava, et al. (2010). "Diagnostic criteria and yield of real-time transcranial Doppler monitoring of intra-arterial reperfusion procedures." Stroke 41(4): 695-699.
17. Sastry, S., A. MacNab, et al. (2009). "Transcranial Doppler detection of venous-to-arterial circulation shunts: criteria for patent foramen ovale." J Clin Ultrasound 37(5): 276-280.
18. Byrd-Raynor SA, Smith WB. (2010). Transcranial duplex imaging. In Zierler RE (Ed.), Strandess's duplex scanning disorders in vascular diagnosis 4th ed. (101-113).Philadelphia Wolters Kluwer Lippincott Williams & Wilkins.
19. Kassab, MY, Majid A, et al. (2007). "Transcranial Doppler: an introduction for primary care physicians." J Am Board Fam Med 20(1): 65-71.
20. Alexandrov, AV, Sloan MA, et al. (2010). "Practice Standards for Transcranial Doppler (TCD) Ultrasound. Part II. Clinical Indications and Expected Outcomes." J Neuroimaging. Epub ahead of print.
21. Spencer Vascular. (n.d.). Grading of Right-to-Left Shunt Conductance. Retrieved from http://spencervascular.com.
22. Nicholls SC. (2010). Transcranial Doppler monitoring for carotid interventions. In Zierler RE (Ed.), Strandess's duplex scanning disorders in vascular diagnosis 4th ed. (123-130).Philadelphia Wolters Kluwer Lippincott Williams & Wilkins
23. Nicholls SC. (2005). Transcranial Doppler: technique and application. In Mansour MA, Labropoulos N. (Eds.), Vascular Diagnosis, (113-129). Philadelphia: Elsevier Saunders
24. Bill, O., Lambrou, D., Sotomayor, G.T. et al. Predictors of the pulsatility index in the middle cerebral artery of acute stroke patients. Sci Rep 10, 17110 (2020). https://doi.org/10.1038/s41598-020-74056-2
25. Transcranial Doppler Monitoring in Subarachnoid Hemorrhage J Neurosonol Neuroimag. 2022;14(1):1-9. Published online June 30, 2022. DOI: https://doi.org/10.31728/jnn.2022.00115
26. Reeves SL, Madden B, Freed GL, Dombkowski KJ. Transcranial Doppler Screening Among Children and Adolescents With Sickle Cell Anemia. JAMA Pediatr. 2016;170(6):550–556. doi:10.1001/jamapediatrics.2015.4859
27. Nelson, S. E., & Nyquist, P. A. (2020). Neurointensive Care Unit: Clinical Practice and Organization (Current Clinical Neurology) (1st ed. 2020 ed.). Springer
28. Bellner J., Romner B., Reinstrup P., Kristiansson K.-A., Ryding E., Brandt L. (2004). Transcranial Doppler sonography pulsatility index (PI) reflects intracranial pressure (ICP). Surg. Neurol. 62 45–51. 10.1016/j.surneu.2003.12.007
29. Zhao L, Barlinn K, Sharma VK, Tsivgoulis G, et.al. (2011). Velocity Criteria for Intracranial Stenosis Revisited An International Multicenter Study of Transcranial Doppler and Digital Subtraction Angiography. Stroke. 42 3429–3434.
30. Transcranial Doppler Monitoring in Subarachnoid Hemorrhage J Neurosonol Neuroimag. 2022;14(1):1-9. Published online June 30, 2022. DOI: https://doi.org/10.31728/jnn.2022.00115
31. Rynkowski, Carla & Caldas, Juliana. (2022). Ten Good Reasons to Practice Neuroultrasound in Critical Care Setting. Frontiers in Neurology. 12. 10.3389/fneur.2021.799421.
32. Neulen, A., Kunzelmann, S., Kosterhon, M., Pantel, T., Stein, M., Berres, M., Ringel, F., Brockmann, M. A., Brockmann, C., & Kantelhardt, S. R. (2020). Automated Grading of Cerebral Vasospasm to Standardize Computed Tomography Angiography Examinations After Subarachnoid Hemorrhage. Frontiers in neurology, 11, 13. https://doi.org/10.3389/fneur.2020.00013
33. Razumovsky, AY, Jahangiri, FR, Balzer, J, et al. ASNM and ASN joint guidelines for transcranial Doppler ultrasonic monitoring: An update. J Neuroimaging 2022; 32: 781– 797. https://doi.org/10.1111/jon.13013
34. Reference: Palazzo, P., Ingrand, P., Agius, P., Belhadj Chaidi, R., & Neau, J. P. (2019). Transcranial Doppler to detect right-to-left shunt in cryptogenic acute ischemic stroke. Brain and behavior, 9(1), e01091. https://doi.org/10.1002/brb3.1091

ARTERIAL TESTING
16. Lower Extremity ABI and Analog Pedal Artery Waveforms

Definition

A non-invasive physiological test comparing the systolic pressure at the level of the ankle to the systolic pressure at the level of the brachial artery. Continuous-wave (CW) analog Doppler waveforms are recorded to support the pressure information.

The ABI only evaluates the presence and severity of disease.

Rationale

Doppler-derived pressure measurements can identify the location of a significant obstruction in an arterial segment and define the resulting decrease in terms of pressure. The term "obstruction" is used to describe either a stenosis or an occlusion of an artery.

When narrowing of the arterial lumen reaches a critical level, distal arterial flow and pressure decrease significantly. Ankle brachial indices (ABI) define the resulting decrease in blood flow to the extremity at the ankle level.

Etiology

- Atherosclerosis
- Embolization
- Thrombus
- Intimal hyperplasia
- Trauma
- Traumatic occlusion
- Extrinsic compression
- Vasculitis
- Pseudoaneurysm
- Aneurysm
- AV fistula (abnormal connection between an artery and a vein)

Risk Factors

- Age (increased risk with age)
- Coronary artery disease
- Diabetes
- Family history
- Hyperlipidemia
- Hypertension
- Obesity
- Smoking
- Sedentary lifestyle
- Previous history of CVA or MI
- Elevated levels of homocysteine
- Excessive levels of C-reactive protein
- History of radiation

Indications for Exam

- Claudication (exercise-related limb pain)
- Follow-up of an abnormal ABI
- Limb pain at rest
- Absent peripheral pulses
- Extremity ulcer
- Gangrene
- Pre-operative assessment of healing potential
- Digital cyanosis
- Cold sensitivity
- Arterial aneurysm
- Trauma to an artery
- Follow-up after revascularization procedure

Contraindications/Limitations

- Calcified vessels which will falsely elevate pressure measurements (typically encountered in patients with diabetes or end-stage renal disease).
- Significant lesions with excellent collateral circulation, which may result in normal distal pressures and waveforms at rest.
- Patients with acute clot or venous thrombosis in the lower extremities should not have pressure cuffs inflated over their thrombus.
- Patients with extensive bandages or casts which are not removable.
- Any site of trauma, surgery, ulceration or graft placement which should not be compressed by the pressure cuff.
- Pressure measurements are typically prohibited on ipsilateral side of mastectomy or AVG/AVF.

Mechanism of Disease

There are two major mechanisms that cause reduced arterial blood supply to the lower extremity: atherosclerotic plaque and embolism. Of these, atherosclerosis is more common.

- **Atherosclerosis** is the most common arterial disease. Atherosclerotic plaque forms in the artery to blocking flow by either narrowing the arterial lumen (arterial stenosis) or totally blocking the artery (arterial occlusion). The term "hemodynamically significant obstruction" refers to either a stenosis or an occlusion that results in a decrease in blood pressure or flow distal to the obstruction. Typically, a stenosis must narrow the diameter of the artery by at least 50% to decrease pressure and flow distally. An arterial occlusion is typically seen from one major branch to the next.
- **Emboli** is the embolization of contents of a plaque and/or fragments of an organized thrombus from the heart or proximal aneurysm which become lodged in a distant blood vessel.[1]
- **Extrinsic compression** from tumors, hematoma, etc., can result in stenosis or occlusion by placing enough pressure on arterial walls to compromise blood flow.[2]
- **Vasospasm** is a temporary constriction of the arteries (typically digital arteries) that may cause significant discomfort to the patient.[3]
- **Pseudoaneurysm (PA)** or "false aneurysm" forms due to trauma to all three layers of the arterial wall. The "false aneurysm" is actually a hematoma, receiving its blood supply via communication with an artery through a patent "neck."[4]
- **Arteriovenous fistula** or abnormal connection between artery and vein can result from trauma or complications during invasive procedures (e.g., cardiac catheterization). In such cases, blood flows directly from the artery into the venous system without passing through the tissues and capillary bed.[5]
- **Aneurysmal disease** results from weakening of the structural proteins (elastin and collagen) within the medial layer of the arterial wall. Aneurysmal disease typically does not obstruct flow, but carries the risk of rupture and/or emboli.[6]

Location of Disease

- Arterial disease can be focal or diffuse and affect any level or multiple levels.
- The most common location of obstruction in the lower extremities is the superficial femoral artery at the adductor canal.
- Arterial bifurcations and the popliteal artery are other common locations of obstruction.

Patient History
- Claudication (exercise related)
- Pain or rest pain
- Paralysis (weakness)
- Paresthesia ("pins and needles")
- Poikilothermia (ice-cold limbs)
- Previous ulceration/gangrene of feet/toes
- Previous therapeutic vascular procedure (e.g., bypass, stenting)

Physical Examination
- Pulselessness
- Pallor
- Cyanosis
- Dependent rubor
- Bruit (abnormal sound heard through auscultation caused by vibration of tissue from turbulent flow)
- Marked temperature difference between extremities
- Gangrene/necrosis (tissue death)
- Palpable thrill (vibration caused by turbulent blood flow as seen in AV fistulas)

Ankle-Brachial Indices Protocol
- Rest the patient for 5-10 minutes before beginning the exam in order for blood pressures to stabilize after "exercise" (walking into the exam room). You may use this time to obtain a patient history, including symptoms and risk factors, explain the procedure, and to place cuffs.
- Appropriately wrap blood pressure cuffs on the limbs. Cuffs should be placed "straight" rather than angled. All cuffs should fit snugly so that inflation of the bladder transmits the head of pressure into the tissue rather than into space between the bladder and the limb, producing falsely elevated readings.
  » Apply cuffs with a 10-12cm bladder (in width) 2-3cm above the medial malleolus, bilaterally.
  » Apply same sized cuffs on the arm to obtain brachial pressures.
- Pressure measurements should be taken in the supine position with the extremity at the same level as the heart.
- Pressures recorded while the patient is sitting will be falsely elevated due to the effects of hydrostatic pressure.
- If pressures can only be obtained while the patient is sitting, use the same method for follow-up exams for accurate comparison.
- Do not take a blood pressure over a bypass graft or dialysis access conduit or fistula without first consulting your medical director. Do not take a blood pressure on the arm of a patient with a history of mastectomy.
- Locate the posterior tibial arterial (PTA) signal posterior to the medial malleolus using a high frequency (8MHz) CW Doppler transducer. (Use a lower frequency transducer (e.g., 4MHz) on obese patients or for deeper vessels when needed.).
  » Angle between 45-60°, pointing the transducer towards the heart.
  » Place enough pressure on the transducer to stay in place without compressing the artery.
  » Manipulate the transducer slightly to obtain the strongest arterial signal. Resting the hand on the foot is helpful in holding the transducer in place during cuff inflation.
  » Record several representative PTA waveforms. If no arterial signal is identified at the ankle, you can try for a signal more proximally along the medial calf. You may also have to reposition your pressure cuff higher on the leg. In such cases, document what level the pressure was taken.

- When testing with an automatic cuff inflator or standard manometer:
  » Inflate the air cuff 20-30mmHg above the last audible arterial signal heard using the Doppler transducer.

For patients with irregular heart beats decrease deflation speeds.

  » Deflate the cuff slowly (at a rate of 2-4mmHg per second). The systolic pressure is recorded in mmHg as soon as the first audible arterial Doppler signal returns. There should be a period of silence after inflation prior to hearing the return of the first pulse to be sure the cuff was inflated beyond the local arterial pressure. The Doppler pulse must continue after hearing the first pulse to assure there is an actual pulse rather than motion artifact.

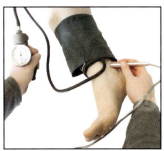 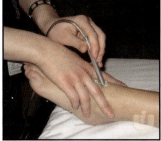

Fig. 16-1: *Have the patient externally rotate their calf to help find the PTA.*

Fig. 16-2: *Place your fingers on the ankle bones to help locate the DPA.*

- Locate the dorsalis pedis arterial (DPA) signal and repeat the procedure using CW Doppler on the dorsum of the foot (about halfway between the toes and ankle). Record several representative waveforms. Avoid sampling too close to the toes, or you will likely be listening to the plantar arch or a digital vessel instead of the DPA (which may be receiving blood from the posterior tibial artery if the DPA or anterior tibial is occluded). If the signal is damped, retrograde or absent, move to the anterior ankle area and search for the anterior tibial (ATA) signal. If no arterial signal is identified, locate the peroneal artery (PerA) slightly anterior to the lateral malleolus.
- If a pressure measurement needs to be repeated, the cuff should be fully deflated for approximately one minute prior to the repeat measurement. The systolic pressure is recorded as the pressure at which the first audible arterial Doppler signal returns.
- Obtain bilateral brachial artery (BrA) pressures. When testing with an automatic cuff inflator or standard manometer:
  » Inflate the cuffs wrapped around the mid upper arms 20-30mmHg above the last audible arterial signal using a Doppler transducer.

Document brachial pressure differences >20mmHg or if brachial waveforms are different. Check for the presence of subclavian steal by sampling vertebral flow direction.

- Calculate the ankle-brachial index (ABI) by dividing the pedal pressure by the highest brachial pressure:

$$\frac{\text{pedal pressure}}{\text{highest brachial pressure}} = \text{ABI}$$

- Repeat on the contralateral leg when indicated.
- Determine severity of disease according to laboratory diagnostic criteria.

Table 16-1: ABI Protocol Summary

- Wrap pressure cuffs around the limbs
    - » Arm
    - » Leg-ankle level
- Using CW Doppler, record representative waveforms
    - » DPA
    - » PTA
    - » BrA (when indicated)
- Inflate cuff 20-30mmHg beyond the last audible arterial signal heard using a Doppler transducer on the appropriate artery distal to the cuff.
- Deflation of the cuff should be at a rate of 2-4mmHg per second. The pressure is recorded as soon as the first continuous audible arterial Doppler signal returns.
- Calculate the ABI:

$$\frac{\text{pedal pressure}}{\text{highest brachial pressure}} = \text{ABI}$$

- Determine classification of disease according to laboratory diagnostic criteria.

Ankle-Brachial Pressure Worksheet

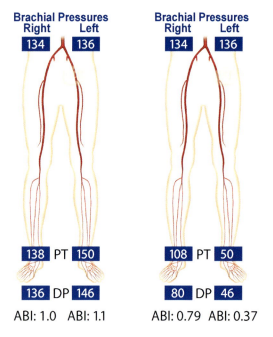

Fig. 16-3: *Normal ABI report   Abnormal ABI report*

The diagnostic criteria used to determine the severity of abnormal lower extremity ankle-brachial indices varies across institutions.

PRINCIPLES OF INTERPRETATION

Pressures

Pressure measurements should be taken in the supine position with the extremity at the same level as the heart. Pressures recorded with the patient sitting will be falsely elevated due to hydrostatic pressure. For every 10 inches the heart is elevated above the ankle level, pressure increases 18.67mmHg. Since the heart level is 34 inches from the ankle on the average person while sitting, the ankle pressure will be affected about 63mmHg (3.4 x 18.67mmHg). If you can only get pressures with the patient sitting, note the position and know that this pressure will be significantly lower than if the pressure was taken while supine. You can also try placing the foot on a chair to get it closer to the heart. Remember to use the same method for follow-up exams for accurate comparison.

Arterial Waveform Terminology

The terminology used to describe arterial waveforms is not consistent across laboratories. A consensus document was published in 2020 by the Society of Vascular Ultrasound and the Society for Vascular Medicine regarding the terminology and interpretation of peripheral arterial and venous waveforms. *See the Arterial Hemodynamics chapter for more detail on arterial waveforms.*

Spectral Doppler Waveforms

Any change in spectral waveform analysis depends on the terminology used by the lab; from triphasic to monophasic or changes in resistance may be significant.

Interpretation/Diagnostic Criteria

Normal

Pressures

- Leg pressures are normally higher than the highest brachial pressure. According to research, the normal pressure difference between the arm and ankle is between 12 (±8) to 24 (±9)mmHg. [7]

- If the ABI is ≥1.0, the presence of a hemodynamically significant stenosis or occlusion is unlikely between the arm and ankle cuffs. The upper and lower limits of normal varies within the literature and is thought to depend on whether the patient is hypertensive or hypotensive.[8] An ABI >0.97 is often considered normal. [9] The ABI typically is no less than 0.92 in a normal limb. [7]

Spectral Doppler Waveforms

- A waveform with a sharp, quick upstroke followed by a brisk downstroke with reversed flow direction in early diastole and another forward phase in late diastole is termed *triphasic*. This is considered a normal finding in the peripheral arteries.

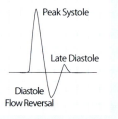
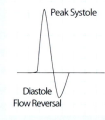

Fig. 16-4: *Normal, triphasic Doppler waveform*   **Fig. 16-5:** *Doppler waveform missing the third component of flow above the baseline.*

- A waveform with a sharp upstroke followed by reversed flow that crosses the zero baseline and contains both forward and reverse components is termed *biphasic* or "multiphasic."

- Some labs have adopted terminology that recognizes any reversed flow as normal by using an abbreviation NR for "normal-reversed" whether or not the third phase is present, in order to avoid the confusing use of "triphasic" and "biphasic" terms. [16]

- Arterial waveforms without a reversed flow component can be a normal finding for some patients, such as the elderly. If arterial pressures are normal, consider the possibility that the signal may also be normal. [9]

The third phase of the triphasic waveform may be missing in older patients with less vessel compliance.

Abnormal

Pressures

The reason for decreased ankle pressures is almost always a hemodynamically significant proximal lesion. [7]

- As the ABI lowers to 90% of the arm pressure, it is likely that a hemodynamically significant obstruction is present in the lower extremity above the level of the ankle. [10]
- A patient with claudication is likely to have an ABI <0.80. [14]
- A patient with rest pain is likely to have an ABI of <0.40. [9]
- An ABI <0.50 suggests multiple levels of disease. [7,9,10]
- The difference in ankle pressure between the dorsalis pedis and posterior tibial arteries in the same limb should be within 10mmHg. [7] A difference in ABI >15mmHg suggests a proximal obstruction. [7,9,11]
- A change in the ABI of ≥0.15 from one study to the next is significant. [7,9,10]

ABI may be combined with exercise stress testing to uncover obstructions unrecognizable at rest that become significant with exercise.

- A foot ulcer is unlikely to heal if the ankle pressure is <80mmHg in a diabetic patient. [15]
- An ABI of >1.3 suggests calcific disease and is considered non-diagnostic. As an alternative means of estimating disease severity, use a toe/brachial index. A diagnosis of disease severity (normal, mild, moderate, severe, critical) can also be made based solely on waveform analysis when calcific disease is present. [7,9]

Spectral Doppler Waveforms

- As the obstruction becomes more severe, changes in the spectral waveform are expected before a stenosis or occlusion, at the point of greatest stenosis and after a stenosis/occlusion as described in the *Arterial Physiology* chapter. These changes are important to note in the interpretation of the vascular exam.
- *Monophasic* arterial Doppler waveforms reflect low resistance and are characterized by a slow upstroke, low amplitude, and broad peak with continuous forward flow in diastole that does not cross the zero baseline. The upstroke has a general direction of being tipped to the right. Monophasic waveforms are typically present distal to an occlusion or a very high-grade stenosis. [7,9,16]

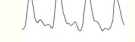

Fig. 16-6: *Multiphasic CW arterial Doppler signals*

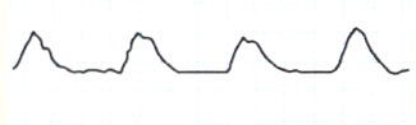

Fig. 16-7: *Monophasic CW arterial Doppler signals*

- *Parvus tardus* is an alternative term for "monophasic" used by some laboratories to describe a waveform with continuous forward flow and a slow, blunted systolic component. [15]

- **Occlusion:** An absent or non-pulsatile Doppler signal suggests occlusion at the site of interrogation. [7,12-14]

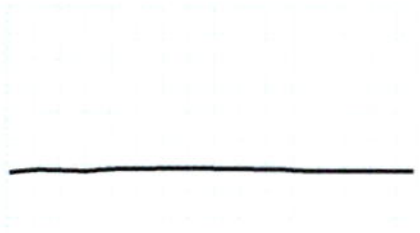

Fig. 16-8: *Absent pulsatility*

Table 16-2: Diagnostic Criteria for ABI

ABI	Comment
≥1.0	Normal
0.90 to <1.0	Mild disease
0.50-0.90	Claudication
0.30-0.50	Severe occlusive disease
<0.30	Ischemia

Source: AbuRahma AF. (2000). Segmental Doppler pressures and Doppler waveform analysis in peripheral vascular disease of the lower extremities. In AbuRahma AF, Bergan JJ (Eds). *Non-invasive Vascular Diagnosis.* (213-229). London: Springer.

Table 16-3: University of Chicago Diagnostic ABI Criteria

ABI	Severity
≥1.0-0.95	Normal
0.80-0.94	Mild disease
0.50-0.79	Moderate disease
0.30-0.49	Severe disease
<0.29	Critical disease

Source: Internally validated at the University of Chicago Medical Center Vascular Laboratory.

Table 16-4: ABI Symptoms

ABI	Symptom
≥1.0	Normal
<0.80	Claudication
<0.40	Rest pain
<0.20	Impending gangrene

Source: Modified from Yao JST. (1970). Hemodynamic studies in peripheral arterial disease. Br J Surg. 57:761.

Differential Diagnosis
- Spinal stenosis
- Venous thrombosis
- Restless leg syndrome
- Compartment syndrome
- Nocturnal leg cramps
- Neuropathy
- Muscle/tendon strains
- Arthritis
- Abnormalities of adrenergic receptor/sympathetic nervous system
- Connective tissue disease (scleroderma)

Correlation
- Duplex ultrasound
- Spiral CT scan
- MRA
- Arteriography

Medical Treatment

- Modify risk factors (e.g., reduce cholesterol, manage HTN and DM, smoking cessation)
- Exercise regimen
- Antiplatelet medication (e.g., aspirin)
- Anticoagulation (warfarin)

Surgical Treatment

- Bypass grafting
- Endarterectomy
- Direct focal repair
- Resection (aneurysmal disease)
- Sympathectomy
- Amputation

Endovascular Treatment

- Angioplasty
- Stent
- Intra-arterial directed thrombolysis (acute blockage)
- Atherectomy

REFERENCES

1. Fecteau SR, Darling III RC, Roddy SP. (2005). Arterial thromboembolism. In *Rutherford Vascular Surgery 6th edition.* (971-986). Philadelphia. Elsevier Saunders.
2. Sumner DS, Zierler RE. (2005). Vascular physiology: essential hemodynamic principles. In *Rutherford Vascular Surgery 6th edition.* (75-123). Philadelphia. Elsevier Saunders.
3. Shepard RFJ. (2005). Raynaud's syndrome: vasospastic and occlusive arterial disease involving the distal upper extremity. In *Rutherford Vascular Surgery 6th edition.* (1319-1346). Philadelphia: Elsevier Saunders.
4. Casey, PJ, LaMuraglia GM. (2005). *Anastomotic aneurysms. In Rutherford Vascular Surgery 6th edition.* (894-902). Philadelphia. Elsevier Saunders.
5. Rutherford RB. (2005). *Diagnostic evaluation of arteriovenous fistulas and vascular anomalies. In Rutherford Vascular Surgery 6th edition.* (1602-1612). Philadelphia. Elsevier Saunders.
6. Dawson DL, Lee ES, Lindholm K. (2010). Aortic and peripheral aneurysms. In Zierler RE (Ed.), *Strandess's duplex scanning disorders in vascular diagnosis 4th ed.* (157-168). Philadelphia: Wolters Kluwer Lippincott Williams & Wilkins.
7. Zierler RE, Sumner DS. (2005). Physiologic assessment of peripheral arterial occlusive disease. . In *Rutherford Vascular Surgery 6th edition.* (197-222). Philadelphia. Elsevier Saunders.
8. Nicolaides AN. (2003). Basic and practical aspects of peripheral arterial testing. In Bernstein EF (Ed.), *Vascular Diagnosis* (481-485). St. Louis: Mosby.
9. Carter SA. (2003). Role of pressure measurements. In Bernstein EF (Ed.), *Vascular Diagnosis* (486-512). St. Louis: Mosby.
10. Zierler, RE, (2005). Nonimaging Physiologic Tests for Assessment of Lower Extremity Arterial Occlusive Disease. In Zwiebel WJ, Pellerito JS (Eds.), *Introduction to Vascular Ultrasonography.* (275-295). Philadelphia: Elsevier Saunders.
11. Nordness PJ, Money SR. (2005). In Mansour MA, Labropoulos N. (Eds.), *Vascular Diagnosis,* (207-214). Philadelphia: Elsevier Saunders.
12. Needham T. (2005). In Mansour MA, Labropoulos N. (Eds.), *Vascular Diagnosis,* (215-222). Philadelphia: Elsevier Saunders.
13. AbuRahma AF. (2000). Segmental Doppler pressures and Doppler waveform analysis in peripheral vascular disease of the lower extremities. In AbuRahma AF, Bergan JJ (Eds). *Non-invasive Vascular Diagnosis.* (213-229). London: Springer.
14. Yao JST. (1970). *Hemodynamic studies in peripheral arterial disease. Br J Surg. 57:761.*
15. Raines JK, Darling RC, Both K et al. (1976). *Vascular laboratory criteria for the management of peripheral vascular disease of the lower extremities. Surgery 79:21-29,*
16. Kim ES, Sharma AM, Scissons R, et al. *Interpretation of peripheral arterial and venous Doppler waveforms: A consensus statement from the Society for Vascular Medicine and Society for Vascular Ultrasound. Vascular Medicine.* 2020;25(5):484-506. doi:10.1177/1358863X20937665

ARTERIAL TESTING

17. Lower Extremity Segmental Pressures and Doppler Waveforms

Definition
Systolic blood pressures and Doppler waveforms are compared at different segments of the lower extremities to identify the general location of a hemodynamically significant arterial obstruction. The term "obstruction" is used to describe either a stenosis or an occlusion of an artery. These techniques also define the resulting decrease in blood flow in terms of pressure and general perfusion of the lower extremity.

Etiology
- Atherosclerosis
- Embolization
- Thrombus
- Intimal hyperplasia
- Trauma
- Traumatic occlusion
- Extrinsic compression
- Vasculitis
- AV fistula (abnormal connection between an artery and a vein)
- Radiation arteritis

Indications for Exam
- Claudication (exercise-related limb pain)
- Follow-up of a previously abnormal segmental exam
- Limb pain at rest
- Absent peripheral pulses
- Extremity ulcer
- Gangrene
- Pre-operative assessment of healing potential
- Digital cyanosis
- Cold sensitivity
- Aneurysmal disease
- Dependent rubor
- Trauma to an artery
- Follow-up after revascularization procedure

Risk Factors
- Age (increased risk with age)
- Coronary artery disease
- Diabetes
- Family history
- Hyperlipidemia
- Hypertension
- Obesity
- Smoking
- Sedentary lifestyle
- Previous history of CVA or MI
- Elevated levels of homocysteine
- Excessive levels of C-reactive protein
- History of radiation

Patient History
- Claudication (exercise-related)
- Rest pain
- Paralysis (weakness)
- Paresthesia ("pins and needles")
- Poikilothermia (ice-cold limbs)
- Previous ulceration/gangrene of feet/toes
- Previous therapeutic vascular procedure (e.g., bypass, stenting)

Physical Examination
- Pulselessness
- Pallor
- Cyanosis
- Dependent rubor
- Bruit (abnormal sound heard through auscultation caused by vibration of tissue from turbulent flow)
- Marked temperature difference between extremities
- Gangrene/necrosis (tissue death)
- Palpable thrill (vibration caused by turbulent blood flow as seen in AV fistulas)

Contraindications/Limitations
- Calcified vessels which will falsely elevate pressures (typically encountered in patients with diabetes or end-stage renal disease). The possibility/presence of upper extremity atherosclerotic disease may also be a consideration.
- Significant lesions with excellent collateral circulation, which may result in normal distal pressures and waveforms at rest.
- Pressure cuffs may not fit around very large thighs. Cuffs which are too small can elevate pressures considerably.
- Patients with acute clot or venous thrombosis in the lower extremities should not have pressure cuffs inflated over their clot.
- Patients with extensive bandages or casts which are not removable.
- Any site of trauma, surgery, ulceration or graft placement which should not be compressed by the pressure cuff.
- Pressure measurements typically prohibited on ipsilateral side of mastectomy or AVG/AVF.

Mechanism of Disease
There are two major mechanisms that cause reduced arterial blood supply to the lower extremity; atherosclerotic plaque and embolism. Of these, atherosclerosis is more common.

- **Atherosclerosis** is the most common arterial disease. Atherosclerotic plaque forms in the artery to blocking flow by either narrowing the arterial lumen (arterial stenosis) or totally blocking the artery (arterial occlusion). The term "hemodynamically significant obstruction" refers to either a stenosis or an occlusion that results in a decrease in blood pressure or flow distal to the obstruction. Typically, a stenosis must narrow the diameter of the artery by at least 50% to decrease pressure and flow distally. An arterial occlusion is typically seen from one major branch to the next.
- **Emboli:** embolization of contents of a plaque and/or fragments of an organized thrombus from the heart or proximal aneurysm which become lodged in a distant blood vessel. [2]
- **Extrinsic compression** from tumors, hematoma, etc., can result in stenosis or occlusion by placing enough pressure on arterial walls to compromise blood flow. [1]
- **Vasospasm:** is a temporary constriction of the arteries (typically digital arteries) that may cause significant discomfort to the patient (uncommon).[3]
- **Pseudoaneurysm (PA):** or "false aneurysm" forms due to trauma to all three layers of the arterial wall. The "false aneurysm" is actually a hematoma, receiving its blood supply via communication with an artery through a patent "neck." [4]
- **Arteriovenous fistula:** an abnormal connection between artery and vein can result from trauma or complications during invasive procedures (e.g., cardiac catheterization). In such cases, blood flows directly from the artery into the venous system without passing through the tissues and capillary bed. [5]
- **Aneurysmal disease** results from weakening of the structural proteins (elastin and collagen) within the medial layer of the arterial wall. Aneurysmal disease typically does not obstruct flow, but carries the risk of rupture and/or emboli. [4]

Location of Obstructive Disease

- Arterial disease can be focal or diffuse and affect any level or multiple levels.
- The most common location of obstruction in the lower extremities is the distal superficial femoral artery at the adductor canal.
- Arterial bifurcations and the popliteal artery are other common locations of obstruction.

Lower Extremity Segmental Pressures and Spectral Doppler Waveforms Protocol

Pressure measurements should be taken in the supine position with the extremity at the same level as the heart. Pressures recorded while the patient is sitting will be falsely elevated due to the effects of hydrostatic pressure.

- Rest the patient for 5-10 minutes before beginning the exam in order for blood pressures to stabilize after "exercise" (walking into the exam room). You may use this time to obtain a patient history, including symptoms and risk factors or wrap cuffs.
- Cuff positions may include:
  » Thigh, calf and ankle (a.k.a. "3-cuff method")
  » High thigh, low thigh, calf, and ankle a.k.a. "4-cuff method")

The 4-cuff method offers more information than the 3-cuff method; distinguishing inflow from femoral disease.

- Choose appropriately sized pneumatic cuffs for each section of the limb:
  » 18-20cm width on thigh (for 3-cuff method)
  » 12cm width on upper/lower thigh (for 4-cuff method)
  » 12cm width on arm, calf and ankle. Some labs prefer a 10cm cuff at the arm and ankle. *The cuff width should be at least 20% greater than the diameter of the limb.*

Using too narrow a cuff for the width of the limb will result in higher pressures due to cuff artifact. [7,10,11]

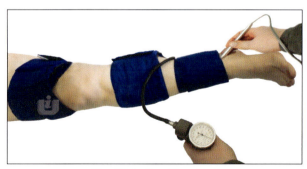

Fig. 17-1: *3-cuff method*

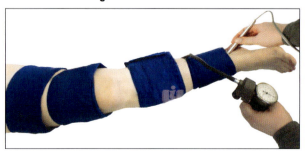

Fig. 17-2: *4-cuff method*

- Appropriately wrap blood pressure cuffs on the limb. Cuffs should be placed "straight" rather than angled. All cuffs should fit snugly, so that inflation of the bladder transmits the head of pressure into the tissue rather than into space between the bladder and the limb, producing falsely elevated readings particularly if they are to be used for the VPR technique following the pressures exam.
- Place the thigh cuff as high as possible on the thigh, the low thigh cuff above the knee, the calf cuff just below the knee and the ankle cuff just above the medial malleolus.
- Arterial physiologic exams are traditionally performed using a continuous wave (CW) Doppler. However, waveforms can be obtained at the same sites using a spectral Doppler. The CW Doppler is recommended for segmental pressure measurement due to its capabilities for a larger sampling region. Use a high frequency (8MHz) CW Doppler transducer to locate arterial signals. Alternate transducers including a lower frequency transducer (e.g., 4MHz) may be needed for obese patients or for deeper vessels.

Segmental Doppler Waveforms

- Place the Doppler transducer on the limb using a 45°-60° angle to the skin with enough pressure to keep contact, but not so much pressure that the artery is compressed by the transducer:
- Document several representative Doppler waveforms at the following levels after moving or angling the transducer appropriately to optimize the signal:
  » Dorsalis pedis artery*
  » Posterior tibial artery*
  » Popliteal artery

If the venous signal is interfering with the arterial waveform, try a slightly more proximal or distal location or manually compress the proximal limb to temporarily stop venous return.

  » Superficial femoral (avoiding the deep femoral artery)
  » Common femoral artery

If neither pedal artery is audible, try to obtain a waveform of the peroneal artery by placing the transducer superior to the lateral malleolus, pointing inward.

Segmental Pressures

- Locate the best arterial signal at the ankle or use the popliteal signal for the thigh pressure(s) and the pedal arteries only for the calf and ankle pressures.

The following instructions can be used when testing with an automatic cuff inflator or standard manometer:

- Inflate cuffs 20-30mmHg above the last audible arterial signal heard using the Doppler transducer.
- There should be a period of silence after inflation and prior to hearing the first pulse to be sure the cuff was inflated beyond the local arterial pressure. The Doppler pulse must continue after hearing the first pulse to assure there is an actual pulse rather than motion artifact.

For patients with irregular heart beats, decrease deflation speeds.

- Deflate the cuff slowly (at a rate of 2-4mmHg per second). The systolic pressure is recorded as soon as the first audible arterial Doppler signal returns.
- If a pressure measurement needs to be repeated, the cuff should be fully deflated for approximately one minute prior to the repeat measurement.

Do not take a blood pressure over a bypass graft or dialysis access conduit or fistula without first consulting your medical director. Do not take a blood pressure on the arm of a patient with a history of mastectomy.

- The pressure is recorded in "mmHg" as soon as the first audible Doppler arterial signal returns at each level indicated; ankle, calf, low thigh and/or high thigh.
- Obtain bilateral brachial artery (BrA) pressures.

If brachial pressures differ by >20mmHg or if the brachial waveforms are different, the vertebral arteries should be examined for flow direction. Retrograde flow in the vertebral artery ipsilateral to the arm with the lower brachial pressure is indicative of subclavian steal syndrome.

- Calculate ankle, calf, low-thigh, high-thigh brachial indices by dividing the systolic pressure at the particular level by the highest brachial pressure.
- Repeat for the contralateral leg when indicated.

Studies have demonstrated that when patients have an SFA occlusion, efforts to address a stenosis in the proximal deep femoral artery may increase blood flow enough to relieve distal ischemia. (Note: Alternate terminology for the DFA is profunda femoral)

- A profundapopliteal collateral index (PPCI) is used to predict whether collateral flow might be adequate enough to heal distal ischemia.[13]

$$PPCI\ (mmHg) = \frac{\text{Above knee - Below knee pressure}}{\text{Above knee pressure}}$$

Table 17-1: Lower Extremity Segmental Pressures Protocol Summary

- Apply appropriately sized pneumatic cuffs for each section of the limb:
  » For 3-cuff method: 18-20cm width; thigh, 12cm width; arm, calf and ankle*
  » For 4-cuff method: 12cm width; arms, thigh, calf and ankle*
- Record representative spectral Doppler waveforms for all lower extremity levels.
- Inflate each cuff 20-30mmHg beyond the last audible arterial signal using a Doppler transducer on the appropriate artery distal to the cuff.
- Deflation of the cuff should be at a rate of 2-4mmHg/s
- The pressure is recorded as soon as the first audible arterial Doppler signal returns.
- Obtain a pressure at each cuff consecutively and calculate the index at each level:

$$\frac{\text{pedal, calf, thigh pressure}}{\text{highest brachial pressure}}$$

- Determine classification of disease according to laboratory diagnostic criteria.
- Repeat for the contralateral side.

(Some labs use a 10cm cuff at the ankle)

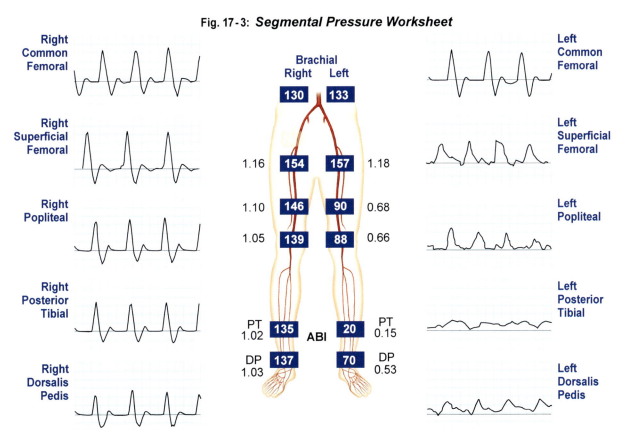

Fig. 17-3: *Segmental Pressure Worksheet*

Normal *segmental pressures and waveforms documented of the right lower extremity.*

Abnormal *pressures and waveforms on the left suggest arterial obstruction at the femoral and tibial levels.*

PRINCIPLES OF INTERPRETATION

Segmental Pressures

Pressure measurements should be taken in the supine position (the extremity at the same level as the heart). Pressures recorded with the patient sitting will be falsely elevated due to hydrostatic pressure. For every 10 inches the heart is elevated above the ankle level, pressure increases 18.67mmHg. Since the heart level is 34 inches from the ankle on the average person while sitting, the ankle pressure will be affected about 63mmHg (3.4 x 18.67mmHg). If you can only get pressures with the patient sitting, note the position and know that this pressure will be significantly lower than if the actual pressure taken while supine. You can also try placing the foot on a chair to get it closer to the heart. Remember to use the same method for follow-up exams for accurate comparison.

Arterial Waveform Terminology

The terminology used to describe arterial waveforms is not consistent across laboratories. A consensus document was published in 2020 by the Society of Vascular Ultrasound and the Society for Vascular Medicine regarding the terminology and interpretation of peripheral arterial and venous waveforms. *See the Arterial Hemodynamics chapter for more detail on arterial waveforms.*

sAny change in spectral waveform analysis depends on the terminology used by the lab; from triphasic to monophasic or changes in resistance may be significant.

Interpretation/Diagnostic Criteria

Normal

Segmental Pressures

- Leg pressures are normally higher than the highest brachial pressure. According to research, the normal pressure difference between the arm and ankle is between 12 (±8) to 24 (±9)mmHg.[7]
- If using the 4-cuff method with a 12cm thigh cuff, the upper thigh pressure is normally 30-40mmHg higher than the arm pressure due to cuff artifact.[5-7]
- Segmental pressure ratios (leg pressure ÷ arm pressure) of the lower thigh, calf and ankle should be =1.0 at all levels.[5] There is normally no significant decrease in pressure (<20mmHg) between the cuffs.[5-8]
- The high thigh ratio using a 12cm cuff is normally =1.2-1.4.[5,7,9]
- A produndapopliteal collateral index (PPCI) of less than 0.25 suggests that there is enough collateral support to carry blood flow to the popliteal run-off vessels in patients with SFA obstruction.[13]

Spectral Doppler Waveforms

- A waveform with a sharp, quick upstroke followed by a brisk downstroke with reversed flow direction in early diastole and another forward phase in late diastole is termed *triphasic*. This is considered a normal finding in the peripheral arteries.

- A waveform with a sharp upstroke followed by reversed flow that crosses the zero baseline and contains both forward and reverse components is termed *biphasic* or "multiphasic."

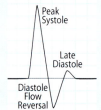

Fig. 17-4: *Normal, triphasic waveform*

- Some labs have adopted terminology that recognizes any reversed flow as normal by using an abbreviation NR for "normal-reversed" whether or not the third phase is present, in order to avoid the confusing use of "triphasic" and "biphasic" terms.[12]
- Arterial waveforms without a reversed flow component can be a normal finding for some patients, such as the elderly. If arterial pressures are normal, consider the possibility that the signal may also be normal.[6]

The third phase of the triphasic waveform may be missing in older patients with less vessel compliance.

Abnormal

Segmental Pressures

- A leg/brachial ratio <1.0 (or <1.2-1.4 at the upper thigh level) is abnormal and indicates a significant stenosis or occlusion at/ or proximal to the cuff.[5,9]
- If the ABI is <0.92 it is likely that a hemodynamically significant obstruction is present in the lower extremity above the level of the ankle.[5,7,9]
- A drop in pressure >20-30mmHg between adjacent cuffs (proximal to distal) indicates significant obstruction between these levels.[6-8,11]
- Significant collateral blood flow may result in a false negative pressure gradient of less than 20mmHg between segments or a normal upper thigh brachial ratio.[8]
- A change in the ABI of ≥0.15 from one study to the next is significant.[8,9]
- A calf pressure ≥65-70mmHg is typically needed to heal a below-knee amputation.[7,8]

If the ankle pressure is significantly higher than the calf, it is likely that calcification is causing a falsely high ankle pressure and should not be used for interpretation.[7,10]

- An ABI >1.3 suggests calcific disease and is considered non-diagnostic.[6,10] As an alternative means of estimating disease severity, use a toe-brachial index.[6,10] A toe-brachial index <0.70 is abnormal.[10]
- A PPCI > 0.25 is abnormal; fixing deep femoral artery obstruction may not be enough to help blood flow reach collateral and popliteal run-off vessels.[13]

Spectral Doppler Waveforms

- As the obstruction becomes more severe, changes in the spectral waveform are expected before a stenosis or occlusion, at the point of greatest stenosis and after a stenosis/occlusion as described in the *Arterial Physiology* chapter. These changes are important to note in the interpretation of the vascular exam.
- *Monophasic* arterial waveforms reflect low resistance and are characterized by a slow upstroke, low amplitude, and broad peak with continuous forward flow in diastole that does not cross the zero baseline. The upstroke has a general direction of being tipped to the right. Monophasic waveforms are typically present distal to an occlusion or a very high-grade stenosis.[11,12]
- *Parvus tardus* is an alternative term for "monophasic" used by some laboratories to describe a waveform with continuous forward flow and a slow, blunted systolic component.[12]
- **Occlusion:** An absent or non-pulsatile Doppler signal suggests occlusion at the site of interrogation.[7,9]

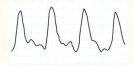

Multiphasic | Monophasic

Fig. 17-5: *Continuous wave arterial Doppler signals*

Distinguishing between multiphasic vs monophasic Doppler waveforms is important, especially at the common femoral and pedal levels.

Table 17-2: Findings of the Lower Extremities and Level of Disease

Level of Disease	Findings
Aortoiliac	High thigh/brachial index <1.0 bilaterally
Iliac	High thigh/brachial index <1.0 unilaterally
Femoral disease	Gradient between high and low thigh cuffs
Distal SFA/popliteal	Gradient between thigh and calf cuffs
Infrapopliteal	Gradient between calf and ankle cuffs

Table 17-3: Diagnostic Criteria for ABI Severity

ABI	Severity
≥1.0	Normal
0.90 to <1.0	Mild disease
0.50-0.90	Claudication
0.30-0.50	Severe occlusive disease
<0.30	Ischemia

Source: AbuRahma AF. (2000). Segmental Doppler pressures and Doppler waveform analysis in peripheral vascular disease of the lower extremities. In AbuRahma AF, Bergan JJ (Eds). *Non-invasive Vascular Diagnosis.* (213-229). London: Springer.

Table 17-4: Diagnostic Criteria for Occlusive Disease by Segmental Arterial Pressure Indices

One primary arterial occlusion

Ankle-brachial index is typically between 0.50-0.80 (Consider highest ABI)

Multilevel occlusive disease

Ankle-brachial index is typically <0.50 (Consider highest ABI)

Source: Zierler RE, Sumner DS. (2005). Physiologic assessment of peripheral arterial occlusive disease. In *Rutherford Vascular Surgery 6th edition.* (197-222). Philadelphia. Elsevier Saunders.

Differential Diagnosis

- Spinal stenosis
- Venous thrombosis
- Restless leg syndrome
- Compartment syndrome
- Nocturnal leg cramps
- Neuropathy
- Muscle/tendon strains
- Arthritis
- Abnormalities of adrenergic receptor/sympathetic nervous system
- Connective tissue disease (scleroderma)

Correlation

- Duplex ultrasound
- Spiral CT scan
- MRA
- Arteriography

Medical Treatment

- Modify risk factors (e.g., reduce cholesterol, manage HTN and DM, smoking cessation)
- Exercise regimen
- Antiplatelet medication (e.g., aspirin)
- Anticoagulation (warfarin)
- Thrombolysis (acute blockage)

Surgical Treatment

- Bypass grafting
- Atherectomy
- Endarterectomy
- Direct focal repair
- Resection (aneurysmal disease)
- Sympathectomy
- Amputation

Endovascular Treatment

- Angioplasty
- Stent
- Atherectomy
- Intra-arterial directed thrombolysis (acute blockage)

REFERENCES

1. Sumner DS, Zierler RE. (2005). Vascular physiology: essential hemodynamic principles. In *Rutherford Vascular Surgery 6th edition.* (75-123). Philadelphia. Elsevier Saunders.
2. Fecteau SR, Darling III RC, Roddy SP. (2005). Arterial thromboembolism. In *Rutherford Vascular Surgery 6th edition.* (971-986). Philadelphia. Elsevier Saunders.
3. Shepard RFJ. (2005). Raynaud's syndrome: vasospastic and occlusive arterial disease involving the distal upper extremity. In *Rutherford Vascular Surgery 6th edition.* (1319-1346). Philadelphia. Elsevier Saunders.
4. Dawson DL, Lee ES, Lindholm K. (2010). Aortic and peripheral aneurysms. In Zierler RE (Ed.), *Strandess's duplex scanning disorders in vascular diagnosis 4th ed.* (157-168). Philadelphia Wolters Kluwer Lippincott Williams & Wilkins.
5. Zierler RE, Sumner DS. (2005). Physiologic assessment of peripheral arterial occlusive disease. In *Rutherford Vascular Surgery 6th edition.* (197-222). Philadelphia. Elsevier Saunders.
6. Carter SA. (2003). Role of pressure measurements. In Bernstein EF (Ed.), Vascular Diagnosis (486-512). St. Louis: Mosby.
7. Zierler, RE, (2005). Nonimaging Physiologic Tests for Assessment of Lower Extremity Arterial Occlusive Disease. In Zwiebel WJ, Pellerito JS (Eds.), *Introduction to Vascular Ultrasonography.* (275-295). Philadelphia: Elsevier Saunders
8. Hallett, JW, Brewster DC, Rasmussen TE, (2001) Non-invasive Vascular Testing, In *Handbook of Patient Care in Vascular Diseases,* (29-49). Philadelphia: Lippincott Williams & Wilkins.
9. Moneta GL, Zacardi MJ, Olmsted KA. (2010). Lower extremity arterial occlusive disease. In Zierler RE (Ed.), Strandess's duplex scanning disorders in vascular diagnosis 4th ed. (133-147).Philadelphia Wolters Kluwer Lippincott Williams & Wilkins.
10. Zwiebel, WJ, Pellerito JS. (2005). Basic concepts of Doppler frequency spectrum analysis and ultrasound blood flow imaging. In Zwiebel WJ, Pellerito JS (Eds.), *In Introduction to Vascular Ultrasonography 5th ed,* (61-89). Philadelphia: Elsevier Saunders.
11. Needham T. (2005). In Mansour MA, Labropoulos N. (Eds.). *Vascular Diagnosis,* (215-222). Philadelphia: Elsevier Saunders.
12. Kim ES, Sharma AM, Scissons R, et al. *Interpretation of peripheral arterial and venous Doppler waveforms: A consensus statement from the Society for Vascular Medicine and Society for Vascular Ultrasound. Vascular Medicine.* 2020;25(5):484-506. doi:10.1177/1358863X20937665
13. Boren, C. H., Towne, J. B., Bernhard, V. M., & Salles-Cunha, S. (1980). Profundapopliteal collateral index. A guide to successful profundaplasty. *Archives of surgery* (Chicago, Ill. : 1960), 115(11), 1366-1372.

ARTERIAL TESTING
18. Volume Pulse Recording

Definition

Volume pulse recording (VPR) uses air plethysmography to detect volume changes related to blood flow. VPR determines whether peripheral arterial disease is present, if there are any effects on arterial perfusion to the extremity, and the segmental location of the obstruction. When ABIs are questionable, VPR can be used to confirm a decrease in perfusion and identify general location of an obstruction.

Rationale

Each arterial pulse creates a change in volume under a pressure cuff. These limb volume changes result in proportional changes in the air pressure in the cuffs. The air pressure changes are monitored by a pressure transducer in the VPR instrument and recorded as a waveform.

VPR waveforms are not affected by calcified vessels. [5,6]

Etiology of Disease

- Atherosclerosis
- Embolization
- Thrombus
- Extrinsic compression
- Intimal hyperplasia
- Trauma
- Traumatic occlusion

Risk Factors

- Age (increased risk with age)
- Coronary artery disease or MI
- Diabetes
- Family history
- Hyperlipidemia
- Hypertension
- Obesity
- Smoking
- Sedentary lifestyle
- Previous history of CVA
- Elevated levels of homocysteine
- Excessive levels of C-reactive protein
- History of radiation
- Occupational exposure to toxic substances

Indications for Exam

- Claudication (exercise-related limb pain)
- Abnormal ABI
- Limb pain at rest
- Absent peripheral pulses
- Extremity ulcer
- Gangrene
- Aneurysmal disease
- Trauma to an artery
- Follow-up after revascularization procedure
- Popliteal artery entrapment

Contraindications/Limitations

- Patients with acute venous thrombosis (there is a slight risk of embolization using the pressure cuff).
- VPR cannot be performed over extensive bandages or casts which are not removable.
- Any site of trauma, recent surgery, ulceration or graft placement which should not be compressed by the pressure cuff.
- Good collaterals around a short occlusion may normalize the VPR waveform.

The VPR amplitude is influenced by a number of physiologic variables including cardiac stroke volume, blood pressure, blood volume, vasoconstriction, motor tone, loose cuff application and size of limb. [5]

Mechanism of Disease

- **Atherosclerosis** [1] is the most common arterial disease. Atherosclerotic plaque forms in the artery blocking flow by either narrowing the arterial lumen (arterial stenosis) or totally blocking the artery (arterial occlusion). The term "hemodynamically significant obstruction" refers to either a stenosis or an occlusion that results in a decrease in blood pressure or flow distal to the obstruction. Typically, a stenosis must narrow the diameter of the artery by at least 50% to decrease pressure and flow distally. An arterial occlusion is typically seen from one major branch to the next.
- **Emboli** may occur as contents of a plaque or fragments of an organized thrombus from the heart or aneurysm loosen and flow downstream. Emboli become lodged in a distant blood vessel, causing arterial occlusion and reduction of flow. [1]
- **Vasospasm** is a temporary constriction of the arteries (typically digital arteries) that may cause significant discomfort to the patient or be a sign of a more serious underlying disease. [2]
- **Extrinsic compression** from tumors, hematoma, etc., can result in stenosis or occlusion by placing enough pressure on arterial walls to compromise blood flow. [1]

Location of Disease

- Location of disease can be focal or diffuse and affect any level or multiple levels.
- The most common location of obstruction in the lower extremities is the superficial femoral artery at the adductor canal.
- The popliteal artery is another common location.
- Arterial bifurcations
- Subclavian artery, palmar arch and/or digital arteries

Patient History

- Claudication (exercise related)
- Rest pain
- Acute occlusion
  - » Pain
  - » Paralysis (weakness)
  - » Paresthesia ("pins and needles")
  - » Poikilothermia (ice-cold limb)
  - » Pulselessness
  - » Pallor
- Previous ulceration/gangrene of feet/toes or hands/digits
- Previous therapeutic vascular procedure (e.g., bypass, stenting)

Physical Examination

- Pulselessness
- Pallor
- Gangrene/necrosis (tissue death)
- Cyanosis
- Dependent rubor
- Bruit (abnormal sound heard through auscultation caused by vibration of tissue from turbulent flow)
- Marked temperature difference between extremities, especially if one is ice cold
- Palpable thrill (vibration caused by turbulent blood flow as seen in AV fistulas)

Volume Pulse Recording Protocol

- Rest the patient for 5 minutes before beginning the exam in order for blood pressures to stabilize after "exercise" (walking into the exam room). You may use this time to obtain a patient history, including symptoms and risk factors, explain the procedure, and wrap the cuffs.
- Patient is examined in the supine position. Elevating the foot onto a pillow or towel momentarily may make it easier to wrap cuffs around the leg for a lower extremity exam, but be careful not to hyperextend the knee during testing and risk possibly compressing the popliteal artery.
- Cuffs should be placed "straight" rather than angled. Choose appropriately sized pneumatic cuffs for each section of the limb:
  - » 12cm width used for the arm, thigh, calf and ankle

    Place the cuffs with equal snugness on the limb; this will affect the height of the VPR waveform.

  - » Most labs use two 12cm cuffs on the thigh, but some may choose to use one 18cm cuff on the thigh instead. Also, some labs prefer a 10cm cuff at the arm and ankle. Whichever you chose, the suggestion is to use the same size cuff on both the arm and ankle.

    Ask the patient to lay as still as possible to eliminate motion artifact on the tracings.

  - » 7cm width; used for the hand/foot
  - » 1.9-2.5cm width; used for digital. A 2.5cm cuff is highly preferred if the cuff will also be used for digital pressures.
  - » Place the cuffs with equal snugness on the limb; the volume of air needed to obtain the appropriate pressure will affect the height of the VPR waveform. If one cuff is very loosely applied, it will take more air to fill the cuff, affecting the wave height. Ask the patient if the cuffs feel equally snug and adjust as necessary.
- Whenever adjustments are made, you must be consistent with these settings on the contralateral leg at the same level:
  - » An obese thigh will create a VPR waveform with a lower amplitude than normal, but may still demonstrate a normal contour. Note this for the interpreting physician and make an interpretation based on a change in the waveform shape rather than a change in amplitude from one level to the next.
  - » During the exam, cuffs will be inflated at each level according to the pressure indicated by the manufacturer of the VPR unit. *See Tables 18-1 and 18-2 for typical settings.* This will ensure appropriate contact is made with the limb to transfer the volume pulse from the limb to the cuff. A volume pulse tracing is then recorded using the indicated gain settings for the extremity.
  - » Record VPR waveforms at each level using the appropriate gain settings. Consider the factory suggested settings for the VPR equipment being used.

- » The size of the VPR tracing in the lower extremities may need to be adjusted during testing to account for the decrease in distal tissue volumes. The calf tracing typically augments 25% in normal limbs and may bound off the chart. (If the size was decreased for the calf, remember to turn the gain back to initial settings for the ankle.)
- When assessing for popliteal artery entrapment syndrome, place the patient's heel up on a firm pillow or roll of towels to create a hyperabduction of the knee. Have the patient slowly plantar and dorsiflex their foot. A resting plantarflexion and dorsiflexion VPR waveform should be documented.
- The VPR trace setting for "size" in the upper extremity is usually consistent for each level (see recommended factory settings for the VPR equipment being used). If you need to change the size of the tracing (i.e., the amplitude of the trace bounds off the chart at any level), remember to be consistent and use the same size for the rest of the levels.
- Determine severity of disease according to shape and relative amplitude of the tracings. Use comparisons between "typical" normal, the tracing of proximal segments and the contralateral limb. [3]

Table 18-1: Typical VPR Settings for Upper Extremities

Cuff Level	Cuff Size	Pressure	Gain
Arm	10-12cm	65mmHg	2.5
Forearm	10-12cm	65mmHg	2.5
Hand	7cm	65mmHg	6.0
Finger	2.5cm	40mmHg	10.0

Table 18-2: Typical VPR Settings for Lower Extremities

Cuff Level	Cuff Size	Pressure	Gain	Size
*High Thigh	12cm	65mmHg	2.5	3
*Low Thigh	12cm	65mmHg	2.5	3
Calf	10cm	65mmHg	2.5	3
Ankle	10cm	65mmHg	2.5	3
Foot	7cm	65mmHg	2.5	6

* Both a high-thigh and low-thigh cuff are used for the "four cuff method." Only one 18cm wide thigh cuff is used for the "three-cuff method."

Table 18-3: Volume Pulse Recording Protocol Summary

- Wrap appropriately sized pneumatic cuffs for each section of the limb:
  - » 12cm width; arm, thigh, calf and ankle*
  - » 7cm width; hand/foot
  - » 1.9-2.5cm width; digital **
- Inflate cuffs at each level according to the pressure and gain settings indicated by the manufacturer of the VPR unit. Refer to tables 17-1 and 17-2. Record representative VPR waveforms.
- Determine classification of disease according to laboratory diagnostic criteria.

* Most labs use two 12cm cuffs on the thigh, some may choose to use one 18cm cuff on the thigh instead. Other labs prefer a 10cm cuff at the arm and ankle. Whichever you chose, the suggestion is to use the same size cuff on both the arm and ankle.

** A 2.5cm cuff is highly preferred if the cuff will also be used for digital pressures.

PRINCIPLES OF INTERPRETATION

- The volume pulse waveform is primarily interpreted by the contour (shape) and amplitude (height) of the tracing relative to the amplitude of the adjacent proximal cuff.
- The tracings are described as being normal, mildly abnormal, moderately abnormal or severely abnormal:

Normal

- Sharp upstroke
- Sharp systolic peak
- Gradual downslope bowing towards baseline
- Dicrotic notch, however some patients may have inward bowing on the downslope

Mildly Abnormal

- Sharp upstroke
- Rounded systolic peak
- Loss of dicrotic notch
- Downslope bends slightly away from the baseline

Moderately Abnormal

- Prolonged upstroke
- Rounded systolic peak
- Loss of dicrotic notch
- Relatively low amplitude compared to normal and proximal tracings
- Upslope and downslope time nearly equal

- sVery prolonged upstroke
- Rounded systolic peak
- No dicrotic notch
- Upslope, downslope time nearly equal
- Very low amplitude or flat, non-pulsatile tracing

Interpretation/Diagnostic Criteria

Normal

- VPR may be helpful in assessing a patient for popliteal entrapment syndrome; the ankle VPR tracing will be normal at rest and flatten with plantarflexion or dorsiflexion with knee hyperextension as the gastrocnemius contracts and compresses the popliteal artery. [7]
- The normal VPR waveform has a quick upstroke, sharp peak and a dicrotic notch on its downslope or bows toward the baseline when the dicrotic notch is absent. [4,5]
- The presence of the dicrotic notch eliminates the possibility of significant arterial occlusive disease. [5]

The absence of a dicrotic notch is less important since it may not be present even in normal patients when resistance is lowered, such as after exercise. [4]

- The calf tracing should be approximately 25% larger than the thigh tracing. [5,6]
- The thigh tracing should generally be the same amplitude as the ankle tracing. [4,5]

Table 18-4: Normal Amplitudes for Lower Extremity VPR

Level	Amplitude
Thigh	>15mm
Calf	>20mm
Ankle	>15mm

Source: Sumner DS, Zierler RE. (2005). Physiologic assessment of peripheral arterial occlusive disease. In Rutherford Vascular Surgery 6th edition. (197-222). Philadelphia. Elsevier Saunders.

Abnormal

- Abnormal VPR waveforms occur distal to the obstructed arterial segment. [4,6]
- The abnormal VPR has a slower upstroke, rounded peak and a downslope that bows away from the baseline. [4]
- The dicrotic notch disappears. [5]

Tremors can cause waveform artifact. [4]

- As disease progresses, the VPR waveform becomes more rounded and loses amplitude. [3,5,6]
- An aortoiliac obstruction produces abnormal VPR waveforms at all levels, though the calf amplitude can be greater than at the thigh. [4,5]
- A low amplitude, abnormally shaped thigh VPR may indicate aortoiliac or proximal SFA obstruction. [4]
- A calf VPR amplitude that is equal to or lower than the ipsilateral thigh VPR amplitude with the same settings is the most indicative finding of superficial femoral artery (SFA) disease. [4,5]
- Tibial artery obstruction will result in normal calf augmentation but demonstrate an abnormal ankle VPR waveform. [6]
- Significant decrease or obliteration of the VPR waveform will occur during provocative maneuvers if a patient has popliteal artery entrapment. [7]

Good collateralization can normalize the VPR waveform in a short occlusion. [5]

Table 18-5: Lower Extremity VPR Waveforms Based on Location of Disease

Level of Disease	PVR Amplitude		
	Thigh	Calf	Ankle
Aoil stenosis*	Abnormal	Abnormal	Abnormal
Aoil occlusion*	Abnormal	Abnormal	Abnormal
Low SFA occlusion	Normal	Abnormal	Abnormal
High SFA occlusion w/o AI disease	Abnormal	Abnormal	Abnormal
Aoil + SFA disease	Abnormal	Abnormal	Abnormal
Tibial disease	Normal	Normal	Abnormal
Small vessel disease	Normal	Normal	Normal

* open distal system

Source: Modified from Raines JK. (1993). The pulse volume recording in peripheral arterial disease. In Bernstein EF (Ed). Vascular Diagnosis 4th ed. (p. 538). St Louis: Mosby.

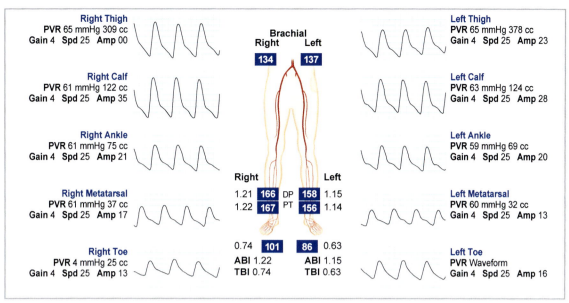

Fig. 18-1: *Normal VPR examination of the lower extremity*

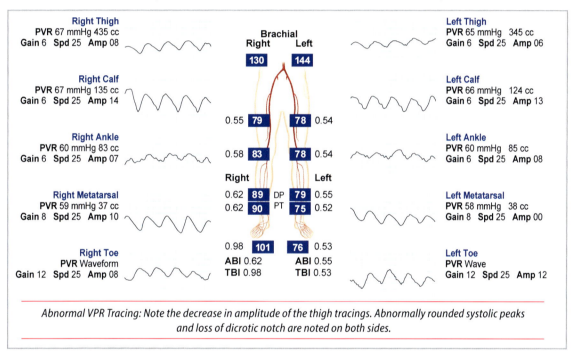

Abnormal VPR Tracing: Note the decrease in amplitude of the thigh tracings. Abnormally rounded systolic peaks and loss of dicrotic notch are noted on both sides.

Fig. 18-2: *Abnormal VPR examination of the bilateral lower extremities*

Differential Diagnosis
- Spinal stenosis
- Venous thrombosis causing pain
- Restless leg syndrome
- Compartment syndrome
- Nocturnal leg cramps
- Neuropathy
- Muscle/tendon strains
- Arthritis
- Abnormalities of adrenergic receptor/sympathetic nervous system
- Connective tissue disease (scleroderma)

Correlation
- Duplex ultrasound
- MRA
- Spiral CT scan
- Arteriography

Medical Treatment
- Modify risk factors (e.g., cessation of tobacco usage, avoidance of cold)
- Antiplatelet medication (e.g., aspirin)
- Anticoagulation (warfarin)

Surgical Treatment
- Bypass grafting
- Atherectomy
- Endarterectomy
- Direct focal repair
- Resection (aneurysmal disease)
- Sympathectomy
- Amputation

Endovascular Treatment
- Angioplasty
- Stent
- Intra-arterial directed thrombolysis (acute blockage)

REFERENCES
1. 1 Sumner DS, Zierler RE. (2005). Vascular physiology: essential hemodynamic principles. In Rutherford Vascular Surgery 6th edition. (75-123). Philadelphia. Elsevier Saunders
2. 2 Shepard RFJ. (2005). Raynaud's syndrome: vasospastic and occlusive arterial disease involving the distal upper extremity. In Rutherford Vascular Surgery 6th edition. (1319-1346). Philadelphia. Elsevier Saunders
3. 3 Talbot, SR, Zwiebel WJ. (2005). Assessment of Upper Extremity Arterial Occlusive Disease. In Zwiebel WJ. Pellerito JS (Eds.), Introduction to Vascular Ultrasonography 5th ed. (297-323). Philadelphia: Elsevier Saunders
4. 4 Kempczinski RE. (1982). Segmental volume plethysmography: The pulse volume recorder. In: Kempczinski RF and Yao SJS. Practical Noninvasive Vascular Diagnosis. (105--117). Chicago: Yearbook Medical.
5. 5 Sumner DS, Zierler RE. (2005). Physiologic assessment of peripheral arterial occlusive disease. In Rutherford Vascular Surgery 6th edition. (197-222). Philadelphia. Elsevier Saunders.
6. 6 Raines JK. (1993). The pulse volume recording in peripheral arterial disease. In Bernstein EF (Ed) Vascular Diagnosis 4th ed. (534-553). St Louis: Mosby
7. 7 Hallett JW, Brewster DC, Rasmussen TE. (2001). Noninvasive vascular testing. In: Handbook of Patient Care in Vascular Diseases. (29-49). Philadelphia Lippincott Williams & Wilkins.

ARTERIAL TESTING

19. Lower Extremity Digital Evaluations: Toe Pressures (TBI) and Photoplethysmography (PPG)

Definition
Noninvasive physiological tests which study blood flow at the terminal portion of the digits. The systolic pressure of the brachial artery is compared to the systolic pressure of the digital arteries in order to calculate a toe-brachial index (TBI). Another component of this exam detects arterial pulsations in the terminal portions of the digits using photoplethysmography (PPG).

Rationale
The sensors of a PPG transducer consist of an infrared light-emitting diode and a phototransistor. Infrared light is transmitted into the superficial tissue and a reflection is received by the phototransistor. The signal received relates to the quantity of red blood cells in the cutaneous circulation. Each arterial pulse creates a change in blood volume under the sensor. These cutaneous volume changes result in a proportional change in the reflection of the infrared light from the tissue. The changes in reflection are monitored in the instrument and recorded as a pulse waveform when the instrument is set in arterial or AC mode. If set in the venous or DC mode, the PPG can be used to monitor slower volume changes related to venous reflux, as opposed to quick changes seen during the arterial pulse cycle.

Falsely elevated digital pressures due to calcified arteries are rarely a problem.

Etiology
- Atherosclerosis
- Trauma
- Embolization
- Thrombus
- Aneurysm
- Pseudoaneurysm
- Intimal hyperplasia
- Traumatic occlusion
- Extrinsic compression
- AV fistula (abnormal connection between an artery and a vein)
- Buerger's disease
- Vasculitis
- Radiation arteritis
- Vasospasm

Risk Factors
- Age (increased risk with age)
- Coronary artery disease
- Diabetes
- Family history
- Hyperlipidemia
- Hypertension
- Smoking
- Obesity
- Aneurysm
- History of radiation
- Fibromuscular dysplasia
- Occupational exposure to toxic substances

Digital analysis should be routinely performed on all diabetics, symptomatic toes and in patients with calcified ankle pressures.

Indications for Exam
- Exercise-related pain (claudication symptoms)
- Limb or digital pain at rest
- Extremity ulcer/gangrene
- Digital cyanosis
- Cold sensitivity
- Absent peripheral pulses
- Arterial trauma and aneurysms
- Bruit
- Raynaud's syndrome/phenomenon

Contraindications/Limitations
- Skin integrity of the digit must be intact to properly assess digital circulation.
- Significant lesions with excellent collateral circulation, which may result in normal distal pressures and waveforms.
- Pressure cuffs may not fit well around very large or very small digits.
- Any site of trauma, surgery or ulceration which should not be compressed by the pressure cuff.
- Patients with extensive bandages or casts.

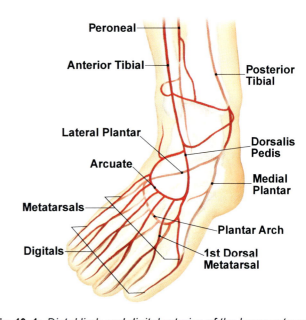

Fig. 19-1: *Distal limb and digital arteries of the lower extremity*

Mechanism of Disease
There are two major mechanisms that cause reduced arterial blood supply to the lower extremity; obstruction from atherosclerotic plaque and embolism. Of these, atherosclerosis is more common.

- **Atherosclerosis** is the most common arterial disease. Atherosclerotic plaque forms in the artery which blocks flow by either narrowing the arterial lumen (arterial stenosis) or totally blocking the artery (arterial occlusion). The term "hemodynamically significant obstruction" refers to either a stenosis or an occlusion that results in a decrease in blood pressure or flow distal to the obstruction. Typically, a stenosis must narrow the diameter of the artery by at least 50% to decrease pressure and flow distally. An arterial occlusion is typically seen from one major branch to the next.
- **Emboli:** embolization of contents of a plaque and/or fragments of an organized thrombus from the heart or proximal aneurysm which become lodged in a distant blood vessel. [2]

A patient presenting with an embolic event such as "blue toe syndrome" should be worked up for an abdominal aortic aneurysm. Embolization is associated with abdominal aortic aneurysm.

- **Vasospasm** is a temporary constriction, typically of the digital arteries, that may cause significant discomfort to the patient.
- **Extrinsic compression** from tumors, hematoma, etc., can result in stenosis or occlusion by placing enough pressure on arterial walls to compromise blood flow. [1]

Patient History
- Claudication (exercise related)
- Pain or rest pain
- Paralysis (weakness)
- Paresthesia ("pins and needles")
- Poikilothermia (ice cold limbs)
- Previous ulceration/gangrene of feet/toes
- Previous therapeutic vascular procedure (e.g., bypass, stent)

Physical Examination
- Pulselessness
- Cyanosis
- Gangrene/necrosis (tissue death)
- Pallor
- Dependent rubor
- Marked temperature difference between digits and/or extremities
- Bruit (abnormal sound heard through auscultation caused by turbulent flow)
- Palpable thrill (vibration caused by turbulent blood flow as seen with an AV fistula)

Exposure to cold conditions or stressful situations can exacerbate digital symptoms.

Lower Extremity Digital Evaluation Protocol
- Obtain a patient history to include symptoms and risk factors. Explain the procedure to the patient.
- Patient is examined in a warm room in the supine position to eliminate the effects of hydrostatic pressure.
- Digits should be room temperature for accurate data collection. Use hot packs or warming devices with care as necessary.
- Apply a 2-2.5cm cuff around the digit to be studied while avoiding cuff placement over the bony joint. Smaller cuffs will result in falsely elevated pressures due to the narrow cuff width. Follow up studies should use the same width cuff for comparison.

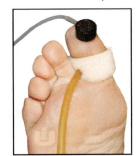

Use a towel to cover the foot to eliminate any room light which may cause an artifact in the PPG tracing.

Fig. 19-2: Lower Extremity TBI and PPG Evaluation Placement of the Digital Cuff and PPG Sensor

- Attach the PPG photocell to the pad of the digit using double-stick tape placed between the photocell and the skin. Avoid taping the entire digit like a cuff since a tightly placed PPG could obliterate a low-pressure pulse. Alternative sensors used by some labs include a digital clip similar to a pulse-oximeter which eliminates the need for tape or Velcro to keep the sensor in place.
- Run the PPG recording at high speed (25mm/s) to record the shape of the digital waveform at rest, ensuring that the PPG tracing is centered on the paper or monitor. Ideally the baseline tracing consists of a series of horizontal pulses.

The size control on the PPG device is kept at "10" for standardization of tracings. If the waveform "goes off" the strip chart recording paper, the size is reduced to "5" and the change is documented.

- Reduce the PPG recording speed to 5mm/s and inflate the pressure cuff on the digit until the PPG waveforms are no longer visible.
- Slowly deflate the cuff at rate of 2-4mmHg/s until the PPG waveforms return. Note the pressure when the first pulse returns, but be sure that the pulse is continuous. If the pulse does not continue, consider that this was not a true pulse, but rather a motion artifact.
- If data is abnormal at rest, consider warming the affected toes for several minutes and repeating the measurements. False-positive results may occur if the digits are cold during testing.
- Repeat the procedure on other digits as necessary.
- Repeat on the contralateral leg.
- Apply pressure cuffs with 10-12cm bladder (in width) on the mid upper arms.
- Locate the brachial artery (BrA) near the antecubital fossa using a Doppler transducer.
- Inflate the cuff on the mid arm 20-30mmHg beyond the last audible arterial Doppler signal.
- Deflate the cuff slowly at a rate of 2-4mmHg per second. The systolic pressure is recorded as soon as the first audible Doppler arterial signal returns.
- Calculate the toe-brachial index (TBI) by dividing the digital pressures by the highest brachial artery pressure.

$$\text{toe pressure} \div \text{highest brachial pressure} = \text{TBI}$$

- Determine severity of disease according to laboratory diagnostic criteria.

Table 19-1: Lower Extremity Digital Protocol Summary

- Wrap pressure cuffs around toes.
- Secure the PPG sensor to the bottom pad of the digit.
- Record representative tracing of PPG waveforms.
- Inflate the digital cuff 20-30mmHg beyond the last visualized PPG tracing. Be sure that a couple seconds pass before the first pulse reappears.
- Deflate cuff at a rate of 2-4mmHg per second. The pressure is recorded as soon as the PPG waveforms return. Check for subsequent pulses to confirm it was a "first pulse" rather than motion artifact.
- Wrap a pressure cuff around the mid upper arms for a brachial pressure.
- Inflate cuff 20-30mmHg beyond the last audible Doppler arterial signal.
- Calculate toe-brachial indices using the highest brachial pressure.

$$\text{toe pressure} \div \text{highest brachial pressure} = \text{TBI}$$

- Determine severity of disease according to laboratory diagnostic criteria.

Table 19-2: Lower Extremity TBI Symptoms

TBI Range	Symptoms
0.80 – 0.90	Normal
0.35 + 15	Claudication
0.11 + 10	Rest pain/ulceration

Source: Zierler, RE, (2005). Nonimaging physiologic tests for assessment of lower extremity arterial occlusive disease. In Zwiebel WJ, Pellerito JS (Eds.), *Introduction to Vascular Ultrasonography* 5th ed. (275-295). Philadelphia: Elsevier Saunders.

PRINCIPLES OF INTERPRETATION

Pressures

- Digital pressures are compared to the highest brachial pressure and are typically lower than the ankle pressures.

PPG Digital Waveforms

- The PPG waveform from any digit is categorized as pulsatile, reduced or non-pulsatile based on the upstroke (amplitude) of the waveform and downslope.
- There may be a dicrotic notch or secondary upstroke in the downslope of the tracing which corresponds to the increased aortic pressure and closure of the aortic valve.

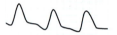

Fig. 19-3: *Normal Pulsatility* **Fig. 19-4:** *Reduced Pulsatility* **Fig. 19-5:** *Absent Pulsatility*

Interpretation/Diagnostic Criteria

Normal

Pressures

- If the TBI is >0.70, the presence of a hemodynamically significant stenosis or occlusion is unlikely from the heart to the digits in the lower extremities. [3]

PPG Digital Waveforms

- Normal PPG waveforms exclude the presence of significant disease. Normal PPG waveform characteristics include: [4]
  » Short onset to peak (subjective)
  » Downslope that bows toward the baseline
  » A dicrotic notch in the downslope

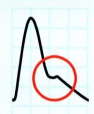

Fig. 19-6: *Dicrotic notch*

Abnormal

Pressures

- A difference in systolic pressures between the ankle and toe indicates pedal or digital artery obstruction. An abnormal difference is >44mmHg in younger patients and >64mmHg in older patients. [4]
- A TBI of <0.60 in the toes indicates a decrease in perfusion at the digital level due to a significant obstruction at or proximal to the digits. [5]
- A toe pressure >30mmHg is associated with healing. With a toe pressure <30mmHg, healing is doubtful. [7,8]
- An absolute toe pressure of <20mmHg is associated with toe ischemia. [4,6]

PPG Digital Waveforms

- Abnormal ("reduced") PPG waveform characteristics (secondary to obstruction) include: [4]
  » Prolonged onset to peak (subjective)
  » Rounded peak
  » Loss of the dicrotic notch in the downslope
  » Downslope that bows away from the baseline
- An "absent" or non-pulsatile digital waveform is reported when the PPG tracing reflects a flat-line.

Digits with pressures of less than 20mmHg may not produce a waveform.

Table 19-3: Diagnostic Criteria for Lower Extremity Digital Testing

Normal: no hemodynamically significant disease
- TBI ≥0.70
- Normal waveform characteristics include:
  » Short onset to peak (subjective)
  » Downslope that bows toward the baseline or
  » A dicrotic notch in the downslope

Abnormal: hemodynamically significant disease
- TBI <0.60
- Pressure difference between the ankle and toes (>44mmHg in younger patients and >64mmHg in older patients)
- Abnormal waveform characteristics include:
- Prolonged onset to peak (subjective)
  » Rounded peak
  » Downslope that bows away from the baseline
  » Absence of tracing
- Absolute pressure <20mmHg (toe ischemia)
- Absent or non-pulsatile waveform pattern

Table 19-4: University of Chicago Lower Extremity TBI Diagnostic Criteria

Severity	Toe Brachial Index (TBI)
Normal	>0.70
Mild	0.60-0.69
Moderate	0.59-0.40
Severe	<0.39

Source: Internally validated at the University of Chicago Medical Center Vascular Laboratory

Differential Diagnosis

- Buerger's disease
- Scleroderma
- Connective tissue disorders
- Abnormalities of adrenergic receptor/sympathetic nervous system
- Neuropathy
- Muscle/tendon strains
- Arthritis

Correlation

- Duplex ultrasound
- Transcutaneous oxygen pressure (TcPO2) testing
- Spiral CT scan
- MR Angiography
- Arteriography

TcPO2 testing is a non-invasive test to measure skin oxygentation and is often used to assess blood flow disorders of the foot in diabetic patients. The information can help physicians decide whether revascularization will be helpful or what level of amputation might be necessary when revascularization is not an option. [10]

Medical Treatment

- Risk factor management (e.g., smoking cessation)
- Cold temperature avoidance
- Antiplatelet medication (e.g., aspirin)
- Anticoagulation (warfarin)
- Thermal biofeedback
- Thrombolysis (acute blockage)

Surgical Treatment

- Sympathectomy
- Endarterectomy
- Bypass grafting
- Direct focal repair
- Resection (aneurysmal disease)
- Amputation

REFERENCES

1. Sumner DS, Zierler RE. (2005). Vascular physiology: essential hemodynamic principles. In *Rutherford Vascular Surgery 6th edition.* (75-123). Philadelphia. Elsevier Saunders.
2. Fecteau SR, Darling III RC, Roddy SP. (2005). Arterial thromboembolism. In *Rutherford Vascular Surgery 6th edition.* (971-986). Philadelphia. Elsevier Saunders.
3. Needham T. (2005). Peripheral atherosclerotic occlusive disease. In Mansour MA, Labropoulos N. (Eds.), *Vascular Diagnosis,* (215-222). Philadelphia: Elsevier Saunders.
4. Zierler RE, Sumner DS. (2005). Physiologic assessment of peripheral arterial occlusive disease. In *Rutherford Vascular Surgery 6th edition.* (197-222). Philadelphia. Elsevier Saunders.
5. Bridges RA, Barnes RW. (1982). Segmental limb pressures. In: Kempczinski RF and Yao SJS. *Practical Noninvasive Vascular Diagnosis.* (79-93). Chicago: Yearbook Medical.
6. Carter SA, Lezack JD. (1971). Digital systolic pressures in the lower limb in arterial disease. *Circulation.* 43: 905-913.
7. Hallett JW, Brewster DC, Rasmussen TE. (2001). Noninvasive vascular testing. In: *Handbook of Patient Care in Vascular Diseases.* (29-49), Philadelphia Lippincott Williams & Wilkins.
8. Ramsey DE, Manke DA, Sumner DS. (1983). Toe blood pressure. A valuable adjunct to ankle pressure measurement for assessing peripheral arterial disease. *J Card Surg.* Jan-Feb;24(1):43-8.
9. Zierler, RE, (2005). Nonimaging physiologic tests for assessment of lower extremity arterial occlusive disease. In Zwiebel WJ, Pellerito JS (Eds.), *Introduction to Vascular Ultrasonography 5th ed.* (275-295). Philadelphia: Elsevier Saunders.
10. Got I. (1998). La pression transcutanée D'oxygène (TcPO2): intérêts et limites [Transcutaneous oxygen pressure (TcPO2): advantages and limitations]. Diabetes & metabolism, 24(4), 379–384.

ARTERIAL TESTING
20. Exercise and Stress Testing of the Extremities

Definitions

Exercise or stress testing can be performed in different ways in the vascular laboratory. Patients can walk on a treadmill, walk a set distance in the hallway or perform exercises with their feet/toes to simulate what happens when they walk/exercise. Reactive hyperemia is another type of stress test that can be used when patients are unable to perform exercise protocols. The main types of exercise and stress testing are discussed in this chapter.

Treadmill testing evaluates the arterial hemodynamics of the lower extremities and determines the functional significance of disease by evaluating walking distance limitations and whether walking induced pain is secondary to nonvascular conditions, such as musculoskeletal or cardiopulmonary disease that may affect exercise performance.

Post-occlusive reactive hyperemia (PORH) is a form of stress testing used on patients with contraindications to other forms of stress testing (e.g., patients with amputation, physical disability, etc.). In this method, exercise is simulated by inflating an arterial cuff (usually placed on the thigh) above the suprasystolic pressure for 3-5 minutes to create a brief period of distal limb ischemia.

Rationale

Exercise increases blood flow which will exaggerate a pressure gradient that may not be appreciated at rest according to Poiseuille's Law ($Q = \Delta P \div R$). After exercise, an individual's distal vascular bed vasodilates, decreasing resistance and increasing blood flow in response to the demand. If a patient cannot exercise, the reactive hyperemia technique is an alternative means of increasing blood flow in order to elicit a pressure gradient that is not present at rest. The ankle pressure will decrease in the presence of increased flow demand and a significant arterial obstruction.

Indications for Exam

- Claudication (exercise-related limb pain) in the presence of normal ABI's at rest
- PORH is useful when a patient cannot exercise via treadmill or toe raises.

Contraindications/Limitations

- Calcified vessels which will falsely elevate pressures (typically encountered in patients with diabetes or end-stage renal disease).
- PORH protocol may be difficult to perform on some patients due to marked numbness and discomfort that the patient experiences from temporary ischemia or from the cuff pressure itself. The technique is not typically used when resting measurements are abnormal, but is only used in selected patients when stress testing with walking cannot be done and is necessary to fully assess the patient's condition.
- Avoid reducing flow further by doing treadmill testing or PORH on patients with rest pain, gangrene, or ulceration.
- Patients with acute venous thrombosis
- Any site of trauma, surgery, ulceration or graft placement which should not be compressed by the pressure cuff.
- Patients with extensive bandages or casts which are not removable.
- Pressures typically prohibited on ipsilateral side of mastectomy or AVG/AVF.

Specific Treadmill Limitations

- Patients with lower extremity amputation
- Inability of the patient to walk (e.g., arthritis, joint disease, stroke, obesity)
- History or suggestion of angina, myocardial infarction (MI) or need to carry nitroglycerin on order of a personal physician
- Significant shortness of breath at rest

Mechanism of Reduction in Peripheral Vascular Resistance

- Muscular vessels dilate and divert blood away from the cutaneous tissue in response to exercise, increasing oxygen to the muscles and reducing oxygen levels in the tissues. Unless arterial inflow is compromised, this reduction will not be measurable. [1]
- An oxygen shortage (hypoxia) is created during cuff occlusion with a build-up of vasodilator metabolites, such as adenosine, prostycyclin, nitrous oxide, and potassium. [2,11]
- Dilatation of arterioles (vasodilation) results, decreasing vascular resistance. [2]
- Once cuff occlusion is released, flow increases creating a hyperemic state. [2]
- When flow is increased, a significant decrease in pressure may occur distal to an arterial obstruction in diseased limbs during the hyperemic period. [2]
- Once tissues reoxygenate, vasodilator metabolites are excreted from the tissue resulting in a return to baseline resistance. [2]

Location of Disease

- Location of disease can be focal or diffuse and affect any level or multiple levels.

Patient History

- Claudication (exercise-related)
- Rest pain

Physical Examination

- Pulselessness
- Pallor
- Gangrene/ulceration
- Dependent rubor
- Bruit

Treadmill Testing Protocol

- Rest the patient for 5-10 minutes before beginning the exam in order for blood pressures to stabilize after "exercise" (walking into the exam room). You may use this time to obtain a patient history, including symptoms and risk factors and to place cuffs. It also helps to fully explain the procedure to the patient and possibly demonstrate how they will walk on the treadmill and then move quickly back to the bed.
- Before starting the exercise portion of the examination, baseline pressures are taken while the patient is in the supine position.
- Appropriately wrap blood pressure cuffs on the limbs (arm and ankle). All cuffs should be placed "straight" rather than angled with the bladder of the cuff over the artery. Apply the ankle cuff with a 10-12cm bladder (in width) 2-3cm above the medial malleolus.

- All cuffs should fit snugly so that inflation of the bladder transmits the head of pressure into the tissue rather than into space between the bladder and the limb, producing falsely elevated readings.
- Obtain resting ankle-brachial indices (ABI) for comparison to post-exercise values. *Refer to the chapter on "ABI and Analog Pedal Artery Waveforms" for detailed instructions.*

Take the pressures in the symptomatic extremity or the extremity with the lower ABI at rest first.

- The following instructions can be used when testing with an automatic cuff inflator or standard manometer:
  » Inflate cuffs 20-30mmHg above the last audible arterial Doppler signal using a Doppler transducer.
  » Deflation of the cuff should be at a rate of 2-4mmHg per second. The pressure is recorded as soon as the first continuous, audible Doppler arterial signal returns. The Doppler pulse must continue after hearing the first pulse to assure there is an actual pulse rather than motion artifact.
  » If a pressure measurement needs to be repeated, the cuff should be fully deflated for approximately one minute prior to the repeat measurement.
  » The ankle cuffs and the cuff on the arm with the higher brachial pressure remain on the patient (tape ends of cuff if necessary). Prepare continuous-wave Doppler and recording equipment for immediate use after completion of the exercise.

Marking the location of the arteries with an indelible marker helps to locate the arterial signals quicker after exercise.

- A treadmill with speed variability and a changeable grade or elevation is preferred. A stopwatch, watch or clock with a second hand is also needed.
- The treadmill grade is initially set at 10%, at a speed of 2 miles/hour.

Treadmill settings may be altered to accommodate the needs of the patient. Any changes should be documented in the exam report.

- Record the exercise start time. As the patient walks on the treadmill, ask periodically if symptoms have improved, worsened or remained unchanged. Record what interval of time has passed when any symptoms begin (*initial claudication*). Also record the time at which the patient can no longer continue walking (*absolute claudication*). Note other pertinent observations (e.g., complaints of shortness of breath). Record the time exercise ends. The patient will not need to walk longer than 5 minutes.
- Stop the treadmill. The patient returns promptly to the supine position on the bed or stretcher after exercise. Obtain ABI measurements within the first minute post-exercise.
- Retake the ankle and brachial pressures every 2 minutes until they return to within 10mmHg of the baseline pressure or for approximately 5-10 minutes (whichever comes first). If the ABIs immediately after exercise are equal to or greater than the resting pressures, no additional pressures are taken.

If a treadmill cannot be utilized, exercise may consist of walking a predetermined distance down the hallway.

Table 20-1: Treadmill Testing Protocol Summary

- Apply pneumatic cuffs on the arm and ankle.
- Measure pre-exercise ankle-brachial indices (ABI).
- Have the patient walk on the treadmill at a 10% grade and speed of 2 mph for 5 minutes or until claudication or other restrictions occur.
- Quickly re-measure ABIs within the first minute post-exercise.
- Retake the ABIs every 2 minutes until ankle pressures return to within 10mmHg of the baseline pressure or for 5-10 minutes (whichever comes first).
- Determine classification of disease according to laboratory diagnostic criteria.
- Calculate the pressure drop after exercise:
  (1 - (post exercise pressure ÷resting pressure)) x 100

Fig. 20-1: *Exercise pressure measurement report example*

	Rest	Imm	1	2	3	4	5
R Ankle:	130	134	135	132	130	131	132
L Ankle:	128	60	62	64	63	64	62
Brachial:	126	129	130	128	127	127	128
R ABI	1.03	1.04	1.04	1.03	1.02	1.03	1.03
L ABI	1.02	0.47	0.48	0.50	0.50	0.50	0.48

■ R Ankle   ● L Ankle   ✕ Brachial

Calculate Exercise Pressure Drop:

(1 - (post exercise pressure ÷ resting pressure)) x 100

RIGHT	LEFT
134 ÷ 130 =1.03 (rounded to 1)	60÷126 = 0.48
1 - 1 = 0	1 - 0.48 = 0.52
0 x 100 = 0%	0.52 x 100 = 52%
Sustained drop is normal	Sustained drop is abnormal

- Consider the change in the ankle pressure before and after exercise. Calculate the % pressure change before/after exercise to determine whether the drop in pressure was significant.

Alternative Exercise Testing (Toe-up)

"Toe-up" exercises are an alternative stress testing method when treadmill testing or PORH is not possible. Although this method is not as quantifiable as the other methods, it is a form of exercise and stress, especially at the calf levels. A fairly normal achievement is 100 toe-ups; however, this is variable. To perform:

- The patient stands facing the side of the bed, balancing their hand on the examination table for support.

- At a moderate speed, the patient rises onto the toes as much as possible, then drops down to a flat-footed position. Performing this maneuver along with the patient can help the patient maintain a moderate speed.

- Record post-exercise ABI measurements as described.

Reactive Hyperemia Testing Protocol

This procedure places uncomfortable pressure on the limb, and may result in numbness and pain in the extremity for 3-5 minutes. This should be thoroughly explained to the patient before the exam begins.

Try making small talk with the patient during the procedure in order to take their mind off the discomfort.

- Obtain a patient history to include symptoms and risk factors.
- Patient is examined in the supine position.
- Since the response to reactive hyperemia typically has a very short duration after release of the cuff, it is important to take the first ankle pressure within the first minute after deflation. Perform this procedure on only one limb at a time.
- Appropriately wrap blood pressure cuffs on the limbs (arm, thigh and ankle). All cuffs should be placed "straight" rather than angled with the bladder of the cuff over the artery. Apply the thigh cuff as high as possible on the thigh. Apply the ankle cuff with 10-12cm bladder (in width) 2-3cm above the medial malleolus.
- Obtain baseline ankle-brachial indices (ABI). *Refer to the chapter on "ABI and Analog Pedal Artery Waveforms" for detailed instructions.*
- Rapid deflation of the cuff should be at a rate of 2-4mmHg per second. The pressure is recorded as soon as the first continuous, audible Doppler arterial signal returns.
- Inflate the thigh cuff 40-50mmHg above the highest brachial systolic pressure for approximately 3-5 minutes.
- Be sure to monitor the pressure in the cuff during the occlusion period to make sure that the suprasystolic pressure is maintained for the full 3-5 minute period.
- Rapidly deflate the thigh cuff and quickly re-measure the ABI.

For patients with irregular heart beats, decrease deflation speeds for exercise or stress testing.

- Retake the ankle and brachial pressures every minute until the ankle pressure returns to within 10mmHg of the baseline pressure or for approximately 5 minutes (whichever comes first) since the recovery time is faster than treadmill testing.
- Determine classification of disease according to laboratory diagnostic criteria.
- If necessary, repeat on the contralateral side.

Table 20-2: Post-Occlusive Reactive Hyperemia Protocol Summary

- Apply pneumatic cuffs on the arm, thigh and ankle.
- Measure baseline ankle-brachial indices (ABI).
- Inflate thigh cuff 40-50mmHg above the highest brachial systolic pressure for 3-5 minutes.
- Rapidly deflate the thigh cuff and quickly re-measure ABI.
- Retake the ABI every minute until the ankle pressure returns to within 10mmHg of the baseline pressure or for 5 minutes (whichever comes first).
- Determine classification of disease according to laboratory diagnostic criteria.

PORH for Subclavian Steal

PORH has also been used to diagnose subclavian steal syndrome in the upper extremity when the vertebral artery demonstrates pendulum (to and fro) flow direction or has questionable reversed flow direction present. To perform:

- Inflate a pressure cuff over the brachial artery (30mmHg above the highest brachial pressure) for 5 minutes to cause temporary ischemia in the arm.

- After cuff deflation, investigate the flow direction of the ipsilateral vertebral artery using the duplex scanner as you would during a carotid exam.

If the flow direction of the vertebral artery is retrograde, this finding suggests a subclavian steal on that side. [10]

PRINCIPLES OF INTERPRETATION

- When interpreting the results of a treadmill exam, the distance a patient can walk and the absolute pressure drop relates to the severity of disease. [1,3] For example, patients with multilevel disease will walk for a shorter distance and there will be a greater pressure decrease. [1]
- Changes in absolute pressure are the most important factors when interpreting the results of treadmill and PORH testing.
- The changes in ABI during PORH testing are similar to those observed during treadmill testing in patients with arterial disease, though recovery is typically much faster. [1,9]

Interpretation/Diagnostic Criteria

Treadmill Testing

Normal

- There should be little to no drop in ankle pressure after 5 minutes of exercise. [1,3] The ABI may even increase. [1] The drop in post-exercise systolic ankle pressure should be <20% of the resting pressure and should return to baseline within approximately 3 minutes after exercise. [4]
- Brachial pressures should increase post-exercise. [1]

Table 20-3: Lower Arterial Exam with Exercise Report

Ankle/Toe Pressures

Location		Press	BI	Waveforms
Right	Brachial	116		
	Dor. Pedis	90	0.71	Triphasic
	Post. Tibial	94	0.75	Triphasic
	Great Toe			
Left	Brachial	126		
	Dor. Pedis	82	0.65	Triphasic
	Post. Tibial	90	0.71	Triphasic
	Great Toe			

Post-Exercise Pressures

	Right			Left		
	Brachial	Ankle	ABI	Brachial	Ankle	ABI
0 min	152	58	0.38		42	0.28
2 min	128	58	0.45		42	0.33
5 min	120	58	0.48		42	0.35
10 min	110	64	0.58		56	0.51
Rec. Time	>10 min			>10 min		
% DROP	49%			61%		

Onset of Symptoms
45 sec.

Symptoms
Lt. buttock pain after 45 sec. on treadmill.
Rt calf pain after 1.5 min. on treadmill.
Lt. calf pain after 2.5 min. of walking

Walking Duration
4 min.

This abnormal treadmill exam reports a significant pressure drop in both legs, post-exercise. The recovery time was >10 minutes suggesting the presence of multilevel disease.

Abnormal

- An immediate drop in ankle pressure post-exercise >20% of the resting pressure indicates significant arterial obstruction involving the arteries which supply the gastrocnemius and soleal muscles. [1]
- A difference between brachial-ankle pressure ≥20mmHg indicates significant arterial disease. [1]
- The drop in post-exercise systolic ankle pressure is >20% of the resting pressure and takes >3 minutes to return to baseline after exercise. [4]
- A recovery time between 2-6 minutes suggests single level disease. Multilevel disease typically requires 6-12 minutes before pressures return to baseline levels. [5,6]

Arterial obstructions involving the tibial arteries may not result in claudication or a decrease in post-exercise pressures. [1]

Reactive Hyperemia

Normal

- A 17-34% drop in ankle pressure is normal after release of the cuff occlusion. [5,7]
- Pressures should return to 90% of their baseline value within the first 60 seconds after release of the cuff occlusion. [1,7]

Abnormal

- Pressure drops >35% of the baseline pressure immediately after occlusion are abnormal. [8]
- Ankle pressures do not return to baseline within 1 minute after cuff deflation. [1,7]
- Single-level arterial disease usually results in a <50% drop in ankle pressure. [5,7]
- Multi-level arterial disease usually results in a >50% drop in ankle pressure. [5,7]

Table 20-4: Diagnostic Criteria for Post-Treadmill Exercise Ankle-Brachial Indices and Recovery Times

Recovery Time	Classification
<3 minutes *	Normal
2-6 minutes **	Single-level disease
6-12 minutes **	Multi-level disease
>15 minutes **	Severe occlusive disease

* The post-exercise systolic ankle pressure drops <20% compared to the resting systolic pressure.

** The post-exercise systolic ankle pressure drops >20% compared to the resting systolic pressure.

Source: Modified from Strandess DE, Zierler RE. (1993). Exercise ankle pressure measurements in arterial disease. In Bernstein EF (Ed.), Vascular Diagnosis (54 553). St. Louis: Mosby.

Table 20-5: Diagnostic Criteria for Post-Reactive Hyperemia Ankle-Brachial Index

% Pressure Decrease	Classification
17-34%	Normal
35-50%	Single-level disease
>50%	Multi-level disease

Source: Strandess DE, Zierler RE. (1993). Exercise ankle pressure measurements in arterial disease. In Bernstein EF (Ed.), Vascular Diagnosis (547-553). St. Louis: Mosby

The initial drop in pressure was once thought to be the most important measurement post-occlusion. [5,7] Other research suggests that post-occlusive ABIs have a greater sensitivity (90%) for detecting obstruction compared to the percentage drop in the ankle pressure (52% sensitivity). [12]

Differential Diagnosis

- Spinal stenosis
- Venous thrombosis
- Restless leg syndrome
- Compartment syndrome
- Nocturnal leg cramps
- Neuropathy
- Muscle/tendon strains
- Arthritis

Correlation

- Duplex ultrasound (measuring changes in arterial flow velocity pre/post occlusion)
- Spiral CT scan
- MRA
- Arteriography
- Near-infrared spectroscopy

Medical Treatment

- Modify risk factors (e.g., reduce cholesterol, manage HTN and DM, smoking cessation)
- Exercise regimen
- Antiplatelet medication (e.g., aspirin)
- Anticoagulation (warfarin)

Surgical Treatment

- Bypass grafting
- Atherectomy
- Endarterectomy
- Direct focal repair
- Amputation

Endovascular Treatment

- Angioplasty
- Stent
- Atherectomy
- Intra-arterial directed thrombolysis (acute blockage)

REFERENCES

1. Zierler RE, Sumner DS. (2005). Physiologic assessment of peripheral arterial occlusive disease. In Rutherford Vascular Surgery 6th edition. (197-222). Philadelphia. Elsevier Saunders.
2. Sumner DS, Zierler RE. (2005). Vascular physiology: essential hemodynamic principles. In *Rutherford Vascular Surgery 6th edition.* (75-123). Philadelphia. Elsevier Saunders.
3. Baker JD. (2005). The role of noninvasive procedures in the management of extremity arterial disease. In Zwiebel WJ. Pellerito JS (Eds.), Introduction to Vascular Ultrasonography 5th ed. (254-260). Philadelphia: Elsevier Saunders.
4. Zaccardi MJ, Olmsted KA. (2002) Peripheral arterial evaluation, In Strandess DE. (Ed.). *Duplex Scanning Disorders 3rd edition.* (253-266). Philadelphia: Lippincott Williams & Wilkins.
5. Strandess DE, Zierler RE, (1993) Exercise ankle pressure measurements in arterial disease. In Bernstein EF (Ed.), *Vascular Diagnosis* (547-553). St. Louis: Mosby.
6. Leon, Labropoulos, N, Mansour MA. (2005). Hemodynamic principles as applied to diagnostic testing. In Mansour MA, Labropoulos N. (Eds.), Vascular Diagnosis, (7-21). Philadelphia: Elsevier Saunders.
7. Zierler, RE. (2005). Nonimaging physiologic tests for assessment of lower extremity arterial occlusive disease: In Zwiebel WJ, Pellerito JS (Eds.). *Introduction to Vascular Ultrasonography 5th ed.* (275-295). Philadelphia: Elsevier Saunders.
8. Baker DJ, (1982) Stress Testing. In Kempczinski RF & Yao JST (Eds.), *Practical Noninvasive Vascular Diagnosis.* (93-103). Chicago: Year Book Medical Publishers.
9. Gerlock A, Giyanani VL, Krebs C (1988): Noninvasive assessment of the lower extremity arteries. In Gerlock A, Giyanani VL, Krebs C (Eds.) Applications of Noninvasive Vascular Techniques. (310). Philadelphia: WB Saunders.
10. Longo MG, Pearce WH, Sumner DS. (2005). Evaluation of upper extremity ischemia. In Rutherford Vascular Surgery 6th edition. (1274-1293). Philadelphia. Elsevier Saunders.
11. Rosenberry R, Nelson MD. (2020). Reactive hyperemia: a review of methods, mechanisms, and considerations. American Journal of Physiology-Regulatory, Integrative and Comparative Physiology. 318:3, R605-R618.
12. Rosenberry R, Nelson MD. (2020). Reactive hyperemia: a review of methods, mechanisms, and considerations. *American Journal of Physiology-Regulatory, Integrative and Comparative Physiology.* 318:3, R605-R618.

ARTERIAL TESTING
21. Lower Extremity Arterial Duplex

Definition

The combination of real time B-mode imaging with spectral and color flow Doppler (duplex scan) to evaluate the lower extremity arteries.

Arterial duplex ultrasound can identify the presence, exact location, extent and severity of disease. The course of the arteries, collaterals and disease can be visualized using B-mode and color while the measurement of Doppler velocity and spectral waveform changes can estimate the severity of obstructions and flow direction.

Etiology

- Atherosclerosis
- Embolization
- Thrombus
- Pseudoaneurysm
- Aneurysm
- Intimal hyperplasia
- Trauma
- Traumatic occlusion
- Extrinsic compression
- External radiation
- AV fistula (abnormal connection between an artery and a vein)
- Popliteal entrapment (extrinsic compression of the popliteal artery)

Risk Factors

- Age (increased risk with age)
- Coronary artery disease
- Diabetes
- Family history
- Hyperlipidemia
- Hypertension
- Obesity
- Smoking
- Sedentary lifestyle
- Previous history of CVA or MI
- Elevated levels of homocysteine
- Excessive levels of C-reactive protein
- Post-op cardiac catheterization

Indications for Exam

- Claudication (exercise-related leg pain)
- Limb pain at rest
- Extremity ulcer
- Gangrene
- Absent peripheral pulses
- Digital cyanosis
- Arterial trauma
- Abnormal ABI
- Aneurysmal disease
- Dependent rubor
- Evaluation prior to dialysis access
- A decrease in ankle-brachial index (ABI) >0.15 compared to the previous exam

Contraindications/Limitations

- Patients with extensive bandages or casts.
- Poor visualization due to vessel depth secondary to obesity/ severe leg edema.
- Diffuse arterial wall calcification (such as in diabetics and end-stage renal failure patients) may interfere with acquisition of duplex information.
- Patients who cannot be adequately positioned.

Mechanism of Disease

- **Atherosclerosis** is the most common arterial disease. Atherosclerotic plaque forms in the artery blocking flow by either narrowing the lumen (arterial stenosis) or totally blocking the artery (arterial occlusion). The term "hemodynamically significant obstruction" refers to either a stenosis or an occlusion that results in a decrease in blood pressure or flow distal to the obstruction. Typically, a stenosis must narrow the diameter of the artery by at least 50% to decrease pressure and flow distally. [1] An arterial occlusion is typically seen from one major branch to the next.

Besides atherosclerosis, narrowing of an arterial lumen can result from intimal hyperplasia or cellular damage after radiation therapy. [23,24]

- **Emboli** may occur as contents of a plaque or fragments of an organized thrombus from the heart or aneurysm loosen and flow downstream. Emboli become lodged in a distant blood vessel, causing arterial occlusion and reduction of flow. [1]
- **Vasospasm** is a temporary constriction of the arteries (typically digital arteries) that may cause significant discomfort to the patient or be a sign of a more serious underlying disease. [2]
- **Extrinsic compression** from tumors, musculoskeletal configuration, hematoma, etc. can result in stenosis or occlusion by placing enough pressure on arterial walls to compromise blood flow. [1]
- **Entrapment syndrome** occurs in certain leg positions, when the gastrocnemius muscle compresses the popliteal artery resulting in the loss of distal pulses. [3]
- **Aneurysmal disease** results from weakening of the structural proteins (elastin and collagen) within the medial layer of the arterial wall. [4]
- A **pseudoaneurysm** (PA) or "false aneurysm" forms due to trauma to all three layers of the arterial wall. The "false aneurysm" is actually a hematoma, receiving its blood supply via communication with an artery through a patent "neck." [5]
- An **arteriovenous fistula** or abnormal connection between artery and vein can be congenital or result from trauma or complications during invasive procedures (e.g., cardiac catheterization). In such cases, blood flows directly from the artery into the venous system without passing through the tissues and capillary bed. [6] The AVF can be congenital, iatrogenic, as a result of trauma or surgically created.
- **Arterial dissections** are caused by tears in the intimal layer of the arterial wall and allow blood flow to access the media. Dissection between the medial and adventitial layers may result in true and false lumens. The false lumen can progressively dilate into a pseudoaneurysm. [7]

Location of Disease

- Location of disease can be focal or diffuse and affect any level or multiple levels.
- The most common location of atherosclerotic obstruction in the lower extremities is the distal superficial femoral artery.
- Arterial bifurcations and the popliteal artery are other common locations of obstruction.
- The popliteal artery can also be affected by entrapment syndrome.

Patient History

- Claudication (exercise-related limb pain)
- Limb pain at rest
- Paralysis (weakness)
- Paresthesia ("pins and needles")
- Poikilothermia (ice-cold limb)
- Ulceration/gangrene of feet/toes
- Previous therapeutic vascular procedure (e.g., bypass, stent)

Physical Examination

- Pulselessness
- Cyanosis
- Pallor
- Dependent rubor
- Bruit (abnormal sound heard through auscultation caused by turbulent flow)
- Pulsatile mass
- Marked temperature difference between extremities
- Gangrene/necrosis (tissue death)
- Palpable thrill (vibration caused by turbulent blood flow as seen in an AV fistula)

Lower Extremity Arterial Duplex Protocol

- Obtain a patient history to include symptoms, risk factors, past vascular interventions, and the general dates. Explain the procedure to the patient.
- Obtain bilateral ankle-brachial indices (ABI's) using the posterior tibial and dorsalis pedis arteries. *Refer to the chapter on ABI and Analog Pedal Artery Waveforms for more detail.*
- The patient is examined in the supine position with the leg externally rotated.
- Some patients may require the use of a range of transducers, including high-frequency (5-7 MHz) (8-15 MHz) transducers and a lower frequency (1-4 MHz) transducer to assist in the Hunter's canal.
- Locate the common femoral artery and vein at the groin in the transverse (short axis) plane. Rotate your transducer onto the common femoral artery in the longitudinal (sagittal) plane. As you move the transducer distally down the leg and then moving the transducer behind the knee, obtain and record B-mode images in longitudinal view of the following:
    » Common femoral artery (CFA)
    » Deep femoral artery (DFA)
    » Superficial femoral artery (SFA)
    » Popliteal artery (POPA)

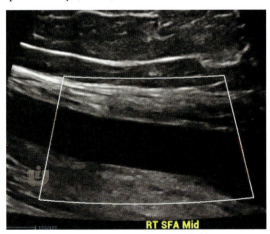

Fig. 21-1: *Normal, clear arterial lumen*

- Scan distally (or begin from the ankle and scan proximally) to record additional B-mode images from the tibial arteries when indicated. Color Doppler will be a useful guide to help identify these arteries. Locate the artery and veins in the transverse plane and rotate the transducer longitudinally onto the artery and document.

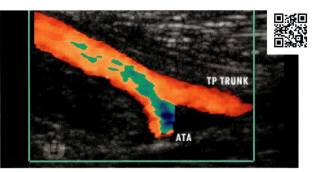

Fig. 21-2: *Bifurcation of the popliteal artery into the anterior tibial artery and tibioperoneal trunk.*

- Position the transducer in the abdomen to record additional B-mode images from the abdominal aorta, common iliac (CIA) and external iliac (EIA) arteries when indicated. Color Doppler will be a useful guide to help identify these arteries. Locate the artery and vein in the transverse plane and rotate the transducer longitudinally onto the artery for documentation.
- Measure and record the peak systolic velocity (PSV) in longitudinal view of the following using spectral Doppler (60° Doppler angle or less, with the angle cursor parallel to the vessel walls in the center of the flow stream):
    » Common femoral artery (CFA)
    » Proximal deep femoral artery (DFA)
    » Proximal, mid and distal superficial femoral artery (SFA)
    » Popliteal artery (POPA)
    » Dorsalis pedis (DPA) and posterior tibial (PTA) arteries
    » Highest obtainable velocity through any area(s) of stenosis
    » Proximal and distal to any stenosis
    » Abdominal aorta, common iliac (CIA), external iliac (EIA), anterior tibial and peroneal arteries (when indicated)

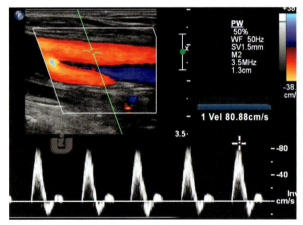

Fig. 21-3: *Measure the PSV in the superficial femoral artery.*

- Document B-mode and color images in areas of suspected stenosis. Measure lumenal reduction, especially caused by a hemodynamically significant lesion to provide supporting documentation for the velocity data.

Color flow can obscure the true lumenal reduction if the color gain is set too high. Measure lumenal reduction in B-mode whenever possible.

- Determine classification of stenosis according to laboratory diagnostic criteria *(see criteria tables)*.
- Document any additional abnormal findings with B-mode and color imaging (e.g., aneurysmal formation, plaque, thrombus, wall irregularity, aneurysm, AV fistula, etc.). Retrograde arterial flow direction is another possible abnormal finding that requires additional documentation.

Decrease color and velocity scales to detect low velocity flow and confirm occlusion.

- When arterial occlusion is suspected, document the lack of flow with spectral Doppler and any visualized collateral branches using color and spectral Doppler. Also note the anatomic level of flow reconstitution when visualized.
- Repeat protocol for the contralateral extremity when indicated.

Duplex Evaluation for Popliteal Entrapment Syndrome

- Ask the patient to lie on his/her side for best access to the popliteal during the positional maneuvers required for this exam.
- Measure and record the PSV in longitudinal view of the distal popliteal artery at the level of the gastrocnemius muscle heads using spectral Doppler (60° Doppler angle or less, with the angle cursor parallel to the vessel walls in the center of the flow stream).
- Document B-mode images of the popliteal artery at rest and measure anterior-posterior (AP) and transverse diameter measurements.
- Instruct the patient to hyperextend the knee and point the foot downward (plantarflexion).
- Re-measure AP and transverse diameter measurements on images of the popliteal artery taken while the foot is pointed downward.
- Repeat the spectral Doppler measurements while the patient hyperextends the knee and points their toes upward (dorsiflexion).

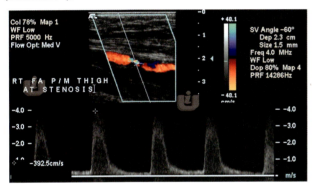

Fig. 21-4: *Abnormal, stenotic arterial waveform noted with elevated PSV*

Table 21-1: Lower Extremity Arterial Duplex Protocol Summary

Scan longitudinal (sagittal) view with B-mode, color and spectral Doppler

1. CFA	• Measure and record the peak systolic velocity (PSV) for all segments.
2. Proximal DFA	
3. Proximal SFA	• When an area of stenosis is identified, "walk" the sample gate through the area of stenosis and obtain representative waveforms at the narrowest point of stenosis, as well as proximal and distal to the stenosis.
4. Mid SFA	
5. Distal SFA	
6. POPA	
7. PTA *	
8. DPA *	• Calculate the velocity ratio (Vr):
9. EIA (optional)	PSV (V$_2$) distal ÷ PSV (V$_1$) proximal
10. ATA (optional)	• Determine classification of stenosis according to laboratory diagnostic criteria.
11. PerA (optional)	

PRINCIPLES OF INTERPRETATION

B-mode Imaging and Color Doppler

Assess all arteries for intraluminal echoes. Determine plaque location and plaque characteristics:

- **Diffuse plaque**: Long segment of the artery lined with plaque, but <50% diameter reduction at any point.
- **Stenotic**: Lumen is narrowed and velocity increases. A hemodynamically significant stenosis typically occurs when narrowing results in a >50% diameter reduction (75% area reduction). A stenosis can be focal or involve a long segment.
- **Calcific**: Highly reflective plaque(s) with acoustic shadowing

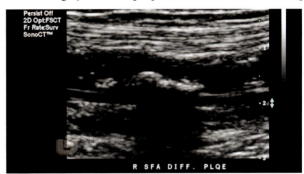

Fig. 21-5: *Abnormal artery: lumenal reduction and calcific plaque noted on B-mode image*

- **Occluded**: Complete occlusion of the vessel
- **"Moving"/"Mobile"**: Debris within the lumen is poorly adhered to the vessel wall, e.g., moving thrombus.
- Color flow is used to show patency of the arterial lumen, the degree of narrowing when there is disease and flow direction.
- Measure lumenal reductions in multiple planes to get the full effect of any plaque:
  » Transverse
  » Longitudinal-anterior/posterior
  » Longitudinal-lateral
  » The most difficult point to define is the true lumen. Look for a black line separating the wall from any plaque.
  » Place calipers on the anterior-inner lumen and the posterior inner lumen.
  » Calculate and report the average of 2-3 measurements.
  » Use color only if needed to clearly define edges of plaque, and update with B-mode frequently to avoid color overgain.

Arterial Waveform Terminology

The terminology used to describe arterial waveforms is not consistent across laboratories. A consensus document was published in 2020 by the Society of Vascular Ultrasound and the Society for Vascular Medicine regarding the terminology and interpretation of peripheral arterial and venous waveforms. *See the Arterial Hemodynamics chapter for more detail on arterial waveforms.*

Spectral Doppler Waveforms

Any change in spectral waveform analysis depends on the terminology used by the lab; from triphasic to monophasic or changes in resistance may be significant.

Flow Velocities

- Determine peak systolic velocity (PSV) and flow direction
- Calculate the velocity ratio (Vr)= V_2/V_1, where V_2 represents the maximum PSV of a stenosis and V_1 is the PSV of the proximal normal segment.

- Calcific shadowing can prohibit Doppler and color flow analysis of a specific arterial segment. Use indirect signs to evaluate hemodynamically significant lesions:
  » Comparing the Doppler waveform proximal and distal to the calcified segment can point to a hemodynamically significant obstruction under the calcific shadowing.
  » If severe post-stenotic turbulence is present distal to the shadowing, there could be a stenosis in the calcified segment, or conversely, if there is essentially no change in the waveform pattern, it is unlikely that a significant obstruction exists under the calcific area.
  » Compare the arterial waveform in the contralateral extremity at the same site.

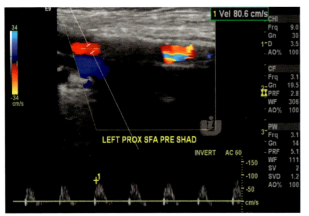

Fig. 21-6: *Spectral Doppler pre-shadowing*

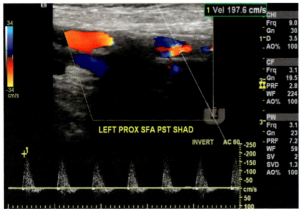

Fig. 21-7: *Spectral Doppler post-shadowing; significant Vr >2.0, suggests a significant stenosis (198 ÷ 81cm/s = 2.4)*

Interpretation/Diagnostic Criteria

Normal

(Absence of a hemodynamically significant stenosis, <50%)
B-mode Imaging and Color Doppler
- The artery is free of intralumenal echoes. [9]
- When utilized, color Doppler fills the entire arterial lumen and is in the appropriate direction for each artery. [9]

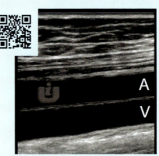
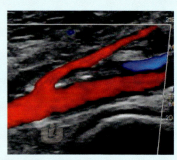

Fig. 21-8: *Normal, clear arterial lumen on a B-mode image.*
Courtesy of Philips Healthcare

Fig. 21-9: *Normal color filling in a popliteal artery*

Spectral Doppler Waveforms

- A waveform with a sharp, quick upstroke followed by a brisk downstroke with reversed flow direction in early diastole and another forward phase in late diastole is termed *triphasic*. This is considered a normal finding in the peripheral arteries.

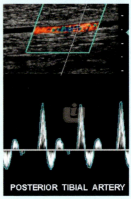
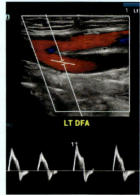

Fig. 21-10: *Triphasic arterial waveform*

Fig. 21-11: *Multiphasic arterial waveform*

- A waveform with a sharp upstroke followed by reversed flow that crosses the zero baseline and contains both forward and reverse components is termed *multiphasic* or *biphasic* by some labs.

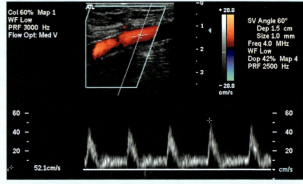

Fig. 21-12: *Biphasic arterial waveform*

- Some labs have adopted terminology that recognizes any reversed flow as normal by using an abbreviation NR for "normal-reversed" whether or not the third phase is present, in order to avoid the confusing use of "triphasic" and "biphasic" terms. [28]

Flow Velocities

PSV and Vr are relatively uniform throughout the sampled arterial segment. [8]

Table 21-2: **Normal PSV of Lower Extremity Arteries**

Artery	PSV cm/s (angle-corrected)
EIA	119 ± 22
CFA	114 ± 25
SFA (proximal)	91 ± 14
SFA (distal)	94 ± 14
PopA	69 ± 14

Source: Modified from Jager KA, Ricketts HJ, Strandess DE Jr. (1985). Duplex scanning for the evaluation of lower limb arterial disease. In Bernstein EF (Ed.), Noninvasive diagnostic techniques in vascular disease. St. Louis: Mosby

Abnormal

B-mode Imaging and Color Doppler

- Intralumenal echoes are visualized within the artery resulting in a measurable lumenal reduction.
- When utilized, color Doppler does not fill the entire arterial lumen. A color jet can be visualized through the narrowed lumen and a mosaic color pattern can be observed due to turbulent flow in the post-stenotic region.[9,10,12]
  » For increased accuracy when assessing disease, consider B-mode reduction measurements together with Doppler velocity and ratios.

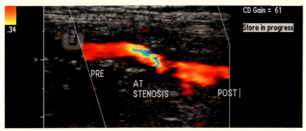

Fig. 21-13: Color changes through a stenotic area

Color Doppler can over/underestimate plaque and diameter reductions if gain settings are not optimized.

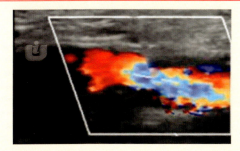

Fig. 21-14: Mosaic color pattern post-stenosis

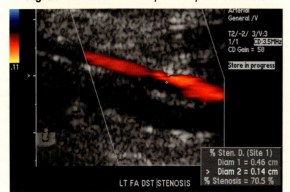

Fig. 21-15: Lumenal reduction of the superficial femoral artery

Spectral Doppler Waveforms

- As the obstruction becomes more severe, changes in the spectral waveform are expected before a stenosis or occlusion, at the point of greatest stenosis and after a stenosis/occlusion as described in the *Arterial Physiology* chapter. These changes are important to note in the interpretation of the vascular exam.
- *Spectral broadening* represents the wide range of velocities usually present when there is disturbed, non-laminar flow. This waveform change occurs in the early stages of arterial disease. The normally clear window below the systolic peak begins to fill in.

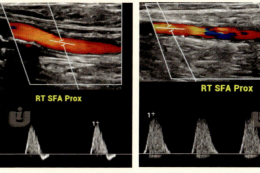

Fig. 21-16: Samples of waveforms with spectral broadening. Note: the space under the systolic peak starts to fill in.

- *Monophasic* arterial Doppler waveforms reflect low resistance and are characterized by a slow upstroke, low amplitude, and broad peak with continuous forward flow in diastole that does not cross the zero baseline. The upstroke has a general direction of being tipped to the right. Monophasic waveforms are typically present distal to an occlusion or a very high-grade stenosis.[9-11,14]

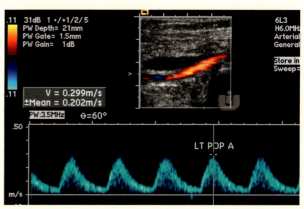

Fig. 21-17: Monophasic popliteal arterial waveform

- A high-resistance waveform with a sharp upstroke and brisk downstroke will be noted in a stenotic region. There may or may not be flow reversal in diastole.[28] When there is a diastolic component, it may be elevated or absent depending on the degree of downstream resistance.
- *Parvus tardus* is an alternative term for "monophasic" used by some laboratories to describe a waveform with continuous forward flow and a slow, blunted systolic component.[15]
- Turbulent waveforms or "post-stenotic turbulence" are indicative of chaotic flow reflecting how blood moves in many directions just past the stenosis.

Monophasic CFA waveforms combined with a PSV <45cm/s is highly indicative of ipsilateral iliac artery occlusion.[26]

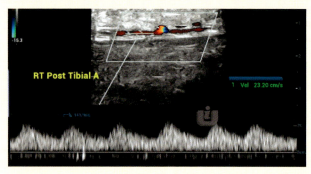

Fig. 21-18: *Monophasic flow in the posterior tibial artery*

- **Staccato:** A "spiked" high-resistant waveform with a short upstroke/downstroke and little to no diastolic component is often a signal of impending occlusion.

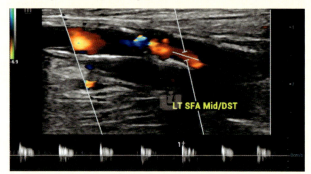

Fig. 21-19: *Staccato arterial waveform (noted pre-occlusion)*

- **Occlusion:** An occlusion of the artery is present when no flow is detected by spectral Doppler. Determine the extent (length) of the occlusion.[8,9,12]

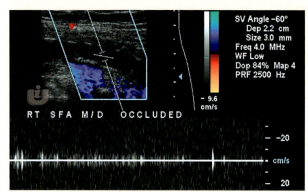

Fig. 21-20: *Absent waveform through a segment with an arterial occlusion*

> *Use flow in the adjacent vein as a guide to identify an occluded artery. Always confirm flow by placing the Doppler sample volume in the vessel lumen.*

» Often a large collateral can be identified at the proximal and distal ends of the occlusion. These collaterals often exit and enter the artery at 90° angles.

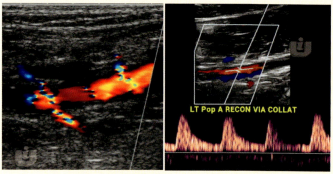

Fig. 21-21: *Collaterals and spectral Doppler after flow reconstitution*

» Blood flow may reverse in arteries supplying collateral flow, especially near arterial bifurcations when the proximal artery is occluded (e.g., retrograde arterial flow from the DFA will supply the SFA in cases of CFA occlusion).[17]

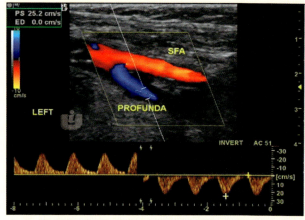

Fig. 21-22: *Doppler waveforms documenting forward flow direction in the SFA and reversed flow direction of the DFA*

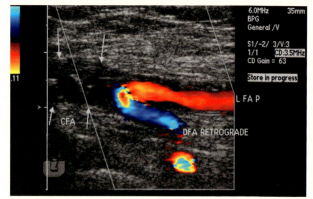

Fig. 21-23: *Retrograde deep femoral arterial flow noted by color Doppler feeding the SFA in cases of CFA occlusion*

Flow Velocities

- A hemodynamically significant lesion (>50%) will result in a focal velocity increase (at least double the velocity in the proximal arterial segment), change in spectral waveform (including *spectral broadening* where the clear window under the spectral waveform is filled in), post-stenotic turbulence and a possible color bruit.[8,10,11,13,16]
- A hemodynamically significant lesion (>70%) will result in a focal velocity increase at least triple the velocity in the proximal arterial segment.[13]

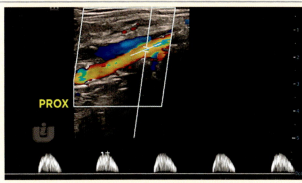

Fig. 21-24: *Monophasic waveform proximal to a severe stenosis*

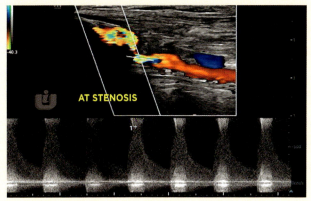

Fig. 21-25: *Hemodynamically significant stenosis: note the aliasing by color flow.*

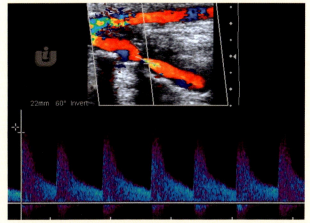

Fig. 21-26: *Spectral waveforms distal to a significant stenosis with post-stenotic turbulence*

The criterion for abnormal lower extremity arterial duplex varies across institutions.

Table 21-3: University of Chicago Arterial Duplex Diagnostic Criteria

% Stenosis	Waveform	Velocity Ratio	Spectral Broadening	Distal Waveform
Normal	Triphasic	0-2.0	None	Normal, triphasic
1-49%	Triphasic	0-2.0	Minimal	Normal, triphasic
50-99%	Bi/monophasic	>2.1	Pronounced, significant spectral broadening	Bi/monophasic
Occluded	Absent	None	None	Collateral flow (monophasic) or absent flow

Source: Modified from Vandenberghe, NJ. (1994). Duplex scan assessment of arterial occlusive disease. Journal of Vascular Technology. 18:287-293.

Table 21-4: Duplex Imaging Diagnostic Criteria

% Stenosis	Peak Velocity	Velocity Ratio
Normal	<150cm/s	<1.5: 1
30-49%	150-200cm/s	1.5:1-2:1
50-74%	200-400cm/s	2:1-4:1
>75-99%	>400cm/s	>4:1
Occlusion	No color saturation	NA

Source: Cossman DV, Ellison JE, et al (1989). Comparison of contrast arteriography to arterial mapping with color flow duplex imaging in the lower extremity *The Journal of Vascular Surgery*, Nov; 10(5):522-8; discussion 528-9.

Table 21-5: University of Washington Arterial Duplex Diagnostic Criteria

% Stenosis	Waveform	Spectral Broadening	Velocity/Ratio	Distal Waveform
Normal	Triphasic	None	None	Normal
1-19%	Triphasic	Minimal spectral broadening	<30% increase in PSV from proximal segment	Waveforms remain normal proximally and distally
20-49%	Tri/biphasic	Prominent spectral broadening	30-100% increase in PSV from proximal segment	Waveforms remain normal proximally and distally
50-99%	Monophasic	Extensive spectral broadening	>100% increase in PSV from proximal segment	Waveform becomes monophasic distally
Occlusion	No flow (pre-occlusive thump may be heard proximal to occluded segment)	None	None	Collateral waveforms are monophasic with reduced PSV

Source: Moneta GL, Zacardi MJ, Olmsted KA. (2010). Lower extremity arterial occlusive disease. In Zierler RE (Ed.), *Strandess's duplex scanning disorders in Vascular Diagnosis 4th ed.* (133-147). Philadelphia: Wolters Kluwer Lippincott Williams & Wilkins.

Other Pathology

Arteriovenous fistula (AVF) [27]

- An arteriovenous fistula between any artery and an adjacent vein is characterized by color bruit on duplex image along with high velocity, low-resistance spectral waveforms at the same site by spectral Doppler. [7]
- The arterial waveforms proximal to the AVF typically demonstrate a low resistant flow pattern as the arterial flow feeds the low resistance vein. The venous segment immediately proximal to the AVF will demonstrate a pulsatile, turbulent waveform.

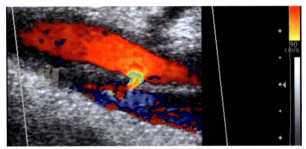

Fig. 21-27: *Arteriovenous fistula by color duplex*

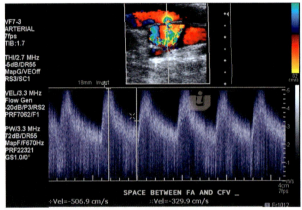

Fig. 21-28: *Doppler waveforms at the site of an arteriovenous fistula.*

- **Pseudoaneurysm (PA):** A pulsatile mass observed communicating with a native artery is indicative of a pseudoaneurysm. A to-and-fro Doppler flow pattern will be apparent within the "neck" of the PA. The size of a pseudoaneurysm varies in diameter, but is typically between 1-5cm. [18]

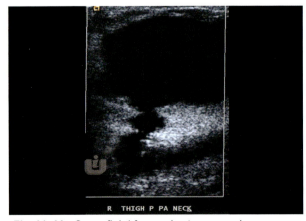

Fig. 21-29: *Superficial femoral artery pseudoaneurysm*

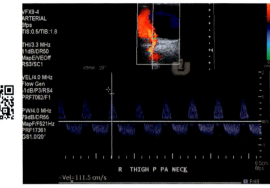

Fig. 21-30: *Pseudoaneurysm: characteristic "to-and-fro" waveform*

- **Aneurysm:** An aneurysm is defined as a focal enlargement of an artery at least twice the diameter of the proximal segment. Intralumenal thrombus may be observed and is a possible source of distal emboli. [12] PSV are typically reduced with abnormal flow patterns within an aneurysm. [10]
  - » **Arteriomegaly:** The term used to describe a uniform arterial dilation throughout an artery. [19]
  - » An artery can also be described as "**ectatic**" (dilatation of a circular tube) when diameters are somewhat larger through a segment, though not yet aneurysmal. The dilated areas of the artery may or may not be uniform.

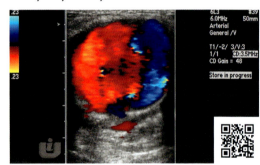

Fig. 21-31: *Superficial femoral artery aneurysm: transverse plane*

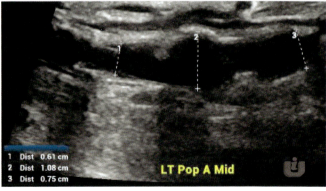

Fig. 21-32: *"Ectatic" popliteal artery since the larger diameter is not 2x the proximal segment*

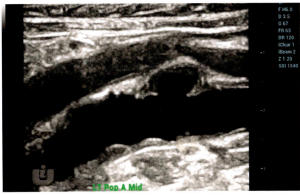

Fig. 21-33: *Popliteal artery saccular aneurysm longitudinal plane*

An important complication of popliteal artery aneurysms is emboli from intramural thrombus, not rupture. [25]

» The most common peripheral artery aneurysm is in the popliteal artery. Approximately 64% of male patients with a popliteal artery aneurysm will have an abdominal aortic aneurysm. [19]

» Popliteal aneurysms usually occur bilaterally. [25]

» 3% of patients with a femoral artery aneurysm also have a popliteal artery aneurysm. [25]

- **Arterial dissection:** A dissection of the arterial lumen is recognized by two distinct flow channels by B-mode and/or color Doppler separated by the dissected intima seen as a white line within the lumen. One lumen is known as the "true lumen" while the other is referred to as the "false lumen." Each lumen has a distinctly different flow pattern or one lumen may be occluded. [7] Waveform patterns in the false lumen will be turbulent, irregular and/or bidirectional compared to the more "normal" or expected waveform in the true lumen.

- **Popliteal entrapment syndrome:** A reduction in arterial diameter while the patient points their foot downward with resulting stenosis or loss of arterial pulse may indicate popliteal entrapment syndrome. [10,20]

The use of duplex testing to diagnose popliteal entrapment syndrome is controversial. Some believe the reduction in arterial diameter is a normal response when pointing the foot downward.

- **Adventitial cystic disease (ACD):** Duplex findings of ACD include focal stenosis or occlusion of the popliteal artery and observance of compression on the arterial lumen by the cyst. [20,21]

Differential Diagnosis
- Spinal stenosis
- Venous thrombosis
- Restless leg syndrome
- Compartment syndrome
- Nocturnal leg cramps
- Neuropathy
- Muscle/tendon strains
- Arthritis
- Cystic disease (such as popliteal)

Correlation
- Spiral CT scan
- MRA
- Arteriography

Medical Treatment
- Modify risk factors (e.g., reduce cholesterol/HTN, manage DM, smoking cessation)
- Exercise regimen
- Antiplatelet medication (e.g., aspirin)
- Botox (for popliteal entrapment)
- Anticoagulation (warfarin)

Surgical Treatment
- Bypass grafting
- Endarterectomy
- Direct focal repair
- Amputation

Endovascular Treatment
- Angioplasty
- Stent
- Atherectomy
- Intra-arterial directed thrombolysis

REFERENCES

1. Sumner DS, Zierler RE. (2005). Vascular physiology: essential hemodynamic principles. In *Rutherford Vascular Surgery 6th edition*. (75-123). Philadelphia. Elsevier Saunders.
2. Shepard RFJ. (2005). Raynaud's syndrome: vasospastic and occlusive arterial disease involving the distal upper extremity. In *Rutherford Vascular Surgery 6th edition*. (1319-1346). Philadelphia. Elsevier Saunders.
3. Levien IJ. (2005). Nonatheromatous causes of popliteal artery disease. In *Rutherford Vascular Surgery 6th edition*. (1236-1255). Philadelphia. Elsevier Saunders.
4. Schermerhorn ML, Cronenwett JL. (2005). Abdominal aortic and iliac aneurysms. In *Rutherford Vascular Surgery 6th edition*. (1408-1452). Philadelphia. Elsevier Saunders.
5. Casey, PJ, LaMuraglia GM. (2005). Anastomotic aneurysms. In *Rutherford Vascular Surgery 6th edition*. (894-902). Philadelphia. Elsevier Saunders.
6. Rutherford RB. (2005). Diagnostic evaluation of arteriovenous fistulas and vascular anomalies. In *Rutherford Vascular Surgery 6th edition*. (1602-1612). Philadelphia. Elsevier Saunders.
7. Baker JD. (2005). The role of noninvasive procedures in the management of extremity arterial disease. In Zwiebel WJ. Pellerito JS (Eds.), *Introduction to Vascular Ultrasonography 5th ed*. (254-260). Philadelphia: Elsevier Saunders.
8. Moneta GL, Zacardi MJ, Olmsted KA. (2010). Lower extremity arterial occlusive disease. In Zierler RE (Ed.), *Strandess's duplex scanning disorders in Vascular Diagnosis 4th ed*. (133-147). Philadelphia Wolters Kluwer Lippincott Williams & Wilkins.
9. Zierler RE. (2005). Ultrasound assessment of lower extremity arteries. In Zwiebel WJ, Pellerito JS (Eds.), *Introduction to Vascular Ultrasonography 5th ed*. (341-356). Philadelphia: Elsevier Saunders.
10. Thrush A, Hartshorne, T. (2005). "Duplex assessment of lower limb arterial disease" In *Peripheral Vascular Ultrasound, How Why and When, 2nd ed*. (111-131). Edinburgh: Elsevier Churchill Livingstone.
11. Kohler TR. (1993). Duplex scanning for the evaluation of lower limb arterial disease. In Bernstein EF (Ed.). *Vascular Diagnosis 4th ed*. (520-526). St. Louis: Mosby.
12. Kerr TM, Bandyk DF. (1993). Color duplex imaging of peripheral arterial disease before angioplasty or surgical intervention. In Bernstein EF (Ed.). *Vascular Diagnosis 4th ed*. (527-533). St. Louis: Mosby.
13. Ascher E, Salles-Cunha SX, Hingorani A, Markevich N. (2005). Duplex ultrasound and arterial mapping before infrainguinal revascularization. In *Mansour MA, Labropoulos N. (Eds.), Vascular Diagnosis*. (237-246). Philadelphia: Elsevier Saunders.
14. Zierler RE, Sumner DS. (2005). Physiologic assessment of peripheral arterial occlusive disease. In *Rutherford Vascular Surgery 6th edition*. (197-222). Philadelphia. Elsevier Saunders
15. Armstrong PA, Bandyk DF. (2010). Vascular laboratory: arterial duplex scanning . In *Rutherford Vascular Surgery 7th edition*. (Chapter 15). Philadelphia. Elsevier Saunders.
16. Rzucidlo EM, Zwolak RM. (2005). Arterial duplex scanning. In *Rutherford Vascular Surgery 6th edition*. (233-253). Philadelphia. Elsevier Saunders.
17. Kalman PG. (2005). Profundaplasty: isolated and adjunctive applications. In *Rutherford Vascular Surgery 6th edition*. (1174-1180). Philadelphia. Elsevier Saunders.
18. Burke BJ, Friedman SG. (2005). Ultrasound in the diagnosis and management of arterial emergencies. In Zwiebel WJ. Pellerito JS (Eds.), *Introduction to Vascular Ultrasonography 5th ed*. (254-260). Philadelphia: Elsevier Saunders.
19. Cronenwett JL. (2005). Abdominal aortic and iliac aneurysms. In *Rutherford Vascular Surgery 6th edition*. (1408-1452). Philadelphia. El Sevier Saunders.
20. Levien IJ. (2005). Nonatheromatous causes of popliteal artery disease. In *Rutherford Vascular Surgery 6th edition*. (1236-1255). Philadelphia. Elsevier Saunders.
21. Flanigan DP, Burnham SJ, Goodreau JJ, Bergan JJ. *Summary of cases of adventitial cystic disease of the popliteal artery*. Ann Surgery 1979 Feb: 189 (2): 165-75.
22. Cossman DV, Ellison JE, et al (1989). Comparison of contrast arteriography to arterial mapping with color flow duplex imaging in the lower extremity *The Journal of Vascular Surgery*, Nov; 10(5):522-8; discussion 528-9.
23. Davies MG. (2005). Intimal hyperplasia: basic response to arterial and vein graft injury and reconstruction. In *Rutherford Vascular Surgery 6th edition*. (149-172). Philadelphia. El Sevier Saunders
24. Shepard RJ, Rooke T. (2005). Uncommon arteriopathies. In *Rutherford Vascular Surgery 6th edition*. (453-474). Philadelphia. Elsevier Saunders.
25. Van Bockel JH, Hamming JF. (2005). Lower extremity aneurysms. In *Rutherford Vascular Surgery 6th edition*. (1534-1551). Philadelphia. El Sevier Saunders
26. Shaalan WE; French-Sherry, F; Castilla MS; Lozanski L; Bassiouny Hisham S. (2003). Reliability of common femoral artery hemodynamics in assessing the severity of aortoiliac inflow disease *The Journal of Vascular Surgery*, May; 37(5):960-9.
27. Brawley JG, Modrall JG. (2005). Traumatic arteriovenous fistulas. In *Rutherford Vascular Surgery 6th edition*. (1619-1626). Philadelphia. El Sevier Saunders.
28. Kim ES, Sharma AM, Scissons R, et al. Interpretation of peripheral arterial and venous Doppler waveforms: A consensus statement from the Society for Vascular Medicine and Society for Vascular Ultrasound. Vascular Medicine. 2020;25(5):484-506. doi:10.1177/1358863X20937665

ARTERIAL TESTING
22. Bypass and Stent Surveillance Duplex Ultrasound

Definition
The use of a combination of real time B-mode imaging with spectral and color flow Doppler (duplex scan) to evaluate the patency of bypass grafts or stents in the upper or lower extremities. Spectral Doppler velocity and spectral waveform changes can estimate the severity of obstructions.

Etiology
- Intimal hyperplasia
- Atherosclerosis
- Thrombosis
- Aneurysm
- Pseudoaneurysm
- Embolization
- Trauma
- Traumatic occlusion
- Extrinsic compression
- AV fistula (abnormal connection between an artery and a vein)

Risk Factors
- Age (increased risk with age)
- Coronary artery disease
- Diabetes
- Family history
- Hyperlipidemia
- Hypertension
- Obesity
- Smoking
- Sedentary lifestyle
- Previous history of CVA or MI
- Elevated levels of homocysteine
- Excessive levels of C-reactive protein

Indications for Exam
- Post-operative follow-up exams
- New symptoms of claudication, pain, ulcer/gangrene post-intervention
- A decrease in ankle-brachial index (ABI) >0.15 compared to the previous exam
- Absent peripheral pulses
- Pulsatile mass near an anastomotic or intervention site
- Digital cyanosis
- Dependent rubor

Contraindications/Limitations
- Patients with extensive bandages or casts
- Obesity/severe edema may cause poor visualization due to vessel depth
- Diffuse arterial wall calcification (often seen in diabetics and end-stage renal failure patients) may interfere with acquisition of duplex information
- Patients who cannot be adequately positioned

Graft Location
Bypass grafts can be located between any two vessels and are named for the two arteries they connect. Examples of typical arterial grafts encountered for surveillance include:
- Aorto-Iliac (abdominal aorta to unilateral or bilateral iliac)
- Aorto-Fem (abdominal aorta to unilateral or bilateral femoral)
- Ax-Fem (axillary to common femoral, axillary to superficial femoral or axillary to deep femoral)
- Fem-Fem (right common femoral artery to left common femoral artery or vice versa)
- Fem-Pop (common or superficial femoral artery to proximal or distal popliteal artery)
- Fem-Tib (common or superficial femoral artery to any one of the tibial arteries)

Graft Types (Graft Conduits)
- Dacron and PTFE (Polytetrafluoroethylene) grafts are easily differentiated from each other by their unique ultrasound pattern; PTFE has a bright double line on B-mode image and Dacron a single line with a "saw tooth" or wavy appearance.

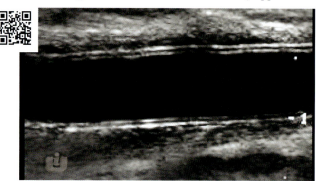

Fig. 22-1: *PTFE with bright double line along the walls (non-ringed)*

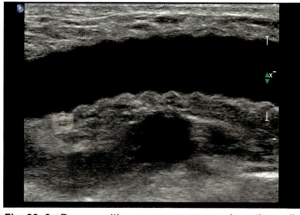

Fig. 22-2: *Dacron with wavy appearance along the walls*

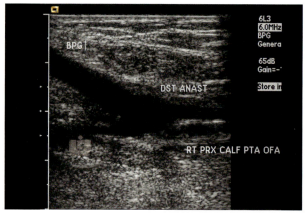

Fig. 22-3: *Vein bypass graft*

- Immediate post-operative duplex scanning of a prosthetic bypass graft (e.g., PTFE, Dacron) can be technically difficult due to air within the walls of the graft, which ultrasound cannot penetrate. [3] This limitation is temporary.

Types of Lower Extremity Bypass Graft Material

Synthetic
- PTFE
- Dacron

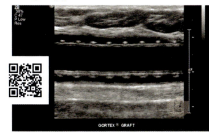

Fig. 22-4: *PTFE (ringed)*
Courtesy of Philips Healthcare

Autogenous: originating from a source within the same individual, e.g., using one of your veins for a bypass

Autogenous (a.k.a. autologous)
Vein bypasses using any of the following:
- In-situ vein (vein left in original anatomic location with valves cut and branches ligated)

In-situ vein grafts have more problems than reverse saphenous vein grafts due to size mismatch and valve site trauma. [11]

- Reversed vein (vein is ligated, reversed and attached to arteries)
- Autogenous conduit originates from a source within the same individual, (e.g. using one of your veins for a bypass conduit).
- Autogenous veins commonly used:
  » Great saphenous vein
  » Small saphenous vein
  » Basilic vein
  » Cephalic vein
- Modified biologic grafts
  » Human umbilical vein
  » Cryopreserved saphenous vein
  » Bovine

Composite
An example of a composite graft is a synthetic graft connected to an autogenous vein.

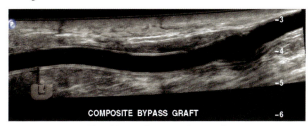

Fig. 22-5: *Composite graft*

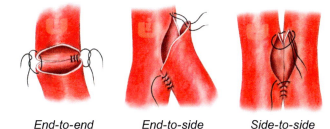

End-to-end   End-to-side   Side-to-side

Fig. 22-6: *Types of Bypass Graft Anastomoses*

Types of Stents

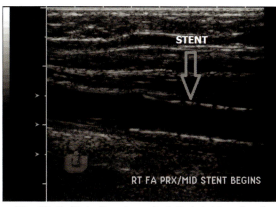

Fig. 22-7: *Note the characteristic bright walls of the stent in this superficial femoral artery.*

Types of stents include (but not limited to):
- Drug-eluting stents (coated with a drug that should decrease the chance of intimal hyperplasia)
- Self-expanding Nitinol stents
- Balloon expanding stents
- Covered stents (graft material covers the stent to exclude the severely diseased native arterial lumen)

Mechanism of Graft Failure
- Early graft failure (<30 days) is most likely due to technical errors in construction of the bypass (e.g., poor choice of inflow or outflow vessels, retained valves, clamp injury etc.). [1,2,3]
- Hemodynamically significant graft stenoses resulting from intimal hyperplasia often occurs between one month and 2 years of graft placement. [1,2,4]
- Hemodynamically significant graft stenoses resulting from atherosclerotic progression in the inflow/outflow beds often occurs in grafts older than 2 years. [1,2,4]
- Patient has undiagnosed hypercoagulable disorder. [3,4]
- Graft infection is possible though rare, occurring in 0.2-5% of operations. [4,5]
- Aneurysmal degeneration can occur in mature vein grafts. [2]
- Trauma to the graft can result in thrombosis. [4]
- Thromboembolism [1-4]
- Early graft failure can occur even without an identifiable mechanical defect or cause. [2,3]

Mechanism of Stent Failure
- Stenting is increasingly being used to treat more complicated lesions and technical failures may occur acutely (<30 days post-op). Technical failure is more common after percutaneous transluminal angioplasty for an occlusion than for stenosis. [1,6]
- Recurrent arterial re-stenosis is believed to be the cause for failures occurring >30 days post-operatively. [6]

Iliac angioplasty has a longer patency rate than femoral-popliteal arterial angioplasty. [6]

Location of Disease
- Location of disease can be focal or diffuse and affect any level or multiple levels.
- Common locations of graft obstruction:
  » Valve sites (vein grafts)   » Outflow arterial tract
  » Graft anastomoses   » Graft kink
  » Inflow arterial tract

- Common locations for disease requiring stent placement:
  - » Iliac arteries
  - » Femoral-popliteal arteries
  - » Tibial arteries (less often)

Below the iliacs, angioplasty is more successful in patients experiencing claudication and there is good distal arterial flow. Angioplasty is less successful for longer lesions and occlusions.[2] Studies suggest that stenting often does not improve long-term patency of lesions.[10]

Patient History
- Claudication (exercise-related)
- Rest pain
- Paralysis
- Paresthesia
- Poikilothermia
- Current and previous ulceration of feet/toes
- Any vascular therapeutic procedures (e.g., bypass, stenting)

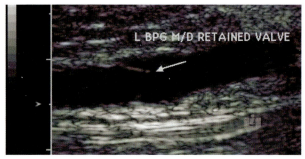

Fig. 22-8: *Vein graft with retained valve cusp noted*

Physical Examination
- Pulselessness
- Cyanosis
- Pallor
- Dependent rubor
- Bruit (abnormal sound heard through auscultation caused by turbulent flow)
- Significant temperature difference between extremities
- Palpable thrill (vibration caused by turbulent blood flow as seen in AV fistula)
- Ulceration
- Gangrene/necrosis (tissue death)
- Pulsatile mass

Arterial Bypass Graft/Stent Surveillance Protocol
- Obtain a patient history to include symptoms, risk factors and past vascular interventions and general dates. This will assist in locating the graft, particularly when multiple grafts are present.
- Obtain past surgical reports/records, including type of bypass graft or stent placed and general date of surgery if available. Explain the procedure to the patient.
- Patient is typically examined in the supine position for grafts and stents. A prone position may be useful to study a stent or graft at or below the knee.
- Obtain bilateral ABI's (never put a blood pressure cuff over a bypass graft or stent without first consulting the medical director of the lab or according to lab protocol).

It may be contraindicated to place a blood pressure cuff over a graft due to the high risk of occluding the graft. Check the laboratory protocol or with the Medical Director for guidance.

- Some patients may require the use of a range of transducers, including high-frequency (5-7 MHz) (8-15 MHz) transducers and a lower frequency (1-4 MHz) transducer for deeper structures, for example the distal anastomosis.
- Evaluate for graft or stent abnormalities while scanning (e.g., thrombosis, stenosis, valves, aneurysm, kinks, intimal hyperplasia, perigraft fluid, etc.).

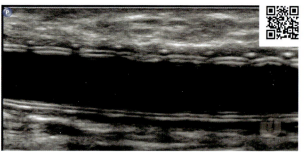

Fig. 22-9: *Normal graft lumen clear of any echogenic material*

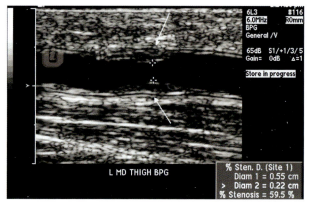

Fig. 22-10: *Lumenal reduction within the graft by B-mode image measuring nearly 60%*

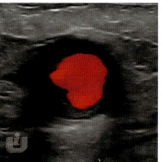 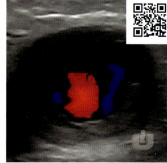

Fig. 22-11: *Transverse color images of a bypass with aneurysmal dilatation. aneurysm. Note diameter change between images and intraluminal thrombosis.*

The majority of infrainguinal bypass grafts use autogenous vein as conduit.[1] Look for incision scars on the extremity to give you a hint what type of graft there is or where the graft anastomosis might be if a report of the operation is unavailable. Do not confuse incisions from vein harvesting with bypass graft incision sites.

Transverse Scan and Images

- Scanning the limb in the transverse (short-axis) plane assists in locating the anastomotic sites, gives information about the length of the graft or stent and locates any previously occluded grafts.
- Once the location of the graft/stent is determined, record transverse B-mode images with and without color flow Doppler of the:
  » Inflow/proximal native artery
  » Proximal anastomosis
  » Proximal graft or stent
  » Mid graft or stent
  » Distal graft or stent
  » Distal anastomosis
  » Outflow/distal native artery
- Color Doppler can overestimate diameter reductions due to bleeding of the color flow over plaque or vessel walls. For increased accuracy, measure in B-mode whenever possible or carefully set color to avoid bleeding over B-mode echoes.

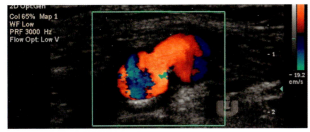

Fig. 22-12: *Transverse bypass graft anastomosis*

Longitudinal Scan and Images

- Record images in a longitudinal (sagittal) view with and without color flow of the:
  » Inflow/proximal native artery
  » Proximal anastomosis
  » Proximal graft or stent
  » Mid graft or stent
  » Distal graft or stent
  » Distal anastomosis
  » Outflow/distal native artery

Disturbed flow may occur at anastomotic sites, areas of valve cusps and vessel diameter changes.

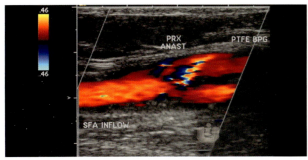

Fig. 22-13: *Proximal anastomosis*

Spectral Doppler Waveforms

Early post-operative flow patterns (within the first 2 months) may not be triphasic due to reactive hyperemia. The waveform will demonstrate a low resistance pattern with forward flow throughout diastole during initial scans that eventually changes to triphasic in follow-up scans.

- Scroll or "walk" the Doppler sample gate through the bypass graft/stent checking for focal changes in velocity and waveform configuration.

- Record and measure the peak systolic velocity (PSV) in longitudinal view using spectral Doppler (≤60° Doppler angle with the angle cursor parallel to the vessel walls and sample volume within the center of the flow stream) at the following levels:
  » Inflow/proximal native artery, at least 2cm proximal to the anastomosis
  » Proximal anastomosis
  » Proximal graft or stent
  » Mid graft or stent
  » Distal graft or stent
  » Distal anastomosis
  » Outflow/distal native artery

- When an area of stenosis is identified, "walk" the sample gate through the area of stenosis and obtain representative waveforms within 2cm proximal to the stenosis, at the highest point of velocity within the stenosis and distal to the stenosis. Post-stenotic turbulence, spectral broadening and color bruit should be documented when present. Measure any lumenal reductions in the longitudinal and sagittal planes when possible to support the spectral Doppler data.

Graft flow velocity (GFV) is an average of peak systolic velocities measured from 3-4 non-stenotic graft segments. Normal GFV ranges from 40-45cm/s, though larger diameter grafts may average less (30-50cm/s). [13]

- Note that longer bypass grafts need B-mode and spectral Doppler waveforms recorded at additional locations. Consider that a thorough femoral-distal tibial bypass graft, for example, requires documentation including:
  » Inflow/proximal native artery
  » Proximal anastomosis
  » Proximal thigh graft
  » Mid thigh graft
  » Distal thigh graft
  » Graft at knee level
  » Proximal calf graft
  » Mid calf graft
  » Distal calf graft
  » Distal anastomosis
  » Outflow/distal native artery

- Repeat protocol for other grafts/stents if necessary.

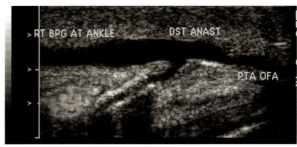

Fig. 22-14: *Longitudinal view of a distal anastomosis near the ankle level*

Preliminary Analysis of Data

- Determine classification of stenosis according to laboratory diagnostic criteria.

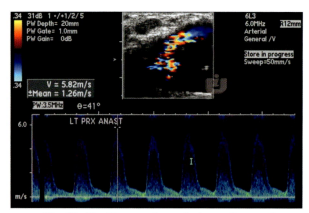

Fig. 22-15: *Abnormal spectral waveforms of bypass graft (anastomotic stenosis)*

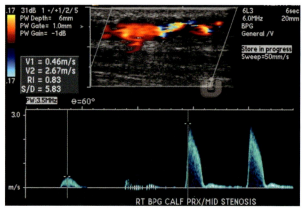

Fig. 22-16: *"Pre" and "at" stenosis spectral waveforms in a bypass graft*

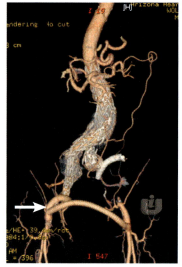

Fig. 22-17: *CTA showing fem-fem bypass*

Table 22-1: Arterial Bypass Graft or Stent Surveillance Protocol Summary

Scan transverse (short-axis) view with B-mode and color flow

- Inflow/proximal native artery
- Proximal anastomosis
- Proximal graft or stent
- Mid graft or stent
- Distal graft or stent
- Distal anastomosis
- Outflow/distal native artery

Scan longitudinal (sagittal) view with B-mode, color flow and spectral Doppler

- Inflow/proximal native artery*
- Proximal anastomosis*
- Proximal graft or stent*
- Mid graft or stent*
- Distal graft or stent*
- Distal anastomosis*
- Outflow/distal native artery*
- Proximal, at and distal to any stenosis*

- Record and measure the peak systolic velocity (PSV). Include additional locations for longer grafts as described in the protocol section.
- Evaluate for graft or stent abnormalities on B-mode and color images.
- Determine classification of stenosis according to laboratory diagnostic criteria.

PRINCIPLES OF INTERPRETATION

- Compare duplex exam findings to the ankle-brachial indices (ABI) or wrist-brachial indices (WBI).
- Explain reasons why the image and velocity data may not agree (for example, elevated velocities with a clear vessel lumen may occur if there is a size "mismatch" between the distal graft and native outflow artery).

Duplex scanning has been shown to be more reliable than ABI's alone for predicting graft failure, though studies have shown how important the ABI remains in graft surveillance exams.

B-mode Imaging and Color Doppler

- Assess the walls of the bypass material for wall irregularity, plaque or thrombus. Document any other abnormal findings (e.g., kink, aneurysmal formation, etc.).
- Assess the inflow/outflow vessels of the bypass using B-mode and color flow for the presence of intralumenal echoes, vessel diameter changes or other unusual pathology.

Plaque and Lesion Descriptions/Characteristics:

- **Diffuse plaque:** long segment of the artery lined with plaque, but <50% diameter reduction at any point.
- **Stenotic:** lumen is narrowed and velocity increases. A hemodynamically significant stenosis typically occurs when narrowing results in a >50% diameter reduction (75% area reduction). A stenosis can be focal or involve a long segment.
- **Calcific:** highly reflective plaque(s) with acoustic shadowing
- **Occluded:** complete occlusion of the vessel

- **"Moving"/"Mobile"**: debris within the lumen is poorly adhered to the vessel wall, e.g., moving thrombus.
- Color flow is used to show patency of the arterial lumen, the degree of narrowing when there is disease and flow direction.

Arterial Waveform Terminology
The terminology used to describe arterial waveforms is not consistent across laboratories. A consensus document was recently endorsed in 2020 by the Society of Vascular Ultrasound and the Society for Vascular Medicine regarding the terminology and interpretation of peripheral arterial waveforms. *See the Arterial Hemodynamics chapter for more detail on arterial waveforms.*

Spectral Doppler Waveforms
Any change in spectral waveform analysis depends on the terminology used by the lab; from triphasic to monophasic or changes in resistance may be significant.

Flow Velocities
- Determine peak systolic velocity (PSV) and flow direction
- Calculate the velocity ratio:

$$Vr = V_2 \div V_1$$

V_2 = Maximum PSV of a stenosis
V_1 = PSV of the proximal normal segment

Interpretation/Diagnostic Criteria

Normal
(absence of a hemodynamically significant stenosis, <50%)

B-mode and Color Doppler
- Normally, there is no echogenic material within the native arterial, graft or stent lumen. [7]
  - Synthetic grafts have a characteristic "double-line" appearance on B-mode image.
  - Stent walls can typically be seen within the lumen of clearly visualized arteries, though deeper stents may be difficult to identify with certainty.
- Color fills the lumen wall-to-wall in transverse and longitudinal views with appropriate settings.

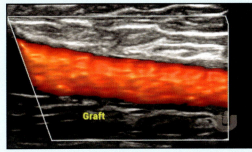

Fig. 22-18: *Normal color flow in a bypass graft*

Spectral Doppler Waveforms
Generally:
- A waveform with a sharp, quick upstroke followed by a brisk downstroke with reversed flow direction in early diastole and another forward phase in late diastole is termed *triphasic*. This is considered a normal finding in the peripheral arteries.
- A waveform with a sharp upstroke followed by reversed flow that crosses the zero baseline and contains both forward and reverse components is termed *multiphasic* or *biphasic* by some labs.

- Some labs have adopted terminology that recognizes any reversed flow as normal by using an abbreviation NR for "normal-reversed" whether or not the third phase is present, in order to avoid the confusing use of "triphasic" and "biphasic" terms. [14]

In addition to general waveform considerations, assess each section of the bypass with the following considerations in mind:
- **Inflow artery:** Normal inflow artery waveform configuration is triphasic.
- **Proximal anastomosis**: Waveforms may demonstrate the typical disturbed flow patterns seen at bifurcations/branches or areas of angulation. [7] These changes are focal at the anastomosis and normalize distally. The image should be scrutinized for the presence of intralumenal echoes.
- **Body of graft/stent:** Waveform configurations remain essentially the same as in the inflow artery throughout a non-obstructed conduit, unless the bypass graft was placed very recently and hyperemic flow is present throughout the graft. [7]
- **Distal anastomosis:** In a bypass graft, there is often a size change between the wider bypass graft and smaller diameter native artery which results in waveform configuration changes caused by disturbed flow due to vessel angulation and size change. [7]
- **Outflow artery:** Flow direction may normally be retrograde in the native artery proximal to the distal anastomosis. [7]

Flow Velocities
- **Inflow artery:** Velocity ratios are less than 2.0 in the inflow or outflow tracts. [8]
- **Proximal anastomosis**: Normal velocity ratios (Vr) are less than 2.0. [4] A large inflow artery feeding a small diameter graft may result in a higher velocity ratio due to the size change. The image should be scrutinized for the presence of intralumenal echoes.

Body of graft/stent
- PSV are <180cm/s and Vr <2.0 throughout the graft body. [4,9]
- PSV are at least >40-45cm/s in vein grafts measuring ≤4mm in diameter.
- Larger conduits (e.g., PTFE conduits or veins measuring >4mm) may demonstrate lower velocities [7]; approximately 35cm/s in a normal setting. [9]
- PSV <190cm/s and Vr <1.5 are normally expected in a superficial femoral artery stent. [10]

- **Distal anastomosis:** In a bypass graft, there is often a size change between the wider bypass graft and smaller diameter native artery which results in a velocity increase. A normal distal anastomosis demonstrates a velocity ratio <3.0. The image should be scrutinized for the presence of intralumenal echoes.
- **Outflow artery:** Velocities remain fairly constant with Vr <2.0.

Abnormal

B-mode Imaging and Color Doppler
- Echogenic material within the native arterial, graft or stent lumen suggests lumenal reduction (intimal hyperplasia, for example). [7] Duplex images may demonstrate echogenic material at the point of highest velocity.
- Moving or frozen, residual valve cusps can also be identified by B-mode imaging. [7]
- Aneurysmal dilatations and intralumenal thrombus may be observed as a graft ages. [7]

- Color does not fill the lumen wall-to-wall in transverse and longitudinal views with appropriate settings. Color flow aliasing will be noted in stenotic segments. [7]
- For increased accuracy when assessing disease, consider B-mode reduction measurements together with Doppler velocity and ratios.

Spectral Doppler Waveforms

Generally:

- As the obstruction becomes more severe, changes in the spectral waveform are expected before a stenosis or occlusion, at the point of greatest stenosis and after a stenosis/occlusion as described in the *Arterial Physiology* chapter of this text. These changes are important to note in the interpretation of the vascular exam.
- *Spectral broadening* represents the wide range of velocities usually present when there is disturbed, non-laminar flow. It is a waveform change in the early stages of arterial disease. The normal systolic peak begins to fill in.
- *Monophasic* arterial Doppler waveforms reflect low resistance and are characterized by a slow upstroke, low amplitude, and broad peak with continuous forward flow in diastole that does not cross the zero baseline. The upstroke has a general direction of being tipped to the right. Monophasic waveforms are typically present distal to an occlusion or a very high-grade stenosis. [7,8,14]
- A high-resistance waveform with a sharp upstroke and brisk downstroke will be noted in a stenotic region. There may or may not be flow reversal in diastole. [14] When there is a diastolic component, it may be elevated or absent depending on the degree of downstream resistance.
- *Parvus tardus* is an alternative term for "monophasic" used by some laboratories to describe a waveform with continuous forward flow and a slow, blunted systolic component. [14]
- **Staccato:** A "spiked" high-resistant waveform with a short upstroke/downstroke and little to no diastolic component is often a signal of impending occlusion.

In addition to general waveform considerations, assess each section of the bypass with the following considerations in mind:

Inflow artery
- Monophasic waveforms in the inflow artery would suggest significant obstruction >50% in the proximal arterial segment.

Proximal anastomosis
- Stenotic waveform patterns, spectral broadening (where the clear window under the spectral waveform is filled in) and post-stenotic turbulence indicate a hemodynamically significant stenosis (≥50%). [7]

Body of graft/stent
- Monophasic waveforms in the graft (blunted, slow upstroke with or without diastolic flow) indicate an obstruction in the inflow tract.
- Depending on the terminology used by the lab waveform changes from triphasic to biphasic or monophasic indicate a hemodynamically significant stenosis (≥50%). [8]
- **Distal anastomosis**: Post-stenotic turbulence and distal waveform pattern changes compared to the pre-anastomotic waveform patterns that accompany increased velocity ratios indicate a hemodynamically significant stenosis (≥50%). [7]

- **Outflow artery:** There is a change in the waveform configuration proximal and distal to any segment with increased velocity which can point to a hemodynamically significant obstruction.

Flow Velocities

Inflow artery
- Velocity ratios >2.0 within the inflow artery that accompany post-stenotic turbulence and waveform changes indicate a hemodynamically significant stenosis (≥50%). [8]

Proximal anastomosis
- Velocity ratios >2.0 (or >3.0 if the graft has a much smaller diameter than the inflow vessel) with elevated velocities, indicate a hemodynamically significant stenosis (≥50%) especially when accompanied by stenotic waveform patterns, spectral broadening and post-stenotic turbulence. [7]

Body of graft/stent
- PSV >180cm/s in a graft that result in a Vr >2.0 indicates a moderately significant (≥50%) stenosis. [9]
- PSV >300cm/s and a Vr >3.5 indicates a high-grade stenosis (>70%) in any graft body. [1,9,11,12]
- PSV >190cm/s in a superficial femoral artery stent that result in a Vr >1.5 indicates a >50% stenosis.
- PSV >275cm/s and a Vr ≥3.5 indicates an >80% stenosis in the stent. [10]
- Generally, PSV <40-45cm/s throughout a normally sized vein graft (<4mm in diameter) are associated with impending graft failure. [1,7,11]

- **Distal anastomosis**
  - » A velocity ratio >3.0 is indicative of a hemodynamically significant stenosis (≥50%), particularly if post-stenotic turbulence is present and the waveform pattern changes distally compared to the pre-anastomotic waveform pattern. [7]

It is important to look at the images for intralumenal defects at the anastomosis or marked diameter changes that may account for velocity increases. [7]

- **Outflow artery:** Vr >2.0 suggest a hemodynamically significant stenosis. In the absence of intralumenal echoes at the distal anastomotic site, a velocity increase due to size mismatch between the bypass and outflow artery should be considered.

Other Pathology

» **Pseudoaneurysm**: A pseudoaneurysm is diagnosed when a pulsatile mass is identified by color and Doppler flow (often near an anastomotic site) which is observed communicating with the bypass or native artery through a patent "neck." [7] The neck must demonstrate to and fro (pendulum) Doppler flow patterns to indicate a pseudoaneurysm.

» **Aneurysmal dilatation**: Arterial diameters that show a focal enlargement twice the proximal arterial segment indicate significant aneurysmal dilatation. Intramural thrombus may be observed within the aneurysm. [7]

» **Graft entrapment** can occur at the knee. Normal flow is recorded with the leg slightly bent (flexion). However, when the knee is straightened, no flow will be detected in the graft by Doppler or color flow. [7]

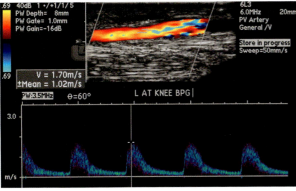

Fig. 22-19: Bypass waveforms with the leg slightly bent

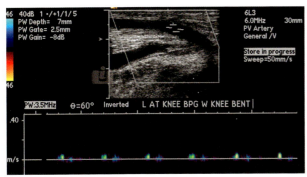

Fig. 22-20: The same graft in Fig. 22-19 occludes with flexion of the knee

» **Perigraft fluid** is suspected when any anechoic, fluid-filled structures appear to surround the bypass conduit. Ultrasound cannot determine the exact fluid substance which may be related to infection, hematoma, etc.

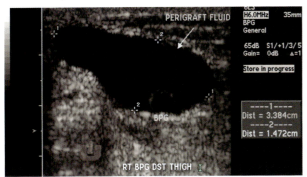

Fig. 22-21: Transverse image of perigraft fluid surrounding the graft

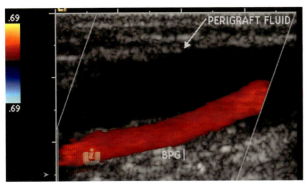

Fig. 22-22: Longitudinal image of a graft with evidence of perigraft fluid

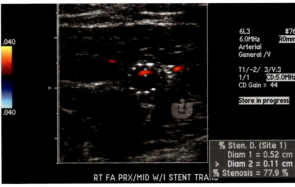

Fig. 22-23: Transverse lumenal reduction of a stent by color flow

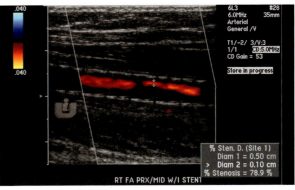

Fig. 22-24: Longitudinal lumenal reduction of a stent by color flow

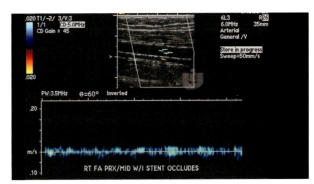

Fig. 22-25: Absent flow through the stent by spectral Doppler

Table 22-2: Duplex Diagnostic Criteria for In-Stent Restenosis of the Superficial Femoral Artery

	PSV	Vr
≥50% stenosis	≥190cm/s	>1.5
≥80% stenosis	≥275cm/s	≥3.5

- Significant decrease in ABI >0.15 was also useful to predict restenosis

Source: Baril DT, et al, Duplex criteria for determination of in-stent restenosis after angioplasty and stenting of the superficial femoral artery. *J Vasc Surg.* 2009, Jan:49(1): 133-8

Table 22-3: Diagnostic Criteria for Prosthetic Graft Surveillance

	Peak Systolic Velocity (PSV)	Velocity Ratio (Vr)
Normal	<180cm/s	<2.0
Moderate stenosis	180-300cm/s	>2.0
High grade stenosis*	PSV >300cm/s	>3.5
Impending graft failure*	PSV <45cm/s	NA
Occlusion	No flow signal or color saturation identifiable	

* A decrease in ABI >0.15 supports the presence of significant disease progression.

Source: Modified from Bandyk DF, Armstrong PA. (2010). Surveillance of infrainguinal bypass grafts. In Zierler RE (Ed.), *Strandess's Duplex Scanning Disorders in Vascular Diagnosis 4th ed.* (341-349).Philadelphia Wolters Kluwer Lippincott Williams & Wilkins.

Table 22-4: Diagnostic Criteria for Vein Graft Surveillance

	PSV	Vr
Normal	>45cm/s	<2.0
Moderate stenosis	250-300cm/s	>3.0
High grade stenosis*	>350cm/s	>3.5
Occlusion	No flow signal or color saturation identifiable	

* A decrease in ABI >0.15 supports the presence of significant disease progression.

Source: Modified from Mofidi R, Kelman J, Bennett BS, Murie JA, Dawson ARW. (2007). Significance of the early post-operative duplex result in infrainguinal vein bypass surveillance. Eur J Vasc Endovasc Surg. Sep: 34, 327-332.

Table 22-5: Diagnostic Criteria for Femoropopliteal Arterial Duplex After Endovascular Intervention

	PSV	Vr
<50% stenosis	<180cm/s	<2.5
>50% stenosis	>180cm/s	>2.5
>70% stenosis	>300cm/s	

- For patients suffering from rest pain or non-healing ulceration; a lower PSV >240cm/s is the threshold for consideration of re-intervention.
- Significant decrease in ABI >0.15 was also useful to predict restenosis.

Source: Shames ML. (2007). Duplex surveillance of lower extremity endovascular interventions. *Perspectives in Vascular Surgery and Endovascular Therapy.* Dec. 19(4), 370-374.

Differential Diagnosis
- Spinal stenosis
- Venous thrombosis
- Restless leg syndrome
- Compartment syndrome
- Nocturnal leg cramps
- Neuropathy
- Muscle/tendon strains
- Arthritis

Correlation
- Spiral CT scan
- MRA
- Arteriography

Medical Treatment
- Modify risk factors (e.g., smoking cessation, etc.)
- Antiplatelet medication (e.g., aspirin)
- Anticoagulation (warfarin)

Surgical Treatment
- Balloon catheter thromboembolectomy
- Open surgical endarterectomy
- Graft revision (e.g., "jump graft" where another bypass is created to flow around a troubled area of the original bypass)
- Direct focal repair
- Amputation

Interventional Treatment
- Angioplasty, with or without stenting
- Intra-arterial directed thrombolysis
- Mechanical clot-removing endoluminal devices (i.e., Angiojet)
- Aspiration thromboembolectomy

Intraoperative duplex can identify technical defects resulting in hemodynamically significant lesions in bypass grafts. Immediate correction of these defects can occur in the operating room to prevent a graft thrombosis which might have occurred. [3,9]

REFERENCES

1. Mills JL. (2005). Infrainguinal bypass. In *Rutherford Vascular Surgery 6th edition.* (1154-1174). Philadelphia. Elsevier Saunders.
2. Veith FJ, Lipsitz EC, Gargiulo NJ, Ascher E. (2005). Secondary arterial reconstruction in the lower extremity. In *Rutherford Vascular Surgery 6th edition.* (1181-1191). Philadelphia. Elsevier Saunders.
3. Walsh D. (2005). Post-operative graft thrombosis: prevention and management. In *Rutherford Vascular Surgery 6th edition.* (938-957). Philadelphia. Elsevier Saunders.
4. Pomposelli FB, LoGerfo FW. (2005). The autogenous vein. In *Rutherford Vascular Surgery 6th edition.* (695-715). Philadelphia. Elsevier Saunders.
5. 5 Bandyk DF, Back MR. (2005). Infection in prosthetic vascular grafts. In *Rutherford Vascular Surgery 6th edition.* (875-894). Philadelphia. Elsevier Saunders.
6. Schneider PA. (2005). Endovascular surgery in the management of chronic lower extremity ischemia. In *Rutherford Vascular Surgery 6th edition.* (1192-1222). Philadelphia. Elsevier Saunders.
7. Thrush A, Hartshorne T. (2005). Graft surveillance and preoperative vein mapping for bypass surgery. In *Peripheral Vascular Ultrasound, How Why and When, 2nd ed.* (207-224). London: Elsevier Chruchill Livingstone.
8. Zwiebel, WJ (2005). Ultrasound assessment of lower extremity arteries. In Zwiebel WJ, Pellerito JS (Eds.), *Introduction to Vascular Ultrasonography 5th ed,* (341-356). Philadelphia: Elsevier Saunders.
9. Bandyk, DF, (2005). Ultrasound assessment during and after peripheral intervention. In Zwiebel WJ, Pellerito JS (Eds.), *Introduction to Vascular Ultrasonography 5th ed,* (357-379). Philadelphia: Elsevier Saunders.
10. Baril, DT, Rhee RY, Kim J, Mararoun MS, Caer RA, Marone LK (2009). Duplex criteria for in-stent restenosis after angioplasty and stenting of the superficial femoral artery. J Vasc Surg. Jan: 49(1) 133-8.
11. Patel, ST, Mills Sr, JL. (2005). The preoperative, intraoperative and post-operative noninvasive evaluation of infrainguinal vein bypass grafts. In Mansour MA, Labropoulos N. (Eds.), *Vascular Diagnosis,* (277-292). Philadelphia: Elsevier Saunders.
12. Mofidi R, Kelman J, Bennett BS, Murie JA, Dawson ARW. (2007). Significance of the early post-operative duplex result in infrainguinal vein bypass surveillance. Eur J Vasc Endovasc Surg. Sep: 34, 327-332.
13. Tinder CN, Bandyk DF. (2009). Detection of imminent vein graft occlusion: what is the optimal surveillance program. *Seminars in Vasc Surgery,* Dec. 22(4) (252-260).
14. Kim ES, Sharma AM, Scissons R, et al. Interpretation of peripheral arterial and venous Doppler waveforms: A consensus statement from the Society for Vascular Medicine and Society for Vascular Ultrasound. Vascular Medicine. 2020;25(5):484-506. doi:10.1177/1358863X20937665

ARTERIAL TESTING
23. Upper Extremity Segmental Pressures and Doppler Waveforms

Description
A non-invasive physiological test comparing the systolic pressure at the level of the brachial artery to the systolic pressure at the level of the forearm/wrist. Continuous-wave (CW) analog Doppler waveforms are recorded to support the pressure information.

Rationale
Doppler-derived pressure measurements can identify the location of a significant obstruction in an arterial segment and define the resulting decrease in terms of pressure. The term "obstruction" is used to describe either a stenosis or an occlusion of an artery.

When narrowing of the arterial lumen increases beyond the critical level, distal arterial flow and pressure decrease significantly. Segmental pressures define the level of disease using a comparison of the brachial pressure to the forearm/wrist pressures, known as wrist-brachial index (WBI). A *pressure gradient* (pressure difference) of 20-30mmHg indicates a significant stenosis or occlusion between cuff levels.

Etiology
- Atherosclerosis
- Embolization
- Thrombus
- Intimal hyperplasia
- Trauma
- Traumatic occlusion
- Extrinsic compression
- Vasculitis
- AV fistula (abnormal connection between an artery and a vein)
- External radiation
- Radiation arteritis

Risk Factors
- Age (increased risk with age)
- Coronary artery disease
- Diabetes
- Family history
- Hyperlipidemia
- Hypertension
- Obesity
- Smoking
- Sedentary lifestyle
- Previous history of CVA or MI
- Elevated homocysteine
- Excessive levels of C-reactive protein
- Post-op cardiac catheterization through the brachial artery
- History of radiation
- Occupational exposure to toxic substances

Indications for Exam
- Claudication
- Follow-up of a previously abnormal pressure index
- Limb pain at rest
- Absent peripheral pulses
- Extremity ulcer
- Gangrene
- Pre-operative assessment of healing potential
- Pre-operative assessment prior to creation of dialysis access
- Pre-operative assessment prior to radial artery harvest for CABG
- Abnormal vertebral artery waveforms
- Bruit
- Digital cyanosis
- Cold sensitivity
- Aneurysmal disease
- Trauma to an artery
- Raynaud's syndrome/phenomenon
- Thoracic outlet symptoms
- Abnormal arterial arm pressures, including BP differential of >20mmHg between arms

Contraindications/Limitations
- Calcified vessels which will falsely elevate pressures (typically encountered in patients with diabetes or end-stage renal disease).
- Significant lesions with excellent collateral circulation, which may result in normal distal pressures and waveforms.
- Patients with acute clot or venous thrombosis in the upper extremities should not have pressure cuffs inflated over their clot.
- Any site of trauma, surgery, ulceration or graft placement which should not be compressed by the pressure cuff.
- Patients with extensive bandages or casts which are not removable.
- Pressures typically prohibited on ipsilateral side of a mastectomy or dialysis AVG/AVF.
- Patient intolerance of cuff pressures.
- Exposure to cold conditions or stressful situations can exacerbate digital symptoms.

Mechanism of Disease
- **Atherosclerosis** is the most common arterial disease. Atherosclerotic plaque forms in the artery to blocking flow by either narrowing the arterial lumen (arterial stenosis) or totally blocking the artery (arterial occlusion). The term "hemodynamically significant obstruction" refers to either a stenosis or an occlusion that results in a decrease in blood pressure or flow distal to the obstruction. Typically, a stenosis must narrow the diameter of the artery by at least 50% to decrease pressure and flow distally. An arterial occlusion is typically seen from one major branch to the next.
- **Emboli** may occur as contents of a plaque or fragments of an organized thrombus from the heart or aneurysm loosen and flow downstream. Emboli become lodged in a distant blood vessel, causing arterial occlusion and reduction of flow. [1]

The source of embolic disease in the upper extremities can be from a cardiac source, the subclavian artery or a proximal aneurysm.

- **Vasospasm** is a temporary constriction of the arteries (typically digital arteries) that may cause significant discomfort to the patient or be a sign of a more serious underlying disease. [2]
- **Extrinsic compression** from tumors, musculoskeletal configuration, hematoma, etc. can result in stenosis or occlusion by placing enough pressure on arterial walls to compromise blood flow. [1]
- **Mechanical compression** in the thoracic outlet region of the subclavian vein, artery or brachial plexus. One cause may be an anatomical defect such as congenital abnormalities of the first rib or fracture of the clavicle, which acts a source of compression. [3] *More details about this condition known as thoracic outlet syndrome can be found in the Arterial Diseases chapter of this book.*
- A **pseudoaneurysm** (PA) or "false aneurysm" forms due to trauma to all three layers of the arterial wall. The "false aneurysm" is actually a hematoma, receiving its blood supply via communication with an artery through a patent "neck." [4]

- An **arteriovenous fistula** or abnormal connection between artery and vein can result from trauma or complications during invasive procedures (e.g., cardiac catheterization). In such cases, blood flows directly from the artery into the venous system without passing through the tissues and capillary bed.[5]

Location of Disease
- Location of disease can be focal or diffuse and affect any level or multiple levels
- Subclavian artery, palmar arch and/or digital arteries
- Axillary artery
- Arterial bifurcations

Patient History
- Claudication (exercise-related)
- Rest pain
- Acute occlusion
  » Pain or rest pain
  » Paralysis (weakness)
  » Paresthesia ("pins and needles")
  » Poikilothermia (ice-cold limb)
  » Pulselessness
  » Pallor
- Ulceration/gangrene of hands/digits
- Previous therapeutic vascular procedure (e.g., bypass, stenting)

Physical Examination
- Pulselessness
- Cyanosis
- Pallor
- Dependent rubor
- Bruit (abnormal sound heard through auscultation caused by turbulent flow vibration)
- Marked temperature difference between hand/fingers, especially if one is ice cold.
- Gangrene/necrosis (tissue death)
- Palpable thrill (vibration caused by turbulent blood flow as seen in AV fistula)

Arterial disease in the upper extremity is uncommon, accounting for less than 5% of patients presenting with extremity ischemia.[8] When disease is present, it is more likely to be small vessel disease (e.g., digital) rather than large vessel disease.[9]

Upper Extremity Segmental Pressures and Doppler Waveforms Protocol
- Obtain a patient history to include symptoms, risk factors and general dates of past vascular interventions. Obtain past surgical reports/records, including type of bypass graft or stent placed and general date of surgery if available. Explain the procedure to the patient.
- Patient is examined in the supine position. The patient can also sit in a chair with their arm extended on a pillow if unable to lie down for the exam.
- Apply cuffs with a 10-12cm bladder (in width) on the mid arm and forearm. All cuffs should be placed "straight" rather than angled. All cuffs should fit snugly.
- The bladder of the cuff must compress soft tissue, not bony structures. Failure to adhere to these guidelines will produce falsely elevated pressure readings.

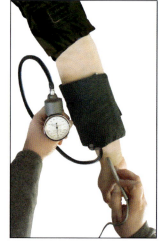

Fig. 23-1: Segmental pressure of the radial artery

The WBI only identifies presence and severity of obstructive disease. To determine location of disease, WBI should be combined with segmental pressures, VPR, Doppler waveforms, or duplex imaging.

- Arterial physiologic exams are traditionally performed using a continuous wave (CW) Doppler. However, waveforms can be obtained at the same sites using a spectral Doppler. The CW Doppler is recommended for segmental pressure measurement due to its capabilities for a larger sampling region.
- Use a high frequency (8MHz) CW Doppler transducer to locate arterial signals. Alternate transducers, including a lower frequency transducer (e.g., 4MHz), may be needed for obese patients or for deeper vessels.
- Place the Doppler transducer on the limb using a 45-60° angle to the skin, with enough pressure to keep contact but not so much pressure that the artery is compressed by the transducer.
- Locate the brachial artery (BrA) near the antecubital fossa. Record several representative Doppler waveforms. If the signal is damped, retrograde or absent at this level, move proximally and search for a better signal to be used for the brachial pressure.
- When testing with an automatic cuff inflator or standard manometer:
  » Inflate the cuffs wrapped around the mid upper arms 20-30mmHg above the last audible arterial signal using a Doppler transducer.

For patients with irregular heart beats, decrease deflation speeds.

  » Deflate the cuff slowly (at a rate of 2-4mmHg per second). The brachial systolic pressure is recorded as soon as the first audible arterial Doppler signal returns. There should be a period of silence after inflation and prior to hearing the first pulse to be sure the cuff was inflated beyond the local arterial pressure. When using a computerized system, move the cursor back to the first pulse.
  » The Doppler pulse must continue after hearing the first pulse to assure there is an actual pulse rather than motion artifact.
  » If a pressure measurement needs to be repeated, the cuff should be fully deflated for approximately one minute prior to the repeat measurement.
  » Locate the radial artery (RA) along the lateral (thumb) side of the arm using the Doppler transducer. Record several representative Doppler waveforms. If the signal is damped, retrograde or absent at this level, move proximally and search for a better signal.
  » Inflate the cuff wrapped on the mid forearm 20-30mmHg beyond the last audible radial artery signal heard using a Doppler transducer. Deflate the cuff slowly. The systolic pressure is recorded as soon as the first audible arterial Doppler signal returns.
  » Repeat procedure using the ulnar arterial (UA) signal found along the medial (pinky) side of the arm.
  » Repeat on the contralateral arm when indicated.
- Record additional representative waveforms proximally in the subclavian and axillary arteries when indicated.
- Determine classification of disease according to laboratory diagnostic criteria.

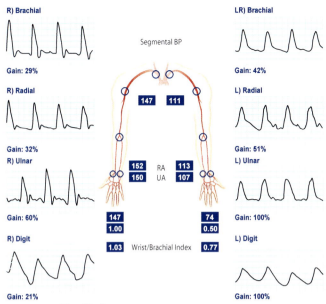

Fig. 23-2: *Abnormal WBI and DBI Physiologic Report on the left. The right arm is normal.*

Table 23-1: Upper Extremity Segmental Pressures and Doppler Waveforms Protocol Summary

- Wrap pressure cuffs around limb:
  » Arm
  » Forearm
- Record representative Doppler waveforms at the following levels:
  » Brachial Artery
  » Radial Artery
  » Ulnar Artery
  » Subclavian Artery (when indicated)
  » Axillary Artery (when indicated)
- Inflate each cuff 20-30mmHg beyond the last audible arterial signal heard using a Doppler transducer on the appropriate artery distal to the cuff.
- Deflation of the cuff should be at a rate of 2-4mmHg/s.
- The pressure is recorded as soon as the first audible, continuous arterial Doppler signal returns.
- Calculate the pressure index at each level:

  brachial, wrist pressure ÷ highest brachial pressure
- Repeat for the contralateral side.
- Determine classification of disease according to laboratory diagnostic criteria.

Spectral Doppler on a duplex scanner can be used to obtain arterial waveforms.

PRINCIPLES OF INTERPRETATION

Segmental Pressures
- Pressure measurements of the arm, forearm and digital cuffs are compared.
- It is very helpful to compare the right and left sides when evaluating pressure changes in the upper extremities.

Arterial Waveform Terminology
The terminology used to describe arterial waveforms is not consistent across laboratories. A consensus document was published in 2020 by the Society of Vascular Ultrasound and the Society for Vascular Medicine regarding the terminology and interpretation of peripheral arterial and venous waveforms. *See the Arterial Hemodynamics chapter for more detail on arterial waveforms.*

Spectral Doppler Waveforms
Any change in spectral waveform analysis depends on the terminology used by the lab; from triphasic to monophasic or changes in resistance may be significant.

- A specific WBI criterion is not well established. Many labs use the same criteria to classify WBI as ABI values.

Interpretation/Diagnostic Criteria

Normal

Segmental Pressures
- There should be <20mmHg difference between the right and left brachial pressures. [6,7]
- If the WBI is ≥1.0, the presence of a hemodynamically significant stenosis or occlusion is unlikely between the arm and forearm cuffs. [6,8]
- There is normally no decrease in pressure between the arm and forearm cuffs. [6]

Spectral Doppler Waveforms
- A waveform with a sharp, quick upstroke followed by a brisk downstroke with reversed flow direction in early diastole and another forward phase in late diastole is termed *triphasic*. This is considered a normal finding in the peripheral arteries.

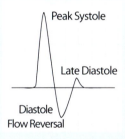

Fig. 23-3: *Normal, triphasic waveform*

- A waveform with a sharp upstroke followed by reversed flow that crosses the zero baseline and contains both forward and reverse components is termed *multiphasic* or *biphasic* by some labs.
- Some labs have adopted terminology that recognizes any reversed flow as normal by using an abbreviation NR for "normal-reversed" whether or not the third phase is present, in order to avoid the confusing use of *triphasic* and *biphasic* terms. [11]
- Arterial waveforms without a reversed flow component can be a normal finding for some patients, such as the elderly. If arterial pressures are normal, consider the possibility that the signal may also be normal. [6]

The third phase of the triphasic waveform may be missing in older patients with less vessel compliance.

Abnormal

Segmental Pressures

- An absolute pressure difference between the right and left brachial cuffs >20mmHg indicates a hemodynamically significant obstruction on the side with the lower pressure. [6,9,10]
- A WBI of <1.0 indicates that disease exists somewhere between the forearm cuffs and the wrist. [8]
- The pressure difference between the brachial-forearm and forearm-digital levels exceeds 15mmHg. [6,8]
- A difference of 10-30mmHg between radial and ulnar artery pressures suggests obstruction in the vessel with the lower pressure. A difference >30mmHg confirms obstruction in the vessel with the lower pressure. [10]
- A change in the WBI of ≥0.15 from one study to the next is significant.
- A WBI ≥1.3 suggests calcific disease and is considered non-diagnostic. As an alternative means of estimating disease severity, use the digital-brachial index.

Two primary limitations to the WBI test are: calcified vessels (e.g., diabetics, end-stage renal disease and general atherosclerosis) and functionally significant lesions with good collateral circulation. Doppler waveforms should be obtained to ensure accuracy of WBI in calcified vessels.

Spectral Doppler Waveforms

- As the obstruction becomes more severe, changes in the spectral waveform are expected before a stenosis or occlusion, at the point of greatest stenosis and after a stenosis/occlusion as described in the *Arterial Physiology* chapter. These changes are important to note in the interpretation of the vascular exam.
- *Monophasic* arterial waveforms reflect low resistance and are characterized by a slow upstroke, low amplitude, and broad peak with continuous forward flow in diastole that does not cross the zero baseline. The upstroke has a general direction of being tipped to the right. Monophasic waveforms are typically present distal to an occlusion or a very high-grade stenosis. [6-8,11]
- *Parvus tardus* is an alternative term for "monophasic" used by some laboratories to describe a waveform with continuous forward flow and a slow, blunted systolic component. [11]
- **Occlusion:** An absent or non-pulsatile Doppler signal suggests occlusion at the site of interrogation. [12, 13]

Multiphasic   *Monophasic*

Fig. 23-4: *Continuous wave arterial Doppler signals*

Other Pathology

Subclavian Steal Syndrome

- Subclavian steal results in a significant difference in brachial artery pressures >20-30mmHg
- Arterial waveforms will demonstrate decreased resistance (e.g., monophasic) and retrograde vertebral artery flow will be evident on the side with the decreased pressure.
- If the lower extremities are free of disease, the ankle pressures may be compared to the upper extremity for an arterial ratio. [6]

Differential Diagnosis

- Spinal stenosis
- Venous thrombosis
- Thoracic outlet syndrome
- Neuropathy
- Muscle/tendon strains
- Cervical arthritis
- Abnormalities of adrenergic receptor/sympathetic nervous system
- Connective tissue disease (scleroderma)

Correlation

- Duplex ultrasound
- Spiral CT scan
- MRA
- Arteriography

Medical Treatment

- Modify risk factors (e.g., reduce cholesterol, manage HTN and DM, smoking cessation)
- Exercise regimen
- Antiplatelet medication (e.g., aspirin)
- Anticoagulation (warfarin)
- Cold temperature avoidance

Surgical Treatment

- Bypass grafting
- Endarterectomy
- Atherectomy
- Direct focal repair
- Resection (aneurysmal disease)
- Amputation

Endovascular Treatment

- Angioplasty
- Stent
- Atherectomy
- Intra-arterial directed thrombolysis (acute blockage)

REFERENCES

1. Sumner DS, Zierler RE. (2005). Vascular physiology: essential hemodynamic principles. *In Rutherford Vascular Surgery 6th edition.* (75-123). Philadelphia. Elsevier Saunders
2. Shepard RFJ. (2005). Raynaud's syndrome: vasospastic and occlusive arterial disease involving the distal upper extremity. In *Rutherford Vascular Surgery 6th edition.* (1319-1346). Philadelphia. Elsevier Saunders
3. Kreienberg PB, Shah, DM, Darling III, RC, Change BB, Paty SK, Roddy SP, Ozsvath KJ, Manish,, (2005). Thoracic Outlet Syndrome. In *Mansour MA, Labropoulos N. (Eds.),* Vascular Diagnosis, (517-522). Philadelphia,; Elsevier Saunders.
4. Casey, PJ, LaMuraglia GM. (2005). Anastomotic aneurysms. *In Rutherford Vascular Surgery 6th edition.* (894-902). Philadelphia. Elsevier Saunders
5. Rutherford RB. (2005). Diagnostic evaluation of arteriovenous fistulas and vascular anomalies. *In Rutherford Vascular Surgery 6th edition.* (1602-1612). Philadelphia. Elsevier Saunders
6. Longo MG, Pearce WH, Sumner DS. (2005). Evaluation of upper extremity ischemia. In *Rutherford Vascular Surgery 6th edition.* (1274-1293). Philadelphia. Elsevier Saunders.
7. Talbot, SR, Zwiebel WJ. (2005). Assessment of upper extremity arterial occlusive disease. In Zwiebel WJ. Pellerito JS (Eds.), *Introduction to Vascular Ultrasonography 5th ed.* (297-323). Philadelphia: Elsevier Saunders.
8. Moneta GL, Partsafas A, Zacardi M. (2010). Noninvasive diagnosis of upper extremity arterial disease. In Zierler RE (Ed.), *Strandess's duplex scanning disorders in vascular diagnosis 4th ed.* (149-156). Philadelphia Wolters Kluwer Lippincott Williams & Wilkins.
9. Talbot, SR, Zwiebel WJ. (2005). Assessment of upper extremity arterial occlusive disease. In *Introduction to Vascular Ultrasonography 5th ed.* (297-323). Philadelphia: Elsevier Saunders.
10. Myers K, Clogh A, (2004). Disease of vessels to the upper limbs. In *Making Sense of Vascular Ultrasound.* (227-254). London: Hodder Arnold.
11. Kim ES, Sharma AM, Scissons R, et al. *Interpretation of peripheral arterial and venous Doppler waveforms: A consensus statement from the Society for Vascular Medicine and Society for Vascular Ultrasound.* Vascular Medicine. 2020;25(5):484-506. doi:10.1177/1358863X20937665
12. Moneta GL, Zacardi MJ, Olmsted KA. (2010). Lower extremity arterial occlusive disease. In Zierler RE (Ed.), *Strandess's duplex scanning disorders in Vascular Diagnosis 4th ed.* (133-147).Philadelphia Wolters Kluwer Lippincott Williams & Wilkins.
13. Kerr TM, Bandyk DF. (1993). Color duplex imaging of peripheral arterial disease before angioplasty or surgical intervention. In Bernstein EF (Ed.). *Vascular Diagnosis 4th ed.* (527-533). St. Louis: Mosby.

ARTERIAL TESTING

24. Upper Extremity Digital Evaluations: Pressure (DBI) and Photoplethysmography (PPG)

Definition
This non-invasive physiological test detects arterial pulsations in the terminal portions of the digits using photoplethysmography (PPG). A ratio known as the digital brachial index (DBI) is calculated by dividing the systolic pressure at the level of the digits in the hand by the highest systolic brachial artery pressure.

Rationale
The sensors of a photoplethysmograph (PPG) consist of an infrared-light-emitting diode and a phototransistor. Infrared light is transmitted into the superficial tissue and a reflection is received by the phototransistor. The signal received relates to the quantity of red blood cells in the cutaneous circulation. Each arterial pulse creates a change in blood volume under the sensor. These cutaneous volume changes result in proportional changes in the reflection of the infrared light from the tissue. The changes in reflection are monitored in the instrument and recorded as a pulse waveform when the instrument is set in arterial or AC mode. If set in the venous or DC mode, the PPG can be used to monitor slower volume changes related to venous reflux, as opposed to quick changes seen during the arterial pulse cycle.

Calcified digital artery pressures are rarely a problem.

Etiology
- Atherosclerosis
- Buerger's disease

Buerger's disease is an inflammatory condition of the arteries and veins, also called thromboangiitis obliterans. Symptoms mimic arterial insufficiency and can progress to gangrene This disease in most common in younger males and smoking is a risk factor in the development of Buerger's disease.

- Embolization
- Vasculitis
- Vasospasm (e.g., Raynaud's phenomenon)
- Trauma
- Connective tissue disease (e.g., scleroderma)
- Traumatic-occupational occlusion (e.g., hypothenar hammer syndrome)
- Vascular steal related to dialysis arteriovenous fistula/graft
- Radiation arteritis
- Thrombus

Risk Factors
- Age (increased risk with age)
- Coronary artery disease
- Diabetes
- Family history
- Smoking
- Hypertension
- Hyperlipidemia
- Post-op cardiac catheterization through the brachial artery
- History of radiation
- Fibromuscular dysplasia
- Occupational exposure to toxic substances
- Arteriovenous fistula or graft for kidney dialysis

Indications for Exam
- Exercise-related pain (claudication symptoms)
- Limb or digital pain at rest
- Extremity ulcer/gangrene
- Digital cyanosis
- Cold sensitivity
- Absent peripheral pulses
- Arterial trauma and aneurysms
- Bruit
- Raynaud's syndrome/phenomenon
- Abnormal vertebral artery waveforms
- Thoracic outlet symptoms
- Abnormal arterial arm pressures, including BP differential of >20mmHg between arms
- Steal syndrome (dialysis patients)

Contraindications/Limitations
- Although rare, calcified vessels which will falsely elevate pressures (typically encountered in arteries proximal to the digits in patients with diabetes or end-stage renal disease).
- Significant lesions with excellent collateral circulation, which may result in normal distal pressures and waveforms
- Any site of trauma, surgery, ulceration or graft placement which should not be compressed by the pressure cuff
- Patients with extensive bandages or casts

Skin integrity of the digit must be intact to properly assess digital circulation.

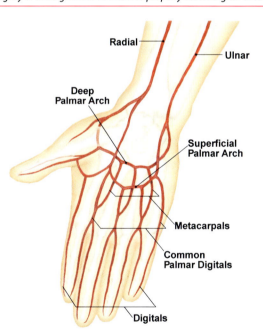

Fig. 24-1: *Upper Extremity Anatomy: Hand and Digital Arteries*

Mechanism of Disease
There are two major mechanisms that cause reduced arterial blood supply to the upper extremity; atherosclerotic plaque and embolism.

- **Atherosclerosis:** The most common arterial disease. Atherosclerotic plaque forms in the artery to blocking flow by either narrowing the arterial lumen (arterial stenosis) or totally blocking the artery (arterial occlusion). The term "hemodynamically significant obstruction" refers to either a stenosis or an occlusion that results in a decrease in blood

pressure or flow distal to the obstruction. Typically, a stenosis must narrow the diameter of the artery by at least 50% to decrease pressure and flow distally. An arterial occlusion is typically seen from one major branch to the next.
- **Emboli**: embolization of contents of a plaque and/or fragments of an organized thrombus from the heart or proximal aneurysm which become lodged in a distant blood vessel. [2]
- **Mechanical compression** in the thoracic outlet region of the subclavian vein, artery or brachial plexus. One cause may be an anatomical defect such as congenital abnormalities of the first rib or fracture of the clavicle, which acts a source of compression. [3] *More details about this condition known as Thoracic Outlet Syndrome can be found in the Arterial Diseases chapter.*
- **External compression** is a much less common cause of obstruction in the upper extremity arteries. Extrinsic compression from tumors, hematomas, etc. can result in stenosis and/or occlusion by placing enough pressure on arterial walls to compress blood flow. [1]
- **Vasospasm** causes obstruction to digital flow and is typically intermittent and associated with Raynaud's disease/phenomenon and is characterized as a primary or secondary condition.
  » *Primary* Raynaud's syndrome is intermittently vasospastic in nature and has no underlying condition or disease. [1]
  » *Secondary* Raynaud's syndrome/phenomenon is associated with an underlying disease such as scleroderma and also involves a fixed arterial obstruction. [1]
  » Digital smooth muscle cells constrict in an abnormal response to cold or stress stimuli.

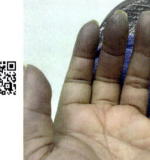

Fig. 24-2: *Upper extremity digital ischemia*
Courtesy of Heather Hall MD

Patient History
- Claudication (exercise related)
- Pain
- Paralysis (weakness)
- Paresthesia ("pins and needles")
- Poikilothermia (ice cold limbs)
- Previous ulceration/gangrene of hands/fingers

Exposure to cold conditions or stressful situations can exacerbate digital symptoms. [7]

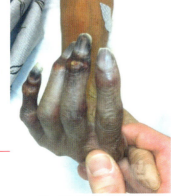

Fig. 24-3: *Gangrene of the hand*

Physical Examination
- Pulselessness
- Cyanosis
- Pallor
- Gangrene/necrosis (tissue death)
- Marked temperature difference between hand/fingers
- Rubor
- Bruit (abnormal sound heard through auscultation caused by turbulent flow)
- Palpable thrill (vibration caused by turbulent blood flow as seen in AV fistula)

Upper Extremity Digital Evaluation Protocol
- Obtain a patient history to include symptoms and risk factors. Explain the procedure to the patient.
- Patient is examined in the supine position, in a warm room. Exposure to cold conditions or stressful situations can exacerbate digital symptoms. [7]

The size control on the PPG device is kept at "10" for standardization of tracings. If the waveform "goes off" the strip chart recording paper, the size is reduced to "5" and the change is documented.

Upper Extremity DBI and PPG Evaluation
- Secure a 2-2.5cm cuff around the mid phalanx of the digit to be studied while avoiding cuff placement over the bony joint. Smaller cuffs will result in falsely elevated pressures due to the narrow width of the cuff. Follow up studies should use same width cuff for comparison.
- Attach the PPG photocell to the pad of the digit using double-stick tape placed between the photocell and the skin. Avoid taping the entire digit like a cuff since a tightly placed PPG could obliterate a low-pressure pulse. Alternative sensors used by some labs include a digital clip similar to a pulse oximeter which eliminates the need for tape or Velcro to keep the sensor in place.
- Run the PPG recording at high speed (25mm/s) to record the shape of the digital waveform at rest, ensuring that the PPG tracing is centered. Center the PPG tracings on the paper or monitor. Ideally the baseline tracing consists of a series of horizontal pulses.

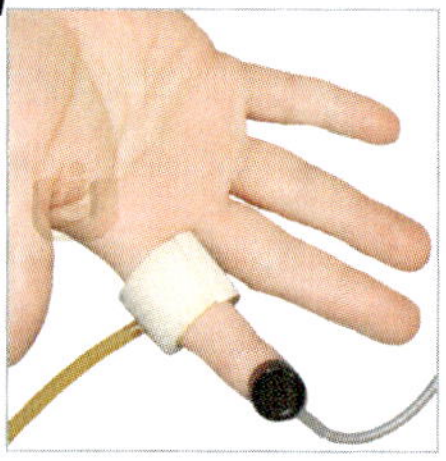

Fig. 24-4: *Digital cuff and PPG sensor placement on the finger*

Use a towel to cover the hand to eliminate any room light which may cause an artifact in the PPG tracing

- Reduce PPG recorder speed to 5mm/s and inflate the pressure cuff on the digit until the PPG waveforms are no longer visible.
- Slowly deflate the cuff (at rate of 2-4mmHg/sec) until the PPG waveforms return. Note the pressure in mmHg when the first pulse returns, but be sure that the pulse continues. If the pulse does not continue, consider that this was not a true pulse, but rather a motion artifact. There should be a flat tracing for a period of time after inflation before seeing the first return. This ensures the cuff was inflated beyond the local arterial pressure.
- If data is abnormal at rest, consider warming the affected fingers for several minutes and repeating the measurements. False positive results will occur if the digits are cold during testing.
- Repeat procedure on other digits as necessary.
- Repeat on the contralateral arm.
- Apply pressure cuffs with 10-12cm bladder (in width) on the mid-arms.

- Locate the brachial artery (BrA) near the antecubital fossa using a Doppler transducer.
- Inflate the cuff on the mid-arm 20-30mmHg beyond the last audible arterial Doppler signal.
- Deflate the cuff slowly (at a rate of 2-4mmHg per second). The systolic pressure is recorded as soon as the first audible Doppler arterial signal returns.
- Calculate the digital-brachial index (DBI)

$$DBI = \frac{\text{digital pressure}}{\text{highest brachial pressure}}$$

- Determine severity of disease according to laboratory diagnostic criteria.

Upper Extremity Palmar Arch Evaluation

The superficial palmar arch is incomplete in 1 of 5 patients.

- Evaluate the palmar arch of the hand using the PPG transducer on either the thumb or index finger and the fifth digit. (CW Doppler of the digital pulse with an analog waveform may also be used).
- Run the PPG recording at low speed (5mm/sec).
- With your hand, compress the radial artery (RA) and ulnar artery (UA) simultaneously, resulting in a flat-line PPG tracing, to verify that the compressions are being performed properly (create a complete cessation of flow). This is best achieved by placing your hand under the wrist and compressing the RA and UA with your index finger and thumb.
- Release compression of the RA and observe for return of the PPG pulse waveform.
- Compress the RA again to be sure that flow stops while still compressing the UA. Release compression of the UA and observe for return of the waveform.

Table 24-1: Upper Extremity Digital Protocol Summary

- Wrap pressure cuffs around digits of hand.
- Secure a PPG sensor to digit.
- Record representative tracing of PPG waveforms.
- Inflate digital cuff 20-30mmHg beyond the last visualized PPG tracing.
- Deflate cuff at a rate of 2-4mmHg per second. The pressure is recorded as soon as the PPG waveforms return. Be sure that a couple seconds pass before the first pulse and check for subsequent pulses to confirm it was a "first pulse" rather than motion artifact.
- Wrap pressure cuff around the mid arm for a brachial pressure.
- Inflate cuff 20-30mmHg beyond the last audible Doppler arterial signal.
- Calculate digital-brachial indices

$$DBI = \frac{\text{digital pressure}}{\text{highest brachial pressure}}$$

- Determine severity of disease according to laboratory diagnostic criteria.

PRINCIPLES OF INTERPRETATION

Digital Pressures

- Digital pressures are compared to the highest brachial pressure and are typically lower than the wrist pressures.

PPG Digital Waveforms

- The PPG waveform from any digit is categorized as *pulsatile, reduced* or *non-pulsatile* based on the upstroke (amplitude) of the waveform and downslope.
- There may be a dicrotic notch or secondary upstroke in the downslope of the tracing which corresponds to the increased aortic pressure and closure of the aortic valve.

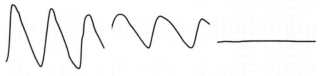

Normal Pulsatility   Reduced Pulsatility   Absent Pulsatility

Fig. 24-5: *PPG Digital Waveforms*

The combination of upper extremity arterial and digital artery examinations will differentiate between large and small vessel disease. [7]

Interpretation/Diagnostic Criteria

Normal

Digital Pressures

- An absolute pressure ≥70mmHg is normal for a digit. [4]
- If the DBI is ≥0.80, the presence of a hemodynamically significant stenosis or occlusion is unlikely between the arm and digital pressure cuffs in the upper extremities. [5,6]
- Normal digital artery pressures are within 20-30mmHg of the brachial pressures in the arms. [5-7]

Digital Waveforms

- Normal waveforms exclude the presence of significant disease. [8] Normal PPG waveform characteristics include: [4,6,7,9]
  » Short onset to peak (subjective)
  » Downslope that bows toward the baseline
- A dicrotic notch in the downslope
  » During palmar arch evaluation, if the PPG trace remains during alternate compression of the ulnar and radial arteries, the palmar arch is complete. [4,10] One artery may appear more "dominant" than the other when the amplitude of the PPG tracing increases with compression.

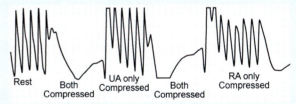

Rest | Both Compressed | UA only Compressed | Both Compressed | RA only Compressed

Fig. 24-6: *CW Doppler analysis recorded at 5cm/s demonstrating a complete palmar arch.*

Flow in the hand is tremendously variable because of the large number of arteriovenous shunts in the skin of the fingertips. [6]

Abnormal

Digital Pressures

- Decreased digital pressures in the presence of otherwise normal arm pressures indicates palmar or digital obstruction. [4]
- An absolute pressure <70mmHg is abnormal for a digit. [4]

- A DBI <0.80 indicates a significant obstruction at or proximal to the digits and indicates a decrease in perfusion at the digital level. [5,6]
- Equally decreased finger pressures in a hand indicate disease in the distal radial and ulnar arteries or the palmar arch. [4]
- A pressure difference >15mmHg is abnormal between fingers. [4]
- When pressures are decreased on only one side of the hand, palmar arch disease is present. [4]

Digital Waveforms

Digital disease can affect a single digit or multiple digits at a time.

- Abnormal ("reduced") PPG waveform characteristics (secondary to obstruction) include: [4,6,9]
    » Prolonged onset to peak (subjective)
    » Rounded peak
    » Downslope that bows away from the baseline
- A PPG waveform with a "double peak" (or early anacrotic notch with high dicrotic notch) is often seen in patients with Raynaud's disease. [4,7-9]

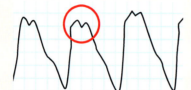

Fig. 24-7: *Abnormal double peaked waveform*

- During palmar arch evaluation, if the PPG tracing remains flat-lined or the waveform amplitude significantly decreases after release of UA or RA compressions, the palmar arch is incomplete. [4,10] Specifically:
    » A flat PPG tracing with radial artery (RA) compression (while the UA is not compressed) suggests the RA alone is feeding the palmar arch. [4]
    » A flat PPG tracing with ulnar artery (UA) compression (while the RA is not compressed) suggests the UA alone is feeding the palmar arch. [4]

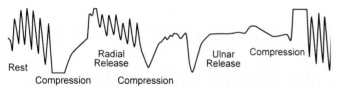

Fig. 24-8: *CW Doppler analysis recorded at 5cm/s demonstrating an incomplete palmar arch fed by the radial artery*

- An "absent" or non-pulsatile digital waveform is reported when the PPG tracing reflects a flat-line. An obstruction is suspected. [4]

Differential Diagnosis

- Buerger's disease
- Scleroderma
- Connective tissue disorders
- Neuropathy
- Abnormalities of adrenergic receptor/sympathetic nervous system
- Muscle/tendon strains
- Arthritis

Correlation

- Duplex ultrasound
- Spiral CT scan
- MR Angiography
- Arteriography

Medical Treatment

- Risk factor management (e.g., smoking cessation)
- Cold temperature avoidance
- Antiplatelet medication (e.g., aspirin)
- Anticoagulation (warfarin)
- Thermal biofeedback
- Thrombolysis (acute blockage)

Surgical Treatment

- Sympathectomy
- Endarterectomy
- Bypass grafting
- Direct focal repair
- Resection (aneurysmal disease)
- Amputation

Digits with pressures of less than 20mmHg may not produce a pulsatile waveform.

Table 24-2: Diagnostic Criteria for Upper Extremity Digital Testing

Normal: No hemodynamically significant disease
- Absolute pressure ≥70mmHg
- DBI ≥0.80
- Digital artery and brachial pressures are within 20-30mmHg of each other.
- Normal waveform characteristics include:
    » Short onset to peak (subjective)
    » Downslope that bows toward the baseline or a dicrotic notch in the downslope
- Complete palmar arch (PPG pulse wave remains or increases with compression)

Abnormal: Hemodynamically significant disease
- Absolute pressure <70mmHg
- DBI <0.80
- Pressure difference >15mmHg between fingers
- Abnormal waveform characteristics include:
    » Prolonged onset to peak (subjective)
    » Rounded peak
    » Downslope that bows away from the baseline
    » Absence of tracing (obstruction)
    » Double-peaked tracing (Raynaud's disease)
- Incomplete palmar arch (PPG pulse wave remains flat-lined or decreases with compression)

REFERENCES

1. Sumner DS, Zierler RE. (2005). Vascular physiology: essential hemodynamic principles. In *Rutherford Vascular Surgery 6th edition.* (75-123). Philadelphia. Elsevier Saunders.
2. Fecteau SR, Darling III RC, Roddy SP. (2005). Arterial thromboembolism. In *Rutherford Vascular Surgery 6th edition.* (971-986). Philadelphia. Elsevier Saunders.
3. Eskandari MK, Yao JST. (10-30-2009). Upper extremity occlusive disease: workup. *eMedicine.* Retrieved from: http://emedicine.medscape.com/article/462289-overview. (12-10-2010).
4. Longo MG, Pearce WH, Sumner DS. (2005). Evaluation of upper extremity ischemia. In Rutherford Vascular Surgery 6th edition. (1274-1293). Philadelphia. Elsevier Saunders.
5. Karkoski JK, Johnson B, Dalman RL. (2005). Upper extremity ischemia: diagnosis techniques and clinical applications. In Mansour MA, Labropoulos N. (Eds.), Vascular Diagnosis, (325-330). Philadelphia. Elsevier Saunders.
6. Moneta GL, Partsafas A, Zacardi M. (2010). Non-invasive diagnosis of upper extremity arterial disease. In Zierler RE (Ed.), *Strandess's duplex scanning disorders in vascular diagnosis 4th ed.* (149-156). Philadelphia Wolters Kluwer Lippincott Williams & Wilkins.
7. Edwards JM, Porter JM. (1998). Upper extremity arterial disease: Etiologic considerations and differential diagnosis. (60-68). Seminars in Vascular Surgery. Vol 11(2).
8. Edwards JM, Porter JM. (1993). Evaluation of upper extremity ischemia. In Bernstein EF (ed).*Vascular Diagnosis 4th ed.* (630-640). St. Louis: Mosby.
9. Sumner DS, Zierler RE. (2005). Physiologic assessment of peripheral arterial occlusive disease. In Rutherford *Vascular Surgery 6th edition.* (197-222). Philadelphia. Elsevier Saunders.
10. Zaccardi MJ, Mokadam NA. (2005). Radial artery evaluation before coronary artery bypass grafts. In Zierler RE (Ed.), *Strandess's duplex scanning disorders in vascular diagnosis 4th ed.* (385-398).Philadelphia Wolters Kluwer Lippincott Williams & Wilkins.

Definition
Non-invasive physiological testing used to detect cold-induced vasospasm by comparing digital pressures, waveforms and temperatures (optional) at rest to those obtained after immersion in an ice bath. Cold immersion testing can also be referred to as cold stress testing.

Rationale
In the presence of Raynaud's disease, digits take longer to increase their blood flow after exposure to cold due to prolonged arterial vasospasm and there is a greater recovery time for fingers to rewarm back to baseline temperatures compared with normal subjects.

A sensor in a photoelectric plethysmography (PPG) uses infrared light-emitting diode and a phototransistor receiver. Infrared light is transmitted into the superficial tissue and a reflection from the tissue is received by the phototransistor. The signal received relates to the quantity of red blood cells in the cutaneous circulation. Each arterial pulse creates a change in the volume of red blood cells reflecting the light. These changes are monitored by the PPG instrument and recorded as a pulse waveform when the instrument is set in arterial or AC mode.

Etiology
- Atherosclerosis
- Buerger's disease
- Vasculitis
- Trauma
- Embolization
- Thrombus
- Aneurysm
- Pseudoaneurysm
- Intimal hyperplasia
- Traumatic occlusion
- Extrinsic compression
- AV fistula (abnormal connection between an artery and a vein)
- Radiation arteritis

Risk Factors (increased risk for Raynaud's)
- Atherosclerosis
- Age (increased risk with age)
- Female
- Family history
- Smoking
- Inhabitants of colder climates
- Occupational exposure to toxic substances
- Occupational stress (those who use vibrating tools, for example)
- Immunology and connective tissue disorders
- Obstructive arterial disease
- Drug-induced Raynaud's syndrome

Indications for Exam
- Intermittent digital pallor, cyanosis and/or rubor
- Cold sensitivity
- Raynaud's disease
- Thoracic outlet symptoms

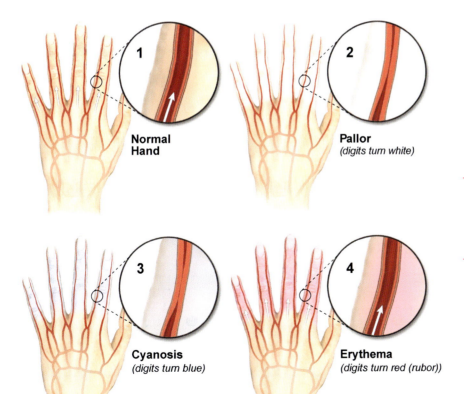

Fig. 25-1: *Raynaud's Phenomenon: Illustration of digital color changes due to stress: white to blue to red*

In Raynaud's syndrome, digits display episodes of cyanosis or pallor due to vasoconstriction of the small, digital arteries or arterioles during times of cold or emotional stress.

Contraindications/Limitations

- Digital ulceration or gangrene
- Severe rest pain
- Intolerance to the ice bath used during this examination
- Severely abnormal pressure values at rest, indicating a fixed obstruction
- DO NOT conduct a cold-immersion test on a patient with ulcerations or other signs of severe Raynaud's disease or phenomenon (unless followed up with sympathectomy), since it may be difficult to reverse the resulting vasospasm. [2]

Mechanism of Disease

- Current theory suggests the amount of receptors responsible for controlling body temperature on smooth muscle cells affect cold sensitivity. *Refer to Raynaud's Syndrome in the Arterial Vascular Disease chapter.*
- Cold sensitivity due to Raynaud's phenomenon is caused by vasospasm in addition to an underlying fixed vessel obstruction. [1]
  - » Digital symptoms that involve pain and/or color changes may be due to obstructive arterial disease and/or vasospastic disease. Arterial obstruction should be ruled out first by completing an upper extremity exam at rest including digital brachial pressures and digital waveform analysis (*see chapter on Upper Extremity Digital Evaluations*).
  - » If digital brachial pressure indices (DBI) and PPG waveforms are abnormal at rest, obstructive arterial disease is probably the cause and the cold immersion test is unnecessary.
- Raynaud's disease/phenomenon is characterized as a primary or secondary condition.
  - » *Primary* Raynaud's syndrome is intermittently vasospastic in nature and has no underlying condition or disease. [1]
  - » *Secondary* Raynaud's syndrome/phenomenon is associated with an underlying disease such as scleroderma and also involves a fixed arterial obstruction. [1]

Patients can suffer from either Raynaud's disease or Raynaud's phenomenon. It is unlikely that cold immersion testing is needed for a patient with Raynaud's symptoms where fixed arterial obstructions are evident at rest, (secondary, Raynaud's phenomenon).

Cold stress evaluations cannot differentiate between the two types of Raynaud's disease.[1]

Location of Vasospastic Disease

- Palmar arch arteries
- Digital vasospasm
- Location of disease can be focal and/or diffuse and affect any arterial level(s).

The most frequent cause of upper extremity ischemia is small artery occlusive disease of the palmar and digital arteries.

Patient History

- Pain
- During stress, digits change colors; from white to blue to red

Physical Examination (all may be intermittent)

- Cyanosis
- Rubor
- Pallor
- Significant temperature difference between digits/extremities
- Pulselessness possible with proximal obstruction

Cold Immersion Testing Protocol

- Obtain a patient history to include symptoms and risk factors. Explain the procedure to the patient (especially the ice bath portion).
- Patient is examined in the supine or sitting position.
- Appropriately wrap a 10-12cm bladder (in width) on the mid arm. The cuff should be placed "straight" rather than angled and fit snugly so that inflation of the bladder transmits the head of pressure into the tissue rather than into space between the bladder and the limb, producing falsely elevated readings.
- Locate the brachial artery (BrA) near the antecubital fossa with the Doppler transducer.
- Inflate the pressure cuff on the mid-arm 20-30mmHg beyond the last audible arterial signal using a Doppler transducer. Deflate the cuff slowly and record the brachial systolic pressure as soon as the first audible Doppler arterial signal returns. The Doppler pulse must continue after hearing the first pulse to assure there is an actual pulse rather than motion artifact.
- Obtain the brachial pressure on the contralateral arm using the same technique.
- Use the highest brachial artery pressure to calculate the pre-submersion digital-brachial index (DBI).

Use a towel to cover the hand to eliminate any light artifact which may disrupt the PPG tracing.

- Apply a 2.0-2.5cm digital cuff around the mid-phalanx of the digit to be studied while avoiding cuff placement over the bony joint. Smaller cuffs will result in falsely elevated pressures due to the narrow width of the cuff.
- Attach the PPG photocell to the pad of the first digit to be examined using double-stick tape placed between the photocell and the skin. Avoid taping the entire digit like a cuff since a tightly placed PPG could obliterate a low-pressure pulse.
- Alternative sensors used by some labs include a digital clip similar to a pulse oximeter which eliminates the need for tape or Velcro to keep the sensor in place.

Skin integrity of the digit must be intact to properly assess digital circulation and properly place the PPG sensor.

- Initiate the PPG (AC coupled) device with strip chart recorder or computer monitor. Make sure the exam room is warm and comfortable so the patient is not cold or stressed before testing.
- Start the PPG recording at low speed (5mm/s) to ensure that the tracing is centered. Ideally the baseline tracing consists of a series of horizontal pulses. When ready, change the recording speed to 25mm/s and document the shape of the waveform. Reduce the recorder speed to 5mm/s again.
- Inflate the pressure cuff around the finger until the PPG waveforms are flat (no longer visible) and then inflate another 20-30mmHg.
- Slowly deflate the cuff (at rate of 2-4mmHg/s) until the PPG waveforms return. Note the pressure in mmHg when the first pulse returns, but be sure that the pulse continues. If the pulse does not continue, consider that this was not a true pulse, but rather a motion artifact. There should be a flat tracing for a period of time after inflation before seeing the first return. This ensures the cuff was inflated beyond the local arterial pressure. When using a computerized system, move the cursor back to the first pulse.
- Repeat this procedure on remaining digits.

- Repeat this procedure on contralateral digits for comparison, especially on any symptomatic contralateral digits. The asymptomatic digits/hand can be used as a baseline or for comparison to the symptomatic digits/hand.
- In addition, thermometry can be used to measure baseline digital temperatures with the use of a temperature transducer sensitive for temperatures ranging from 0-55° C, placed on the tip of the finger.
- Immerse digits in an ice bath (approx. 1° C) for 1-3 minutes if able. Record the amount of time tolerated by the patient.
- Remove the hand promptly. Quickly pat the fingers dry. Do not attempt to warm the fingers with the towel.

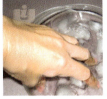

You can place the hand in a plastic bag before the ice bath to keep the hand dry.

- Promptly determine post-submersion digital waveforms, digital pressures and/or digital temperatures.
- Repeat digital pressure, waveforms and/or digital temperature measurements every 2-3 minutes until baseline values return, or for 10 minutes. Record the length of time spent on the post-submersion study.
- Calculate the digital-brachial index

$$DBI = \frac{\text{Digital pressure}}{\text{Highest brachial pressure}}$$

Cold immersion testing can also be performed on toes.

Table 25-1: Cold Immersion Protocol Summary

- Wrap pressure cuffs around:
  » Brachial artery
  » Digits
- Secure a PPG sensor to digit.
- Record representative digital PPG waveforms from tips of fingers (or toes).
- Determine pre-submersion digital-brachial indices (DBI)
  » Inflate cuffs 20-30mmHg beyond the last audible Doppler brachial artery signal and visualized PPG waveform(s).
  » Slowly deflate cuff (rate of 2-4mmHg per second). Record the systolic pressure as soon as the PPG waveform or brachial artery Doppler signal returns.
- Obtain baseline temperatures (optional).
- Immerse digits in an ice bath for 1-3 minutes.
- Record post-submersion digital waveforms and pressures (temperature-optional).
- Repeat post-submersion digital waveforms and pressures every 2-3 minutes for 10 minutes or until baseline values return (temperature optional).
- Determine classification of disease according to lab diagnostic criteria.
- Calculate the DBI:

$$DBI = \frac{\text{digital pressure}}{\text{highest brachial pressure}}$$

PRINCIPLES OF INTERPRETATION

Pressures and Digital Temperatures
- Digital pressures are compared to the highest brachial pressure and are typically lower than the wrist pressures.
- Changes in absolute pressure are important factors when interpreting the results of cold immersion testing.
- The asymptomatic hand can be used as a baseline or comparison to the symptomatic hand.
- Digital temperatures at rest are compared to those taken after immersion in an ice bath.

PPG Digital Waveforms
- The PPG waveform from any digit is categorized as *pulsatile, reduced or non-pulsatile* based on the upstroke (amplitude) of the waveform and downslope.

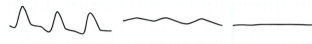

Fig. 25-2: *Normal Pulsatility*   Fig. 25-3: *Reduced Pulsatility*   Fig. 25-4: *Absent Pulsatility*

- There may be a dicrotic notch or secondary upstroke in the downslope of the tracing which corresponds to the increased aortic pressure and closure of the aortic valve.

Interpretation/Diagnostic Criteria

Normal

Pressures and Digital Temperatures
- Absolute digital artery pressure only decreases 16mmHg ±3% at a skin temperature of 10° C. [4]

PPG Digital Waveforms
- Normal waveforms are typically lower in amplitude following immersion, but it is most important to check that the waveforms, pressures and temperatures return to baseline values within 10 minutes of cold immersion. [1-3]

Fig. 25-5: *Normal PPG tracing with a dicrotic notch*

- Normal baseline PPG waveforms characteristics include: [4-7]
  » Short onset to sharp peak (subjective)
  » Downslope that bows toward the baseline
  » A dicrotic notch in the downslope

Normal recovery and response time

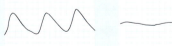

Fig. 25-6: *Pre-immersion tracing 2nd digit; 110mmHg*   Fig. 25-7: *Immediate post-immersion tracing 2nd digit 104mmHg*   Fig. 25-8: *5 minutes post-immersion tracing 2nd digit 108mmHg*

Abnormal

Pressure and Digital Temperatures
- Digital pressures are typically lower than the wrist pressure.
- Baseline finger pressures, and temperatures return in >10 minutes. [1,4]

- A digital pressure drop of greater than 17% from baseline indicates a significant digital artery vasospasm. [8]

PPG Digital Waveforms
- Baseline waveforms return in >10 minutes. [1,4]
- Abnormal ("reduced") baseline PPG waveform characteristics (secondary to obstruction, not vasospasm) include: [4,5,7]
  » Prolonged onset to peak (subjective)
  » Rounded peak
  » Downslope that bows away from the baseline

Digits with pressures of <20mmHg may not produce a pulsatile waveform.

- An "absent" digital waveform is reported when the PPG tracing reflects a flat-line after stress testing. This is considered a positive study for Raynaud's phenomenon. If the flat-line tracing was pre-immersion, a fixed obstruction would be suspected.

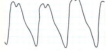

Fig. 25-9: Severely reduced PPG

Fig. 25-10: Obliteration of pulse

Fig. 25-11: Abnormal double peaked waveform

- A PPG waveform with a "double peak" (or early anacrotic notch with high dicrotic notch) are often seen in patients with Raynaud's phenomenon. [4,7] *(Fig. 25-11)*

Recovery time for baseline digital pressures, waveforms and temperatures may be 30 minutes or more in some Raynaud's patients.[1,4]

Table 25-2: Cold Immersion Thermometry Worksheet

	Cold Tolerance Thermometry (°F)					
Digit	Base	1 min	5 min	10 min	15 min	20 min
R 1st	73.8	67.5	65.9	66.2	67.3	67.5
R 2nd	74.4	68.3	67.0	68.0	68.4	69.1
R 3rd	74.4	74.4	67.0	68.6	67.3	67.4
R 4th	74.0	66.9	67.5	67.1	68.4	67.5
R 5th	74.4	65.0	69.1	67.2	68.9	67.9
L 1st	74.7	67.3	67.9	67.4	71.5	68.2
L 2nd	74.6	66.7	68.5	67.5	69.0	69.3
L 3rd	74.2	66.1	67.1	67.5	67.8	68.7
L 4th	74.2	64.2	67.2	66.4	67.8	68.7
L 5th	74.4	65.0	65.7	66.5	68.9	68.4

Interpretation of Worksheet

This abnormal cold stress exam reports a recovery time >10 minutes for finger pressures to return to baseline temperatures bilaterally.

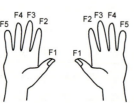

Differential Diagnosis
- Buerger's disease
- Scleroderma
- Connective tissue disorder
- Abnormalities of adrenergic receptor/sympathetic nervous system
- Neuropathy
- Muscle/tendon strains
- Arthritis
- Emboli
- Thoracic outlet syndrome

Correlation
- Duplex ultrasound
- MRA
- Contrast angiography
- Nailfold capillary microscopy

Medical Treatment
- Cold temperature avoidance
- Risk factor management (cessation of tobacco usage, avoidance of cold)
- Calcium channel blocker
- Alpha adrenergic antagonist
- Angiotensin antagonist
- Serotonin uptake inhibitor
- Prostaglandins
- Thermal biofeedback

Surgical Treatment
- Bypass grafting
- Thoracoscopic sympathectomy
- Amputation

A sympathectomy (a nerve block performed to produce vasodilatation and improve blood flow) may be performed in conjunction with a cold stress evaluation. A local anesthetic is injected into a nerve to inactivate its tone. PPG waveforms are repeated and if normal, this suggests vasodilator therapy may be helpful. [2]

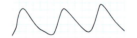

Fig. 25-12: *Pre-immersion tracing*

Fig. 25-13: *Post-immersion and xylocaine injection (The abnormal, flat PPG tracing suggests vasodilator therapy would not be helpful for this patient)*

REFERENCES

1. Shepherd RFJ. (2005). Raynaud's syndrome: vasospastic and occlusive arterial disease involving the distal upper extremity. In Rutherford Vascular Surgery 6th edition. (1319-1346). Philadelphia. Elsevier Saunders.
2. Talbot, SR, Zwiebel WJ. (2005). Assessment of upper extremity arterial occlusive disease. In Zwiebel WJ, Pellerito JS (Eds.), Introduction to Vascular Ultrasonography. (297-323). Philadelphia: Elsevier Saunders.
3. Hallett, JW, Brewster DC, Rasmussen TE. (2001). Upper extremity arterial disease and vasospastic disorder. In Handbook of Patient Care in Vascular Diseases, 4th ed. (238-247). Philadelphia. Lippincott Williams and Wilkins.
4. Longo GM, Pearce WH, Sumner DS. (2005). Evaluation of upper extremity ischemia. In Rutherford Vascular Surgery 6th edition. (1274-1293). Philadelphia. Elsevier Saunders.
5. Moneta GL, Partsafas A, Zacardi M. (2010). Non-invasive diagnosis of upper extremity arterial disease. In Zierler RE (Ed.), Strandess's duplex scanning disorders in vascular diagnosis 4th ed. (149-156). Philadelphia Wolters Kluwer Lippincott Williams & Wilkins.
6. Edwards JM, Porter JM. (1998). Upper extremity arterial disease: Etiologic considerations and differential diagnosis. (60-68). Seminars in Vascular Surgery. Vol 11(2).
7. Sumner DS, Zierler RE. (2005). Physiologic assessment of peripheral arterial occlusive disease. In Rutherford Vascular Surgery 6th edition. (197-222). Philadelphia. Elsevier Saunders.
8. Segall JA, Moneta GL. (2006). Non-invasive diagnosis of upper extremity vascular disease. In AbuRahma AF, Bergan JJ (Eds.), Non-invasive Vascular Diagnosis: A Practical Guide to Therapy. 2nd edition. (317-323). London. Springer-Verlag.
9. www.nytimes.com "Getting to the Root of Raynaud's." New York Times. 4/29/10 by Winnie Yu interviewing Dr. Frederick Wigley.

ARTERIAL TESTING
26. Upper Extremity Arterial Duplex Ultrasound

Definition

The use of a combination of real time B-mode ultrasonography with spectral and color flow Doppler (duplex scan) to evaluate the upper extremity arteries.

Arterial duplex ultrasound can identify the presence, exact location, extent, and severity of disease. The course of the arteries, collaterals and disease can be visualized using B-mode and color, while the measurement of Doppler velocity and waveform changes can estimate the severity of obstructions and flow direction.

Etiology

- Atherosclerosis
- Embolization
- Thrombus
- Intimal hyperplasia
- Pseudoaneurysm
- Aneurysm
- Trauma
- Traumatic occlusion
- Extrinsic compression
- Vasculitis
- AV fistula (abnormal connection between an artery and a vein)
- External radiation
- Radiation arteritis

Risk Factors

- Age (increased risk with age)
- Coronary artery disease
- Diabetes
- Family history
- Hyperlipidemia
- Hypertension
- Smoking
- Obesity
- Post-op cardiac catheterization through the brachial artery
- History of radiation
- Fibromuscular dysplasia
- Occupational exposure to toxic substances
- Previous history of CVA or MI
- Elevated homocysteine
- Excessive levels of C-reactive protein

Indications for Exam

- Absent peripheral pulses
- Abnormal arterial arm pressures, including BP differential of >20mmHg between arms
- Thoracic outlet symptoms
- Cold sensitivity
- Digital cyanosis
- Raynaud's syndrome/ phenomenon abnormal vertebral artery waveforms
- Bruit (abnormal sound heard through auscultation caused by vibration of tissue from turbulent flow)
- Claudication (exercise-related arm pain)
- Rest pain
- Extremity ulcer
- Gangrene
- Trauma to an artery
- Arterial aneurysm

Contraindications/Limitations

- Patients with extensive bandages or casts
- Subclavian or peripheral IV line placements may make it difficult to image an area.

Since the left subclavian artery originates directly from the aortic arch, its origin is often not seen in a routine examination. [9,11]

- Poor visualization due to vessel depth (e.g., near clavicular area)
- Diffuse arterial wall calcification (such as in diabetics and end-stage renal failure patients) may interfere with acquisition of duplex information.

Mechanism of Disease

- **Atherosclerosis** is the most common arterial disease. Atherosclerotic plaque forms in the artery to block flow by either narrowing the arterial lumen (arterial stenosis) or totally blocking the artery (arterial occlusion). The term "hemodynamically significant obstruction" refers to either a stenosis or an occlusion that results in a decrease in blood pressure or flow distal to the obstruction. Typically, a stenosis must narrow the diameter of the artery by at least 50% to decrease pressure and flow distally. [1] An arterial occlusion is typically seen from one major branch to the next.

Besides atherosclerosis, narrowing of an arterial lumen can result from intimal hyperplasia or cellular damage after radiation therapy.

- **Emboli** may occur as contents of a plaque or fragments of an organized thrombus from the heart or aneurysm loosen and flow downstream. Emboli become lodged in a distant blood vessel, causing arterial occlusion and reduction of flow. [1]
- **Vasospasm** is a temporary constriction of the arteries (typically digital arteries) that may cause significant discomfort to the patient or be a sign of a more serious underlying disease. [2]
- **Extrinsic compression** from tumors, musculoskeletal configuration, hematoma, etc. can result in stenosis or occlusion by placing enough pressure on arterial walls to compromise blood flow. [1]
- **Mechanical compression** of arterial vessels in the thoracic outlet can compromise flow. Anatomical defects, such as a congenital abnormality of the first rib or fracture of the clavicle, are examples of possible sources of this compression. [3]
- **Aneurysmal disease** results from weakening of the structural proteins (elastin and collagen) within the medial layer of the arterial wall. [4]
- A **pseudoaneurysm** (PA) or "false aneurysm" forms due to trauma to all three layers of the arterial wall. The "false aneurysm" is actually a hematoma, receiving its blood supply via communication with an artery through a patent "neck." [5]
- An **arteriovenous fistula** or abnormal connection between artery and vein can result from trauma or complications during invasive procedures (e.g., cardiac catheterization). In such cases, blood flows directly from the artery into the venous system without passing through the tissues and capillary bed. [6]
- **Arterial dissections** are caused by tears in the intimal layer of the arterial wall that allows blood flow to access the media. Dissection between the medial and adventitial layers may result in true and false lumens. The false lumen can progressively dilate into a pseudoaneurysm. [7]

Location of Disease

- Location of disease can be focal or diffuse and affect any level or multiple levels.
- At the origin of the great vessels
- Subclavian or axillary artery
- Palmar arch and/or digital arteries

The most common locations for upper extremity atherosclerotic plaques and aneurysms involve the SCA and AXA. [9,11] *Obstruction of the RA and UA is less common, though can result from low-flow states or embolization.* [9]

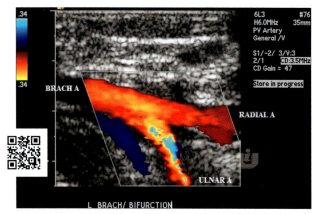

Fig. 26-1: *Bifurcation of the brachial artery into the radial artery and ulnar artery*

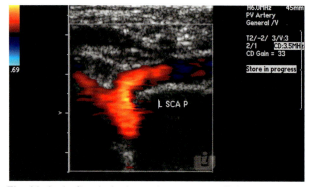

Fig. 26-2: *Left subclavian artery comes off the aortic arch*

Patient History
- Claudication (exercise related limb pain)
- Limb pain at rest
- Paralysis
- Paresthesia
- Poikilothermia
- Previous therapeutic vascular procedure (e.g., bypass, stenting)

Physical Examination
- Pulselessness
- Cyanosis
- Pallor
- Rubor
- Bruit (abnormal sound heard through auscultation caused by turbulent flow vibration)
- Marked temperature difference between hand/fingers
- Palpable thrill (vibration caused by turbulent blood flow as seen in an AV fistula)
- Gangrene/necrosis (tissue death)
- Pulsatile mass

Upper Extremity Arterial Duplex Protocol
- Obtain a patient history to include symptoms, risk factors and past vascular interventions and general dates. Explain the procedure to the patient.
- Patient is examined in the supine position with the arm angled approximately 45-90° and externally rotated away from the body.
- Some patients may require the use of a range of transducers; including high-frequency (5-7 MHz) (8-15 MHz) transducers and a lower frequency (1-4 MHz) transducer for the area around the clavicle.
- Locate the subclavian artery (SCA) and vein in the supraclavicular fossa in the transverse (short axis) plane. Rotate your transducer in the longitudinal (sagittal) plane to follow the artery proximal to its origin. Record B-mode and color images of the proximal SCA in a longitudinal view.
  » The clavicle bone prohibits direct Doppler and color flow analysis of a segment of the subclavian artery. Compare the spectral Doppler waveform above and below the clavicle.
- As you move the transducer distally down the arm, record B-mode and color images in a longitudinal view of the:
  » Right distal innominate artery (optional)
  » Distal SCA (below the clavicle)
  » Axillary artery (AXA)
  » Brachial artery (BrA)
- Record the peak systolic velocity (PSV) in longitudinal view using spectral Doppler (60° Doppler angle or less, with the angle cursor (angle correct) parallel to the vessel walls in the center of the flow stream) in the following:
  » Subclavian artery (SCA)
  » Axillary artery (AXA)
  » Brachial artery (BrA)
  » Radial (RA) artery
  » Ulnar (UA) artery
  » Right distal innominate artery (optional)

The left SCA should be evaluated above the clavicle as proximally as possible.

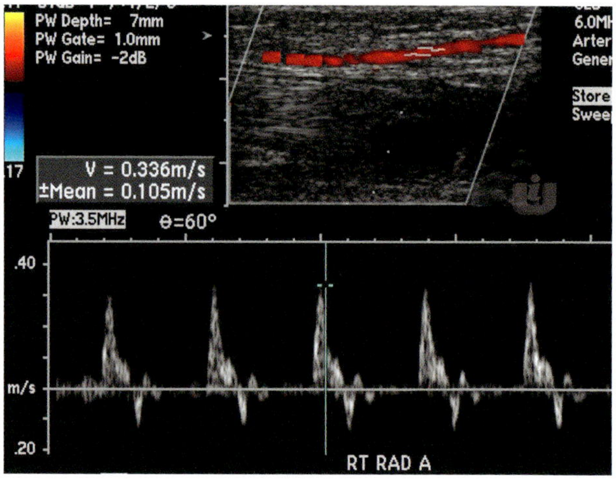

Fig. 26-3: *Normal radial artery waveforms*

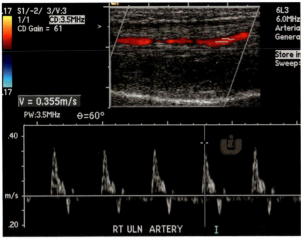
Fig. 26-4: *Normal ulnar artery waveforms*

- Document additional B-mode and color images at areas of suspected stenosis.
  » When an area of stenosis is identified, "walk" the sample gate through the area of stenosis and obtain representative waveforms within 2cm proximal to the stenosis, at the highest point of velocity within the stenosis and distal to the stenosis.
  » Post-stenotic turbulence and color bruit should be documented when present.
  » Measure diameter reduction in longitudinal and/or transverse planes, especially if the lesion is hemodynamically significant.

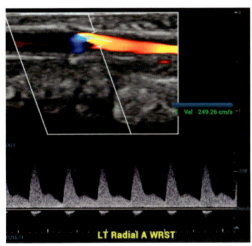
Radal artery stenosis by spectral Doppler

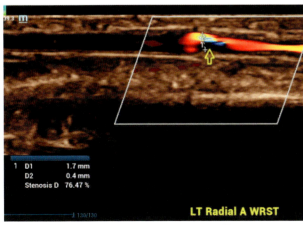
Diameter reduction measured in radial artery

- Document any additional abnormal findings with B-mode and color imaging (e.g., aneurysmal formation, plaque, thrombus, wall irregularity, aneurysm, AV fistula, etc.).
- Repeat for the left side (omitting innominate artery visualization).
- Determine classification of stenosis according to laboratory diagnostic criteria.

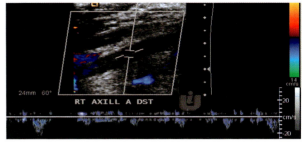
Fig. 26-5: *Occlusion of the AXA by spectral Doppler*

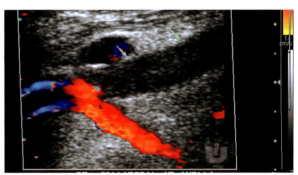
Fig. 26-6: *Arterial occlusion of the SCA by color flow. Note patent collateral*

Subclavian Steal Syndrome Examination

Arterial duplex of the AXA can be used to diagnose subclavian steal syndrome. Patients present with abnormal arterial arm pressures, including a BP differential of >20mmHg between arms. [8]

- Using the duplex scanner, record a waveform in the vertebral artery on the same side as the arm with the lower blood pressure. Note the direction of flow.
- The following additional interrogation may also be performed:
  » Use spectral Doppler to insonate the ipsilateral subclavian artery to identify a significant velocity increase or occlusion proximal to the origin of the vertebral artery.
  » Identify any lumenal reduction by B-mode or color flow in the SCA. (Always use images in combination with PSV documentation).
  » Compare bilateral axillary waveforms using spectral Doppler.
- **Post occlusive reactive hyperemia (PORH)** has also been used to diagnose subclavian steal syndrome when the vertebral artery demonstrates pendulum (to and fro) flow direction or has questionable reversed flow direction present. [8]
  » Inflate a pressure cuff over the brachial artery (30mmHg above the highest brachial pressure) for 5 minutes to cause temporary ischemia in the arm.
  » After cuff deflation, investigate the flow direction of the ipsilateral vertebral artery using the duplex scanner as you would during a carotid exam.

The rate of subclavian steal involving the left arm is 85%. [9]

Table 26-1: Upper Extremity Arterial Protocol Summary

Scan longitudinal (sagittal) view with B-mode, color and spectral Doppler
- SCA
- AXA
- BrA
- Right distal innominate artery (optional)
- RA
- UA
- Record the peak systolic velocity (PSV) for any segment interrogated.
- When an area of stenosis is identified, "walk" the sample gate through the area of stenosis and obtain representative waveforms at the tightest point of stenosis (highest velocity), as well as proximal and distal to the stenosis.
- Calculate the velocity ratio (Vr):

  PSV (V_2) distal ÷ PSV (V_1) proximal

- Determine classification of stenosis according to laboratory diagnostic criteria.

PRINCIPLES OF INTERPRETATION

The criterion for abnormal upper extremity arterial duplex varies across institutions.

B-mode Imaging and Color Doppler
- Measure lumenal reductions in multiple planes to get the full effect of any plaque:
  » Transverse
  » Longitudinal-anterior/posterior
  » Longitudinal-lateral
  » The most difficult point to define is the true lumen. Look for a black line separating the wall from any plaque.
  » Place calipers on the anterior-inner lumen and the posterior inner lumen.
  » Calculate and report the average of 2-3 measurements.
  » Use color only if needed to clearly define edges of plaque, and update with B-mode frequently to avoid color overgain.
- Assess all arteries for intraluminal echoes. Determine plaque location and plaque characteristics:
  » **Diffuse plaque:** Long segment of the artery lined with plaque, but <50% diameter reduction at any point.
  » **Stenotic:** Lumen is narrowed and velocity increases. A hemodynamically significant stenosis typically occurs when narrowing results in a >50% diameter reduction (75% area reduction). A stenosis can be focal or involve a long segment.
  » **Calcific:** Highly reflective plaque(s) with acoustic shadowing
  » **Occluded:** Complete occlusion of the vessel
  » "Moving"/"Mobile": Debris within the lumen is poorly adhered to the vessel wall, e.g., moving thrombus.
- Color flow is used to show patency of the arterial lumen, the degree of narrowing when there is disease and flow direction.

Arterial Waveform Terminology
The terminology used to describe arterial waveforms is not consistent across laboratories. A consensus document was published in 2020 by the Society of Vascular Ultrasound and the Society for Vascular Medicine regarding the terminology and interpretation of peripheral arterial and venous waveforms. *See the Arterial Hemodynamics chapter for more detail on arterial waveforms.*

Spectral Doppler Waveforms
Any change in spectral waveform analysis depends on the terminology used by the lab; from triphasic to monophasic or changes in resistance may be significant.

Flow Velocities
- Determine peak systolic velocity (PSV) and flow direction
- Calculate the velocity ratio (Vr)= V_2/V_1, where V_2 represents the maximum PSV of a stenosis and V_1 is the PSV of the proximal normal segment.
- Calcific shadowing can prohibit Doppler and color flow analysis of a specific arterial segment. Use indirect signs to evaluate hemodynamically significant lesions:
  » Compare the Doppler waveform proximal and distal to the calcified segment can point to a hemodynamically significant obstruction under the calcific shadowing.
  » If severe post-stenotic turbulence is present distal to the shadowing, there could be a stenosis in the calcified segment, or conversely, if there is essentially no change in the waveform pattern, it is unlikely that a significant obstruction exists under the calcific area.
  » Compare the arterial waveform in the contralateral extremity at the same site.

Interpretation/Diagnostic Criteria

Normal

Absence of a hemodynamically significant stenosis, <50%)

B-mode Imaging and Color Doppler
- The artery is free of intralumenal echoes.[9]
- When utilized, color Doppler fills the entire arterial lumen and is in the appropriate direction for each artery.[9]

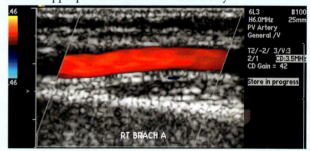

Fig. 26-7: Normal artery showing color filling from wall-to-wall

Spectral Doppler Waveforms
- A waveform with a sharp, quick upstroke followed by a brisk downstroke with reversed flow direction in early diastole and another forward phase in late diastole is termed *triphasic*. This is considered a normal finding in the peripheral arteries.

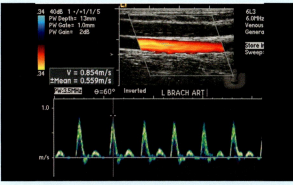

Fig. 26-8: *Triphasic arterial waveforms*

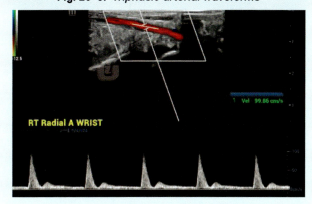

Fig. 26-9: *Multiphasic arterial waveforms may be normal in some patients.*

- A waveform with a sharp upstroke followed by reversed flow that crosses the zero baseline and contains both forward and reverse components is termed *multiphasic* or *biphasic* by some labs.
- Some labs have adopted terminology that recognizes any reversed flow as normal by using an abbreviation NR for "normal-reversed" whether or not the third phase is present, in order to avoid the confusing use of "triphasic" and "biphasic" terms. [13]
- Arterial waveforms without a reversed flow component can be a normal finding for some patients, such as the elderly. If arterial pressures are normal, consider the possibility that the signal may also be normal. [6]

The third phase of the triphasic waveform may be missing in older patients with less vessel compliance.

Flow Velocities

- PSV and Vr are relatively uniform throughout the sampled arterial segment. [8]

Table 26-2: Normal PSV of Upper Extremity Arteries [7]

Artery	PSV (angle-corrected)
SCA and AXA	70-120cm/s
BrA	50-120cm/s
RA and UA	40-90cm/s
Palmar arch and digits	<RA/UA PSV

Source: Baker JD. (2005). The role of non-invasive procedures in the management of extremity arterial disease. In Zwiebel WJ, Pellerito JS (Eds.), Introduction to Vascular Ultrasonography 5th ed. (254-260). Philadelphia: Elsevier Saunders

Abnormal

B-mode Imaging and Color Doppler

- Intralumenal echoes are visualized within the artery resulting in a measurable lumenal reduction.
- When utilized, color Doppler does not fill the entire arterial lumen. A color jet can be visualized through the narrowed lumen and a mosaic color pattern can be observed due to turbulent flow in the post-stenotic region. [9,10,12]
  » For increased accuracy when assessing disease, consider B-mode reduction measurements together with Doppler velocity and ratios.

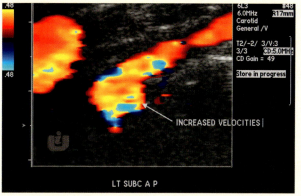

Fig. 26-10: *Significant stenosis of SCA by color Doppler (mosaic pattern)*

Color Doppler can over/underestimate plaque and diameter reductions if gain settings are not optimized.

Spectral Doppler Waveforms

- As the obstruction becomes more severe, changes in the spectral waveform are expected before a stenosis or occlusion, at the point of greatest stenosis and after a stenosis/occlusion as described in the *Arterial Physiology* chapter. These changes are important to note in the interpretation of the vascular exam.
- *Spectral broadening* represents the wide range of velocities usually present when there is disturbed, non-laminar flow. This waveform change occurs in the early stages of arterial disease. The normally clear window below the systolic peak begins to fill in.
- *Monophasic* arterial Doppler waveforms reflect low resistance and are characterized by a slow upstroke, low amplitude, and broad peak with continuous forward flow in diastole that does not cross the zero baseline. The upstroke has a general direction of being tipped to the right. Monophasic waveforms are typically present distal to an occlusion or a very high-grade stenosis. [9-11,14]

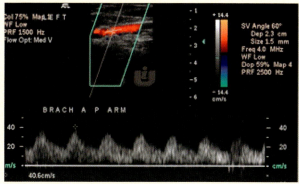

Fig. 26-11: *Abnormal, monophasic arterial waveforms*

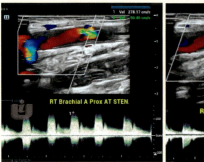
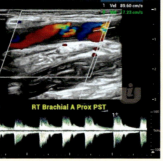

Fig. 26-12: *Hemodynamically significant brachial artery stenosis*

- A high-resistance waveform with a sharp upstroke and brisk downstroke will be noted in a stenotic region. There may or may not be flow reversal in diastole.[28] When there is a diastolic component, it may be elevated or absent depending on the degree of downstream resistance.
- Turbulent waveforms or "post-stenotic turbulence" are indicative of chaotic flow reflecting how blood moves in many directions just past the stenosis.
- *Parvus tardus* is an alternative term for "monophasic" used by some laboratories to describe a waveform with continuous forward flow and a slow, blunted systolic component.[15]
- **Staccato:** A "spiked" high-resistant waveform with a short upstroke/downstroke and little to no diastolic component is often a signal of impending occlusion.

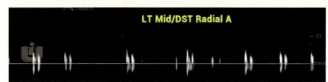

Fig. 26-13: *Staccato waveform of the radial artery*

- **Occlusion:** An occlusion of the artery is present when no flow is detected by spectral Doppler. Determine the extent (length) of the occlusion.[8,9,12]

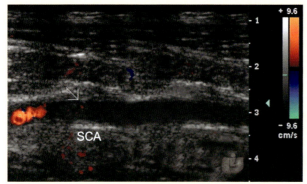

Fig. 26-14: *Abnormal occluded artery; color filling is absent*

> Use flow in the adjacent vein as a guide to identify an occluded artery. Always confirm flow by placing the Doppler sample volume in the vessel lumen.

» Often a large collateral can be identified at the proximal and distal ends of the occlusion. These collaterals often exit and enter the artery at 90° angles.

Flow Velocities

- A hemodynamically significant lesion (>50%) will result in a focal velocity increase (at least double the velocity in the proximal arterial segment), change in spectral waveform (including *spectral broadening* where the clear window under the spectral waveform is filled in), post-stenotic turbulence and a possible color bruit.[8,10,11,13,16]
- A hemodynamically significant lesion (>70%) will result in a focal velocity increase at least triple the velocity in the proximal arterial segment.[13]

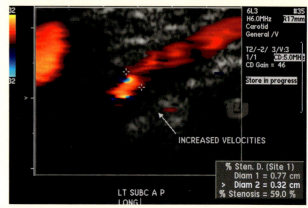

Fig. 26-15: *Lumenal reduction of the SCA by color flow*

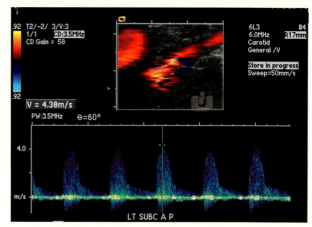

Fig. 26-16: *Spectral Doppler showing significant stenosis of the SCA with a PSV=438cm/s.*

Table 26-3: Diagnostic Criteria for Arterial Stenosis [8,9,11]

- PSV* ratio >2 indicates significant stenosis
- Changes in velocity measurements or waveform shape on serial examinations warrant close interval follow-up

*PSV = Peak systolic velocity

Other Pathology

- **Thoracic outlet syndrome:** The thoracic outlet is comprised of the clavicle, the first rib and the scalene muscle. Compression of the subclavian vessels is a common issue. Complete or partial compression of the vessels is possible, which over time may lead to damage of the arterial wall or formation of thrombus. Oftentimes symptoms are experienced with certain positional changes.[12] (*Refer to the Thoracic Outlet Testing chapter for details on interpretation of this condition.*)

- **Arteriovenous fistula (AVF):** An AVF between any artery and an adjacent vein is characterized by color bruit on duplex image along with high velocity, low-resistance spectral waveforms at the same site by spectral Doppler. [11] The turbulent, pulsatile waveform typically continues for a short distance in the vein proximal to the AVF and slowly loses its pulsatility more proximally. The Doppler signal proximal to the AVF is clearly different than the venous signal distal to the AVF.

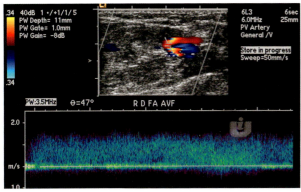

Fig. 26-17: *Typical AVF Doppler waveform*

- **Pseudoaneurysm:** A pulsatile mass observed communicating with a native artery is indicative of a pseudoaneurysm. To-and-fro Doppler flow patterns will be apparent within the "neck" of the PA.[5]

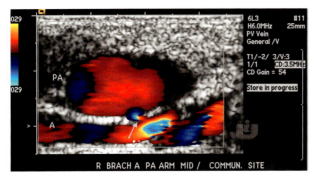

Fig. 26-18: *Brachial artery pseudoaneurysm*

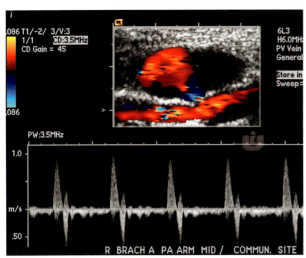

Fig. 26-19: *Spectral Doppler waveforms from a pseudoaneurysm neck*

- **Aneurysm:** Arterial diameters that show a focal enlargement, which is at least 1.5-2 times the size of the proximal arterial segment, indicates significant aneurysmal dilatation. [9] Intralumenal thrombus may be present and is a possible source of distal emboli. [10]
  » The typical shape of an aneurysm in the upper extremity is fusiform. [10]
- **Arteriomegaly:** The term used to describe a uniform arterial dilation throughout an artery. [19]
  » An artery can also be described as "ectatic" (dilatation of a circular tube) when diameters are somewhat larger through a segment, though not yet aneurysmal. The dilated areas of the artery may or may not be uniform.

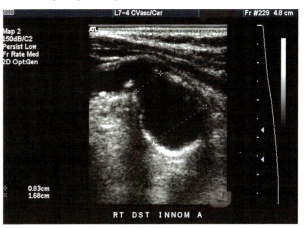

Fig. 26-20: *Innominate artery aneurysm*

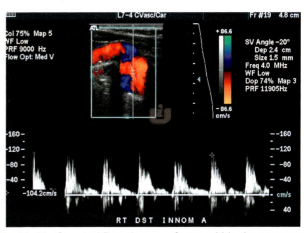

Fig. 26-21: *Spectral Doppler waveforms within the aneurysm*

- **Subclavian steal syndrome:** A significant difference in brachial artery pressures >20-30mmHg warrants additional interrogation of the arm with the lower blood pressure. Arterial flow in the ipsilateral vertebral, subclavian and axillary arteries is considered during interpretation. Reversed flow direction in the vertebral artery, combined with a significant difference in arm pressures, is indicative of a subclavian steal.
  » **By duplex:**
    - A focal velocity increase in the ipsilateral subclavian artery proximal to the origin of the vertebral artery that is at least double the velocity in the proximal arterial segment indicates a hemodynamically significant stenosis (>50%). Additional duplex findings including; changes in spectral waveform (from triphasic to biphasic or monophasic), post-stenotic turbulence and color bruit all support this finding. [8,9]

- No flow detected by color or spectral Doppler (occlusion) in the SCA proximal to the origin of the vertebral artery is another possible abnormal finding. [9,10]
  » **By PORH:** [8]
  - If the flow direction of the vertebral artery becomes retrograde after the PORH technique, this finding suggests a subclavian steal on that side.

- **Arterial dissection:** A dissection of the arterial lumen is recognized by two distinct flow channels by B-mode and/or color Doppler separated by intimal echoes. One lumen is known as the "true lumen" while the other is referred to as the "false lumen." One of the lumens may be occluded or demonstrate reversed or unusual flow direction. [7,11]

- Waveform patterns in the false lumen will be turbulent, irregular and/or bidirectional compared to the more "normal" or expected waveform in the true lumen.

The SCA is the most likely artery of the upper extremity to demonstrate a dissection, though it can occur elsewhere.

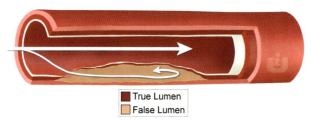

Fig. 26-22: *Artery with a true and false lumen*

A proximal branch of the SCA, the internal thoracic (internal mammary) artery, is frequently used as conduit for cardiac surgery and surgically grafted to the heart. The artery can often be visualized coming off the SCA at a 90° angle to the vessel. [11]

Differential Diagnosis
- Spinal stenosis
- Venous thrombosis
- Thoracic outlet syndrome
- Neuropathy
- Muscle/tendon strains
- Cervical arthritis
- Abnormalities of adrenergic receptor/sympathetic nervous system
- Connective tissue disease (scleroderma)

Correlation
- Spiral CT scan
- MRA
- Arteriography

Medical Treatment
- Modify risk factors, (e.g., smoking cessation, especially for Raynaud's symptoms, reduce cholesterol/HTN, manage DM)
- Antiplatelet medication (e.g., aspirin)
- Anticoagulation (warfarin)
- Steroids
- Cold temperature avoidance

Surgical Treatment
- Bypass grafting
- Embolectomy
- Direct focal repair
- Resection (aneurysmal disease)
- Amputation

Endovascular Treatment
- Angioplasty
- Stent
- Atherectomy
- Intra-arterial directed thrombolysis (acute blockage)

REFERENCES
1. Sumner DS, Zierler RE. (2005). Vascular physiology: essential hemodynamic principles. In Rutherford Vascular Surgery 6th edition. (75-123). Philadelphia. Elsevier Saunders
2. Shepard RFJ. (2005). Raynaud's syndrome: vasospastic and occlusive arterial disease involving the distal upper extremity. In Rutherford Vascular Surgery 6th edition. (1319-1346). Philadelphia. Elsevier Saunders
3. Kreienberg PB, Shah, DM, Darling III, RC, Change BB, Paty SK, Roddy SP, Ozsvath KJ, Manish,, (2005). Thoracic Outlet Syndrome. In Mansour MA, Labropoulos N. (Eds.), *Vascular Diagnosis*, (517-522). Philadelphia,: Elsevier Saunders.
4. Schermerhorn ML, Cronenwett JL. (2005). Abdominal aortic and iliac aneurysms. In *Rutherford Vascular Surgery 6th edition*. (1408-1452). Philadelphia. Elsevier Saunders.
5. Casey, PJ, LaMuraglia GM. (2005). Anastomotic aneurysms. In Rutherford Vascular Surgery 6th edition. (894-902). Philadelphia. Elsevier Saunders
6. Rutherford RB. (2005). Diagnostic evaluation of arteriovenous fistulas and vascular anomalies. In Rutherford Vascular Surgery 6th edition. (1602-1612). Philadelphia. Elsevier Saunders.
7. Baker JD. (2005). The role of non-invasive procedures in the management of extremity arterial disease. In Zwiebel WJ. Pellerito JS (Eds.), Introduction to Vascular Ultrasonography 5th ed. (254-260). Philadelphia: Elsevier Saunders.
8. Longo MG, Pearce WH, Sumner DS. (2005). Evaluation of upper extremity ischemia. In Rutherford Vascular Surgery 6th edition. (1274-1293). Philadelphia. Elsevier Saunders.
9. Talbot SR, Zwiebel WJ. (2005). Assessment of upper extremity arterial occlusive disease. In Zwiebel WJ. Pellerito JS (Eds.), Introduction to Vascular Ultrasonography 5th ed. (297-323). Philadelphia: Elsevier Saunders
10. Moneta GL, Partsafas A, Zacardi M. (2010). Non-invasive diagnosis of upper extremity arterial disease. In Zierler RE (Ed.), Strandess's duplex scanning disorders in vascular diagnosis 4th ed. (149-156). Philadelphia Wolters Kluwer Lippincott Williams & Wilkins.
11. Thrush, A, Hartshorne, T. (2005). Duplex assessment of upper extremity arterial disease. In Peripheral Vascular Ultrasound (2nd ed). (133-144). Philadelphia: Elsevier
12. Myers K, Clough A. (2004). Diseases of vessels to the upper limb. In Making sense of vascular ultrasound: A hands on guide. (227-254). London: Hodder Arnold.
13. Kim ES, Sharma AM, Scissons R, et al. Interpretation of peripheral arterial and venous Doppler waveforms: A consensus statement from the Society for Vascular Medicine and Society for Vascular Ultrasound. Vascular Medicine. 2020;25(5):484-506. doi:10.1177/1358863X20937665

27. Venous Photoplethysmography (PPG)

Definition

Venous photoplethysmography (PPG) is an indirect method used to evaluate the lower extremity veins for evidence of valvular incompetence. Venous PPG can also help differentiate between primary and secondary venous insufficiency to plan treatment options.

Chronic venous disorders are caused by incompetent valves in the superficial, perforators, and/or deep venous systems, resulting in venous hypertension and stasis.

Venous PPG testing involves exercise or manual calf compressions to cause contraction of the calf muscles. These contractions empty the blood out of the veins in the lower leg.

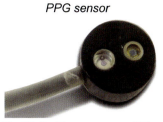

PPG sensor

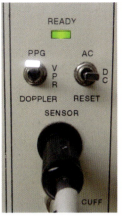

PPG device

Fig. 27-2: *The venous or DC mode on the PPG instrument is used to monitor slow venous changes. The arterial or AC mode is used to monitor the faster volume changes that occur with arterial pulsations.*

Principle

PPG equipment can monitor and display blood volume changes over time.

A PPG sensor consists of infrared light and a receiver attached to the skin approximately 5cm (2in) above the medial malleolus in the gaiter area with double-sided tape or a Velcro strap. The calf muscles normally compress the veins during exercise or manual compression. A rapid decrease in venous blood volume is followed by a slow refilling of the veins via the arteries and capillaries.

After obtaining a baseline for the PPG tracing during testing, the calf veins are emptied through exercise or manual compression, and the leg is rested so the veins can refill.

The PPG tracing demonstrates the volume changes during this venous emptying and filling. The venous filling index (a.k.a., Venous Recovery Time or VRT) can be calculated from this tracing.

Valvular incompetence results in a faster VRT than normal since veins refill via immediate backflow of venous blood past the incompetent valves rather than through the normal course; through artery, arteriole, capillary, venule, and then vein.

Indications for Exam

- Varicose veins
- Chronic edema/swelling which worsens at the end of the day (especially when unilateral)
- Pain, which may be localized to a specific varix or described as a "dull ache."
- Discoloration at the gaiter area
- Ulceration (e.g., gaiter area)
- Venous claudication

Contraindications/Limitation

- PPG testing is a subjective test. Although an actual number is VRT number is calculated, it is an overall measurement of venous refill and not specific to a particular vein.
- Patient's inability to maximally point/flex their foot (manual compression can be used in such cases).
- Patient's inability to sit and hang their limb over the bedside.
- Ulcerations and lack of intact skin prohibits placement of the PPG sensor.
- Patients with extensive bandages or casts

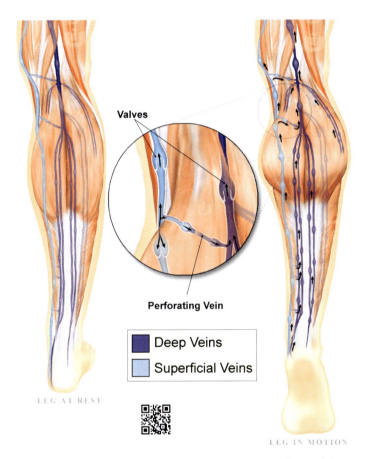

Fig. 27-1: *The calf muscle pump drives venous flow. While walking, muscle contractions squeeze the veins initiating venous blood flow. Venous flow opens the venous valves allowing the blood to flow towards the heart. As the muscle relaxes, valves close to prevent retrograde of blood (reflux).*

Mechanism of Disease

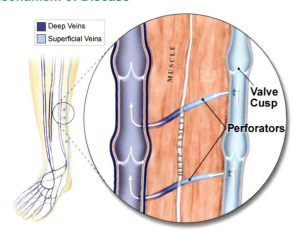

Fig. 27-3: Blood normally flows from the superficial veins via perforators to the deep veins.

Venous Flow with Normal Valve Function
- The direction of normal blood flow in the deep and superficial veins is toward the heart. In the perforating (communicating) veins, blood normally flows from the superficial to the deep veins. [1]
- At various times, the blood may encounter pressure to move in the opposite direction from the heart, e.g., in response to gravity. Normally, flow reversal is prevented by the venous valves, which close in response to pressure from the reversed flow. [1]
- Upon exercise, the action of the calf muscles typically sends blood flow up the leg away from the calf. This action empties the calf veins, reduces blood volume, and reduces venous pressure. [1]

Venous Flow with Abnormal Valve Function
- *Primary* venous insufficiency is thought to have a congenital etiology and involves the superficial more than the deep venous system.
- *Secondary* venous insufficiency is typically an acquired condition (e.g., after venous thrombosis) and can involve the superficial, perforating, and deep venous systems. [8] Secondary venous insufficiency can result from a congenital condition such as an extrinsic compression of an iliac vein by an overlying iliac artery.
- Valvular damage and dysfunction (valvular incompetence) result in venous reflux, which is venous flow in the wrong (or opposite) direction, away from the heart and back into the leg.
- In the perforating veins, blood flows in the wrong direction from the deep to the superficial system.
- Venous reflux creates a high blood volume in the veins distal to the incompetent valve(s). [1]
- High blood volume in a vein causes ambulatory venous pressure or venous hypertension. [1]
- Hypertension will be greatest upon standing due to the effect of hydrostatic pressure from gravity, adding to the increased pressure from volume. [1]
- Normally venous blood volume and pressure are reduced by activating the calf muscle pump upon walking. When the valves are not working, the venous volume and resulting pressure do not decrease sufficiently, and the patient suffers from *ambulatory venous hypertension*. [1]
- Venous hypertension also increases pressure within the venules and capillaries. This high-pressure system encourages fluids to escape into the tissues causing edema. [1]
- Local edema results in a decrease in fluid and protein reabsorption. Fibrinogen and red blood cells (RBC) in the capillaries escape back into the tissues. Proteins organize and form tissue fibrosis, causing hardening of the skin. The RBCs break down and cause hyperpigmentation (causing hardening of the skin). Oxygen intake is decreased in the tissues, causing tissue malnutrition/hypoxia. Ulceration may follow. [1,2,3,4]

Varicose Veins
- Histological studies describe an increase in collagen and fibrous tissue within the layers of the venous wall in varicose vein patients. Collagen bundles disrupt the typical, orderly configuration of smooth muscle cells (SMC) in the medial layer. These SMC are thought to contain an excessive amount of granules, which may secrete collagenase and elastase, resulting in weakening of the venous wall and dilatation. Weakened venous walls allow for dilatation and elongation. [5]
- Varicose veins demonstrate decreased ability to contract normally, and the valves of varicose veins become stretched. [1]
- Tributaries of the great saphenous vein (GSV) are thought to varicose before the main trunk of the GSV because they contain less muscle in their vessel walls and lack support in the subcutaneous fat layer under the skin where they are commonly located. [1]

Pregnancy
- Pregnancy increases the amount of blood circulating in the body and causes veins to enlarge. The pressure of the fetus on the veins can decrease the blood flow back through the pelvic venous system. [1,6,7]

Patient History
- Persistent leg/calf swelling (usually unilateral)
- Previous DVT
- Localized pain, burning, or itching
- Tired, heavy legs after prolonged standing
- Varicose veins
- Skin changes and skin ulcers

Physical Examination
- Edema
- Tenderness, warmth, or redness along the course of a superficial vein or varicosity
- Varicose veins
- Hyperpigmentation, hardened tissue around the ankles
- Ulceration (usually the gaiter area)
- Dermatitis in the gaiter area or area along the course of a superficial vein
- Noticeable telangiectasia
- Venous claudication – severe symptoms of CVI (including those listed above) with pain/aching that worsens when walking and is relieved by elevation of the leg.

Location of Disease
Incompetent valves may be located at any segment of the deep, perforating, or superficial veins but are more commonly found in the superficial venous tributaries. [2]
- Most common location for incompetent perforating veins is the gaiter area – just above the medial malleolus.
- Saphenofemoral junction (SFJ)

Venous PPG Protocol

- Obtain a patient history to include symptoms and risk factors.
- Ensure that the patient is not cold (will result in vasoconstriction).
- Explain the procedure to the patient and ensure they understand their role during the examination.
- Position the patient at the edge of the bed/stretcher with their legs dangling over the side in a non-weight bearing position. Be sure the bed is not compressing the back of the calf.
- Set the PPG monitor to the DC (venous) mode.
- Adhere the PPG sensor to the ankle about 5cm (2") above the medial malleolus (gaiter area) with double stick transparent tape or a Velcro strap. Try not to touch the tape surface under the PPG sensor since fingerprints can degrade the skin/PPG sensor coupling and reduce the signal amplitude. Ensure there will be no movement between the PPG sensor and the skin during the exercise.

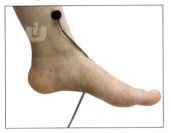

Skin integrity must be checked before placing the PPG sensor. Choose a location that is free of ulceration or hardened skin. Do not place sensor directly on a varicose vein.

Fig. 27-4: Resting venous PPG position

- Turn on the PPG strip chart recorder at a speed of 5mm/sec. Adjust the PPG gain to the machine's midpoint. Set the tracing near the top portion of the chart and establish a stable baseline. Center the PPG tracings on the paper or monitor.
- Ask the patient to begin cycles of plantar flexion (pointing their foot downward) and dorsiflexion (pointing their foot upward). This type of exercise causes contraction of the calf muscles and empties the blood out of the veins in the lower leg.

Demonstrating the exercise for the patient often helps to obtain maximum flexion and correct timing.

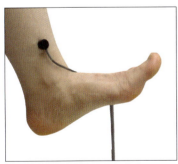 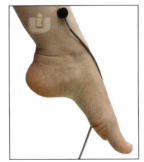

Fig. 27-5: Dorsiflexion of the foot with a PPG sensor.

Fig. 27-6: Plantar flexion of the foot with a PPG sensor.

- If the tracing starts to drift off the page during exercise, readjust the gain and position of the trace.

As an alternative to dorsi- and plantar flexions, manual compressions of the gastrocnemius muscle will empty the blood out of the calf veins. With the patient's legs dangling off the bed, place your thumbs along each side of the tibia and squeeze the back of the patient's calf upward with your remaining fingers. Compress the calf for 1 second, then release the compression for 1 second. Five of these compressions are typically performed.

- The PPG tracing should drop with exercise and then slope slowly upwards once the exercise is completed.
- Let the patient know they can relax while the recording is being taken and analyzed.
- On the tracing, note when the PPG slope either stabilizes by flattening out for at least 5 seconds or peaks and falls slightly. If the tracing is still rising after 20-30 seconds, you can stop the recording since this is past the threshold for reflux.

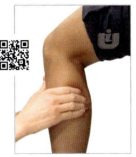

Fig. 27-7: Manual compressions can be used to empty the calf

Remember to keep the speed of the PPG strip chart recorder at 5mm/sec.

- Determine the VRT by calculating the time between the end of the exercise or manual compressions and the peak or beginning of the plateau.

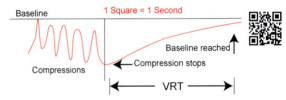

Fig. 27-8: Calculation of a normal VRT (>20 seconds)

- Repeat the exam several times on each leg, with a 1-minute rest period between each attempt. Report the average or mean VRT. The author suggests collecting VRT from three exercises, calculating the sum, dividing this value by 3, and reporting the number as the mean VRT.

If the trace does not oscillate during testing, let the patient rest for about 1 minute and try increasing the gain settings while repeating the exercise. Expect the trace to show "pendulum" flow during exercise.

The next steps of the exam are based on initial VRT results:
- **If the VRT is ≥20 seconds:** Valvular function is normal, and testing is complete.
- **If the VRT is <20 seconds:** Apply a 10-12cm straight pressure cuff (or tourniquet) to the distal thigh to be used to occlude the superficial venous system.
  » Inflate the pressure cuff (or tourniquet) to approximately 50mmHg. This should occlude the GSV in the sitting position while the deep system remains patent.
  » Repeat the exercise and recalculate the VRT.
    - **If the VRT is ≥20 seconds:** testing is complete.

- **If the VRT is <20 seconds:** use a duplex scanner to further evaluate for reflux or apply a 10-12cm straight pressure cuff (or tourniquet) just below the knee to occlude the small saphenous venous system. Repeat the exercise and recalculate the VRT.

Table 27-1: Photoplethysmography Protocol Summary

- Hang the leg over the bedside in a non-weight bearing position. Keep the calf from touching the bed.
- Place the PPG transducer about 5cm (2") above the medial malleolus using double-stick transparent tape or a Velcro strap.
- Turn the recorder on DC (venous) mode and run the PPG tracing at a speed of 5mm/sec.
- Ask the patient to perform 5 cycles of the plantar flexion/dorsiflexion exercise. (Or perform manual compressions if the patient is unable to exercise independently.)
- Wait for the tracing to either rise and plateau, or run for 30 seconds, whichever comes first.
- Calculate the VRT on the recorded trace by counting from the end of the exercise/compression cycle until the tracing reaches a stable baseline or runs for 30 seconds.
- Repeat the exam several times on each leg in order to calculate a mean VRT. Rest about 1 minute between cycles.
- The exam is finished if the mean VRT is ≥20 seconds.

Continue with additional testing or use duplex imaging to further evaluate reflux if the mean VRT is <20 seconds.

- Inflate a pressure cuff (or tourniquet) placed on the distal thigh to 50mmHg.
- Repeat the exercise/compression several times and calculate the mean VRT.
- **The exam is completed if the mean VRT is ≥20 seconds. Continue with additional testing or use duplex imaging to further evaluate reflux if the mean VRT is <20 seconds.**
- Inflate a pressure cuff (or tourniquet) placed on the proximal calf to 50mmHg.
- Repeat the exercise/compression several times and calculate the mean VRT.
- The exam is complete, calculate and report the mean VRT.

PRINCIPLES OF INTERPRETATION

The time it takes is for the calf veins to refill after being emptied (venous recovery time) or VRT is calculated using the PPG tracing by counting the squares on a graph, which each represent 1 second in time.

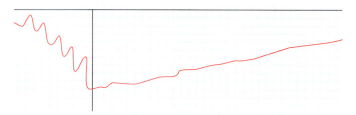

Fig. 27-9: *1 square = 1 second PPG tracing*

Normal

Initial VRT Measurement

VRT ≥20 seconds is considered normal; the venous refill time via the arterial system is within normal limits.

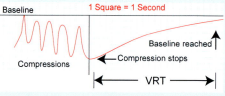

Fig. 27-10: *Calculation of a normal VRT*

Some labs may use normal VRT values as low as 17.

Abnormal

Initial VRT Measurement

- VRT <20 seconds is associated with chronic venous insufficiency (CVI). The calf veins do not empty or fill properly due to venous obstruction and/or incompetent venous valves allowing for retrograde flow (backflow).

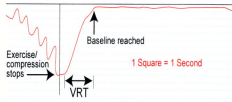

Fig. 27-11: *Calculation of an abnormal VRT (7sec)*

VRT with use of a thigh cuff

- If the mean VRT is <20 seconds without a pressure cuff (or tourniquet) and ≥20 seconds after application of a cuff on the thigh, the diagnosis is primary venous insufficiency or incompetence of the great saphenous system.

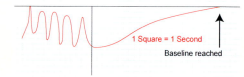

Fig. 27-12: *VRT normalizes with placement of a thigh cuff (20 sec).*

- If the mean VRT remains abnormal <20 seconds with a pressure cuff (or tourniquet) on the thigh, the diagnosis is secondary venous insufficiency or incompetence of the superficial and deep systems.

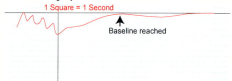

Fig. 27-13: *VRT remains abnormal with placement of a thigh cuff (10 to 11 sec).*

VRT with use of a cuff below the knee

- If the mean VRT <20 seconds with the pressure cuff (or tourniquet) below the knee but ≥20 seconds above the knee, this finding suggests reflux in the small saphenous vein.
- If the mean VRT is <20 seconds with the pressure cuff (or tourniquet) above AND below the knee, venous incompetence is present in the deep venous, great saphenous, and small saphenous.

Table 27-2: Diagnostic Criteria for PPG

Position of pressure cuff or tourniquet	Mean VRT	Location of venous incompetence
None	≥20 sec	None
	<20 sec	Incompetence present (*Test further to determine if superficial or deep)
Distal thigh	≥20 sec	Great saphenous
	<20 sec	Deep and superficial venous system
Proximal calf	≥20 sec	Small saphenous
	<20 sec	Deep and superficial venous systems

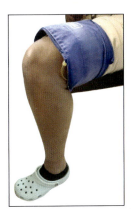 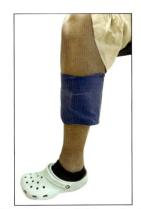

Fig. 27-14: *Pressure cuff positioned on the thigh and calf*

Differential Diagnosis for CVD

- Lymphedema
- Lipedema
- Cellulitis
- Deep venous thrombosis
- Adenopathy
- Arteriovenous fistula
- Direct injury to an extremity
- Mass (including vascularized mass)
- Arteriovenous malformation (AVM)
- Collagen vasculitis
- Abscess
- Peripheral neuritis
- Stasis dermatitis
- Klippel-Trenaunay
- Skin cancer
- Arterial disease

Correlation

- Lower extremity duplex scan for venous insufficiency
- Spectral Doppler reflux testing
- Descending venography

Medical Treatment for CVD

- Promote venous drainage (e.g., elevate legs, wear elastic stockings/support hose)
- Limit long periods of inactivity
- Compression bandaging (for ulceration)
- Proper skin care

Surgical Treatment for CVD

- Ligation (e.g., of saphenofemoral junction)
- Vein stripping
- Subfascial ligation of perforators
- Ambulatory phlebectomy (a.k.a. stab avulsion phlebectomy)

Endovascular Treatment for CVD

- Thermal venous ablation
- Mechanochemical ablation
- Chemical ablation (with visual or ultrasound-guided sclerotherapy)
- Visual or ultrasound-guided sclerotherapy
- Adhesive ablation

REFERENCES

1. Sumner DS, Zierler RE. (2005). Vascular physiology: essential hemodynamic principles. In Rutherford *Vascular Surgery 6th edition*. (75-123). Philadelphia. Elsevier Saunders.
2. Labropoulos N, Leon LR. (2005). Evaluation of chronic venous disease. In Mansour MA, Labropoulos N. (Eds.), Vascular Diagnosis, (447-461). Philadelphia: Elsevier Saunders
3. Zwiebel, WJ (2005). Ultrasound diagnosis of venous insufficiency. In Zwiebel WJ, Pellerito JS (Eds.), Introduction to Vascular Ultrasonography 5th ed, (479-499). Philadelphia: Elsevier Saunders.
4. Meissner MH. (2010). Chronic venous disorders. In Zierler RE (Ed.), Strandess's duplex scanning disorders in vascular diagnosis 4th ed. (223-229).Philadelphia Wolters Kluwer Lippincott Williams & Wilkins.
5. Browse NL, Burnand, KG, Thomas, ML (1988). Disease of the Veins; Pathology, Diagnosis and Treatment, Edward Arnold, a division of Hodder & Stoughton.
6. Meissner MH, Strandess DE. (2005). Pathophysiology and natural history of acute deep venous thrombosis. In *Rutherford Vascular Surgery 6th edition*. (2124-2142). Philadelphia. Elsevier Saunders.
7. Min RJ, Rosenblatt M. US Department of Health and Human Services, Office on Women's Health (2010). Varicose Veins and Spider Veins. Retrieved from http://www.womenshealth.gov/faq/varicose-spider-veins.cfm. (7-7-2010).
8. Eberhardt RT, Raffetto JD. (2005). Contemporary Reviews in Cardiovascular Medicine. Circulation. 111: 2398-2409.

ADDITIONAL REFERENCES

9. Barnes RW, Garrett WV, Hummel BA, et al: (AAMI 13th Annual Meeting, March 1978) Photoplethysmographic assessment of altered cutaneous circulation in the post-phlebitic syndrome. In Technology in Diagnosis and Therapy. (25). Washington, DC.
10. Abramowitz HB., Queral LA., Flinn WR., et al. (1979). The use of photoplethysmography in the assessment of venous insufficiency: a comparison to venous pressure measurements. *Surgery 86*, 434 – 441.
11. Li JM., Anderson FA., Wheeler HB. (1983). Non-invasive testing for venous reflux using photoplethysmography: Standardization of technique and evaluation of interpretation criteria. *Bruit [J Vasc Technol]* 7, 25 – 29.
12. Needham TN., Jury P., Hoare M. (1983). Photoplethysmographic refilling time: The relationship between the initial rate of refilling and venous incompetence. *Bruit [J Vasc Technol]* 7, 18 – 21.

28. Lower Extremity Venous Duplex Ultrasound

Definition
The combination of real time B-mode ultrasonography with spectral Doppler and color flow to evaluate the lower extremity veins for evidence of a venous thrombus or aneurysm. Typically, venous compression studies are a component of these exams.

Venous duplex ultrasound can identify the presence, exact location and extent of venous thrombosis.

Risk Factors
- Age (greater with advanced age)
- Immobilization
- Genetic prothrombotic conditions (clotting disorders, such as Factor V Leiden)
- Post-operative phase (especially after orthopedic surgery)
- Central venous or femoral catheters
- Female
- Pregnancy
- Oral contraceptives
- Estrogen replacement
- Cancer/malignancy
- Previous DVT
- Heart complications (MI, CHF, etc.)
- Obesity

Indications for Exam
- Edema/swelling (especially when unilateral)
- Limb pain/tenderness
- Symptoms of a pulmonary embolism (PE; shortness of breath, chest pain, hemoptysis)
- Ulceration (especially in gaiter area)
- Discoloration in the gaiter area
- Varicose veins
- Hypercoagulable state
- Pallor (phlegmasia alba dolens)
- Cyanosis (phlegmasia cerulea dolens)
- Positive D-dimer test result

Contraindications/Limitations
- Poor visualization due to vessel depth because of obesity or severe edema.
- Open wounds prohibiting ultrasound transducer placement along the length of the vessels.
- Non-removable casts or bandaging that interfere with the placement of the ultrasound transducer.
- Patients who cannot be adequately positioned.

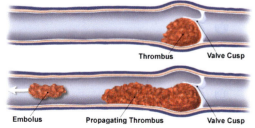

Fig. 28-1: Thrombosis of the vein showing an embolus breaking free.

Mechanism of Disease [1,2]
Three factors: vein wall injury, hypercoagulability and the stasis of blood flow are responsible for venous thrombosis according to Virchow's Triad theory. The presence of one or more of these three factors increases the risk for venous thrombosis.

- There is a balance between coagulation (process to prevent excessive bleeding after injury) and anticoagulation (process to prevent spontaneous intravascular clotting) in normal blood flow.
- The venous endothelial layer is normally antithrombotic. In response to endothelial injury, leukocytes (white blood cells) attach to the vessel wall. A plasma protein known as *prothrombin* is activated. Prothrombin activator catalyzes conversion of prothrombin into thrombin. Thrombin acts as an enzyme to convert fibrinogen into fibrin threads, forming a clot.
- Hypercoagulable states result from genetic mutation or acquired deficiencies that accompany certain diseases (e.g., liver disease). In such cases, naturally occurring anticoagulants (antithrombin, protein C, protein S, etc.) are deficient. For example, the genetic mutation, factor V Leiden, causes resistance to the natural anticoagulant protein C.
- Non-movement of blood flow (stasis) permits coagulation. Platelets are thought to become trapped due to flow recirculation behind the valve cusps. Platelets adhere to the subendothelial (collagen) layer of the venous wall and may aggregate depending on the amount of coagulation and thrombolysis occurring in the body at that time.
- Increased activation of coagulation factors in those suffering from cancer is thought to lead to formation of venous thrombosis. In addition, the levels of coagulation inhibitors normally found in the blood (e.g., proteins C or S) are thought to be reduced in these patients.
- Thrombosis in pregnancy is attributed to a prothrombotic state along with decreased venous outflow by the weight of the fetus. The use of estrogen (in replacement therapy or contraceptives) alters coagulation and may predispose an individual to thrombosis.
- The left leg has a higher incidence of DVT than the right leg. The major reason is that the left common iliac vein crosses under the right common iliac artery, which can compress the vein and cause thrombosis. This is known as *iliac compression syndrome* (formerly May-Thurner). [11]
- Venous aneurysms are a rare condition. Research suggests several possible causes; either an increase or decrease in the fibrous connective tissue and elastic fibers or decreased smooth muscle cells and an increase in fibrous connective tissue. [3]
- Once a thrombus of sufficient size has formed, it can:
  » **Stabilize:** Stabilized thrombi firmly adhere to the vessel wall and do not move or propagate. If a thrombus forms, the most favorable occurrence would be stabilization. This minimizes the risk of embolization and a PE.
  » **Propagate:** Propagation includes "growth of the thrombus" in size or location. Examples of propagation include a thrombus that extends from the superficial system into the deep system or from a calf vein into the popliteal vein.
  » **Embolize:** A portion of a thrombus breaks free and is carried by the flowing blood through the vessels until it becomes lodged in a smaller vessel resulting in an obstruction. Emboli can become wedged in pulmonary vessels, creating an extremely high-risk factor for PE.

Patient History
- Acute onset of leg pain
- Acute onset of swelling
- Persistent leg/calf swelling (usually unilateral, but can be bilateral)
- Symptoms of PE (e.g., shortness of breath, chest pain, hemoptysis)
- Previous DVT
- Clotting issues (e.g., problems with anticoagulation therapy, malignant cancer)
- Recent periods of immobilization (e.g., bed rest, long plane or car ride)
- Post-operative (e.g., orthopedic or neurosurgery; can occur anytime during surgery or the 6 months thereafter)
- Covid-19
- Smoking
- COPD
- Blood type, (highest risk with type-A lowest risk with type-O)
- Trauma
- Antiphospholipid antibodies (e.g., lupus)
- Occupations requiring long periods of standing or sitting
- Varicose veins
- Congenital abnormalities (e.g., Klippel-Trenaunay)
- Inflammatory bowel disease
- Drug abuse
- Cerebrovascular events (stroke, transient ischemic attack (TIA))
- Iliac compression syndrome
- Elevated D-dimer levels (D-dimer is a degradation product of fibrin polymers, biomarker for ongoing thrombus formation and fibrinolysis)

Physical Examination
- Edema or swelling
- Tenderness
- Limb redness or warmth (superficial thrombophlebitis)
- Varicose veins
- Hyperpigmentation, hardened tissue around the ankles
- Ulceration (especially in the gaiter area)
- Pallor (phlegmasia alba dolens)
- Cyanosis (phlegmasia cerulea dolens)

Location of Disease

A thrombus within the deep veins is referred to as a Deep Venous Thrombosis (DVT). A thrombus within the superficial veins is referred to as a superficial venous thrombosis.

Although a thrombus can develop at any venous site, the more common sites are the:
- Muscular veins (gastrocnemius and soleal sinus)
- Valves (behind the cusps)
- Venous confluences
- Inferior vena cava
- Iliac veins
- Deep venous system of the lower extremity: common femoral, deep femoral, femoral, popliteal, peroneal, posterior tibial
- Superficial venous system of the lower extremity (great and small saphenous veins)
- Perforators (especially in the lower extremity)

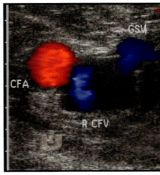
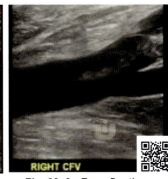

Fig. 28-2: A thrombus in the common femoral vein at the saphenofemoral junction that partially blocks blood flow.

Fig. 28-3: Free-floating venous thrombus: free-floating tail located in the common femoral vein.

Lower Extremity Venous Duplex Protocol
- Obtain a patient history that includes symptoms and risk factors for venous thrombosis. Explain the procedure to the patient.
- Assist the patient as they get into a supine position with their head elevated. Placing the bed in a reverse Trendelenburg position may optimize the exam when visualization is difficult, as it increases the size of the calf veins.

Vessel size can be affected by the incline of the bed and room temperature. Putting a patient in the reverse Trendelenburg position can improve visibility of small veins (e.g., calf veins).

- For some patients it may be necessary to use a range of transducers. Typically, high-frequency (5-7MHz or 8-15MHz) transducers are used in conjunction with low frequency (1-4MHz) transducers.
- It is possible for only one vein of a pair to be thrombosed. For this reason, it is important to make sure all veins are studied carefully.

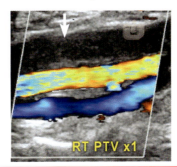

Fig. 28-4: No color flow in the top vein (longitudinal) indicates thrombosis in one of the paired posterior tibial veins.

Superficial venous thrombosis can occur with or without inflammation. There are several terms used to describe venous issues which are sometimes used incorrectly. Thrombophlebitis is defined as inflammation of a vein associated with a blood clot. Phlebitis simply means inflammation of a vein and can exist without thrombus.

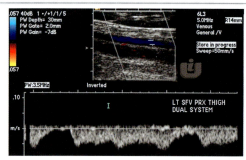

Fig. 28-5: *Spectral Doppler waveform analysis is important for a dual venous system. The waveform for the superior vein is typical for venous blood flow. No color flow is present in the inferior vein suggesting venous occlusion.*

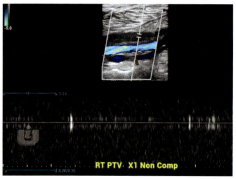

Fig. 28-6: *No color flow or spectral Doppler in one paired vein.*

Transverse Scan and Images

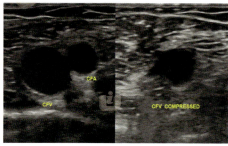

Fig. 28-7: *Compression of a normal common femoral vein. Left: Vein prior to compression. Right: The compressed vein has collapsed.*

Vein compression at the distal thigh is sometimes difficult. Try placing one hand under the thigh while compressing the vein with the transducer or push your hand up against the transducer to compress the vein.

- Compressions should always be performed when imaging in the transverse plane to ensure full compression and to avoid missing duplicated veins. The best B-mode images are obtained when the transducer is kept at a 90° angle to the skin.
- Veins can usually be imaged from a medial view or "window." Move the transducer distally performing venous compression every 2-4cm while watching for the vein to fully collapse.
- Transverse images are to be captured using "dual-screen." Obtain and freeze an image without vein compression on the left side of the screen. Capture an image with vein compression on the right side of the screen. Capture transverse images with and without compressions as described above for the following veins:
  » **Common femoral vein** (CFV): above the saphenofemoral junction. Locate the common femoral vein and artery at the groin above the saphenofemoral junction in the transverse (short axis) plane. A normal vein will collapse with light to moderate transducer pressure, while the artery remains open. Observe for the vein to completely collapse upon compression.
  » **Saphenofemoral junction** (SFJ): image includes the common femoral vein and proximal end of the great saphenous vein (GSV). Continue scanning the GSV down the leg when appropriate.

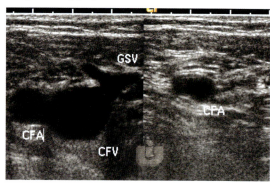

Fig. 28-8: *Compression of the saphenofemoral junction. On the left of the dual screen image is the uncompressed saphenofemoral junction and on the right the veins are compressed.*

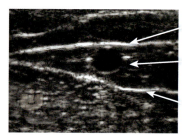

Fig. 28-9: *Fascial components of the saphenous compartment* [8]

Superficial veins course within the superficial compartment, above the deep muscular fascia. A vein located outside of the saphenous compartment is known as a tributary and is not a main vein. It is important for the physician to know whether the vein in question is a tributary or within the saphenous compartment.

  » **Proximal deep femoral vein** (DFV)

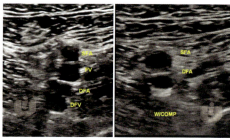

Fig. 28-10: *Compression near the junction of the femoral vein and deep femoral vein. On the left of the dual-screen image are the veins prior to compression. On the right, the femoral veins are compressed.*

» **Proximal femoral vein** (FV)

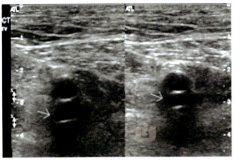

Fig. 28-11: *Compression of a thrombosed femoral vein. The femoral vein is partially incompressible on the right.*

» **Mid femoral vein**
» **Distal femoral vein**: try a medial to posterior window if visualization is difficult with the medial window or change to a lower frequency transducer.

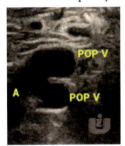

Fig. 28-12: *Duplicated popliteal venous system*

Femoral and popliteal veins are commonly duplicated.

» **Popliteal vein** (PopV): for best visualization move the transducer behind the knee using a posterior approach. To scan the entire popliteal vein, it is often best to start in the middle at the crease of the knee and move proximally to the femoral vein and then distally to the tibial-peroneal confluence.

When scanning the popliteal vein, the patient may be placed in the prone position.

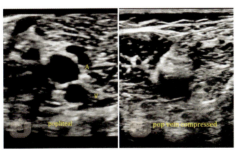

Fig. 28-13: *Compression of the popliteal vein. On the left of the dual screen image is the popliteal vein prior to compression. On the right, the popliteal vein is compressed.*

» **Posterior tibial veins** (PTV): place the transducer posterior to the medial malleolus and use color flow as a guide to locate these veins alongside their artery.

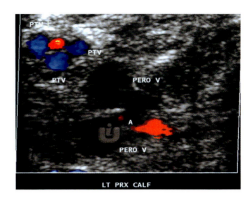

Fig. 28-14: *Color flow is present indicating venous blood flow in the posterior tibial veins. No color is present in one peroneal vein suggesting venous occlusion.*

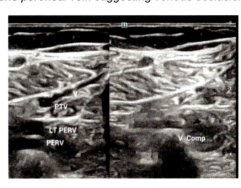

Fig. 28-15: *Compression of the tibial veins. On the left of the dual screen image are the tibial veins prior to compression. On the right, the tibial veins are compressed.*

» **Peroneal veins** (PerV): the peroneal veins can be seen using a medial window superficial to the fibula and deep to the posterior tibial veins. They can also be visualized using a posterolateral approach alongside the fibula.

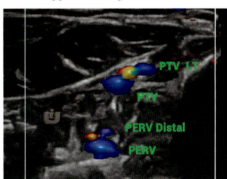

Fig. 28-16: *Color Doppler image of tibial veins and arteries.*

- Images need to be captured for each of the vein segments listed regardless of whether or not they collapse when compressed.
- Documentation of venous compression can also be obtained for the common and external iliac, great and small saphenous, gastrocnemius, soleal or anterior tibial veins when appropriate.

Longitudinal Scan and Images

Use venous presets on the duplex scanner. Low color and Doppler scales will be needed to detect flow.

- On one image, record both a color image of the vein in longitudinal and the spectral Doppler waveform.

- The Doppler sample gate should be set in the center of the flow stream with the gate set approximately 2-4mm wide. Spectral documentation should illustrate spontaneity (automatic Doppler signal), respiratory variation and phasicity (flow increases and decreases with respiration).

Some labs record venous spectral Doppler waveforms without setting an angle since actual velocities are usually not important in a venous exam. If your lab chooses to set an angle, use a Doppler angle ≤60° with the cursor placed parallel to the vessel walls in the center of the flow stream.

- The spectral trace needs to show both non-augmented and augmented flow. Slow the sweep speed down on the spectral trace to capture more information as needed.
- Document venous flow in the following segments:
  » **Common femoral vein:** either above or at the saphenofemoral junction. Augment the signal using a distal compression of the thigh or calf.
  » **SFJ:** Augment the signal using a distal compression of the thigh or calf.
  » **Deep femoral vein:** using a medial approach (patient's leg is turned outward), begin at the distal CFV and move the transducer distally to observe the DFV which lies deep to the femoral vein. Augment the signal using a compression of the thigh (not the calf).
  » **Proximal femoral vein:** using a medial approach and color Doppler, capture an image of the femoral vein alone in the proximal thigh or at the junction of the femoral vein and the DFV. Record a FV Doppler waveform, while augmenting the signal using a compression of the calf.

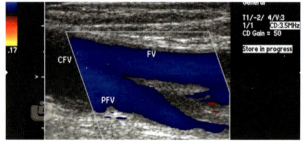

Fig. 28-17: *Femoral vein bifurcation*

  » **Mid and distal femoral vein:** Using a medial approach and color Doppler, capture an image of the femoral vein in the mid and distal thigh. Record a FV Doppler waveforms while augmenting the signal using a compression of the calf.

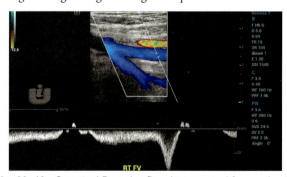

Fig. 28-18: *Spectral Doppler flow in a normal femoral vein.*

  » **Mid popliteal vein:** Use a posterior approach with the transducer behind the knee. Record a mid PopV Doppler waveform while augmenting the signal using a compression of the calf.
- When necessary, you can document patency of the inferior vena cava, the common and external iliac veins, the great saphenous, small saphenous and tibial veins.
- If veins are duplicated, spectral Doppler waveforms may need to be recorded for each vein individually.
- To confirm the absence of flow, use spectral Doppler for each vein segment suspected of being thrombosed. Lack of flow will compliment compression, color flow and B-mode images that indicate the vein is occluded. Accompanying arteries are helpful in locating concomitant occluded veins.
- Repeat for the contralateral extremity if a bilateral exam was ordered.
- If a unilateral exam was requested, B-mode and color flow images of the contralateral CFV with and without compression, as well as spectral Doppler waveforms, should be recorded for comparison purposes.

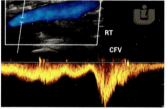 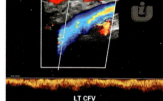

Fig. 28-19: *Comparing the Doppler waveform from the bilateral CFV is important. The right CFV waveform shows normal phasicity and augmentation while the left CFV waveform shows decreased phasicity and no augmentation.*

Include incidental findings, such as tissue edema or enlarged lymph nodes. Findings may be contributing to the patient's symptoms.

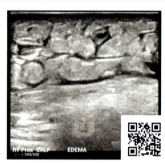 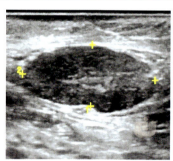

Fig. 28-20: *B-mode image of lower extremity superficial tissue edema.*

Fig. 28-21: *B-mode image of an enlarged lymph node.*

Table 28-1: **Lower Extremity Venous Protocol Summary**

Scan transverse (short axis) with and without compression in B-mode and color flow	Scan longitudinal (sagittal axis) with spectral Doppler and B-mode
• CFV • Saphenofemoral junction • Proximal DFV • Proximal FV • Mid FV • Distal FV • PopV • PTV • PerV	• CFV • DFV • FV • PopV

- Additional documentation of compression and spectral Doppler waveforms may be recorded in additional venous segments such as the GSV.
- If venous compressions are contraindicated due to anatomy or patient discomfort, document patency with color.

PRINCIPLES OF INTERPRETATION

B-mode Imaging
- Use B-mode imaging to determine if a thrombus is present:
  » Confirm the vein collapses completely with light transducer pressure.
  » Look for echogenic material present within the lumen of the vein.
- It is possible for only one vein of a pair to be thrombosed. For this reason, it is important to make sure all veins are studied carefully.

Color Doppler
- Use color Doppler to determine if color flow is present wall-to-wall or if there is a filling defect.

Spectral Doppler Waveforms
Use spectral Doppler to determine if venous flow is:
- **Spontaneous:** Automatically hear a Doppler signal due to blood flow, no compression required
- **Phasic:** Flow increases and decreases with respiration
- **Augmentable:** Flow increases with distal compression
- **Pulsatile:** regular, rhythmic increase and decrease in the flow signal, similar to an arterial pulsation.

Interpretation/Diagnostic Criteria

Normal

B-mode Imaging
- The vein is free of echogenic material and compresses completely when it is technically possible to compress the vein.

Color Doppler
- Wall-to-wall color flow will fill the vein spontaneously and upon distal compression.

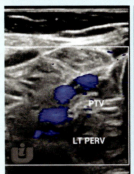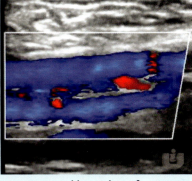

Fig. 28-22: *Transverse and long view of normal tibial veins with color flow.*

Spectral Doppler Waveforms
- **Spontaneous:** Expect to automatically hear a Doppler signal due to blood flow above the knee, (no compression required).
- **Phasicity:** Venous flow is phasic and varies with the respiratory and cardiac cycles. Due to intrathoracic pressure changes during respiration, venous flow decreases during deep inhalation and increases during exhalation. In the calf veins, the absence of phasic flow is a normal finding since blood flow is more dependent on muscle contraction than respiration.

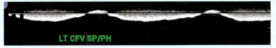

Fig. 28-23: *Normal spectral Doppler waveform with spontaneous and phasic flow.*

- **Augmentation:** Compression of the limb distal to the transducer augments (increases) venous flow at the level of the transducer.

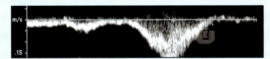

Fig. 28-24: *Distal compression producing augmentation.*

- **Pulsatility:** Absent usually in the lower extremity veins.

Abnormal

Dilatation of the lower extremity venous system can be due to portal hypertension.

B-mode Imaging
- Intralumenal echoes are visualized within the vein and the vein is not completely compressible.
- The vein is partially compressible when the lumen is partially obstructed and incompressible when the lumen is completely obstructed.[12]
- Collapse of the artery with transducer pressure can be a confirmation of an incompressible venous segment.

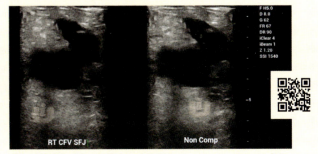

Fig. 28-25: *The CFV and GSV are non-compressible at the SJF in this dual screen image.*

Thrombus

If a thrombus is present, determine
- Location (by B-mode)
- Whether the thrombus is partially or completely occlusive
- Extent (by B-mode and color flow)
- Characteristics of the thrombus by B-mode (echogenicity; acute, chronic, re-canalization free-floating versus attached to the wall, recanalization etc.)

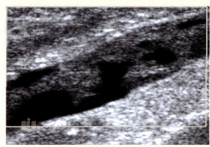

Fig. 28-26: *B-mode image of a venous thrombus which is partially obstructing the vein.*

Age of Thrombus

- **Acute thrombus:** Typical characteristics include medium to lightly echogenic spongy texture, or anechoic, with poor attachment to the vein wall or thrombus that is noted to be "free floating" within the lumen. The moving tail is usually seen at the end of the thrombus. When a vein is fully thrombosed, the cross-sectional area has usually increased, (in an acute event) making the vein larger than the adjacent artery. [1,3,7]

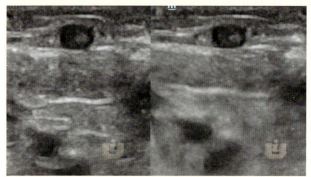

Fig. 28-27: *Incompressible GSV on B-mode image. Aging clot can be difficult if thrombus echogenicity appears mixed and the vein appears only slightly dilated.*

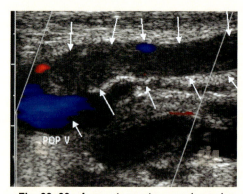

Fig. 28-28: *An acute gastrocnemius vein thrombus extending into the popliteal vein.*

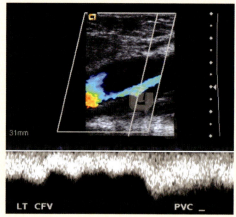

Fig. 28-29: *A longitudinal view of an acute DVT. Partially obstructing blood flow can still produce a spontaneous, phasic signal with augmentation.*

- **Chronic thrombus:** Typical characteristics include brightly echogenic or heterogeneous echoes, irregular surface texture and thrombus that is attached to the venous wall with no signs of floating flaps. The vein can stay the same size as the artery, but often contracts in diameter over time. Collateral veins may be observed adjacent to the affected vein(s) and small irregular flow channels within the thrombus can sometimes be seen with color.

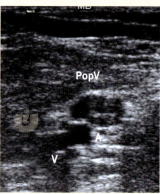
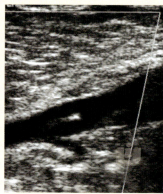

Fig. 28-30: *A transverse view of a partially occlusive chronic DVT in the popliteal vein.*

Fig. 28-31: *A longitudinal view of a chronic DVT in the popliteal that is partially obstructing blood flow.*

The term, chronic postthrombotic change has been suggested as a replacement for "chronic thrombus". The SRU has suggested that only acute events should be referred to as "acute thrombus". When it is technically difficult to determine whether findings are acute/chronic, use the term "indeterminate". [12]

- **Indeterminate age:** Characteristics of both acute and chronic stages may be present, making age difficult to determine. [12] (*Fig. 28-28*).
  » *Subacute* is another term used by some labs. Reports have suggested using this term only to describe thrombus that appears to have changed appearance on B-mode compared to a previous study where the diagnosis of acute DVT was made some weeks earlier.

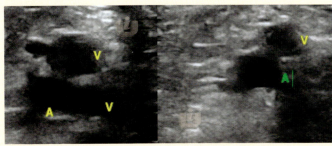

Fig. 28-32: *Indeterminate age of thrombus. The vein is the same size as the artery and the intraluminal echoes appear mixed.*

Table 28-2: **Thrombosis Descriptions and Characteristics**	
Acute	**Chronic**
Light to medium echogenic/anechoic	Bright/heterogeneous echoes
Spongy texture on compression (Homogeneous)	Irregular texture (Heterogeneous)
Poorly attached or free floating	Attached
Dilated vein (if totally occluded)	Same or smaller diameter than that of the artery
	Collateral veins may be observed

- Veins can be partially or totally incompressible in both acute and chronic stages.
- Combination of events can occur (e.g., acute thrombus on top of a chronic thrombus).
- Chronic thrombus with partial recanalization is seen as a thrombus with small color flow channels.
- Age of thrombus is sometimes indeterminate.

Color Doppler
- If a thrombus does not completely inhibit blood flow, color flow will be seen flowing around echogenic material in the vein spontaneously or with distal compression.
- If a totally obstructive thrombus is present, color flow will not be observed even with distal limb compression using the appropriate low-flow machine settings.

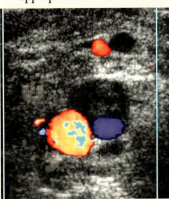

Fig. 28-33: *Color Doppler image of a thrombus in the popliteal vein. Color flow indicates that the thrombus is partially obstructing blood flow.*

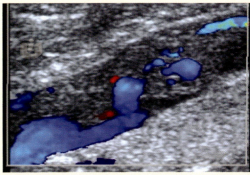

Fig. 28-34: *Color Doppler image of an irregular thrombus in the CFV. Note echogenic material in the CFV by B-mode with color flowing around the thrombus indicating a partial obstruction.*

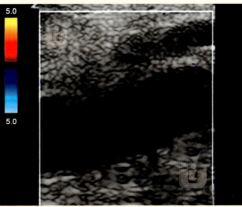

Fig. 28-35: *Color Doppler image of an occluded vein. No color flow indicates that the thrombus has occluded the vein.*

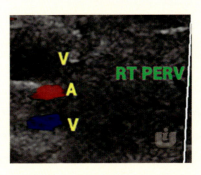

Fig. 28-36: *Transverse view of one of two occluded peroneal veins. The absence of color flow within one vein suggests that the vein has occluded.*

Spectral Doppler Waveforms
- **Spontaneity:** Absence of flow indicates venous obstruction. Use color flow in the adjacent artery as a guide to identify an occluded vein. But always confirm the absence of flow by placing the sample volume in the vessel while using Doppler.
- **Phasicity:** Continuous venous flow (does not vary with respiratory and cardiac cycles) suggests either obstruction from DVT in a proximal venous segment or extrinsic compression of a proximal vein. Partially occlusive thrombus can still produce spontaneous, phasic signals with augmentation.

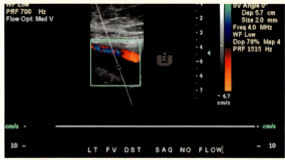

Fig. 28-38: *Color Doppler image and spectral waveform of an occluded vein. The absence of color flow and no spectral waveform (no flow) indicates that the thrombus has totally occluded the vein.*

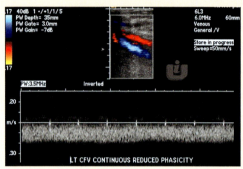

Fig. 28-39: *Spectral Doppler image of the CFV. Continuous venous flow (reduced phasicity) in the CFV indicating proximal obstruction or extrinsic compression.*

- **Augmentation:** If distal compression does not produce augmentation of the venous signal, a total obstruction at or distal to the transducer is suspected. A weak or dampened augmentation suggests there is a venous obstruction distal to the transducer, but it does not occlude the vessel. If the augmentation is weak or undetectable, changing the patient's position and/or compressing a more muscular area of the leg may increase the augmentation. Allow time for venous refill before compressing a second time. A normal Doppler signal can be produced proximal to a dual venous system when only one vein is thrombosed, or if large collateral veins are present.

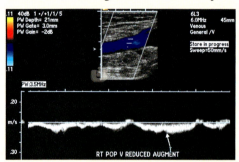

Fig. 28-40: *Spectral Doppler of the popliteal vein. The flow is not augmented by distal compression indicating venous obstruction distal to the transducer.*

- **Pulsatility:** Pulsatile venous flow is present in the legs when right sided heart disease, a distal fistula and/or a hypervolemic state is present.

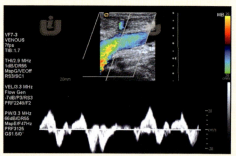

Fig. 28-41: *Spectral Doppler of the CFV with pulsatile venous flow indicating right sided heart disease, a distal fistula and/or a hypervolemic state is present.*

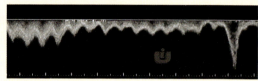

Fig. 28-42: *Pulsatile venous spectral Doppler signal.*

Table 28-3: Venous Duplex Diagnostic Criteria	
Normal	**Abnormal**
Complete collapse of vein walls with light transducer pressure	Lack of complete vein compression
Absent intralumenal thrombus	Intralumenal echoes present (acute thrombus can be echolucent)
Color flow fills the lumen completely	Decrease or absence of color flow
Normal venous Doppler spontaneity, phasicity and augmentation	Abnormal venous Doppler spontaneity, phasicity or augmentation
No venous dilatation	Dilated or contracted veins noted

Other Pathology

Extrinsic Compression

Extrinsic compression by a tumor or pulsations from an adjacent artery can cause a venous stenosis. When high venous velocities are present compared to the proximal segment with a venous velocity ratio >2.5, a venous stenosis >50% secondary to compression is suspected. Post-stenotic turbulence and distal segments with continuous venous waveforms support this finding.[13]

Venous Aneurysms

Venous aneurysm: a region in the vein where the lumen has become significantly larger than that of the proximal segment.[3]

Venous aneurysms are less common in the lower extremity than they are in the upper extremity.[9]

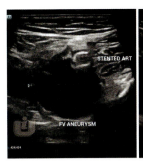
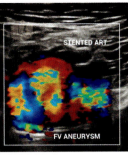

Fig. 28-43: *Venous aneurysm*

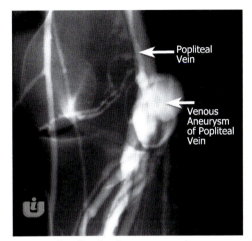

Fig. 28-44: *Popliteal vein aneurysm by venography*

Differential Diagnosis

- Arterial disease
- Lymphedema
- Lipedema
- Cellulitis
- Cysts (e.g., popliteal, Baker's)
- Extrinsic compression
- Hematoma
- Muscle tear
- Joint effusion
- Adenopathy
- Arteriovenous fistula
- Heart failure (edema)
- Direct injury to extremity
- Vascularized mass
- Collagen vasculitis
- Abscess

Correlation

- Venogram
- MRI
- Computed Tomography (CT) scan

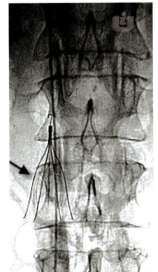

Fig. 28-45: *Inferior vena cavagram showing an IVC filter*

Medical Treatment and Prevention

- Anticoagulation therapy (e.g., heparin, warfarin)
- DVT prophylaxis (e.g., intermittent pneumatic cuff compression)
  » The Caprini Risk Score assesses DVT risk with questions that divide patients into low, moderate, and high risk. Perform the assessment at **caprinirikscore.org**
- Limit long periods of inactivity
- Promote venous return (e.g., elevate legs, wear elastic stockings/support hose)
- Compression bandaging (for ulceration)

Surgical Treatment

- Iliofemoral venous thrombectomy
- Bypass grafting (caval occlusion)
- Surgical ligation/excision/bypass (aneurysms)

Endovascular Treatment

- IVC filter (for acute DVT)
- Catheter-directed thrombolysis with Urokinase, etc. (for acute DVT)
- Balloon venoplasty and stenting (for chronic iliofemoral DVT)
- Mechanical thrombectomy (e.g., Angiojet; acute DVT)

REFERENCES

1. Wakefield TW. (2005). Bleeding and clotting: fundamental considerations. In Rutherford Vascular Surgery 6th edition. (493-511). Philadelphia. Elsevier Saunders.
2. Guyton AC. (1986). Hemostasis and blood coagulation. In Textbook of Medical Physiology 7th edition. (76-86). Philadelphia: WB Saunders.
3. Gillespie DL, Villavicencio JL, Gallagher C, Chang A, Hamelink JK, Fiala LA, O'Donnell SD, Jackson MR, Pikoulis E, Rich, NM. (1997). Presentation and management of venous aneurysms. *J Vasc Surg.* Nov;26(5):845-52.
4. Thrush A, Hartshorne T. (2005). Duplex assessment of deep venous thrombosis and upper limb venous disorders. In Peripheral Vascular Ultrasound, How Why and When, 2nd ed. (189-206). Edinburgh: Elsevier Churchill Livingstone.
5. Zwiebel, WJ (2005). Ultrasound Diagnosis of Venous Thrombosis. In Zwiebel WJ, Pellerito JS (Eds.), *Introduction to Vascular Ultrasonography 5th ed*, (449-465). Philadelphia: Elsevier Saunders.
6. Meissner MH. (2005). Venous duplex scanning. In Rutherford Vascular Surgery 6th edition. (254-270). Philadelphia. Elsevier Saunders.
7. Myers K, Clough A. (2004). Venous thrombosis in the lower limbs. In Making sense of vascular ultrasound: A hands on guide. (181-197). London: Hodder Arnold.
8. Dawson DL, Beals H. (2010). Acute lower extremity deep venous thrombosis. In Zierler RE (Ed.), Strandess's duplex scanning disorders in vascular diagnosis 4th ed. (179-198).Philadelphia Wolters Kluwer Lippincott Williams & Wilkins.
9. Sumner DS, Mattos MA. (1993). Diagnosis of deep vein thrombosis with real-time color and duplex scanning. In Vascular Diagnosis 4th edition. (785-800). St. Louis. Mosby.
10. Gloviczki P, Yao, JST (Eds.) (2001). Handbook of Venous Disorders, 2nd ed. (p. 38) London: Arnold.
11. Gloviczki P, Cho JS. (2005) Surgical treatment of chronic occlusions of the iliac veins and the superior vena cava. In Rutherford Vascular Surgery 6th edition. (2303-2320). Philadelphia. Elsevier Saunders.
12. Needleman, L., Cronan, J. J., Lilly, M. P., Merli, G. J., Adhikari, S., Hertzberg, B. S., DeJong, M. R., Streiff, M. B., & Meissner, M. H. (2018). Ultrasound for Lower Extremity Deep Venous Thrombosis: Multidisciplinary Recommendations From the Society of Radiologists in Ultrasound Consensus Conference. Circulation, 137(14), 1505–1515. https://doi.org/10.1161/CIRCULATIONAHA.117.030687
13. Labropoulos, N., Borge, M., Pierce, K., & Pappas, P. J. (2007). Criteria for defining significant central vein stenosis with duplex ultrasound. Journal of vascular surgery, 46(1), 101–107. https://doi.org/10.1016/j.jvs.2007.02.062

VENOUS TESTING
29. Lower Extremity Venous Insufficiency Duplex

 For more in-depth interpretation, refer to the *Inside Ultrasound Venous Vascular Reference Guide, 2nd Edition.* insideultrasound.com

Definition
The combination of real time B-mode ultrasonography, spectral Doppler and color flow to evaluate the lower extremity veins for evidence of valvular incompetence. Chronic venous insufficiency (CVI) is caused by incompetent valves in the superficial and/or deep venous system and can result in venous hypertension and stasis.

Rationale
Reflux means to "flow backward." Venous reflux is venous flow moving in the wrong direction, either away from the heart or from the deep to the superficial system through the perforating veins. Duplex ultrasound can identify the presence, exact location, extent, and severity of venous reflux.

Approximately 25% of American women and 15% of American men suffer from some type of varicose veins (VV). Higher estimates have also been reported. [12,13]

Etiology of Chronic Venous Insufficiency
- Genetic
- History of venous thrombosis
- Venous hypertension, caused by valve damage or dysfunction

Risk Factors
- Age (greater with advanced age)
- Previous deep vein thrombosis (DVT)
- Female
- Pregnancy
- Obesity
- Family history
- Occupations requiring long period of standing or sitting
- Congenital abnormalities (e.g., Klippel-Trenaunay)

Approximately 2-5% of Americans suffer from venous insufficiency. [14]
Approximately 500,000 Americans suffer from venous ulceration. [10]

Indications for Exam
- Varicose veins
- Chronic edema/swelling which worsens at the end of the day (especially when unilateral)
- Pain, which may be localized to a specific varix or described as a "dull ache"
- Discoloration at the gaiter area
- Ulceration (gaiter area)
- Worsening pain on walking may be venous claudication. (esp. with chronic evidence of any other indications in this list)
- Restless leg syndrome

Venous claudication is pain upon walking, which is relieved with leg elevation.

Contraindications/Limitations
- Poor visualization due to vessel depth because of obesity or severe edema
- Ulcerations prohibiting access by the ultrasound transducer
- Patients with extensive bandages or casts
- Patient's inability to stand for an extended period of time or the inability to place the patient in extreme reversed Trendelenburg position with available equipment

Mechanism of Disease
Venous Flow with Normal Valve Function [1]
- The direction of normal blood flow in the deep and superficial veins is toward the heart. In the perforating (communicating) veins, blood normally flows from the superficial to the deep veins.

Superficial veins course within the superficial compartment, above the deep muscular fascia. A vein located outside of the saphenous compartment is known as a tributary and is not a main vein. It is important for the physician to know whether the vein in question is a tributary or within the saphenous compartment.

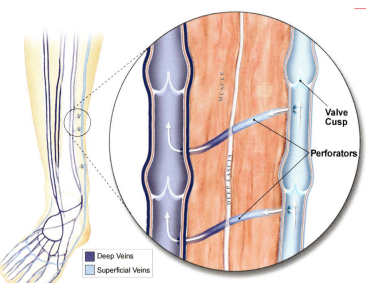

Fig. 29-1: Perforator Venous System (connection between the deep and superficial systems)

Studies have shown that a perforator diameter >3-4mm is indicative of venous incompetence. [10]

- At various times, the blood may encounter pressure to move backwards away from the heart, for example in response to gravity. Normally, flow reversal is prevented by the venous valves which close in response to the pressure from the reversed flow.
- Upon exercise, the action of the calf muscles normally sends blood up the leg away from the calf. This action empties the calf veins, reduces the blood volume and reduces venous pressure.

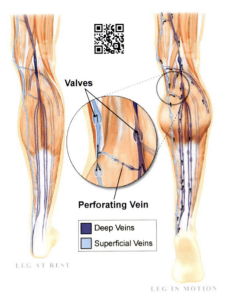

Fig. 29-2: *The calf muscle pump drives venous flow. While walking, muscle contractions squeeze the veins initiating venous blood flow. Venous flow opens the venous valves allowing the blood to flow towards the heart. As the muscle relaxes, valves close to prevent the backward flow of blood (reflux).*

Venous Flow with Abnormal Valve Function

- Valvular damage and dysfunction (valvular incompetence) result in *venous reflux*, which is venous flow in the wrong direction, away from the heart.
- In the perforating veins, blood flows in the wrong direction from the deep to the superficial system.
- Venous reflux creates a high blood volume in the veins distal to the incompetent valve(s).[1] High blood volume in a vein causes increased venous pressure (*venous hypertension*).[1] Hypertension will be greatest upon standing due to the effect of hydrostatic pressure from gravity, adding to the increased pressure from volume.[1]
- Normally, venous blood volume and venous pressure are reduced by activation of the calf muscle pump upon walking. When the valves are not working, the venous volume and resulting pressure do not reduce sufficiently and the patient suffers from *ambulatory venous hypertension*.[1]
- Venous hypertension also increases pressure within the venules and capillaries. This high-pressure system encourages fluids to escape into the tissues causing edema.[1]
- Local edema results in a decrease in fluid and protein reabsorption. Fibrinogen and red blood cells (RBC) in the capillaries escape into the tissues. Proteins organize and form tissue fibrosis (hardening of the skin). The RBC's break down and cause hyperpigmentation (dark tissue discoloration). Oxygen intake is decreased in the tissues, causing tissue malnutrition/hypoxia. Ulceration may follow.[4]

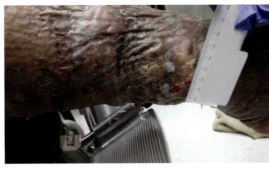

Fig. 29-3: *This venous ulceration measures about 5cm in width. Venous ulceration typically develop on the inner-ankle (gaiter area) as opposed to arterial ulcerations which occur on the outside of the ankle.*

Varicose Veins

- The pathogenesis of primary varicose veins remains unclear. Initially it was thought that varicose veins are due to valvular incompetence.[5,6] However, a current hypothesis states that alterations in vein wall structure (cells and extracellular matrix) cause weakness and altered tone, leading to valvular dysfunction.

Varicose veins can occur anywhere in the body, though are most often located in the legs. Approximately 50% of those over 50 years of age have VV.[7]

  » There is a decrease in the elastin content of varicose vein walls. There is also a change in the ratio of type I to type III collagen with an increase in type I (rigid, provides tensile strength) and a decrease in type III (compliant, increases elasticity). These changes undoubtedly contribute to the weakening of the varicose vein wall.
  » The degradation of the extracellular matrix (ECM) is a function of matrix metalloproteinases and their inhibitors. An increase in matrix degradation would weaken the wall, while a decrease could promote ECM accumulation. Reports have varied on whether their levels remain the same, increase or decrease in varicose vein.[18]
  » Interspersed in varicose veins are thick (two-fold thicker than normal veins) and thin regions (two-fold thinner than normal veins).[19] In the thick regions, smooth muscle cells are no longer organized in circumferential and longitudinal bundles but disrupted by an increased amount of fibrous tissue. The intima is thickened with an increase in smooth muscle cells. In the thin regions, there is a decrease in cell number. The adventitia is thin and lacks vasa vasorum. These regions correspond to areas of dilatation.
- Tributaries of the great saphenous vein (GSV) are thought to varicose before the main trunk of the GSV because they contain fewer smooth muscle cells in their vessel walls and lack support in the subcutaneous fat layer under the skin where they are commonly located.[1]

Pregnancy

- Pregnancy increases the amount of blood circulating in your system and causes veins to enlarge. The pressure of the fetus on the veins can decrease the blood flow back through the pelvic venous system.[1,6,7]
- Birth control pills can increase the risk of varicose/spider veins.[7] Spider veins are not true varicose veins and are oftentimes thought to be related to hormonal changes.
- The number and severity of varicose veins can increase with each additional pregnancy. Varicose veins can improve postpartum.

Location of Disease

Incompetent valves may be located at any segment of the deep, perforating, or superficial veins, but are more commonly found in the superficial venous tributaries. [2]

- Perforating veins in the gaiter area-medial aspect of the leg, just above the medial malleolus (most common)
- Saphenofemoral junction (SFJ)

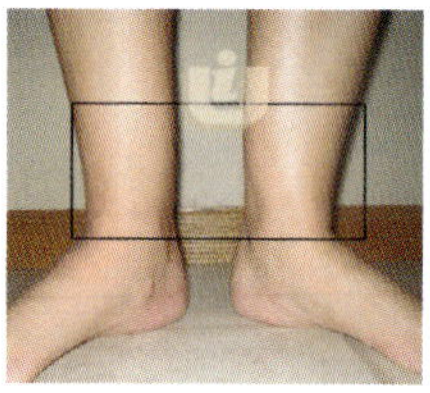

Fig. 29-4: *Gaiter Area*

Patient History

- Persistent leg/calf swelling (usually unilateral)
- Previous DVT
- Localized pain, burning or itching
- Tired, heavy legs after prolonged standing
- Symptoms can increase for women around menstruation.
- Symptoms may increase for pregnant women.
- Symptoms may vary with time of day.
- Patients may present with signs without symptoms or symptoms without signs.

If both parents had VV, there are estimates that there is a 90% chance of developing them. If you are male and only one parent had VV, the chances of developing VV is 25%. If you are female the chances of developing VV is 62%. Even if neither parent had VV, there is still a 20% chance of developing VV. [15]

Physical Examination

- Edema
- Tenderness
- Tenderness, warmth or redness along the course of a superficial vein or varicosity
- Varicose veins
- Hyperpigmentation, hardened tissue around the ankles
- Ulceration (gaiter area)
- Dermatitis
- Noticeable telangiectasia
- Severe, chronic swelling and symptoms of CVI (listed above) with pain/aching that worsens when walking and is relieved by elevation (venous claudication)

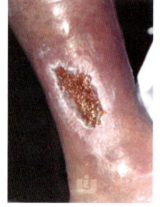

Fig. 29-5: *C6: Active venous ulcer. For more on ulcers, refer to the Venous Diseases chapter.*

The American Venous Forum's Revision of the CEAP CVD Classification
(www.veinforum.org)

CEAP Classification

The American Venous Forum has developed a classification system for chronic venous disease called CEAP which categorizes clinical class (C), etiology (E), anatomic location (A) and pathological mechanism (P). CEAP which categorizes clinical class (C), etiology (E), anatomic location (A) and pathological mechanism (P).

In the CEAP classification system, clinical signs are grouped and numbered, for example: [2,11]

Table 29-1: CEAP: Summary of Clinical (C) Classifications	
C0	No visible or palpable signs of venous disease
C1	Telangiectasias or reticular veins
C2	Varicose veins
C2r	Recurrent varicose veins
C3	Edema
C4	Changes in skin and subcutaneous tissue secondary to CVD
C4a	Pigmentation or eczema
C4b	Lipodermatosclerosis or atrophie blanche
C4c	Corona Phlebictatica
C5	Healed venous ulcer
C6	Active venous ulcer

Lower Extremity Venous Insufficiency Duplex Protocol

- Obtain a patient history to include symptoms and risk factors.
- Patient is examined to rule out venous obstruction in the supine position with the head elevated or in a reversed Trendelenburg position. Explain the procedure to the patient.

Putting a patient in the reverse Trendelenburg position can improve visibility of smaller veins (e.g., calf veins). The size of the superficial veins can be affected by the position of the bed or the room temperature.

- Higher-frequency transducers (5-7 MHz or 8-15 MHz) should work well for visualization of the superficial and perforating veins, including their connection to the deep veins. Some patients may require the use of a range of transducers including a lower frequency (1-4 MHz) transducer for the deep veins.
- Before the assessment for reflux, a standard venous exam to rule out thrombosis is typically performed (see chapter on *Lower Extremity Venous Duplex Ultrasound*).
- The patient must be examined for insufficiency while standing or with the bed in an extreme reverse Trendelenburg position.
  » When standing the patient, use a stool or platform with a handrail. Have the patient hold the handrail and slightly rotate the leg outward. Then have the patient transfer weight onto the opposite leg.
- The calf veins can be examined for reflux while the patient sits with their legs dangling over the side of the bed.
- The *Valsalva maneuver* may be used during testing in order to increase intra-abdominal pressure and interrogate proximal venous valves for competency. This maneuver involves asking the patient to inhale deeply. While holding this breath, the patient will need to contract the abdomen. Ask the patient to release the breath and relax the abdomen after 1-2 seconds.

Deep inspiration followed by "bearing down" (Valsalva maneuver) creates an abrupt cessation of blood flow when valves close properly.

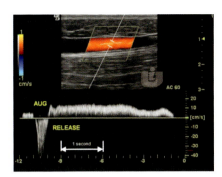

Fig. 29-6: *Venous reflux by spectral Doppler*
Courtesy of GE Healthcare

Most ultrasound machines have a mechanism to measure time in seconds for the purpose of assessing the significance of reflux.

- Record venous flow with color and spectral Doppler waveforms in longitudinal (sagittal axis) view at the following locations: (use the Valsalva maneuver and manual distal leg compressions to try to elicit reflux if it is present. Some laboratories use an automatic cuff inflator to further standardize the distal compression). [5]

Some labs record venous spectral Doppler waveforms without setting an angle since actual velocities are usually not important in a venous exam. If your lab chooses to set an angle, use a ≤60° Doppler angle with the cursor placed parallel to the vessel walls in the center of the flow stream.

» Proximal common femoral vein (above SFJ)
» Saphenofemoral junction (SFJ)
» Distal common femoral vein (below SFJ)
» Proximal GSV
» Proximal femoral vein in the proximal thigh (*Note: there is often a valve just distal to the femoral bifurcation*)
» Multiple levels of the GSV in the proximal, mid, distal thigh, at knee and proximal, mid, distal calf.
» Popliteal vein
» Saphenopopliteal junction (SPJ)
» Multiple levels of the small saphenous vein (SSV)
» Thigh extension of the small saphenous vein (TE-SSV) (when visualized)
» Any visualized perforating veins

You may turn the patient prone while scanning behind the knee. Use a pillow under the shin to put a bend in the knee and reduce pressure on the PopV.

- Additional documentation of reflux can be performed as necessary of the tibial or other veins such as the accessory GSV in the thigh.
- Report the connection between the vein of Giacomini and the deep system when visualized.
- Report the location of any varicosed tributaries and where they connect to the great or small saphenous veins when indicated.

The superficial veins do not have a corresponding artery which makes them easy to distinguish from deep veins. Saphenous diameters help physicians choose between various treatment options.

- Measure several diameters of the main GSV trunk from the groin to the knee (e.g. proximal thigh, mid thigh and at the knee). A diameter at the saphenofemoral junction may also be a requested measurement. If a diameter measurement of the SSV is required, document this about 3cm from either the popliteal crease or the SPJ.
- Physicians may request depth measurements between the main trunk of the GSV and the skin (top of screen) when considering certain treatments, such as radiofrequency ablation.
- Familiarizing yourself with the course of the GSV is crucial. Many times, patients will have had prior interventions and the saphenous vein compartment will still require interrogation. If you are not familiar with the trajectory this vein takes you may move the probe off track.
- Repeat for the contralateral extremity if a bilateral exam was ordered.

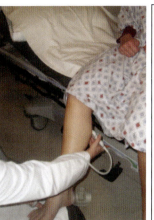
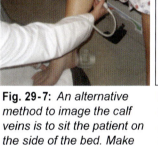
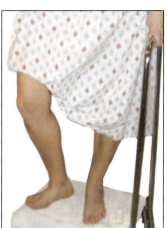

Fig. 29-7: *An alternative method to image the calf veins is to sit the patient on the side of the bed. Make sure the back of the leg or knee is not compressed against the bed.*

Fig. 29-8: *Instruct the patient to stand on a stool with their leg rotated outward and ask the patient to shift their weight onto the contralateral leg while the veins are evaluated for reflux.*

Alternative Testing Method

- Use pressure cuffs, a rapid cuff inflator and air source. Cuffs are inflated at various levels for 3 seconds while continuously recording a spectral waveform using a duplex scanner. Refer to the recommended pressure settings indicated by the manufacturer of the unit.
  » A 12-24cm width cuff is wrapped around the thigh and inflated for 3 seconds around 80mmHg to test for reflux while imaging in the CFV, proximal FV and at the SFJ.
  » A 12cm width cuff is wrapped around the calf and inflated for 3 seconds around 100mmHg to test for reflux in the GSV, mid/distal FV, PopV, perforators and at the SPJ. This cuff is then moved to the ankle level and reinflated for 3 seconds at the same pressure while duplex is used to detect reflux in the PerV, PTV and SSV.
  » A 7cm width cuff is wrapped around the transmetatarsal portion of the foot and inflated for 3 sec around 120mmHg to test for reflux in the PTV, PERV, distal GSV and any distal perforators.

Table 29-2: Lower Extremity Venous Insufficiency Examination Protocol Summary

Scan longitudinal (sagittal axis) with color and Spectral Doppler

- Proximal and distal CFV segments
- Proximal FV
- Saphenofemoral junction
- Proximal, mid, distal thigh and at knee GSV
- Proximal, mid and distal calf GSV
- PopV
- Saphenopopliteal junction
- Thigh extension of the small saphenous vein (when visualized)
- Proximal, mid and distal calf SSV
- Tibial veins (PTV, PerV) (when appropriate)
- Perforator veins (when visualized)
- Note location where varicose tributaries connect with saphenous veins.
- Measure necessary superficial venous diameters according to lab protocol.
- Additional documentation may be recorded as necessary in segments other than those listed above.

PRINCIPLES OF INTERPRETATION

This chapter outlines interpretation of the venous spectral Doppler only. See the LE Venous Duplex chapter for information on how to interpret B-mode images and color flow, which are also important components of venous insufficiency testing.

Spectral Doppler Waveforms

Determine whether venous blood is flowing exclusively back to the heart (normal direction) or flowing backward, down the leg (retrograde direction).

Interpretation/Diagnostic Criteria

Normal

Spectral Doppler Waveforms

- Venous flow should be directed towards the heart (negative deflection of the Doppler tracing)
- The normal response would be no flow detected:
  » During cuff deflation.
  » Both during and after compression of the leg below the transducer
  » During the Valsalva maneuver
  » During manual compression above the transducer
- A brief period of reflux (<0.5 sec) immediately after maneuvers is most likely the normal amount of time for a valve to fully close. [2,9]

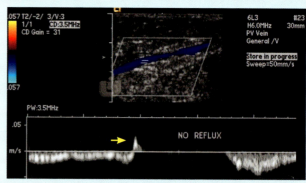

Fig. 29-9: *Normal valve closure results in a brief period of flow reversal*

Abnormal

Spectral Doppler Waveforms

- Venous reflux is caused by incompetent valves allowing both antegrade and retrograde flow direction (negative and positive deflection of the Doppler tracing). Venous reflux (reversed flow direction) may be seen:
  » During manual leg compressions above the transducer
  » Upon release of compression below the transducer
  » During the Valsalva maneuver, indicating reflux
- An abnormal response would be retrograde flow during cuff deflation due to valvular incompetence.

Outward flow may be another term used for reflux.

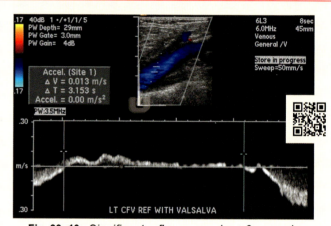

Fig. 29-10: *Significant reflux measuring >3 seconds*

- The diagnostic criteria typically used for clinically significant reflux lasts for more than: [2,8,10,11]
  » 1 second in the deep veins (CFV, FV, POPV)
  » 0.5 second in the tibial veins
  » 0.5 second in the superficial veins
  » 0.5 second in a perforating vein
- If the sum of venous closure time in the FV and PopV is >4 seconds, severe reflux is suggested.

Some labs report reflux in milliseconds instead of seconds.

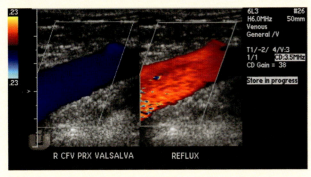

Fig. 29-11: *Venous reflux by color flow*

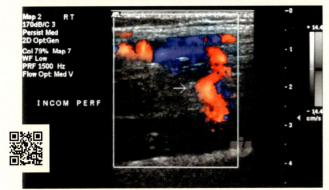

Fig. 29-12: *Perforator reflux-flow away from the deep system*

Table 29-3: Venous Reflux Diagnostic Criteria [2,8,10,11]

	Deep Thigh	Deep Calf	Superficial	Perforator
Normal	<1 sec	<0.5 sec	<0.5 sec	<0.5 sec
Abnormal	>1 sec	>0.5 sec	>0.5 sec	>0.5 sec

Differential Diagnosis

- Lymphedema
- Lipidema
- Cellulitis
- Deep venous thrombosis
- Adenopathy
- Arteriovenous fistula
- Direct injury to extremity
- Mass (including vascularized mass)
- Arteriovenous malformation (AVM)
- Collagen vasculitis
- Abscess
- Peripheral neuritis
- Stasis dermatitis
- Klippel-Trenaunay
- Skin cancer
- Arterial disease

Correlation

- Photoplethysmography for reflux testing
- Continuous wave Doppler reflux testing
- Descending venography

Medical Treatment

- Promote venous drainage (e.g., elevate legs, wear elastic stockings/support hose)
- Limit long periods of inactivity
- Compression bandaging (for ulceration)
- Anti-inflammatory medication
- Injection sclerotherapy
- Ultrasound-guided sclerotherapy
- Laser therapy
- Proper skin care

Surgical Treatment

- Ligation (e.g., of saphenofemoral junction)
- Venous ablation
- Stab avulsion phlebectomy
- Vein stripping
- Subfascial endoscopic perforator vein surgery
- Transverse repair of incompetent valves
- Subfascial ligation of perforators
- Ambulatory phlebectomy

Endovascular Treatment

- Thermal ablation
  » Endovenous LASER ablation
  » Radiofrequency ablation (RFA)
- Chemical ablation, including sclerotherapy
- Adhesive ablation (e.g., cyanoacrylate)

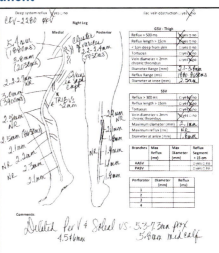

Fig. 29-13: *Due to the complex nature of venous valvular disease, a drawing may be helpful to appreciate branch points, reflux and vein diameters.*

For more in-depth interpretation and worksheet downloads, refer to the *Inside Ultrasound Venous Vascular Reference Guide, 2nd Edition.*
insideultrasound.com

REFERENCES

1. Sumner DS, Zierler RE. (2005). Vascular physiology: essential hemodynamic principles. In Rutherford *Vascular Surgery 6th edition*. (75-123). Philadelphia. Elsevier Saunders.
2. Labropoulos N, Leon LR. (2005). Evaluation of chronic venous disease. In Mansour MA, Labropoulos N. (Eds.), Vascular Diagnosis, (447-461). Philadelphia: Elsevier Saunders
3. Zwiebel, WJ (2005). Ultrasound diagnosis of venous insufficiency. In Zwiebel WJ, Pellerito JS (Eds.), Introduction to Vascular Ultrasonography 5th ed, (479-499). Philadelphia: Elsevier Saunders.
4. Meissner MH. (2010). Chronic venous disorders. In Zierler RE (Ed.), Strandess's duplex scanning disorders in vascular diagnosis 4th ed. (223-229).Philadelphia Wolters Kluwer Lippincott Williams & Wilkins. Oklu et al. (2012). J Vasc Interv Radiol; 23:33–39.
5. Browse NL, Burnand, KG, Thomas, ML (1988). Disease of the Veins; Pathology, Diagnosis and Treatment, Edward Arnold, a division of Hodder & Stoughton.
6. Meissner MH, Strandess DE. (2005). Pathophysiology and natural history of acute deep venous thrombosis. In *Rutherford Vascular Surgery 6th edition*. (2124-2142). Philadelphia. Elsevier Saunders.
7. Min RJ, Rosenblatt M. US Department of Health and Human Services, Office on Women's Health (2010). Varicose Veins and Spider Veins. Retrieved from http://www.womenshealth.gov/faq/varicose-spider-veins.cfm. (7-7-2010).
8. Coleridge-Smith P, Labropoulos N, Partsch H, Myers K, Nicolaides A, Cavezzi A. (2006). Duplex ultrasound investigation of the veins in chronic venous disease of the lower limbs: UIP consensus document. Part I. Basic principles. Eur J Vasc Endovasc Surg 31, 83–92
9. Meissner MH. (2005). Venous duplex scanning. In *Rutherford Vascular Surgery 6th edition*. (254-270). Philadelphia. Elsevier Saunders
10. Cina A, Pedicelli A, Di Stasi C, Pocelli A, Fiorentino A, Cina G, Rulli F, Bonomo L. (2005). Color Doppler sonography in chronic venous insufficiency: what the radiologist should know. Curr Probl Diagn Radiol; 34; 51-62.
11. Pascarella L, Mekenas, L (2006). Ultrasound examination of the patient with primary venous insufficiency. In *The Vein Book*, Philadelphia: Elsevier 171-181.
12. Callam MJ. (1994). Epidemiology of varicose veins. *British Journal of Surgery*, 81:167-173.
13. Varicose veins and venous insufficiency: Interventional radiology nonsurgical outpatient procedure treats varicose veins. (2010). Society of Interventional Radiologists. http://www.scvir.org/patients/varicose-veins/. (12-9-2010).
14. Tessier DJ, Williams RA. (10-5-2006). "Chronic venous insufficiency" Emedicine. Retrieved from: http://emedicine.medscape.com/article/461449-overview (date viewed)
15. Cornu-Thenard A, Boivin P, Baud JM, De Vincenzi I, Carperntier PH. (1994). Importance of the familiar factor in varicose disease. Clinical study of 134 families. *J Dermatol Surg*. 20:318-326.
16. Janniger CK. (3-17-2010). Klippel-Trenaunay-Weber Syndrome. *eMedicine*. Retrieved from http://www.emedicine.com/article/1084257-overview. (12-5-2010).
17. Connors JP, Mulliken JB. (2005). Vascular tumors and malformations in childhood. In *Rutherford Vascular Surgery 6th edition*. (1626-1645). Philadelphia. Elsevier Saunders.
18. Lim and Davies. (2009) Pathogenesis of primary varicose veins British Journal of Surgery; 96: 1231–1242).
19. Badier-Commander et al. (2001). Smooth muscle cell modulation and cytokine overproduction in varicose veins. An in situ study. J Pathol; 193: 398-407.

VENOUS TESTING

30. Venous Ablation Duplex Ultrasound

 For more in-depth information refer to the *Inside Ultrasound Venous Vascular Reference Guide, 2nd Edition*. insideultrasound.com

Definition
Venous duplex ultrasound is the primary diagnostic imaging modality utilized for identifying patients with chronic venous insufficiency (CVI). The combination of real time B-mode imaging with spectral and color flow Doppler (duplex scanning) used during an ablation procedure including vein mapping, vein access, catheter placement and the infusion of perivenous anesthetic.

Etiology of Conditions Treated Using Thermal Ablation
- Congenital
- Primary venous insufficiency
- History of venous thrombosis
  » Secondary venous insufficiency to valve injury, usually due to venous thrombosis
- Venous hypertension, caused by valve damage or dysfunction

Risk Factors
- Genetics (complex, involving many genes)
- Age (greater with advancing age)
- Obesity
- Female gender
- Pregnancy (greater with each pregnancy)
- Previous venous thrombosis
- Occupations requiring long period of standing or sitting

Indications for Venous Ablation Procedure
- Significant volume of reflux in the saphenous venous system with documented valve closure time greater than 500 milliseconds (ms). (Most pathologic reflux is over 1000 ms) in the great saphenous vein, contributing to the development of:
  » Retrograde flow
  » Varicose veins
  » Soft tissue pain or tenderness
  » Edema
  » Venous stasis dermatitis
  » Venous ulceration.
  » Leg fatigue

Contraindications/Limitations
- Pregnancy or breast feeing
- Tortuous veins which cannot be traversed with endovenous glidewire/catheter techniques (rare)
- Obstructed deep venous system resulting in the saphenous veins becoming a major outflow collateral
- Close proximity of the target vein to a nerve
- Obstructed deep venous system
- Anesthetic allergy
- Coagulopathy
- Patient immobility
- Obese patients may have a higher rate of failure for an ablation procedure. The cause may be due to a higher central venous pressure.

Location of Veins (treated with chemical or thermal ablation)
- Great saphenous vein (GSV): most commonly affected
- Small saphenous vein (SSV): second most commonly treated
- Anterior saphenous vein (ASV)
- Posterior accessory saphenous vein (PASV)
- Cranial extension of the small saphenous vein
- Perforators: (rare) including, but not limited to:
  » Posterior tibial
  » Paratibial perforators
  » Perforators in the thigh, buttock and lateral calf may also be treated if clinically indicated.

Patient History
- Leg discomfort, fatigue, heaviness, burning, stinging, pruritus
- Soft tissue leg pain or tenderness
- Lower extremity swelling
- Enlarging varicose veins
- Spontaneous venous hemorrhage
- Symptoms often are worse with dependency or perimenstrual
- Prior endovenous intervention
- Prior deep or superficial vein thrombosis
- Persistent swelling (especially at the end of the day)
- Standing or sitting for prolonged periods of time
- Restless legs

Physical Examination
- Varicose veins
- Tenderness in soft tissue
- Edema
- Hyperpigmentation near the ankles or foot
- Stasis dermatitis
- Superficial thrombophlebitis
- Venous stasis ulceration
- Lipodermatosclerosis
- Corona Phlebectasia
- Venous ulceration
- Active or healed ulcer

There is a high success rate for healing of venous ulceration, post-procedure.

Thermal Ablation
- Thermal ablation is a procedure using heat to remove tissue or destroy its function. Currently, two types of thermal ablation methods are used: endovenous LASER ablation, and radiofrequency ablation. Both methods may be used in an operating room or in an out-patient setting.
- The procedure uses heat to achieve venous closure of the diseased veins, decreasing the risk of complications and symptoms from venous disease.
- Thermal ablation when compared with traditional surgical techniques, is less invasive, offers the same cosmetic results with virtually no scarring, and a faster return to normal activities.

Technique

- The underlying goal for all thermal ablation procedures is to deliver sufficient thermal energy to the wall of an incompetent vein segment to produce irreversible occlusion, fibrosis, and ultimately disappearance of the vein.[8]
- A thermal device is placed into the target vein using ultrasound guidance and positioned at the level of its junction with the deep venous system.
- A local anesthetic is administered between the vein wall and soft tissue, within the saphenous compartment. Then thermal energy is delivered to the diseased vein through the device tip. As the catheter is withdrawn, heat causes the vein to collapse and eventually close.
- Tumescent anesthesia involves the injection of a very dilute local anesthetic solution, into the tissue until it becomes firm and engorged. The technique was initially pioneered in the 1980s for the purposes of liposuction, but its application has since expanded to cover a variety of surgeries.

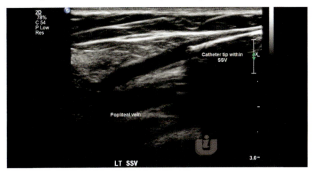

Fig. 30-1: *Catheter tip position*
Image courtesy of Diana L. Neuhardt, BS MBA RVT

Adhesive Ablation

- A procedure using cyanoacrylate to close a vein. Cyanoacrylate (Superglue) is a strong, biodegradable tissue adhesive that polymerizes upon contact with tissues.
- The procedure differs from heat and chemical ablation by leaving the glue in the vein as a medical implant.

 For more in-depth information, including full protocols for these exams, refer to the *Inside Ultrasound Venous Vascular Reference Guide, 2nd Edition*.
insideultrasound.com

Lower Extremity Venous Duplex Protocol for Pre- and Post-Venous Ablation

Most labs schedule 45-90 minutes for each venous ablation procedure.

Pre-procedure Vein Mapping Duplex Protocol

Prior to the ablation procedure, the vein to be treated can be mapped with skin markings.

Essential elements of the mapping include an assessment of:

- » Location of the vein to be treated
- » Maximum diameter (with patient supine)
- » Depth of the vein from the skin surface (vein segments less than 8-10mm below the surface of the skin may develop a tender, palpable cord with hyperpigmentation which slowly resolves and treatment of superficial veins may result in thermal burns of the skin).
- » Tributaries
- » Aneurysmal segments
- » Duplicate vein segments
- » Evidence of challenges to catheterization e.g., obstruction, webs, tortuosity, large tributary veins, the catheter may want to feed into the perforating veins.
- » Areas of hypoplasia and aplasia
- » Determination of the intended vein access site

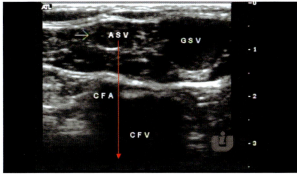

Fig. 30-2: *The arrow demonstrates the anatomical landmark of the Alignment Sign. The ASV is aligned with the femoral artery and vein. Note the vessels are within the saphenous compartment.*
Image courtesy of Jean White-Melendez, Quality Vascular Imaging, Inc.

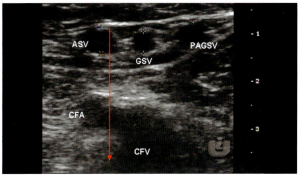

Fig. 30-3: *Unusual variant of the Alignment Sign, the ASV is on the left, GSV in the middle and PAGSV on the right. Note the vessels still are within the saphenous compartment.*
Image courtesy of Jean White-Melendez, Quality Vascular Imaging, Inc.

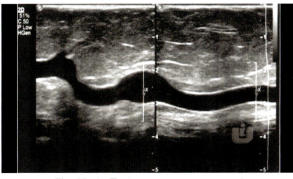

Fig. 30-4: *Tortuous venous segment*
Image courtesy of Paula Heggerick BS RVT RDMS RPhS FSVU

Patient positioning (GSV)

- The exam is best performed with the bed in the reverse Trendelenburg position to facilitate emptying of the veins.
- Leg is externally rotated and slightly bent at the knee.
- Using a straw (or a pencil capable of marking the skin while the gel is still on the skin), the technologist can make skin depressions while mapping vein.

- Depressions will stay visible after gel is removed from the skin.
  » Remove any remaining gel.
  » Use a permanent marker to map the venous pathway and include any areas of interest such as:
    - Large perforators
    - Tortuous segments
    - Chronic disease
- Two access sites should be identified in case one is not able to be used (e.g., due to venous spasm).

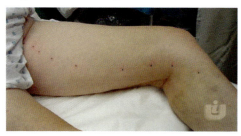

Fig. 30-5: *Initial mapping of the venous pathway using the "straw method"*
Image courtesy of Paula Heggerick BS RVT RDMS RPhS FSVU

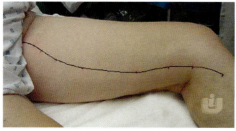

Fig. 30-6: *Final mapping of the venous pathway and areas of interest*
Image courtesy of Paula Heggerick BS RVT RDMS RPhS FSVU

Peri-procedural Ultrasound
During the procedure, B-mode ultrasound is used to:
- Obtain percutaneous vein access.
- Assess for adequate tumescent fluid within the saphenous compartment around the vein being treated (a halo of fluid should completely surround the vein prior to thermal ablation).
- *Tumescent* is a term which describes a fluid mixture that serves as an anesthetic during the ablation procedure. When the tumescence is injected into the tissue, the area becomes swollen and firm or "tumescent."
- Assure that the vein being treated is >1cm from the skin surface (to prevent skin burn)
- Observe the immediate effect of the heat on the treated vein.

Procedural Ultrasound
During the procedure, ultrasound is used to:
- Guide needle access to the vein.
- Guide placement of glidewire and sheath.
- Guide positioning of the LASER fiber tip or the radiofrequency catheter tip in the great saphenous vein (GSV), usually 2.5cm below the deep venous junction.
- Guide infusion of perivenous anesthetic to create a halo of fluid surrounding the target vein.
- Assure that the target vein is at least 8-10mm below the surface of the skin to reduce the likelihood of a palpable visible cord or skin burn post-operatively. Perform a sweep of the entire length of the vein to ensure there is adequate tumescent through the vein segment being treated.

- To maintain a safe and optimal junctional distance, use transverse and longitudinal views to document a final junctional measurement before activation:
  » Typically, somewhere between 2-3cm peripheral to the ostium for the inguinal veins (e.g., great saphenous, anterior saphenous veins).
  » Typically, at the descent of the small saphenous vein before it dives toward the popliteal vein.
- The table is then positioned to 20-30° reverse Trendelenburg.
- Imaging during the procedure will be defined according to the device being used.
- Observe the immediate effect of the heat upon the target vein.

Post-procedural Ultrasound
Most centers evaluate the target vein and the associated deep vein, i.e., great saphenous and common femoral veins or the small saphenous and the popliteal veins 1 to 7 days post-treatment.

Following endovenous treatment, duplex ultrasound is used to evaluate:
- Occlusion of the targeted vein segment
- Secondary thrombosis of associated tributary veins and the target vein above or below the targeted segment

True DVT is a rare finding. Endovenous Heat Induced Thrombosis (EHIT) post-ablation can occur as an extension of the thrombus from the treated area and would typically be limited to the femoral or popliteal regions.

- Endovenous Heat Induced Thrombus (EHIT) described for the great saphenous vein is reported as:
  » **EHIT I:** Confined to the great saphenous vein near the saphenofemoral junction
  » **EHIT II:** Great saphenous vein thrombus extending into the common femoral vein, less than 50% diameter compromise of the CFV
  » **EHIT III:** Great saphenous vein thrombus extending into the common femoral vein, more than 50% diameter compromise of the CFV
  » **EHIT IV:** Occlusion of the common femoral vein

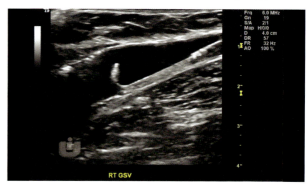

Fig. 30-7: *J-wire placed in the GSV to be treated*
Image courtesy of Patrick Washko, BS RT RDMS RVT

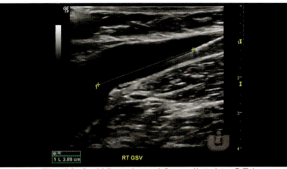

Fig. 30-8: *Wire placed 2cm distal to SFJ*
Image courtesy of Patrick Washko, BS RT RDMS RVT

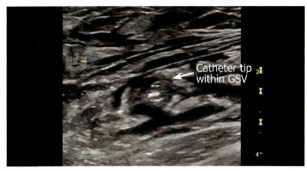

Fig. 30-9: *Tumescent fluid within the saphenous compartment*
Image courtesy of Patrick Washko, BS RT RDMS RVT

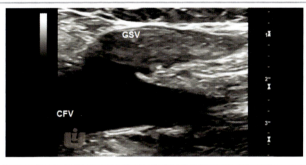

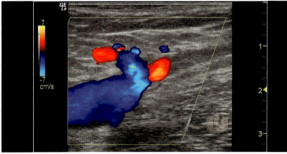

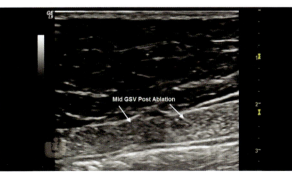

Fig. 30-10: *Post-operative images illustrating absence of flow within the GSV*
Images courtesy of Paula Heggerick BS RVT RDMS RPhS FSVU

Table 30-1: **Protocol Summary for Venous Ablation Duplex Imaging**

Scan pre, peri and post-procedure with B-mode, spectral Doppler and color are complementary

Position the patient in the supine position, with the leg externally rotated and the knee slightly bent. The bed should be in a slight reverse Trendelenburg position.

Pre-procedure

- Determine the source, presence and extent of deep and superficial venous reflux.
- Document the maximum diameter of any superficial veins to be treated.
- Document the depth of any superficial veins to be treated.
- Document location and size of all significant tributaries off any veins to be treated.
- Identify 2 access sites (in case one site is unusable, in the event of venous spasm).
- Document any additional clinically significant observations, including but not limited to aneurysmal segments, duplicated veins, evidence of venous obstruction, etc.

Peri-procedure

- Provide guidance for the physician during wire/catheter placement and make observations to ensure procedure's success:
  » Confirm the catheter tip is distal to the deep system by 1-2.5cm; it should also be distal to the superficial inferior epigastric vein if possible.
  » Assess for adequate perivenous tumescent anesthesia within the saphenous compartment around the treated venous segment (Observe for a halo of fluid surrounding the vein prior to thermal ablation).
  » Assure treated venous segment is >1cm from skin surface.
  » Observe for abnormalities after heat is administered during ablation.

Post-procedure

- Document vein sclerosis/fibrosis of the treated venous segment (non-compressible vein with thickened vein walls and absence of flow by duplex).
- Document absence or presence of deep venous thrombosis in the surrounding venous segments.
- Additional documentation may be recorded as necessary in segments other than those listed above.

Duplex ultrasound at 9-12 months post-procedure ultimately determines the success of the procedure.

PRINCIPLES OF INTERPRETATION

B-mode Imaging

Use B-mode imaging to determine if vein is closed

- Confirm the vein does not collapse completely with light transducer pressure.
- Look for echogenic material present within the lumen of the vein.

Color Doppler
- Use color Doppler to determine if wall-to-wall color flow is present or if there is a filling defect.

Spectral Doppler Waveforms
Use spectral Doppler to determine
- If venous flow can be detected with augmentation
- Flow should increase with distal compression

Interpretation/Diagnostic Criteria

Normal
- The treated vein should be non-compressible
- Treated vein walls should appear thickened
- Absence of flow by color and spectral Doppler in the treated venous segment
- Documented absence of deep venous thrombosis

Abnormal
- Venous thrombosis in the deep and/or untreated superficial segments is an abnormal finding.
- Tissue damage (e.g., thermal or chemical skin burn)
- Ulceration

Most recanalization will occur between 6-12 months post-procedure.

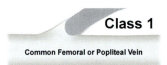

Class 1 — Common Femoral or Popliteal Vein
Venous thrombosis extending to the SFJ/SPJ, but not into the deep system.

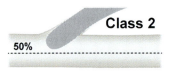

Class 2 — 50%
Non-occlusive venous thrombosis, extending into the deep system. Cross sectional area <50%.

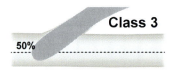

Class 3 — 50%
Non-occlusive venous thrombosis extending into the deep system. Cross sectional area >50%.

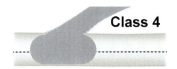

Class 4
Occlusive thrombosis of the deep vein.

Fig. 30-11: Thrombus Extension Classification

For more in-depth information refer to the *Inside Ultrasound Venous Vascular Reference Guide, 2nd Edition*. insideultrasound.com

Correlation
- Venogram
- MR venography
- CT venography

Endovascular Treatment
- Sclerotherapy, with or without US guidance

Surgical Treatment
- Ligation, with or without stripping
- Phlebectomy
- Transilluminated power phlebectomy (Trivex)
- Superficial perforator ligation surgery (SEPS)

Table 30-2: Diagnostic Criteria for Post-Venous Ablation Venous Duplex

Normal
- Complete vein sclerosis/fibrosis of the treated venous segment by B-mode image, spectral Doppler and color flow
- Absence of deep vein thrombosis:
  » Absent intralumenal deep vein thrombus
  » Color flow fills lumen completely
  » Normal venous Doppler spontaneity, phasicity and augmentation of the deep venous system

Abnormal
- Lack of complete vein ablation
- Presence of deep vein thrombosis:
  » Intralumenal echoes (although acute thrombus can be echolucent)
  » Decrease or absence of color flow
  » Abnormal venous Doppler spontaneity, phasicity or augmentation

Table 30-3: Post Ablation Superficial Thrombus Extension (PASTE)[15]

Device Used	Thrombus Extension Terminology
ETA Endovenous Thermal Ablation (ELA, EVLA, EVLT, RFA)	**EHIT** Endovenous Heat Induced Thrombus
UGFS (foam) **UGS** (liquid) **MOCA** (Mechanochemical ablation)	**EFIT** Endovenous Foam Induced Thrombus
EVAA Endovenous Adhesive Ablation	**EGIT** Endovenous Glue Induced Thrombus

REFERENCES
1. Size G.P. (2022). *Inside Ultrasound Venous Vascular Reference Guide 2nd Ed.* Inside Ultrasound. 9-20-2022
2. American College of Phlebology (ACP) www.phlebology.org
3. American Registry for Diagnostic Medical Sonography (ARDMS) www.ardms.org
4. Cardiovascular Credentialing (CCI) www.cci-online.org
5. American Venous Forum (AVF) www.venous-info.com
6. Intersocietal Commission for the Accreditation of Vascular Laboratories (ICAVL) www.icavl.org
7. Society of Vascular Ultrasound (SVU) www.svunet.org
8. Bergan J. (2006). The Vein Book. Elsevier.
9. Gloviczki P. (2009). Handbook of Venous Disorders 3rd edition, Hodder Arnold.
10. Fronek H, Fundamental of Phlebology: Venous disease for clinicians. 2nd edition. Royal Society of Medicine Press 2008
11. Goldman M, Bergan J, Guex JJ. (2007). Sclerotherapy: Treatment of Varicose and Telangiectatic Leg Veins. Mosby.
12. Ricci S, Georgiev M, Goldman, M. (2005). Ambulatory Phlebectomy. 2nd edition. Taylor & Francis Group.
13. Weiss R. (2001). Vein Diagnosis and Treatment. McGraw-Hill.
14. Khilani NM, Elston DM, Khan S, Butler DF, Miller JJ, Crawford GH. (2010). Varicose Vein Treatment with Endovenous Laser Therapy. www.emedicine.medscape.com (accessed 12/4/2011).
15. Passariello, F. (2014). Post-ablation superficial thrombus extension (PASTE) as a consequence of endovenous ablation. An up to- date review. Vascular Medicine 2, 62-66

VENOUS TESTING
31. IVC and Iliac Venous Duplex Ultrasound

Definition

The combination of real time B-mode ultrasonography with spectral Doppler and color flow to evaluate the inferior vena cava (IVC) and iliac veins for evidence of thrombus or external compression.

Venous duplex ultrasound can identify the presence, location and extent of venous thrombosis or external compression. The course of the veins, collaterals and thrombus can be visualized using B-mode and color while the analysis of Doppler waveform changes can confirm occlusion and focal venous stenosis, or indirectly confirm proximal obstruction.

Etiology

- Thrombosis; The theory of Virchow's triad states that venous thrombosis is caused by: venous stasis, vein wall (intimal) injury or a hypercoagulable state.
- Extrinsic compression (e.g., from renal or hepatocellular carcinomas or tumors that have spread to the paracaval lymph nodes for example)

Risk Factors

- Age (greater with advanced age)
- Immobilization
- Genetic prothrombotic conditions (clotting disorders, such as Factor V Leiden)
- Post-operative phase (especially after orthopedic surgery)
- Central venous or femoral catheters
- Female
  » Pregnancy
  » Oral contraceptives
  » Estrogen replacement
- Cancer/malignancy
- Previous DVT
- Heart complications (MI, CHF, etc.)
- Obesity
- Family history
- Smoking
- COPD
- Blood type (highest risk with "type A," lowest risk with "type O")
- Trauma
- Antiphospholipid antibodies (lupus, etc.)
- Occupations requiring long periods of standing or sitting
- Varicose veins
- Congenital abnormalities (Klippel-Trenaunay)
- Inflammatory bowel disease
- Drug abuse
- Cerebrovascular events (stroke, TIA)
- Iliac vein compression syndrome

Indications for Exam

- Edema/swelling (especially when unilateral)
- Limb pain/tenderness
- Symptoms of pulmonary embolism (PE) (shortness of breath, chest pain, hemoptysis)
- Hypercoagulable state
- Duplex-guided filter insertion
- Pre-operative exam for patency prior to placement of caval filter
- Post-operative evaluation of filter device

Perforation of the IVC in the presence of a filter is possible, though uncommon. [7]

- Pallor (phlegmasia alba dolens)
- Cyanosis (phlegmasia cerulea dolens- iliofemoral thrombosis)
- Positive D-dimer test result

Contraindications/Limitations

- Poor visualization due to vessel depth because of obesity, swelling or abdominal gas.
- Compressibility of the IVC and iliac veins can be technically difficult due to the deep location of these veins.

Mechanism of Disease

There are three factors responsible for the formation of venous thrombosis, as outlined in Virchow's Triad (vein wall injury, hypercoagulability and stasis of blood flow). A combination of any of these events may increase the risk of venous thrombosis. [1]

- There is a balance between coagulation (process to prevent excessive bleeding after injury) and anticoagulation (process to prevent spontaneous intravascular clotting) in normal blood flow.
- The venous endothelial layer is normally antithrombotic. In response to endothelial injury, leukocytes (white blood cells) attach to the vessel wall. A plasma protein known as *prothrombin* is activated. Prothrombin activator catalyzes conversion of prothrombin into thrombin. Thrombin acts as an enzyme to convert fibrinogen into fibrin threads, forming a clot. [2,3]
- Hypercoagulable states result from genetic mutation or acquired deficiencies that accompany certain diseases (i.e., liver disease). In such cases, naturally occurring anticoagulants (antithrombin, protein C, protein S, etc.) are deficient. For example, the genetic mutation, factor V Leiden, causes resistance to the natural anticoagulant protein C. [4]
- Non-movement of blood flow (stasis) permits coagulation. Platelets are thought to become trapped by low shear stress (flow) at valve cusps. Platelets adhere to the subendothelial (collagen) layer of the venous wall, and may aggregate depending on the amount of coagulation and thrombolysis occurring in the body at that time.
- Increased activation of coagulation factors in those suffering from cancer is thought to lead to formation of venous thrombosis. In addition, the levels of coagulation inhibitors normally found in the blood (i.e., proteins C or S) are thought to be reduced in these patients. [4]
- Thrombosis in pregnancy is attributed to a prothrombotic state along with decreased venous outflow by the weight of the fetus. The use of estrogen (in replacement therapy or use of contraceptives) alters coagulation and may predispose an individual to thrombosis. [4]
- Extrinsic compression: IVC obstruction can result secondary to an extrinsic compression by a mass or intralumenal tumor. [7,11] Visualization of any echoic structures should be documented. Venous flow signals may be altered depending on the degree of compression.
  » The IVC and iliac veins can become totally thrombosed secondary to the compression. The absence of color flow and spectral Doppler signal using appropriate low-flow duplex settings indicates venous obstruction. [6]
  » Venous stenosis: When continuous flow and increased venous velocities are noted (compared to proximal segments), a venous stenosis secondary to compression is suspected. [6]

Free-floating thrombus in the iliofemoral veins has a higher risk of embolization (60%) than occlusive thrombus (5.5%). [8]

» Extrinsic compression from tumors, enlarged lymph nodes, etc. can result in stenosis or occlusion by placing enough pressure on venous walls to cause venous hypertension distal to the obstruction. [5]

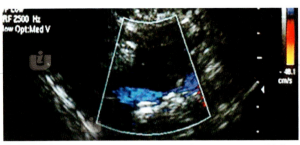

Fig. 31-1: *Extrinsic compression from a tumor which has narrowed the venous lumen by color flow.*

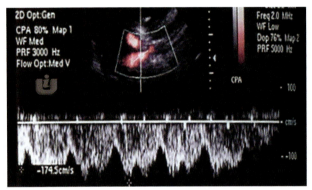

Fig. 31-2: *Increased venous flow velocities as a result of extrinsic compression from a tumor.*

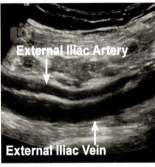 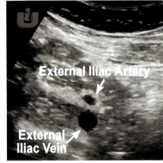

Fig. 31-3: *EIV in longitudinal and transverse views demonstrating pulsatile, repetitive compression of the EIV by the overlying EIA.*

- Once thrombus is formed, it can:
  » **Stabilize**: Stabilization includes adherence of the thrombus to the vessel wall without changing location or propagating. If thrombus has formed, the most favorable occurrence would be to stabilize. This reduces the risk of embolization or PE to the patient.
  » **Propagate**: Propagation includes "growth of thrombus" in size or location. The most notable importance of propagation is the possibility that a superficial system thrombus might propagate into the deep system.
  » **Embolize**: During embolization, a portion of the thrombus breaks free and travels elsewhere within the vascular system. The greatest risk to the patient is that the thrombus travels to the lungs and results in a pulmonary embolus. [2]

Location of Disease

- IVC
- External or internal iliac veins

Anatomic Variations of the IVC

- The IVC can be duplicated, especially in the infrarenal portion of the vein. The iliac veins can continue from the pelvis without joining at an iliac venous bifurcation. Often the two IVC will join at the renal level and then follow a typical course. [6,7]
- Instead of its normal position to the right of the aorta, the IVC may be located on the left side. [13]
- There may be a congenital absence of the IVC at the intrahepatic level. The hepatic vein will be observed draining directly into the right atrium by duplex imaging. [7]
- Membranous obstruction of the IVC is a common cause of hepatic outflow obstruction. In these cases, a visible membrane is noted by ultrasound at the level of the diaphragm, with a reversal of blood flow and significant dilatation noted of the IVC. The right hepatic vein is most commonly obstructed and will appear dilated with slow, continuous flow. Portal hypertension and venous collateralization may also be noted. [7]
- Iliac vein compression syndrome is the pathologic compression of an iliac vein by an overlying iliac artery. This form of extrinsic compression is referred to as a Nonthrombotic Iliac Vein Lesion (NIVL) and can cause lower extremity venous hypertension and/or the development of pelvic varices.

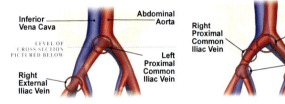

Fig. 31-4: *Most frequently occurring NIVLs*

Fig. 31-5: *Less frequently occurring NIVLs*

Note the slight shift in the position of the aorta and the IVC creating additional sites of potential obstruction.

Patient History

- Acute onset of leg pain
- Acute onset of swelling
- Persistent leg swelling (usually unilateral, but can be bilateral)
- Symptoms of PE (shortness of breath, chest pain, hemoptysis)
- Previous DVT
- Clotting issues (including problems regulating anticoagulation therapy)

Physical Examination

- Edema or swelling
- Tenderness
- Pallor (phlegmasia alba dolens)
- Cyanosis (phlegmasia cerulea dolens)

IVC and Iliac Venous Duplex Protocol

- Patients should be fasting for 6-12 hours to minimize the presence of air/bowel gas in the abdomen. A limited volume of clear liquids may be ingested prior to the examination (e.g., to swallow medications).
- Obtain a patient history to include symptoms and risk factors. Explain the procedure to the patient.
- Patient is examined in the supine position with the head slightly elevated. Explain the procedure to the patient.

- Use a lower frequency (1-4 MHz) curved or sector transducer for most patients. Thinner patients may require the use of a higher frequency (5-7 MHz) transducer.

Transverse IVC

- Locate the IVC in the upper abdomen just below the xiphoid process in the transverse (short axis) plane. It may be possible to compress the vein wall with transducer pressure, though color flow and spectral Doppler waveforms will be the main tools used during this evaluation in most patients.
- For the purposes of the ultrasound examination, the IVC is divided into three regions: [1]
  » **Suprahepatic**: superior to the liver
  » **Intrahepatic**: at the level of the liver; includes tributaries from the liver
  » **Infrahepatic**: inferior to the liver and to the level of the iliac bifurcation

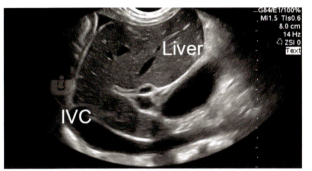

Fig. 31-6: *Proximal IVC; longitudinal plane*

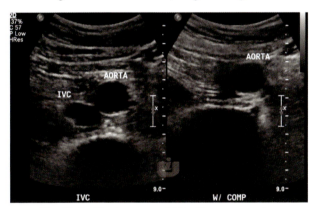

Fig. 31-7: *Dual screen; IVC with compression*

Keep the transducer at a 90° angle to the skin for the best B-mode images.

- Image the IVC to the iliac bifurcation. Document transverse B-mode images of the IVC at the suprahepatic, intrahepatic and infrahepatic levels. Color flow can be added to demonstrate color filling of the vessel.

Longitudinal IVC

- Return the transducer to the xiphoid process and rotate onto the IVC in the longitudinal (sagittal) plane. Record B-mode images of the IVC at the suprahepatic, intrahepatic and infrahepatic levels.
- Record images of the IVC using color Doppler at the suprahepatic, intrahepatic and infrahepatic levels.

Scanning from the right flank is an alternative to the subxiphoid approach.

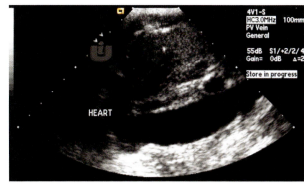

Fig. 31-8: *IVC in longitudinal plane by B-mode image*

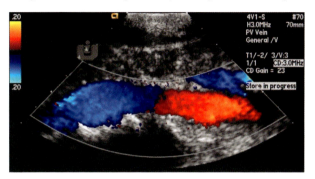

Fig. 31-9: *IVC in with longitudinal plane with color Doppler*

- Document venous flow of the IVC in longitudinal view with spectral Doppler. Some labs record venous spectral Doppler flow without setting an angle since actual velocities are usually not important in a venous exam. (If your lab chooses to set an angle, use a ≤60° Doppler angle with the cursor placed parallel to the vessel walls in the center of the flow stream for spectral waveforms.) Spectral documentation should illustrate spontaneity, respiratory variation and phasicity. Record spectral waveforms in the suprahepatic, intrahepatic and infrahepatic IVC segments.

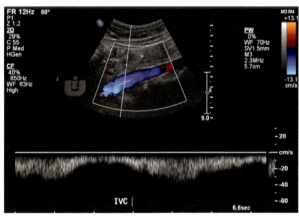

Fig. 31-10: *IVC waveform by spectral Doppler*

Use abdominal and venous presets on the duplex scanner. Low color flow and Doppler scales will be needed to detect venous flow at these depths.

Transverse IVC

- Reposition the transducer in transverse at the infrahepatic IVC and scan distally to the common iliac venous bifurcation. Document a transverse B-mode image of the right and left common iliac veins (CIV) at the bifurcation near the umbilical level. Color flow can be added to demonstrate spontaneous color filling of the vessels.

- Continue distally, using color flow as a guide for the course of the vein. Document a transverse image of the right external (EIV) and internal iliac (IIV) veins at their bifurcation in the pelvis using color flow to demonstrate spontaneous color filling of the vessels.

Longitudinal Iliac Veins

- Return to the common iliac vein bifurcation and rotate onto the right common iliac vein in the longitudinal (sagittal) plane. Record venous flow in the proximal and mid/distal CIV with spectral Doppler. Spectral documentation should illustrate spontaneity and respiratory variation.
- Continue distally, using color flow as a guide. Rotate onto the right EIV in the longitudinal (sagittal) plane. Record venous flow in the proximal and mid/distal EIV with spectral Doppler. Compress the proximal thigh in attempt to elicit augmentation of venous flow. Spectral documentation should illustrate spontaneity, respiratory variation and possibly augmentation of the Doppler signal upon compression.

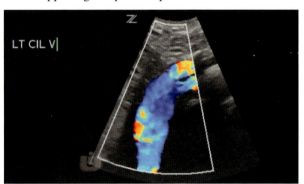

Fig. 31-11: *Longitudinal view of the common iliac vein as it bifurcates into the external and internal iliac veins*

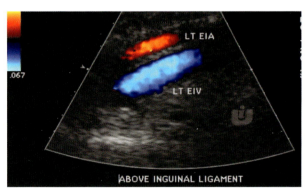

Fig. 31-12: *External iliac vein and artery in the longitudinal plane with color Doppler*

- Additional color and spectral Doppler waveforms may be recorded in the internal iliac venous segment.
- Document any abnormal findings with B-mode and color imaging noted while scanning (e.g., thrombus, wall irregularity, extrinsic masses/tumors, etc.).
- Use spectral Doppler and a large sample gate to analyze absence of flow by placing the Doppler sample volume in any vein segment suspected to be thrombosed. Doppler flow or lack of flow, compliments compression, color flow and B-mode images. Use the adjacent artery as a guide to identify an occluded vein when possible.
- Repeat for the left common and external iliac venous system.
- Compare venous flow in the right and left external iliac veins to evaluate for obstruction at the common iliac level.

The inferior vena cava and common iliac veins do not have valves.

Table 31-1: IVC and Iliac Venous Duplex Protocol Summary

Scan transverse (short axis) in B-mode and color	Scan longitudinal (sagittal axis) with spectral Doppler and color

• IVC
  - Suprahepatic segment
  - Intrahepatic segment
  - Infrahepatic segment
• CIV
• EIV
• IIV (when visualized)
	• IVC
	• CIV (proximal and mid/distal segments)
	• EIV (proximal and mid/distal segments)
	• IIV (when visualized)

- Repeat the exam for the contralateral iliac segment when indicated.
- Additional documentation of compression and spectral Doppler waveforms may be recorded in segments other than those listed during evaluation for thrombus as necessary.

PRINCIPLES OF INTERPRETATION

B-mode Imaging
- Determine whether echogenic material is observed within the lumen of the vein.
- Compressibility: Determine if the vein collapses completely with transducer pressure (when possible).

Color Doppler
- Use color Doppler to determine if color flow is present wall-to-wall or if there is a filling defect.

Spectral Doppler Waveforms
Determine whether venous flow is:
- Spontaneous (automatically heard with Doppler)
- Phasicity increases and decreases with respiration
- Augmentable (increases) with distal compression
- Pulsatile: regular, rhythmic increase and decrease in the flow signal, similar to an arterial pulsation.

Interpretation/Diagnostic Criteria

Normal

B-mode Imaging
- **Compressibility:** The vein is free of thrombus (intralumenal echoes) and compresses completely when technically possible. [6]
- Diameter: The average IVC diameter is 17.2mm just below the renal veins during quiet respiration. The IVC diameter ranges between 5-29mm at rest and increases approximately 10% with inspiration. [7]

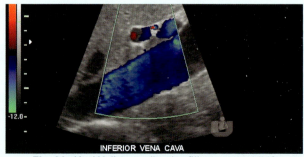

Fig. 31-13: *Wall-to-wall color fills a normal IVC*
Courtesy of Philips Healthcare

Color Doppler
- Wall-to-wall color flow will fill the vein spontaneously or upon distal limb compression. [6]

Spectral Doppler Waveforms
- **Spontaneity:** The vein demonstrates spontaneous flow.
- **Phasicity:** Venous signals are phasic and vary with respiration/cardiac cycle in the distal IVC and iliac veins. During deep inhalation, venous signals decrease or discontinue and increase during exhalation due to changes in intrathoracic pressure during the respiratory cycle. [6,7]
- **Augmentation:** Compression of the limb distal to the transducer can augment or increase venous flow in the external iliac veins. [6]
- **Pulsatility:** Pulsatile venous flow is often present in the proximal inferior vena cava due to its proximity to the heart. [6,7]

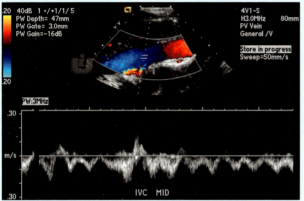

Fig. 31-14: Normal spectral Doppler recorded in the mid IVC
Courtesy of Philips Healthcare

Abnormal

B-mode Imaging
- Intralumenal echoes are visualized within the vein. [8]
- **Compressibility:** Full coaptation of the vein on manual compression (when technically possible in the IVC-iliac segment) is absent or limited due to thrombus. [8] Compression of the artery but not the vein with transducer pressure can be a confirmation of an incompressible venous segment.

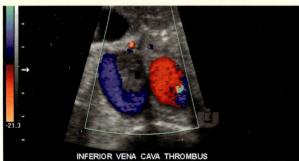

Fig. 31-15: Partial thrombosis of the IVC by color flow in the transverse plane. *Courtesy of Philips Healthcare*

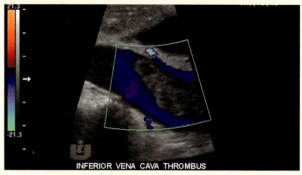

Fig. 31-16: Partial thrombosis of the IVC by color flow in the longitudinal plane. *Courtesy of Philips Healthcare*

Color flow can obscure a partially occlusive thrombus if the color gain is set too high.

Thrombus characteristics: If thrombus is present, determine whether the thrombus is partially or totally occlusive, its location, as well as the extent and characteristics of the thrombus.

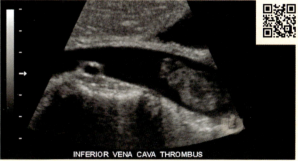

Fig. 31-17: Acute IVC thrombus poorly attached to the wall
Courtesy of Philips Healthcare

» **Acute thrombus:** Characteristics include lightly echogenic or anechoic clot, spongy texture and thrombus which is poorly attached to the venous wall or "free floating" within the lumen. A moving tail may be seen at the end of the thrombus. When a vein is fully thrombosed, the vein is often dilated in diameter. [7,8,9]

» **Chronic thrombus:** Characteristics include brightly echogenic or heterogeneous echoes, irregular surface texture and thrombus which is attached to the venous wall. The vein can stay the same size as the artery, but often contracts in diameter over time. Collateral veins may be observed adjacent to the affected vein(s) and small irregular flow channels can sometimes be seen with color. [8,9]

*The term, **chronic postthrombotic change** has been suggested as a replacement for "chronic thrombus". The SRU has suggested that only acute events should be referred to as " acute thrombus". When it is technically difficult to determine whether findings are acute/chronic, use the term "indeterminate".* [14]

» **Indeterminate age:** Characteristics of both acute and chronic stages may be present, making age difficult to determine. [9,14]
- *Subacute* is another term used by labs. Reports have suggested using this term only to describe thrombus that appears to have changed appearance on B-mode compared to a previous study where the diagnosis of acute DVT was made some weeks earlier.

Color Doppler
- If partially occlusive thrombus is present, color flow will be observed flowing around echogenic material in the vein spontaneously or with distal limb compression. [6,8]

- If totally occlusive thrombus is present, with appropriate low-flow settings no color flow will be observed spontaneously or with distal limb compression. [6,8]

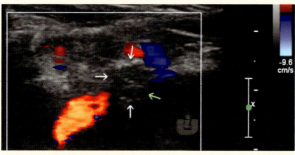

Fig. 31-18: *Total thrombosis of the external iliac vein by color flow in the transverse plane*

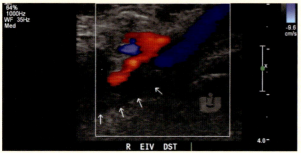

Fig. 31-19: *Total thrombosis of the external iliac vein by color flow in the longitudinal plane*

Table 31-2: Thrombosis Descriptions and Characteristics

Acute	Chronic
Light to medium echogenic/anechoic	Bright/heterogeneous echoes
Spongy texture on compression (homogeneous)	Irregular texture (heterogeneous)
Poorly attached or free floating	Attached
Dilated vein (if totally occluded)	Same size as artery or vein is contracted
	Collateral veins may be noted

- Veins can be partially or totally incompressible in both acute and chronic stages.
- Combination of events can occurs (e.g., acute on top of chronic thrombus).
- Chronic thrombus with partial recanalization is seen as small color flow channels within thrombus.
- Age of thrombus is sometimes indeterminate.

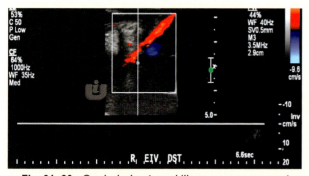

Fig. 31-20: *Occluded external iliac venous segment with absent color and spectral Doppler*

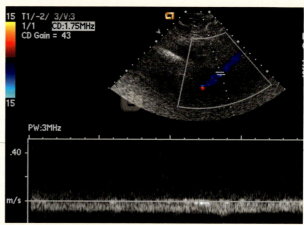

Fig. 31-21: *Continuous venous signal in an external iliac vein*

Spectral Doppler Waveforms

- **Spontaneity:** Absence of flow indicates venous obstruction. [8]
- **Phasicity:** Continuous venous flow (lack of respirophasicty) suggests either obstruction in a proximal venous segment or extrinsic compression of a proximal vein. [6,7]
  - » A comparable difference in external iliac venous signals between limbs suggests a common iliac venous obstruction on the side exhibiting decreased spontaneity or respirophasicty. [6] If both EIV signals are abnormal, this suggests that there may be an IVC obstruction affecting both sides.
- **Augmentation:** If distal compression does not produce augmentation of the venous signal, a total obstruction distal to the transducer is suspected. A weak or dampened augmentation suggests a possible venous occlusion distal to the transducer. [9]
- **Pulsatility:** The absence of pulsatility especially in the proximal inferior vena cava is suggestive of venous obstruction.

Normal Doppler signals may be present when thrombus is partially occlusive. [3]

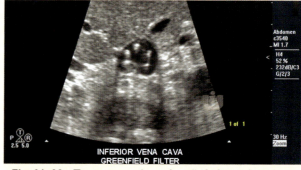

Fig. 31-22: *Transverse view of an IVC Greenfield filter*

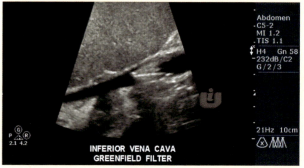

Fig. 31-23: *Longitudinal view of a IVC Greenfield filter*

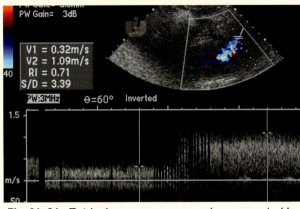

Fig. 31-24: *Extrinsic venous compression suspected by spectral Doppler: increased venous velocities and visualization of a superficial mass*

Use flow in the adjacent artery as a guide to identify an occluded vein. Always confirm absence of flow by placing the sample volume within the vessel walls.

Other Pathology

- **IVC Filter:** IVC filters should be positioned below the level of the renal veins.
  - » Duplex documentation should illustrate patency of the IVC below the filter for a normal result.
  - » Thrombus visualized below the filter is an abnormal finding. [6,7]
- **Extrinsic compression** from tumors, enlarged lymph nodes, etc. can result in stenosis or occlusion by placing enough pressure on venous walls to cause venous hypertension distal to the obstruction. [5]
  - » **Venous stenosis:** When an increased focal venous velocity is noted, with or without provocative positional maneuvers, a venous stenosis is suspected. Some labs use a velocity increase of at least 2.5 times the immediate distal venous segment to diagnose a hemodynamically significant stenosis (venous-velocity ratio of ≥2.5).
  - » **NIVL** (Nonthrombotic Iliac Vein Lesion) is the pathological compression of an iliac vein by an overlying iliac artery.
  - » Extrinsic compression results if partial or complete compression of the vein lumen exists.
  - » Intrinsic obstruction results in wall fibrosis and intraluminal changes caused by the pulsations of an overlying artery.

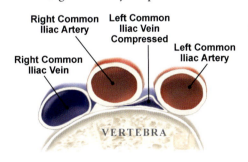

Fig. 31-25: *Cross-section view of the left CIV being compressed by the right and left CIAs. Adapted from www.scgvs.com*

Since thrombus is non-vascularized, echogenic material with color flow is most likely a vascularized mass.

- **Tumor invasion of the IVC:** On rare occasion, the lumen of the IVC can be invaded by a tumor. [6,7] On duplex image, the tumor appears moderately echogenic with diffuse color flow noted (typical characteristic of sarcomas or cancerous tumors). [6]

Differential Diagnosis

- Arterial disease
- Lymphedema
- Lipedema
- Extrinsic compression
- Hematoma, cysts
- Adenopathy
- Arteriovenous fistula
- Heart failure (edema)
- Vascularized mass
- Abscess

Correlation

- CT scan
- MRI
- Venogram

Medical Treatment

- Anticoagulation therapy (e.g., heparin, warfarin)
- DVT prophylaxis (e.g., intermittent pneumatic cuff compression)
- Limit long periods of inactivity
- Promote venous return (e.g., elevate legs, wear elastic stockings/support hose)

Surgical Treatment

- Iliofemoral venous thrombectomy
- Iliocaval or IVC bypass (caval occlusion)

Endovascular Treatment

- IVC filter (acute DVT)
- Catheter directed thrombolysis with Urokinase, etc. (acute DVT)
- Balloon venoplasty and stenting for chronic iliofemoral DVT
- Mechanical thrombectomy, such as Angiojet (acute DVT)

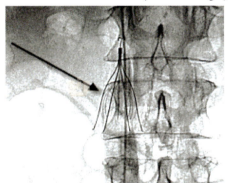

Fig. 31-26: *Inferior vena cavagram showing IVC filter*

REFERENCES

1. Glovicczki P. (2005). Introduction and general considerations. In *Rutherford Vascular Surgery 6th edition.* (2111-2123). Philadelphia. Elsevier Saunders.
2. Guyton AC. (1986). Hemostasis and blood coagulation. In *Textbook of Medical Physiology 7th edition.* (76-86). Philadelphia: WB Saunders.
3. Fareed J, Hoppenstedt DA, Iqbal O, Florian-Kujawski M, Tobu M, Bick, RL, Sheikh T, Jeske W. (2005). Normal and abnormal coagulation. In *Rutherford Vascular Sugery 6th edition.* (493-511). Philadelphia. Elsevier Saunders.
4. Henke PK, Schmaier A, Wakefield TW. (2005). Vascular thrombosis due to hypercoaguable states. In *Rutherford Vascular Sugery 6th edition.* (568-578). Philadelphia. Elsevier Saunders.
5. Sumner DS, Zierler RE. (2005). Vascular physiology: essential hemodynamic principles. In *Rutherford Vascular Sugery 6th edition.* (75-123). Philadelphia. Elsevier Saunders
6. Dawson DL, Beals H. (2010). Acute lower extremity deep venous thrombosis. In Zierler RE (Ed.), *Strandess's duplex scanning disorders in vascular diagnosis 4th ed.* (179-198). Philadelphia Wolters Kluwer Lippincott Williams & Wilkins
7. Zwiebel, WJ (2005). Ultrasound assessment of the aorta, iliac arteries and inferior vena cava. In Zwiebel WJ, Pellerito JS (Eds.), *Introduction to Vascular Ultrasonography 5th ed,* (530-552). Philadelphia: Elsevier Saunders.
8. Meissner MH. (2005). Venous duplex scanning. In *Rutherford Vascular Sugery 6th edition.* (254-270). Philadelphia. Elsevier Saunders.
9. Zwiebel, WJ (2005). Ultrasound Diagnosis of Venous Thrombosis. In Zwiebel WJ, Pellerito JS (Eds.), Introduction to Vascular Ultrasonography 5th ed, (449-465). Philadelphia: Elsevier Saunders.
10. Myers K, Clough A. (2004). Venous thrombosis in the lower limbs. In *Making sense of Vascular ultrasound: A Hands on Guide.* (181-197). London: Hodder Arnold.
11. Bower TC. (2005). Evaluation and management of malignant tumors of the inferior vena cava. In *Rutherford Vascular Sugery 6th edition.* (2245-2357). Philadelphia. El Sevier Saunders.
12. Glovicczki P, Cho JS. (2005) Surgical treatment of chronic occlusions of the iliac veins and the superior vena cava. In *Rutherford Vascular Sugery 6th edition.* (2303-2320). Philadelphia. El Sevier Saunders.
13. Sidawy AN. (2005) Embryology of the vascular system. In *Rutherford Vascular Sugery 6th edition.* (53-62). Philadelphia. El Sevier Saunders.
14. Needleman, L., Cronan, J. J., Lilly, M. P., Merli, G. J., Adhikari, S., Hertzberg, B. S., DeJong, M. R., Streiff, M. B., & Meissner, M. H. (2018). Ultrasound for Lower Extremity Deep Venous Thrombosis: Multidisciplinary Recommendations From the Society of Radiologists in Ultrasound Consensus Conference. Circulation, 137(14), 1505–1515. https://doi.org/10.1161/CIRCULATIONAHA.117.030687

VENOUS TESTING
32. Venous Stent Duplex

Definition
The combination of real-time B-mode ultrasonography with spectral and color Doppler used to diagnose the presence or absence of a hemodynamically significant obstruction, provide ultrasound guidance during stenting procedures, and allow for post-procedure surveillance of the iliac venous segment.

Etiology [1,2,15,16]
- Thrombosis
- Tumors
  » Extrinsic compression by a cell mass or a tumor
  » Tumor invasion of the inferior vena cava (IVC)
- Iliac vein obstruction
  » Thrombotic
  » Nonthrombotic iliac vein lesion (NIVL)
- Congenital anomalies

Risk Factors
- Age
- Immobilization
- Prothrombotic gene mutation (clotting disorders such as factor V Leiden)
- Postoperative phase (especially after orthopedic surgery)
- Peri pregnancy
- Previous deep vein thrombosis (DVT)
- Venous malformations (e.g., Klippel-Trenaunay)
- Mechanical compression of an iliac vein by an overlying artery
- Intraluminal obstruction (thrombosis, scarring, or mass)

Indications for Exam
- History of DVT involving the common femoral veins (CFV) or iliac veins
- History of pulmonary embolus
- Edema involving the upper thigh
- Edema/swelling, especially when unilateral
- Ulceration (especially in gaiter area)
- Discoloration in the gaiter area
- Venous claudication
  » Pain with physical exercise which increases with intensity and feels constrictive in the calf or thigh
  » Results in functional impairment
  » Symptoms only dissipate when the leg is positioned to enhance venous drainage (leg raised)
- History of inferior vena cava (IVC) filter placement
- Asymmetry of the CFV spectral Doppler waveforms observed during lower extremity venous duplex
- Varicose veins, especially reoccurring post previous vein treatment
- Pallor (phlegmasia alba dolens)
- Cyanosis (phlegmasia cerulea dolens)
- Reoccurring lower extremity deep vein thrombosis
- Genital varicosities
- Lower extremity varicosities of pelvic origin (via the pelvic escape points)
- Routine stent surveillance

Contraindications/Limitations
- Morbid obesity
- Open wounds with bandaging that cannot be removed
- Patients who cannot cooperate or cannot be positioned adequately
- Excessive bowel gas
- Dense scar tissue from major abdominal surgery
- Patients with a large amount of peristaltic motion may produce major color and power Doppler artifacts obstructing the visualization of vessels
- Enlarged uterus overlying the IVC or iliac veins

This exam is operator-dependent; its accuracy and success depend upon the level of experience of the sonographer.

Mechanism of Disease
Inferior Vena Cava

Idiopathic/primary obstruction [3]
- Propagation of thrombus from the iliac veins
- Isolated thrombus of the inferior vena cava can occur, even though the incidence is low.

Provoked/secondary obstruction [3]
- Outflow obstruction, e.g., Budd Chiari-Syndrome (obstruction of veins of the liver)
- Extrinsic compression by a mass
- Intrinsic pathology (e.g., IVC filter occlusion or filter migration)
- Tumor invasion of the IVC

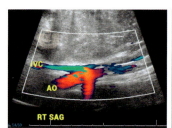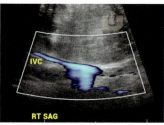

Fig. 32-1: *Extrinsic compression of the IVC by a Wilms tumor, (a rare kidney cancer in children)*

Anatomic variations causing obstruction may include: [4,5]
- **Aplasia:** The failure of the IVC to develop or to function normally
- **Hypoplasia:** Underdevelopment of the IVC
- **Left-sided cava:** Refers to a variant course of the inferior vena cava. It is the most common anomaly of the IVC and occurs due to the persistence of the left supra cardinal vein.
- **Duplication of the IVC**

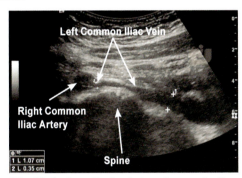

Fig. 32-2: *Color and spectral Doppler tracing of extrinsically compressed EIV. A tumor is compressing and narrowing the lumen. The increased velocities on the spectral Doppler tracing indicate that the vein is extrinsically compressed.*

Native Common and External Iliac Veins (CIV and EIV)
Iliac vein obstruction can occur due to: [2]

- Thrombotic lesions (Can occur after an incidence of DVT and cause an intrinsic obstruction).
- NIVL (non thrombotic vein lesion) is the pathological compression of an iliac vein by an overlying iliac artery.
  » Extrinsic compression results if partial or complete compression of the vein lumen exists.
  » Intrinsic obstruction results in wall fibrosis and intraluminal changes caused by the pulsations of an overlying artery.
- The source of extrinsic compression can also be a cell mass or a tumor.

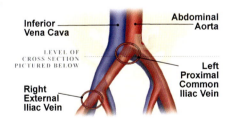

Fig. 32-3: *Longitudinal view demonstrating significant narrowing of the CIV due to the stretching of the vein over the spine.*

Note the slight shift in the position (when comparing Figs. 32-4 and 5) of the aorta and the IVC creating additional sites of potential obstruction.

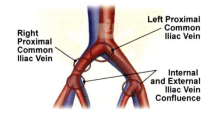

Fig. 32-4: *Most frequently occurring NIVLs*

Fig. 32-5: *Less frequently occurring NIVLs*

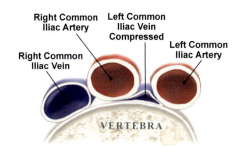

Fig. 32-6: *Cross-section view of the left CIV being compressed by the right and left CIAs.* Adapted from www.scgvs.com

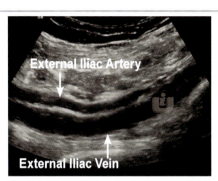

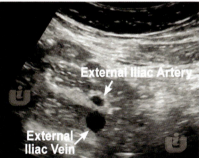

Fig. 32-7: *EIV in longitudinal and transverse views demonstrating pulsatile, repetitive compression of the EIV by the overlying EIA.*

Table 32-1: Areas of Iliac Vein Compression*

Common Iliac Veins
- Right common iliac artery on left common iliac vein
- Right common iliac artery on right common iliac vein
- Left common iliac artery on left common iliac vein

External Iliac Veins
- Right external iliac artery on right external iliac vein
- Right internal iliac artery on right external iliac vein
- Left external iliac artery on left external iliac vein
- Left internal iliac artery on left external iliac vein
- Inguinal ligament on right external iliac vein
- Inguinal ligament on left external iliac vein

*More than one type of compression may exist.

Labropoulos Nicos, Diagnosis of Iliac Vein Obstruction with Duplex Ultrasound Criteria used during duplex ultrasound examination to identify iliac vein obstruction. Endovascular Today, July 2018, Vol. 17, No. 7, page 3

Patient History
- Acute onset of leg pain
- Acute onset of swelling
- Persistent leg/calf swelling (usually unilateral, but can be bilateral)
- Symptoms of PE (e.g., shortness of breath, chest pain, hemoptysis)
- Previous DVT
- Clotting issues (e.g., problems with anticoagulation therapy, cancer)
- Recent periods of immobilization (e.g., bed rest, long plane or car ride)
- Postoperative (e.g., orthopedic or neurosurgery; can occur anytime during surgery or the six months thereafter)
- Venous claudication
- Iliac vein compression
- History of endovascular treatment (angioplasty and/or stent)
- Additional history for patients being considered for stents: A combination of signs and symptoms that have been unresponsive to conservative measures may be a candidate for stenting

Family History
- DVT
- Congenital abnormalities (e.g., Klippel-Trenaunay)
- Iliac vein compression
- Anatomic variations

Physical Examination
- Edema or swelling
- Varicose veins (particularly reoccurring)
- Edema
- Venous origin changes in skin and subcutaneous tissue
- Corona Phlebectatica
- Venous ulcer

Location of Disease
- Inferior Vena Cava (IVC)
- The left common iliac vein (CIV) is the most common to have obstructive pathology
- Compression of the right CIV and bilateral EIVs have been documented

Patient Preparation
If possible, the patients should be fasting for 6 - 12 hours to minimize the presence of air/bowel gas in the abdomen for better visualization. However, the iliac veins can often be visualized without a fasting preparation. Explain the procedure to the patient.

Patient Position
- The patient is in a supine position with the head of the bed slightly raised, arms by their side, or resting on their chest.
- The patient should breathe normally and not talk when spectral Doppler waveforms are obtained (Valsalva should not be used when testing for phasicity).

Scanning Protocol
B-mode imaging and transverse transducer compression maneuvers are often ineffective when evaluating abdominal or pelvic veins. Therefore, color, power Doppler, and spectral Doppler will be the primary modalities for evaluation. Gain settings for color or power Doppler should be adjusted for low flow states; persistence increased, sensitivity set high, velocity scale decreased, filter set low and smooth settings increased.

Inferior Vena Cava
- Locate the IVC in the upper abdomen just below the xiphoid process in the transverse view. Follow the IVC from the xiphoid process to the peripheral abdomen (the level of the confluence of the right and left common iliac veins, record diameters at central, mid, and peripheral abdomen.
- In a transverse view, starting at the xiphoid process, the IVC should appear as an oval; if it is seen nearly round, it may be indicative of right heart congestion or fluid overload.
- Turn the transducer to a longitudinal view and obtain spectral Doppler waveforms.

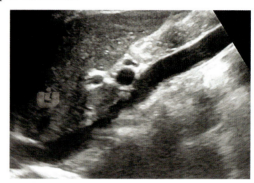

Fig. 32-8: *Longitudinal view of the IVC.*

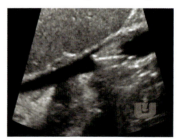

Fig. 32-9: *Longitudinal view of an IVC with a Greenfield filter.*

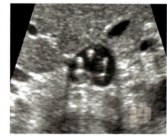

Fig. 32-10: *Transverse view of an IVC with a Greenfield filter.*

Images courtesy of Philips Healthcare

Iliac Veins [5,6,7]
Indirect testing of the iliac veins should be included in all lower extremity venous duplex testing via comparison of the bilateral CFV spectral Doppler waveforms. They should demonstrate phasic symmetrical flow.

When indirect signs are detected, they always indicate some form of obstruction. However, they cannot differentiate between stenosis and occlusion, extrinsic compression, or luminal changes. Therefore, direct imaging of the affected veins is important. The presence of phasic flow and good augmentation cannot exclude obstruction.

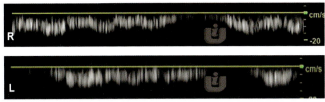

Fig. 32-11: Spectral Doppler demonstrating symmetrical phasicity when comparing the right and left common femoral veins.

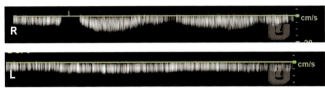

Fig. 32-12: Spectral Doppler demonstrates a total lack of phasicity (aka continuous flow) in the left CFV when compared to the right CFV. This is an indirect indication of a more central obstruction.

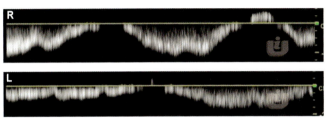

Fig. 32-13: Asymmetry (not just an absence of phasicity) indicates a more central obstruction when comparing the common femoral Doppler waveforms.

- The confluence of the right and left CIV is identified by moving the transducer in transverse orientation caudally to the peripheral IVC at the level of the umbilicus.
- Because the right CIV has a fairly straight course to the IVC, a long view can be obtained by placing the transducer longitudinally just to the right of the umbilicus.
- To establish the long view of the left CIV, the transducer is positioned obliquely.
- The entire length of the iliac veins from the IVC to the inguinal ligament is imaged.

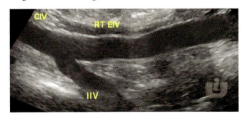

Fig. 32-14: The confluence of the IIV and EIV forms the CIV.

Native Iliac Veins [7,8,9]

- The exam begins at the confluence of the femoral and deep femoral veins and finishes at the inferior vena cava.
- Care should be taken to avoid heavy manual compression; this can create false positive results.
- The majority of the evaluation of the iliac system is performed in a longitudinal view.
- Transverse evaluation of the CIVs and EIVs should be included when they can be well visualized in that view.

- If a significant obstruction is present, the inflow to the iliac veins via the lower extremity and the outflow via the IVC should be imaged to:
  » Assess the veins to determine optimal stent placement from one healthy vein segment to the next
  » Ensure there is adequate inflow which allows for long-term patency of the stent
- B-mode imaging should be used to assess for:
  » Vein diameter
  » Intraluminal changes
  » Spurring/fibrotic changes to the walls
  » Thrombosis (occlusive or nonocclusive)
  » Chronic changes from previous thrombosis (e.g., synechiae, wall thickening)
  » Occlusion
- Color Doppler scale should be adjusted to allow for slow venous flow and is used to assess for:
  » A color jet at the level of stenosis
  » Mosaic color flow pattern due to post stenotic turbulence
  » Direction of flow; particularly in the IIV
  » Retrograde flow in the IIV is often seen in patients with a significant CIV compression

An ideal Doppler angle is 60°, but <60° may be used. Velocity measurements should be obtained using the same angle. .Compare the peripheral velocity with the velocity at the point of compression to obtain the ratio used to detect significant compression.

- Spectral Doppler using an angle of ≤60° is used to assess for:
  » Side-to-side (right-to-left) variability in spectral Doppler waveforms
  » Peak venous velocities when a stenosis is suspected. Velocities are obtained peripheral to and at the level of the stenosis to obtain a velocity ratio.
- B-mode imaging, color, and spectral Doppler image documentation in the longitudinal view should include:
  » The deep femoral and femoral veins just peripheral to their confluence
  » CFV
  » Peripheral EIV
  » Mid EIV
  » Above EIV
  » EIV and IIV confluence
  » Peripheral CIV
  » Mid CIV
  » Central CIV
  » IIV
  » If external compression or luminal changes are present, diameters (anterior to posterior wall) and spectral Doppler peak vein velocity should be documented:
    - Peripheral to the obstruction (pre-stenosis)
    - At the level of obstruction
    - Above the obstruction (post-stenosis)

The term "peripheral" refers to the segment closest to the legs. The term "central" refers to the segment closest to the IVC.

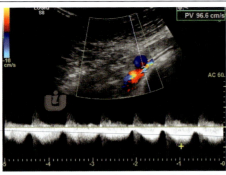

Fig. 32-15: Spectral Doppler of the CIV at the level of compression.

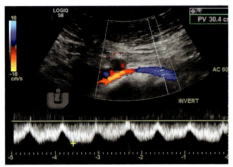

Fig. 32-16: Spectral Doppler of the left CIV within the peripheral segment. These velocities are used to calculate a ratio to determine if there is a significant stenosis. Note that a ≤60° angle is used to obtain accurate velocities. 96.6cm/s *(Fig. 32-15)* ÷ 30.4cm/s *(Fig. 32-16)* = ratio of 3.18

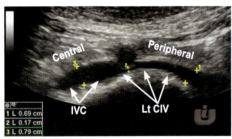

Fig. 32-17: For accurate measurements, diameters are obtained in B-mode to ensure good visualization of the anterior and posterior wall measurements.

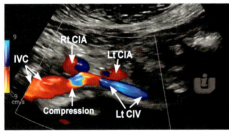

Fig. 32-18: Left CIV as it courses posterior to the right CIA, the point of compression is demonstrated by the decreased diameter in the vein along with color flow aliasing.

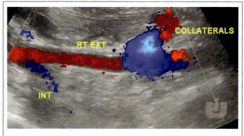

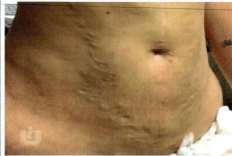

Fig. 32-19: Patients with an IVC and CIV occlusion present with extensive abdominal varices, which are visualized as tributaries of the external iliac vein using duplex ultrasound.

Care should be taken with transducer pressure on the abdomen to not extrinsically compress the CIVs, creating false positives. This most commonly occurs on the left side; however, this should apply to a visibly narrowed right CIV.

Internal Iliac Vein
- The bilateral IIVs should be evaluated with color and spectral Doppler for flow direction and phasicity
- Spontaneous, continuous reflux within the IIV indicates a significant, more central stenosis.[7]

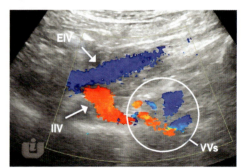

Fig. 32-20: Transabdominal color flow demonstrating varicose veins of the IIV.

Post-Stenting Ultrasound [9, 10, 11]
- Placement and length of a venous stent is based upon provider preference and could be:
  » Limited to the location of the lesion (typically the CIV)
  » Extending along the CIV into the EIV

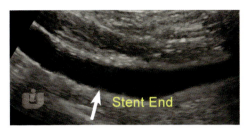

Fig. 32-21: *Peripheral end of a stent that is limited to the CIV, no extension into the EIV.*

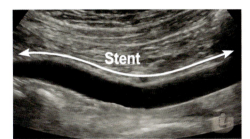

Fig. 32-22: *Left iliac vein stent extending from the IVC into the external iliac vein.*

- Follow the native iliac ultrasound protocol for the post-stenting duplex with the addition of the stent-specific measurements.
- Using B-mode, the stent is assessed along its length in longitudinal and transverse views to evaluate for any mural thrombus, visual narrowing, and intraluminal changes.
- Use color Doppler, with a low scale setting for venous flow in a longitudinal view to assess the length of the stent and its inflow (native vein peripheral to the stent) and outflow (native vein central to the stent) for:
  » A color jet indicating a stenosis
  » A mosaic color flow pattern due to post stenotic turbulence at the following levels.
  » The absence of color flow indicating an occlusion
- Obtain spectral Doppler waveforms in a longitudinal view using a ≤60° angle to evaluate for spontaneous flow in the following areas:
  » Inflow-to-the-stent (peripheral-to-the-stent)
  » Peripheral end-of-the-stent
  » Mid stent
  » Central end-of-the-stent
  » Outflow-of-the-stent (central-to-the-stent)
  » Additionally, peak vein velocities should be obtained at the level of a suspected stenosis, peripheral to the stenosis, and central to the stenosis.

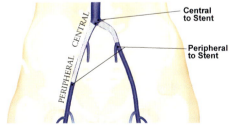

Fig. 32-23: *Spectral Doppler waveforms are obtained within the stent, peripheral and central to the stent. Note that two different lengths of stents are depicted. Stent length is provider-dependent.*

If a significant stenosis is suspected, the patient may have a repeat venogram and IVUS to determine the severity of stenosis, and treat it if needed.

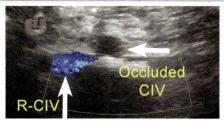

Fig. 32-24: *Occlusion of the left CIV pre-stenting.*

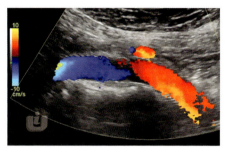

Fig. 32-25: *Resolution of the occlusion of the left CIV post stenting.*

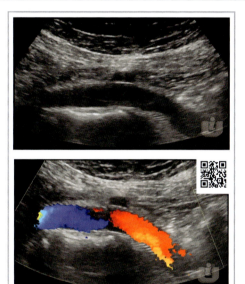

Fig. 32-26: *Cine loop of left CIV stent at the level of the right CIA.*

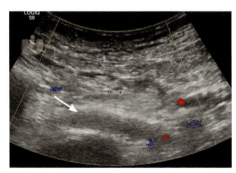

Fig. 32-27: *Longitudinal view demonstrating the absence of color flow in an occluded CIV stent.*

Ideal vein stents have increased wall strength to resist compression and can with stand repetitive motion.

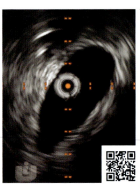

Fig. 32-28: *Cine loop of the IVUS catheter coursing from the peripheral CIV to the IVC. At the .08-second mark, note that the CIV lumen is beginning to narrow. At the .10-second mark, the Rt CIA courses anterior to the CIV, causing near occlusion, and at the .12 sec mark, the vein dilates as the catheter moves beyond the lesion.*

Protocol: Venous Stenting

- Common imaging modalities include venography and Intravascular Ultrasound (IVUS). Local anesthetic or mild IV sedation is administered.

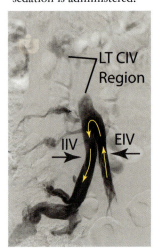

Fig. 32-29: *Contrast is visualized as it moves toward the EIV and IIV confluence. Note the absence of flow centrally toward the IVC, instead, it fills the left IIV. This is indicative of a near or complete occlusion of the CIV.*

- A final venogram is performed to confirm flow and absence of collateral vessels seen before the procedure.
- Stent deployment requires the support of multiple imaging modalities to locate diseased vessels and choose stent type and size to ensure proper deployment.

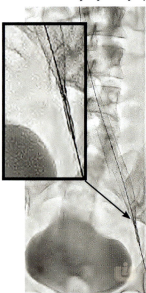

Fig. 32-30: *The stent is deployed and expands as the delivery system is withdrawn.*

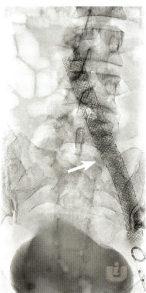

Fig. 32-31: *Fully deployed stent extending from the peripheral EIV to the IVC.*

- It is recommended that there is at least 1cm of overlap when multiple stents are needed to cover the length of a lesion.
  » The entire length of the stent system is re-dilated using the balloon catheter.
  » Self-expanding stents are used with post-placement balloon dilation to ensure that the stent is fully expanded.
- IVUS is used to confirm that the stent system is fully expanded along its length and confirms the location of the peripheral end of the stent.

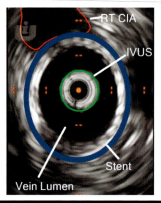

Fig. 32-32: *IVUS demonstrating widely patent stent at the level of the pre-stent lesion.*

Interpretation/Diagnostic Criteria

Normal

Native IVC Iliac and Stent

B-mode Imaging
- The vein/stent is free of echogenic material
- **IVC/Native Iliac:** Variation of diameter is visualized in response to breathing
- **Stent:** No variation of diameter is visualized in response to breathing

Color Doppler

Spontaneous, antegrade color filling of the vein/stent with respiration.

Spectral Doppler Waveforms
- **Spontaneity:** The vein demonstrates spontaneous flow and symmetrical spectral Doppler waveform compared to the contralateral vein.
- **Phasicity:** Venous flow varies with the respiratory and cardiac cycles. Phasicity is symmetrical when compared with the contralateral side.
- In stents, the symmetry from side to side may be slightly decreased due to the rigidity of the stent.

Abnormal [8,9,12,13,6,7,14]

B-mode Imaging
- Indirect signs of central obstruction/occlusion include:
  » Difficulty in compressing the CFV
  » Presence of collateral veins
- Direct signs of iliac/stent obstruction or occlusion
  » Intraluminal changes, which may include thrombus, webbing, and fibrotic changes to the vein wall
  » Visible narrowing on B-mode, measure the pre-stenotic segment and the stenotic segment with calipers

Table 32-2: Diagnostic Criteria for Iliac Vein and Stent Duplex Scan Obstruction

	B-mode	Spectral Doppler	Color Doppler
CIV and EIV	• Visible narrowing of the vein lumen • Presence of collateral veins	• Peak vein velocity ratio >2.5 (point of obstruction ÷ peripheral segment) • Lack of symmetrical and phasic waveforms when comparing left to right	• Absence of color flow • Presence of a color jet at the level of a suspected stenosis • Mosaic color flow pattern due to post stenotic turbulence
Stent	• Visible narrowing of the stent lumen	• Localized increase in peak venous velocity	• Same as above
IIV	• Presence of collateral veins	• Retrograde flow (spontaneous or with provocative maneuvers)	• Reversal of color flow with provocative maneuvers

Color Doppler

Color Doppler scale should be adjusted to allow for slow venous flow.

- Indirect signs of obstruction
  - » Reversal of flow in the ipsilateral IIV
  - » Reversal of flow in the deep external pudendal vein
  - » Cephalad flow in the inferior epigastric
- Direct signs of obstruction
  - » Absence of color flow
  - » Presence of a color jet at the level of a suspected stenosis
  - » Mosaic color flow pattern due to post stenotic turbulence

Spectral Doppler Waveforms

Spectral Doppler scale should be adjusted to allow for slow venous flow.

- Indirect signs
  - » Non-phasic flow in the central CFV
  - » Asymmetrical flow pattern in the CFVs
  - » Non-phasic flow during Valsalva maneuver
  - » Low or no velocity augmentation in CFV during thigh compression or dorsi/plantar flexion
- Direct signs
  - » **Native iliac:** Peak vein velocity ratio of >2.5 when comparing the peak vein velocity of the pre-stenotic (peripheral) segment to the peak vein velocity at the stenosis
  - » **Stented iliac:** Localized increase in peak vein velocity indicates an in-stent stenosis.

At present, there are no published validated diagnostic criteria to determine the severity of an in-stent stenosis.

REFERENCES

1. Raju S. (2013). Best management options for chronic iliac vein stenosis and occlusion. Journal of vascular surgery, 57(4), 1163–1169.
2. Meissner, M. H., Khilnani, N. M., Labropoulos, N., Gasparis, A. P., Gibson, K., Greiner, M., Learman, L. A., Atashroo, D., Lurie, F., Passman, M. A., Basile, A., Lazarshvilli, Z., Lohr, J., Kim, M. D., Nicolini, P. H., Pabon-Ramos, W. M., & Rosenblatt, M. (2021). The Symptoms-Varices-Pathophysiology classification of pelvic venous disorders: A report of the American Vein & Lymphatic Society International Working Group on Pelvic Venous Disorders. Journal of vascular surgery: Venous and lymphatic disorders, 9(3), 568–584.
3. Shi, W., & Dowell, J. D. (2017). Etiology and treatment of acute inferior vena cava thrombosis. Thrombosis research, 149, 9–16. https://doi.org/10.1016/j.thromres.2016.07.010
4. Morita, S., Higuchi, M., Saito, N., & Mitsuhashi, N. (2007). Pelvic venous variations in patients with congenital inferior vena cava anomalies: Classification with computed tomography. Acta Radiologica, 48(9), 974–979. https://doi.org/10.1080/02841850701499409
5. Labropoulos, N., Jasinski, P. T., Adrahtas, D., Gasparis, A. P., & Meissner, M. H. (2017). A standardized ultrasound approach to pelvic congestion syndrome. Phlebology, 32(9), 608–619. https://doi.org/10.1177/0268355516677135
6. Kayıhoğlu, S. I., Köksoy, C., & Alaçayır, İ. (2016). Diagnostic value of the femoral vein flow pattern for detecting an iliocaval venous obstruction. Journal of vascular surgery: Venous and lymphatic disorders, 4(1), 2–8. https://doi.org/10.1016/j.jvsv.2015.08.002
7. Labropoulos N. (2018). Diagnosis of iliac vein obstruction with duplex ultrasound: Criteria used during duplex ultrasound examination to identify iliac vein obstruction. Endovascular Today, 17(7), 50–52.
8. O'Sullivan, G.J. (2020). What is the best method of imaging in iliofemoral venous obstruction? Phlebolymphology, 27(2). 61-69.
9. Labropoulos, N., Borge, M., Pierce, K., & Pappas, P. J. (2007). Criteria for defining significant central vein stenosis with duplex ultrasound. Journal of Vascular Surgery, 46(1), 101–107. https://doi.org/10.1016/j.jvs.2007.02.062
10. Raju, S., Tackett, P., Jr, & Neglen, P. (2009). Reinterventions for nonocclusive iliofemoral venous stent malfunctions. Journal of Vascular Surgery, 49(2), 511–518. https://doi.org/10.1016/j.jvs.2008.08.003
11. Gibson, K. (July 2021). Iliac Vein Stenting: Best Practices for Patient Safety and Successful Outcomes. Endovascular Today. https://evtoday.com/articles/2021-july/iliac-vein-stenting-best-practices-for-patient-safety-and-successful-outcomes
12. Mousa, A. Y., Broce, M., Yacoub, M., & AbuRahma, A. F. (2016). Iliac Vein Interrogation Augments Venous Ulcer Healing in Patients Who Have Failed Standard Compression Therapy along with Pathological Venous Closure. Annals of Vascular Surgery, 34, 144–151.
13. Metzger, P. B., Rossi, F. H., Kambara, A. M., Izukawa, N. M., Saleh, M. H., Pinto, I. M., Amorim, J. E., & Thorpe, P. E. (2016). Criteria for detecting significant chronic iliac venous obstructions with duplex ultrasound. Journal of Vascular Surgery: Venous and Lymphatic Disorders, 4(1), 18–27.
14. MayR., & Thurner, J. (1957). The cause of the predominantly sinistral occurrence of thrombosis of the pelvic veins. Angiology, 8(5), 419–427.
15. Dawson, D.L., Beals, H. (2010). Acute lower extremity deep venous thrombosis. In R.E. Zierler (Ed.), Strandess's duplex scanning disorders in vascular diagnosis (4th ed., pp. 179-198). Philadelphia Wolters Kluwer Lippincott Williams & Wilkins.
16. Zwiebel, W.J. (2005). Ultrasound assessment of the aorta, iliac arteries and inferior vena cava. In W.J. Zwiebel & J.S. Pellerito (Eds.), Introduction to vascular ultrasonography (5th ed., pp. 530-552). Philadelphia: Elsevier Saunders.

VENOUS TESTING

33. Upper Extremity Venous Duplex Ultrasound

Definition

The combination of real time B-mode ultrasonography with spectral Doppler and color flow to evaluate the upper extremity veins for evidence of thrombus.

Venous duplex ultrasound can identify the presence, exact location, extent, and severity of venous thrombosis. The course of the veins, collaterals and thrombus can be visualized using B-mode and color while the analysis of Doppler flow patterns can yield further information regarding flow direction and both local and remote obstructions.

Etiology of Venous Disease

- The theory of Virchow's triad states that venous thrombosis is caused by: venous stasis, vein wall (intimal) injury or a hypercoagulable state.
- Extrinsic compression

Risk Factors

- Age (greater with advanced age)
- Central venous catheters
- Repetitive arm activities (e.g., weight lifting)
- Immobilization
- Genetic prothrombotic conditions (clotting disorders, such as Factor V Leiden)
- Post-operative phase (especially after orthopedic surgery)
- Pregnancy
- Oral contraceptives
- Estrogen replacement
- Cancer/malignancy
- Previous DVT
- Heart complications (e.g., MI, CHF)
- Obesity
- Family history
- Smoking
- COPD
- Blood type (highest risk with type-A, lowest risk with type-O)
- Trauma
- Antiphospholipid antibodies (e.g., lupus)
- Congenital abnormalities
- Drug use
- Cerebrovascular events (stroke, TIA)

Indications for Exam

- Edema/swelling (especially when unilateral)
- Limb pain/tenderness
- Limb redness
- Suspected injury after venous puncture/catheterization, especially of the IJV
- Symptoms of pulmonary embolism (PE) (e.g., shortness of breath, chest pain, hemoptysis)

Contraindications/Limitations

- Anatomical limitations (clavicle and ribs)
- Open wounds prohibiting access by the ultrasound transducer
- Casts that cannot be removed or traction that limits access to the scan areas
- Poor visualization due to vessel depth because of obesity or severe edema
- Patients who cannot be adequately positioned

It is technically difficult to image the neck veins with the patient in a sitting position. The veins sometimes collapse due to compression by atmospheric pressure from the outside.

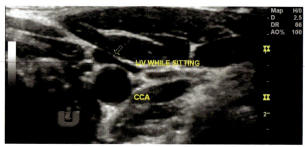

Fig. 33-1: *IJV collapses with patient sitting up*

Mechanism of Disease [1,2]

There are three factors responsible for the formation of venous thrombosis, as outlined in Virchow's Triad: (vein wall injury, hypercoagulability and stasis of blood flow). A combination of any of these events may increase the risk of venous thrombosis.

- There is a balance between coagulation (process to prevent excessive bleeding after injury) and anticoagulation (process to prevent spontaneous intravascular clotting) in normal blood flow.
- The venous endothelial layer is normally antithrombotic. In response to endothelial injury, leukocytes (white blood cells) attach to the vessel wall. A plasma protein known as *prothrombin* is activated. Prothrombin activator catalyzes conversion of prothrombin into thrombin. Thrombin acts as an enzyme to convert fibrinogen into fibrin threads, forming a clot.
- Hypercoagulable, states result from genetic mutation or acquired deficiencies that accompany certain diseases (e.g., liver disease). In such cases, naturally occurring anticoagulants (antithrombin, protein C, protein S, etc.) are deficient. For example, genetic mutation, factor V Leiden, causes resistance to the natural anticoagulant protein C.
- Non-movement of blood flow (stasis) permits coagulation. Platelets are thought to become trapped by low shear stress (flow) at valve cusps. Platelets adhere to the subendothelial (collagen) layer of the venous wall and may aggregate depending on the amount of coagulation and thrombolysis occurring in the body at that time.
- Increased activation of coagulation factors in those suffering from cancer is thought to lead to formation of venous thrombosis. In addition, the levels of coagulation inhibitors normally found in the blood (e.g., proteins C or S), are thought to be reduced in these patients.
- The use of estrogen (in replacement therapy or birth control) alters coagulation and may predispose individuals to thrombosis.
- Venous aneurysms are a rare condition. Research suggests several possible causes; decreased smooth muscle cells and an increase in fibrous connective tissue or either an increase or decrease in the fibrous connective tissue and elastic fibers. [3]
  » Upper extremity venous aneurysm are reported to be more common than lower extremity venous aneurysms, although both are rare. [14]
- Once thrombus is formed, it can:
  » **Stabilize:** Stabilization includes adherence of the thrombus to the vessel wall without changing location or propagating. If thrombus has formed, the most favorable occurrence would be to stabilize. This reduces the risk to the patient.

- » **Propagate:** Propagation includes "growth of the thrombus" in size or location. Examples of propagation may include a thrombus that extends from the superficial system into the deep system.
- » **Embolize:** During embolization, a portion of a thrombus breaks free and travels downstream in the vascular system. The greatest risk to the patient is that the thrombus travels to the lungs and results in a pulmonary embolus.

Upper extremity venous thrombosis is less likely to embolize and cause a symptomatic pulmonary embolism compared to DVT in the lower extremities. [8]

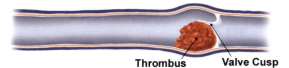

Fig. 33-2: *Thrombosis of vein*

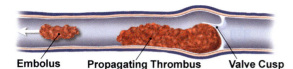

Fig. 33-3: *Embolization of thrombus*

Thrombus located within the deep veins is known as deep venous thrombosis (DVT). Thrombus located within the superficial veins is known as superficial venous thrombosis.

Location of Disease

Although any venous site can develop thrombus, common origins include:
- Valve sites
- Venous confluences
- Superficial venous system (basilic, cephalic, median cubital)
- Deep venous system:
  - » "Central veins" typically refer to the jugular, innominate, subclavian and sometimes axillary veins.
  - » Brachial, radial, ulnar veins

The upper extremity veins contain far fewer venous valves compared to the lower extremity.

The superficial veins of the upper extremity are the primary route of drainage for the arm.

Patient History

- Previous DVT
- Post-operative; orthopedic or neurosurgery for example, (can occur anytime during surgery or for 6 months thereafter)
- Persistent swelling (usually unilateral, but can be bilateral)
- Clotting issues (including problems regulating anticoagulation therapy, malignant cancer)
- Localized pain, burning or itching
- Symptoms of pulmonary embolism (PE) (e.g., shortness of breath, chest pain, hemoptysis)

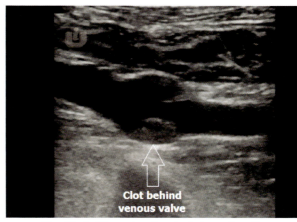

Fig. 33-4: *Thrombus located at a valve site*

Physical Examination

- Edema or swelling
- Tenderness
- Limb redness or warmth
- Dark pigmentation, hardened tissue
- Cyanosis (superior vena cava syndrome)
- Excessive collaterals around area of concern

Upper Extremity Venous Duplex Protocol

- Obtain a patient history to include symptoms and risk factors. Explain the procedure to the patient.
- The patient is examined in the supine position with the head turned slightly to the side and the chin slightly raised.
- Some patients may require the use of a range of transducers; including high-frequency (5-7 MHz) (8-15 MHz) transducers and a lower frequency (1-4 MHz) transducer may be useful around the clavicle.

Use venous presets on the duplex scanner; low color flow and Doppler scales will be needed to detect venous flow.

Use the deep transducer to aid visualization around the clavicle. Compare the waveforms and color from the segments above and below the bone since the segment cannot be directly studied.

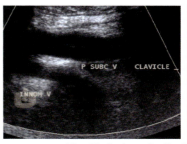 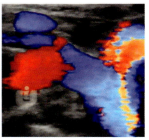

Fig. 33-5: *Longitudinal subclavian vein*

Transverse Scan and Images

Asking the patient to "sniff" will cause compression of the SCV and sometimes results in flow augmentation.

- Perform venous compression in the transverse plane (short axis) every 2-4cm along the limb. This is anatomically difficult and may not be possible near the clavicle. Instead of compressions, have the patient inhale or ask the patient to "sniff, like you're going to sniff a flower."

Compressions should always be performed in the transverse plane to ensure full compression and so duplicated veins are not missed.

Dual Screen Vein Compression

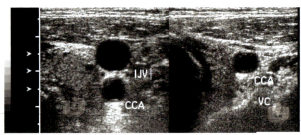

Fig. 33-6: *Dual screen image showing internal jugular vein compressibility*

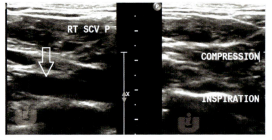

Fig. 33-7: *Dual screen image showing subclavian vein compressibility (demonstrated using the "sniff" technique)*

- Record transverse images using "dual-screen" on the duplex scanner. Obtain and freeze an image without vein compression on the left side of the screen. Capture an image with vein compression on the right side of the screen. Document transverse images of the following veins with and without compressions as described above:
  » Internal jugular vein (IJV)
  » Subclavian vein (if possible)
  » Axillary vein
  » Brachial vein
  » Basilic vein
  » Cephalic vein

Keep the transducer at a 90° angle to the skin for the best B-mode images.

- Additional documentation of compressions can be performed when indicated and anatomically possible to include the cephalic arch, brachiocephalic (innominate), radial, ulnar or median cubital veins.

Dual Screen Image Showing Venous Compressibility

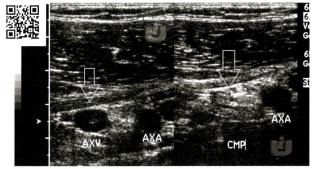

Fig. 33-8: *Dual screen showing axillary vein compressibility*

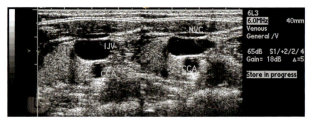

Fig. 33-9: *Dual screen showing internal jugular vein partial compressibility*

Longitudinal Scan and Images

- Record venous spectral waveforms with color Doppler in the longitudinal (sagittal axis) view. If your lab chooses to set an angle, use a ≤60° Doppler angle with the cursor placed parallel to the vessel walls in the center of the flow stream.
- Observe for augmentation of venous flow.
- Documentation should illustrate spontaneity, phasicity, augmentation. Pulsatility should be documented in all but the brachial and superficial veins. Record at the following locations:
  » Internal jugular vein
  » Subclavian vein
  » Axillary vein(s)
  » Brachial vein
  » Cephalic vein
  » Basilic vein

Some labs record venous spectral Doppler waveforms without setting an angle since actual velocities are usually not important in a venous exam.

  » Document spectral waveforms of paired veins individually.
  » Additional documentation of patency can be performed when necessary of the distal brachiocephalic, jugular-subclavian junction, radial, ulnar or median cubital veins.
- Use spectral Doppler to analyze absence of flow by placing an expanded Doppler sample volume in any vein segment suspected to be thrombosed. Doppler flow or lack of flow, compliments compression, color flow and B-mode images. Use the adjacent artery as a guide to identify an occluded vein when possible.

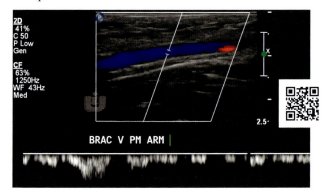

Fig. 33-10: *Normal brachial vein spectral waveform*

- Repeat for the contralateral extremity if a bilateral exam was ordered.
- If only a unilateral exam was requested, documentation of the contralateral subclavian venous spectral waveform is performed for comparison.

The transverse or oblique plane to the body may be better for recording flow in the distal brachiocephalic (innominate) vein.

Table 33-1: Upper Extremity Venous Protocol Summary

Scan transverse (short axis) with and without color compression	Scan longitudinal (sagittal axis) in B-mode and spectral Doppler (color Doppler can be used intermediately)
• Internal jugular vein (IJV) • Subclavian vein (SCV) • Axillary vein (AXV) • Brachial vein (BRV) • Basilic vein (BsV) • Cephalic vein (CV) • Subclavian-jugular confluence (optional) • Distal BCV (optional) • Radial vein (RV) (optional) • Ulnar vein (UV) (optional) • Median cubital vein (MCV) (optional)	• Internal jugular vein (IJV) • Subclavian vein (SCV) • Distal brachiocephalic (BCV) • Axillary vein (AXV) • Brachial vein (BRV) • Cephalic vein (CV) • Basilic vein (BsV) • Subclavian-jugular confluence (optional) • Radial vein (RV) (optional) • Ulnar vein (UV) (optional) • Median cubital vein (MCV) (optional)

- Additional documentation of compression may be recorded in segments other than those listed during evaluation for thrombus as necessary. (Compressions may be anatomically contraindicated, especially near the clavicle. If so, document patency with color flow and spectral waveforms.)
- Document additional spectral Doppler waveforms in all veins when dual (or more) venous systems are present.

PRINCIPLES OF INTERPRETATION

B-mode Imaging
Use B-mode imaging to determine if a thrombus is present:
- Confirm the vein collapses completely with light transducer pressure.
- Look for echogenic material present within the lumen of the vein.

Color Doppler
- Use color Doppler to determine if color flow is present wall-to-wall or if there is a filling defect.

Spectral Doppler Waveforms
Use spectral Doppler to determine if venous flow is:
- **Spontaneous:** Automatically hear a Doppler signal due to blood flow, no compression required
- **Phasic:** Flow increases and decreases with respiration
- **Augmentable:** Flow increases with distal compression
- **Pulsatile:** regular, rhythmic increase and decrease in the flow signal, similar to an arterial pulsation.

Interpretation/Diagnostic Criteria

Normal

B-mode Imaging
The vein is free of echogenic material and compresses completely when it is technically possible to compress the vein.

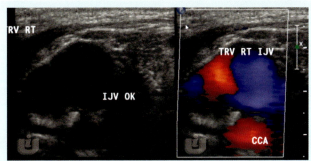

Fig. 33-11: *B-mode and color images of the internal jugular vein in transverse.*

Color Doppler
- Wall-to-wall color flow will fill the vein spontaneously or upon distal limb compression.

Spectral Doppler Waveforms
- **Spontaneity:** The vein demonstrates spontaneous flow, especially in the central veins (jugular, brachiocephalic (innominate), subclavian) and axillary vein. In the distal arm veins, the absence of spontaneous flow can be a normal finding.
- **Phasicity:** Venous signals are phasic and vary with respiration and the cardiac cycle. Cardiac changes are more obvious in the central veins and respiratory changes are more obvious distally, in the axillary veins for example. During deep exhalation, venous signals typically decrease or discontinue and increase with inhalation due to changes in intrathoracic pressures during the respiratory cycle.
- **Augmentation:** Compression of the limb distal to the transducer augments venous flow in the axillary and arm veins.
- **Pulsatility:** Pulsatile venous flow should be present in the upper extremity, especially in the central veins. Compare pulsatility when evaluating the distal brachiocephalic (innominate), subclavian and internal jugular veins. Equally pulsatile BCV, SCV and IJV flow is expected.

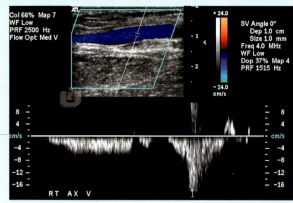

Fig. 33-12: *Normal, axillary spectral waveform. Phasic, non-pulsatile flow, which augments upon distal compression.*

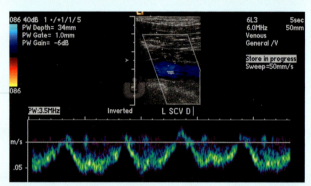

Fig. 33-13: *Normal, pulsatile subclavian spectral waveform*

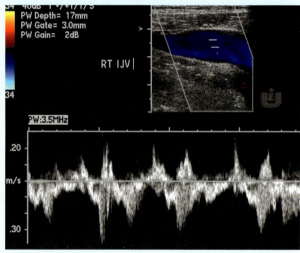

Fig. 33-14: *Normal spectral waveform-central veins (flow is normally spontaneous and pulsatile)*

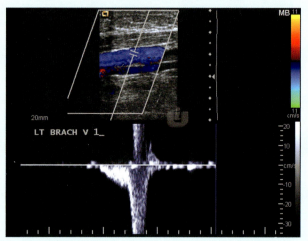

Fig. 33-15: *Normal spectral waveform-arm veins (normal for spontaneity and phasicity to be absent)*

Abnormal

B-mode Imaging

- **Compressibility:** Intralumenal echoes are visualized within the vein and full coaptation of the vein on manual compression is absent or limited due to thrombus.
  - » Compression of the artery with transducer pressure can be a confirmation of an incompressible venous segment.

Color flow can obscure a partially occlusive thrombus if the color gain is set too high.

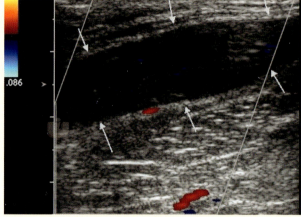

Fig. 33-16: *Longitudinal-totally occlusive thrombus (no color flow, low color scale)*

- It is possible for only one vein of a pair to be thrombosed. For this reason, it is important to make sure all veins are studied carefully.

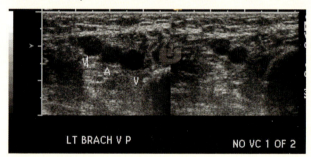

Fig. 33-17: *Dual screen: single brachial vein is incompressible*

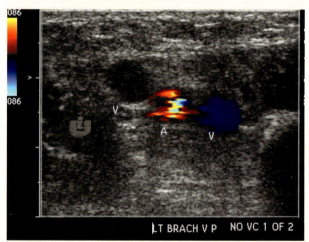

Fig. 33-18: *Single brachial vein without color flow in transverse plane*

- **Thrombus:** If thrombus is present, determine whether the thrombus is partially or totally occlusive, its location and the extent and the characteristics of the thrombus.
  - » **Acute thrombus:** Characteristics include medium to lightly echogenic or anechoic, spongy texture upon compression,

poor attachment to the venous wall or "free floating" within the lumen. A moving tail may be seen at the end of the thrombus. When a vein is fully thrombosed, the vein is often dilated, especially compared to the adjacent artery.

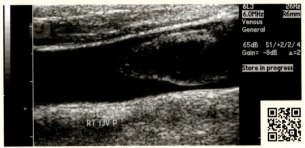

Fig. 33-19: *Free floating, acute thrombus*

» **Chronic thrombus:** Characteristics include brightly echogenic or heterogeneous echoes, irregular surface texture and thrombus which is attached to the venous wall. The vein can stay the same size as the artery, but often contracts in diameter over time. Collateral veins may be observed adjacent to the affected vein(s) and small irregular flow channels within the thrombus can sometimes be seen with color.

The term, chronic postthrombotic change has been suggested as a replacement for "chronic thrombus". The SRU has suggested that only acute events should be referred to as "acute thrombus". When it is technically difficult to determine whether findings are acute/chronic, use the term "indeterminate". [16]

» **Indeterminate age:** Characteristics of both acute and chronic stages may be present, making age difficult to determine (*Fig. 33-23*). [16]
» *Subacute* is another term used by labs. Reports have suggested using this term only to describe thrombus that appears to have changed appearance on B-mode compared to a previous study where the diagnosis of acute DVT was made some weeks earlier.

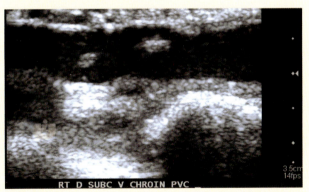

Fig. 33-20: *Chronic thrombus by B-mode image*

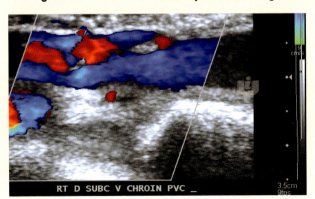

Fig. 33-21: *Color flows around chronic thrombus longitudinal view-irregular flow channel*

Stages of Thrombus: Comparison of Typical Venous Diameter During the Different Stages

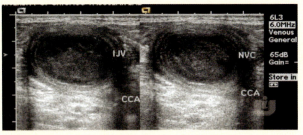

Fig. 33-22: *Acute IJV DVT*

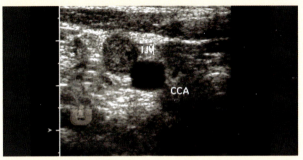

Fig. 33-23: *Indeterminate age: IJV DVT*

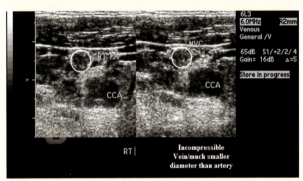

Fig. 33-24: *Chronic IJV DVT*

Color Doppler

» If partially occlusive thrombus is present, color flow will be seen flowing around echogenic material in the vein, spontaneously or with distal limb compression.
» If totally occlusive thrombus is present, no color flow will be observed even with distal limb compression.

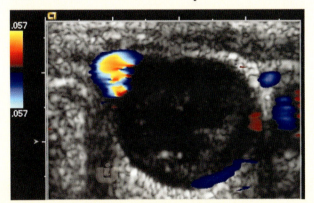

Fig. 33-25: *Transverse vein with minimal color flow around the thrombus*

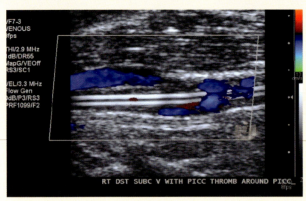

Fig. 33-26: *Longitudinal subclavian vein with color flowing around PICC line thrombus*

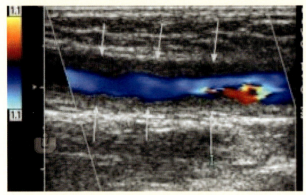

Fig. 33-27: *Longitudinal-partially occlusive thrombus (partial color flow)*

Table 33-2: Thrombosis Descriptions and Characteristics

Acute	Chronic
• Light to medium echogenic/anechoic	• Bright/heterogeneous echoes
• Spongy texture on compression (homogeneous)	• Irregular texture (heterogeneous)
• Poorly attached or free floating	• Attached
• Dilated vein (if totally occluded)	• Same size as artery or vein is contracted
	• Collateral veins may be noted

- Veins can be partially or totally incompressible in both acute and chronic stages.
- Combination of events can occurs (e.g., acute on top of chronic thrombus).
- Chronic thrombus with partial recanalization is seen as small color flow channels within thrombus.
- Age of thrombus is sometimes indeterminate.

Normal Doppler signals may be present when thrombus is partially occlusive.

Spectral Doppler Waveforms

- **Spontaneity:** Absence of flow with appropriate low-flow settings indicates venous obstruction. Use color flow in the adjacent artery as a guide to identify an occluded vein. But always confirm the absence of flow by placing sample volume in the vessel.
- **Phasicity:** Continuous venous flow (non-phasic flow) suggests either obstruction from DVT in a proximal venous segment or extrinsic compression of a proximal vein.
- **Augmentation:** If distal compression does not produce augmentation of the venous signal, a total obstruction distal to the transducer is suspected. It may be helpful to change the patient's position and/or try compressing a more muscular area of the arm after giving time for venous refill.
- **Pulsatility:** The absence of pulsatile venous flow suggests obstruction, especially in the central veins.

Table 33-3: Venous Duplex Diagnostic Criteria

Normal	Abnormal
Complete coaptation of vein walls with light transducer pressure	Lack of complete vein compression
Absent intralumenal thrombus	Intralumenal echoes present (acute thrombus can be echolucent)
Color flow fills the lumen completely	Decrease or absence of color flow
Normal venous Doppler spontaneity, phasicity and augmentation	Abnormal venous Doppler spontaneity, phasicity or augmentation
No venous dilatation	Dilated or contracted veins noted

Other Pathology

- **Extrinsic compression:** Continuous venous flow suggests either obstruction in a proximal venous segment or extrinsic compression of a vein.[11]

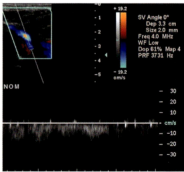
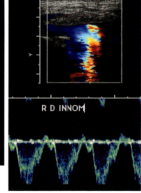

Fig. 33-28: *Abnormal innominate vein: Spectral Doppler with decreased pulsatility*

Fig. 33-29: *Normal innominate vein spectral Doppler*

- **Venous stenosis:** When increased focal venous velocity is noted (compared to distal segments), with or without provocative positional maneuvers, a venous stenosis is suspected. This condition can occur secondary to thoracic outlet syndrome, dialysis access intervention or extrinsic compression. Some labs use a venous-velocity ratio of ≥2.5 (a velocity increase of at least 2.5 times the immediate distal venous segment) to diagnose a hemodynamically significant stenosis.[12]

- **Effort thrombosis:** *Effort thrombosis or Paget-Schroetter syndrome* usually involves the subclavian venous segment. In this syndrome, the subclavian vein (SCV) is compressed between the first rib and scalene muscle (the thoracic outlet), which results in formation of venous thrombus and flow obstruction.[11,13]

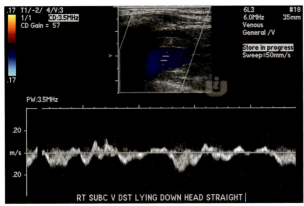

Fig. 33-30: *Normal SCV waveforms at rest*

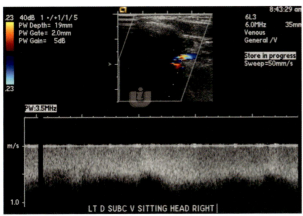

Fig. 33-31: *Increased venous flow with positional changes of the arm*

- **Upper extremity AXV and SCV thrombosis:** divided into two categories:
  » **Primary venous thrombosis:** also known as effort thrombosis or Paget-Schroetter syndrome, results from compression and the repetitive trauma which occurs to the venous segment in the thoracic outlet.
  » **Secondary venous thrombosis:** occurs due to other causes (e.g., insertion of catheters, hemodialysis ports, pacemakers, immobilization, etc.). Secondary thrombosis is more common (80% of cases).[15]

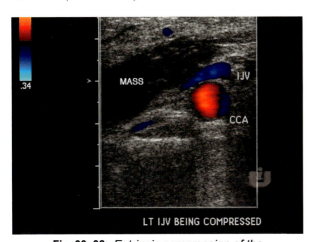

Fig. 33-32: *Extrinsic compression of the vein suspected-transverse view*

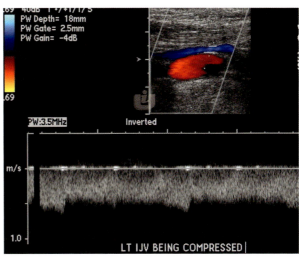

Fig. 33-33: *Venous compression confirmed by spectral Doppler (continuous flow/lacks pulsatility)*

- **Superior vena cava syndrome versus BCV obstruction:** When comparing the distal brachiocephalic (innominate) veins, the absence of pulsatile flow on both sides suggests a proximal obstruction in both innominate veins or in the superior vena cava (SVC syndrome). If the decrease in pulsatility is unilateral, obstruction of that brachiocephalic vein proximally is suspected (BCV obstruction).[8]
- **Venous aneurysm:** is diagnosed when there is an area of significant venous dilatation compared to the adjacent venous segment. Common locations for upper extremity venous aneurysms include the internal jugular and axillary veins. Document the presence of any mural thrombus.[14]
- **Central venous catheters:**[8] A central venous catheter is placed in one of the central veins and used to administer medication, nutrition, dialysis or chemotherapy treatments, etc. The use of central venous catheters has greatly increased in recent years. These lines increase the risk for venous thrombosis.[11]
- Observe the surface of any visualized intravenous catheters for thrombus development. It is possible for the thrombus that forms anywhere along these lines to extend into the more central veins.

  There are several different types of central venous catheters:
  » Tunneled catheters: A catheter that is "tunneled" under the skin makes it more discrete and keeps it in place before the catheter exits through the skin. Common tunneled catheters include *Hickman* and *Groshong* catheters.
  » Implanted ports remain under the skin and medications are injected through the skin into this type of catheter. Though these ports can be used for hemodialysis patients, they are primarily used for cancer treatment.
  » PICC line (*peripherally inserted central catheter*) is a line inserted in an arm vein with a tip that lies in one of the large veins in the chest. It can remain in position for up to six months.

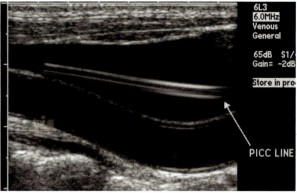

Fig. 33-34: *Upper extremity IJV PICC line without thrombus*

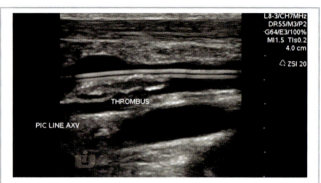

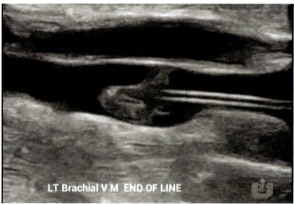

Fig. 33-35: *Upper extremity IJV PICC line with thrombus*

- Superficial tissue edema can helpful for clinicians to understand swelling/edema in the absence of thrombus.

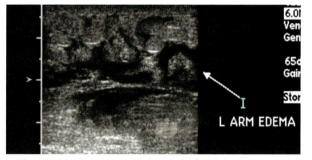

Fig. 33-36: *Upper extremity superficial tissue edema*

Differential Diagnosis

- Arterial disease
- Lymphedema
- Cellulitis
- Cysts
- Extrinsic compression
- Hematoma
- Muscle tear
- Joint effusion
- Adenopathy
- Arteriovenous fistula
- Heart failure
- Direct injury to extremity
- Vascularized mass
- Collagen vasculitis
- Abscess

Correlation

- CT scan
- MRI
- Venogram
- The Caprini Risk Score assesses DVT risk with questions that divide patients into low, moderate, and high risk. Perform the assessment at **capriniriskscore.org**

Medical Treatment and Prevention

- Anticoagulation therapy (e.g., heparin, warfarin)
- Promote venous drainage (e.g., elevate arms, wear elastic/support sleeves)

Surgical Treatment

- IVC filter (acute DVT)
- SVC reconstruction (femoral, spiral saphenous vein, PTFE or cryopreserved grafts)

Endovascular Treatment

- Catheter-directed thrombolysis with urokinase, etc. (acute DVT)
- Mechanical thrombectomy such as angiojet (acute DVT)
- Percutaneous transluminal angioplasty and stenting (SVC syndrome or axillo-subclavian issues)

REFERENCES

1. Wakefield TW. (2005). Bleeding and clotting: fundamental considerations. In Rutherford Vascular Surgery 6th edition. (493-511). Philadelphia. Elsevier Saunders.
2. Guyton AC. (1986). Hemostasis and blood coagulation. In Textbook of Medical Physiology 7th edition. (76-86). Philadelphia: WB Saunders.
3. Gillespie DL, Villavicencio JL, Gallagher C, Chang A, Hamelink JK, Fiala LA, O'Donnell SD, Jackson MR, Pikoulis E, Rich, NM. (1997). Presentation and management of venous aneurysms. *J Vasc Surg*. Nov;26(5):845-52.
4. Thrush A, Hartshorne T. (2005). Duplex assessment of deep venous thrombosis and upper limb venous disorders. In Peripheral Vascular Ultrasound, How Why and When, 2nd ed. (189-206). Edinburgh: Elsevier Churchill Livingstone.
5. Zwiebel, WJ (2005). Ultrasound Diagnosis of Venous Thrombosis. In Zwiebel WJ, Pellerito JS (Eds.), *Introduction to Vascular Ultrasonography 5th ed*, (449-465). Philadelphia: Elsevier Saunders.
6. Meissner MH. (2005). Venous duplex scanning. In Rutherford Vascular Surgery 6th edition. (254-270). Philadelphia. Elsevier Saunders.
7. Myers K, Clough A. (2004). Venous thrombosis in the lower limbs. In Making sense of vascular ultrasound: A hands on guide. (181-197). London: Hodder Arnold.
8. Caps MT, Mraz BA. (2010). Upper extremity venous thrombosis. In Zierler RE (Ed.), Strandess's duplex scanning disorders in vascular diagnosis 4th ed. (199-221).Philadelphia Wolters Kluwer Lippincott Williams & Wilkins.
9. Sumner DS, Mattos MA. (1993). Diagnosis of deep vein thrombosis with real-time color and duplex scanning. In Vascular Diagnosis 4th edition. (785-800). St. Louis. Mosby.
10. Lohr, J (2005). Upper Extremity Venous Duplex Imaging. In Mansour MA, Labropoulos N. (Eds.), *Vascular Diagnosis*, (469-477). Philadelphia: Elsevier Saunders.
11. Green RM. (2005). Subclavian-axillary vein thrombosis. In *Rutherford Vascular Surgery 6th edition*. (1371-1392). Philadelphia. Elsevier Saunders.
12. Leon, LR, Labropoulos, N, Mansour MA. (2005). Hemodynamic principles as applied to diagnostic testing. In Mansour MA, Labropoulos N. (Eds.), *Vascular Diagnosis*, (7-21). Philadelphia: Elsevier Saunders.
13. Kreienberg PB, Shah, DM, Darling III, RC, Change BB, Paty SK, Roddy SP, Ozsvath KJ, Manish M. (2005) Thoracic outlet syndrome: In Mansour MA, Labropoulos N. (Eds.), *Vascular Diagnosis*, (517-522). Philadelphia: Elsevier Saunders.
14. Gillespie DL, Villavicencio JL, Gallagher C, Chang A, Hamelink JK, Fiala LA, O'Donnell SD, Jackson MR, Pikoulis E, Rich, NM. (1997). Presentation and management of venous aneurysms. *J Vasc Surg*. Nov;26(5):845-52.
15. Spiezia L, Simioni P. (2010). Upper extremity deep vein thrombosis. Intern Emerg Med. Apr;5(2):103-9. Epub 2009 Sep 26.
16. Needleman, L., Cronan, J. J., Lilly, M. P., Merli, G. J., Adhikari, S., Hertzberg, B. S., DeJong, M. R., Streiff, M. B., & Meissner, M. H. (2018). Ultrasound for Lower Extremity Deep Venous Thrombosis: Multidisciplinary Recommendations From the Society of Radiologists in Ultrasound Consensus Conference. Circulation, 137(14), 1505–1515. https://doi.org/10.1161/CIRCULATIONAHA.117.030687

VENOUS TESTING
34. Upper and Lower Extremity Venous Duplex Mapping

Definition
The use of real time B-mode ultrasonography to evaluate the suitability of extremity veins for use in dialysis access creation or for bypass conduit.

Risk Factors (requiring intervention using vein)
- Atherosclerosis
- Cardiac disease
- Renal failure
- Trauma
- Aneurysm

Risk Factors (for conditions that would affect venous suitability)
- Previous thrombosis
- Venous injury (e.g., intravenous lines or ports used for cancer treatment)
- Varicosities

Indications for Exam

The GSV has many tributaries and is commonly used as conduit for cardiac and vascular bypass surgeries.

- Severe ischemia of the upper or lower extremities which may require revascularization with autogenous conduit/bypass graft
- Severe ischemia of the heart which may require revascularization with autogenous conduit/bypass graft
- Renal failure requiring fistula placement for hemodialysis
- Request to identify patent veins for intravenous line placement

Marking venous tributaries on the skin for the surgeon helps direct incisions directly over the vein to avoid skin flaps, wound complications and ultimately improves post-operative healing. [3]

Contraindications/Limitations
- Open wounds prohibiting access by the ultrasound transducer
- Casts that cannot be removed or traction that limits access to the scan areas
- Poor visualization due to vessel depth because of obesity or severe edema
- Patients who cannot be adequately positioned
- Anatomical limitations (clavicle and ribs)
- The GSV is often the first choice for an autogenous graft. [3] In some cases, the GSV may be absent, previously used as a bypass, stripped if it was varicosed, not continuous/long enough for the required bypass or unsuitable because of thrombophlebitis. In the absence of great saphenous veins, arm veins become an alternative for autogenous bypass grafts. [1]

Location of Disease
Location of disease can be focal or diffuse and affect any level or multiple levels. Common sites include:

- Valve sites
- The cephalic vein may demonstrate a venous stenosis at its junction with the subclavian vein.

Patient History
- Previous vein harvesting or history of vein stripping
- History of deep or superficial venous thrombosis

Complex and small venous systems can take as long as one hour to map completely.

Physical Examination
Check for these possible contraindications to venous mapping prior to exam:
- Varicose veins
- Scars from previous vein harvesting (look for any missing venous segments proximal, distal, or near the scar)
- Palpable chord, redness or warmth along the superficial venous tract (concerning for acute thrombosis)

Upper and Lower Extremity Venous Duplex Mapping Protocol
- The room and the patient should be warm and comfortable to prevent venous constriction.
- Obtain a patient history to include symptoms and risk factors. Explain the procedure to the patient.
- Patient position should be optimized so that gravity can help dilate the veins. Patient may be examined in one of several positions: while sitting, in the supine position with the head elevated and the arms dependent (upper extremity exams) or placed on a bed in a reverse Trendelenburg position (lower extremity exams).
- Some patients may require the use of a range of transducers for superficial vessels including high-frequency (5-7 MHz) (8-15 MHz) transducers. A lower frequency (1-4 MHz) transducer may be useful around the clavicle.
- Locate the superficial vein of interest in a transverse view (short axis) using B-mode imaging. A gentle tap of the veins, especially in the arm, can facilitate venous dilatation should the veins appear small in diameter. Hand exercises may also help dilate the arm veins.

Placing a tourniquet around the upper arm may help to dilate the veins while imaging. [9]

- Perform venous compression every 2-4cm along the superficial vein in the transverse plane to check for thrombosis. Thrombosed or phlebitic superficial venous segments should be documented since thrombosed veins are not suitable for bypass/access conduit.

Superficial veins run within the superficial compartment above the deep fascia and do not have a corresponding artery, which makes them easy to distinguish from the deep veins.

- Document venous flow by recording a waveform using spectral Doppler in the longitudinal (sagittal) plane.
- Color flow imaging may also be used as additional documentation of patency.

- The anterior-posterior diameter of the vein is measured in the transverse plane with minimal, if any, transducer pressure from outer-wall to outer-wall. Measurements should be taken approximately every 2-3 inches or when a significant change in size is noted. Size changes are frequently observed near a tributary. Report the diameter measurements in millimeters.
- **Record measurements in duplicated systems, especially when diameters are sizable.**

A drawing or diagram may be provided by the technologist to aid the surgeon regarding diameter or course of the vessels.

Cephalic vein

Locate the cephalic vein (CV) at the "snuffbox" (the hollow on the radial aspect of the wrist when the thumb is extended fully). Follow the CV through the forearm. At the antecubital fossa, the CV continues into the (upper) arm. Follow the CV toward the shoulder to the junction with the axillary and subclavian veins, near the clavicle at the deltopectoral groove. Note the presence of any double cephalic venous systems. Record diameter measurements at the following levels:

» At wrist	» Distal arm
» Distal forearm	» Mid arm
» Mid forearm	» Proximal arm
» Proximal forearm	» Cephalic-subclavian vein confluence (cephalic arch)
» Antecubital fossa	

An anastomosis to either the cephalic or basilic veins may be used in the upper extremities to create an arteriovenous fistula for dialysis.[9]

Basilic vein

Locate the basilic vein (BSV) medially in the arm, near the elbow. Follow the BSV superiorly along the medial arm, toward its junction with the axillary or brachial vein. Go back and follow the BSV posteriomedially through the forearm.

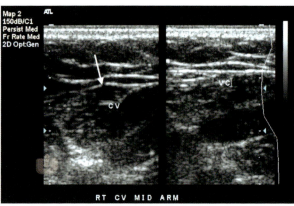

Fig. 34-1: *Dual screen image showing a compressible cephalic vein*

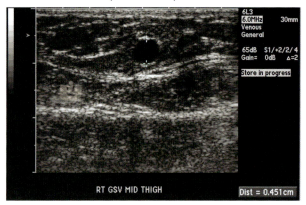

Fig. 34-2: *Lower extremity transverse diameter measurement*

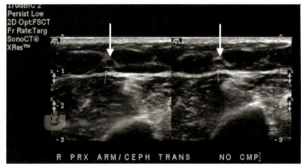

Fig. 34-3: *Dual screen image showing an incompressible cephalic vein*

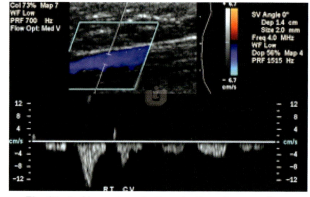

Fig. 34-4: *Normal cephalic vein Doppler waveform*

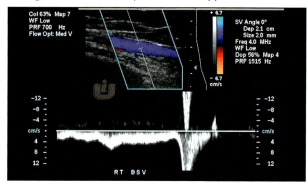

Fig. 34-5: *Normal basilic vein Doppler waveforms*

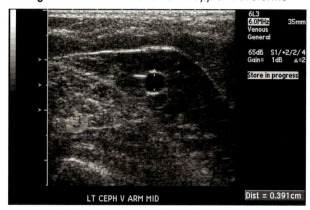

Fig. 34-6: *Upper extremity transverse diameter measurement*

Note the presence of any double basilic venous systems. Record diameter measurements at the following levels:

- » At wrist
- » Distal forearm
- » Mid forearm
- » Proximal forearm
- » Antecubital fossa
- » Distal arm
- » Mid arm
- » Proximal arm
- » Basilic-brachial-axillary vein confluence

Identification of a perforator between the basilic or cephalic and deep veins is important to note when performing a vein mapping for certain endovascular procedures pre-dialysis. Also report whether this perforator has a straight versus tortuous course and measure its distance from the artery.

Median cubital vein

Only one diameter measurement of the median cubital vein (MCV) in the antecubital fossa is usually recorded, since this vein is very short. When indicated, determine the anatomical connections of the MCV and note potential variations in this area, which are common.

Lower Extremity Superficial Veins

Great saphenous vein

- Locate the great saphenous vein (GSV) at the saphenofemoral junction. Follow the vein along the medial aspect of the thigh, calf and ankle. Note the presence of any large great saphenous accessory tributaries. Record diameter measurements at the following levels:

- » Groin (just distal to the saphenofemoral junction)
- » Proximal thigh
- » Mid thigh
- » Distal thigh
- » At knee
- » Proximal calf
- » Mid calf
- » Distal calf
- » At ankle

Small saphenous vein

- Locate the small saphenous vein (SSV) at the saphenopopliteal junction (or its alternative origin). Follow the vein along the posterior aspect of the calf to the ankle. Note the presence of any large small saphenous accessory tributaries. Record diameter measurements at the following levels:

- » Just distal to the saphenopopliteal junction (or at origin in the distal thigh, etc.)
- » Proximal calf
- » Mid calf
- » Distal calf
- » At ankle

Typical Anatomic Variations of the Veins at the Antecubital Fossa

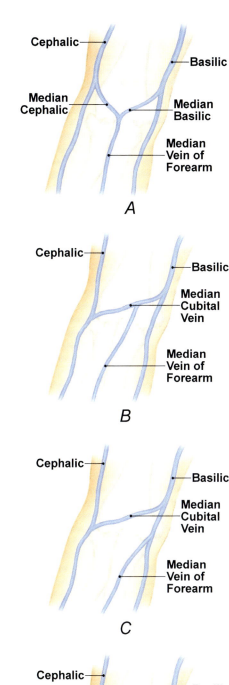

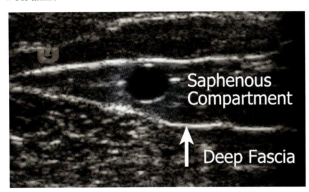

Fig. 34-7: *Great saphenous vein within the saphenous compartment*

Fig. 34-8: *Anatomical variations of the superficial veins in the antecubital fossa. (A) M-shaped configuration, (B and C) N-shaped configurations with the MCV terminating in CV and BSV, respectively, (D) no communication between the CV and BSV.*

Table 34-1: Upper and Lower Extremity Venous Duplex Mapping Protocol Summary

Scan transverse (short axis) with and without compression in B-mode (to check for thrombus) and measure (anterior-posterior) venous diameters (in millimeters) as appropriate at the following levels:

Upper Extremity-Cephalic (CV), Basilic (BSV), Median Cubital (MCV)	Lower Extremity-great Saphenous (GSV) Small Saphenous (SSV)
• Proximal arm (CV/BSV)	• Saphenofemoral junction (GSV)
• Mid arm (CV/BSV)	• Proximal thigh (GSV)
• Distal arm (CV/BSV)	• Mid thigh (GSV)
• Antecubital fossa (CV/BSV/MCV)	• Distal thigh (GSV)
• Proximal forearm (CV/BSV)	• Origin SSV (e.g., saphenopopliteal junction)
• Mid forearm (CV/BSV)	• At knee (GSV/SSV)
• Distal forearm (CV/BSV)	• Proximal calf (GSV/SSV)
• At wrist (CV/BSV)	• Mid calf (GSV/SSV)
• Origin CV, BSV and MCV veins	• Distal calf (GSV/SSV)
	• At ankle (GSV/SSV)

- Document venous flow using spectral Doppler or color flow imaging.
- Measure length of entire continuous venous segment(s) in centimeters (cm).
- Map the vein course using indelible marker when instructed.
- Repeat for the contralateral extremity if necessary.

A vein located outside of the saphenous compartment is known as a tributary and is not a main vein. It is important to note this distinction for the surgeon since most expect reported veins to run in the saphenous compartment.

- Large GSV or SSV tributaries may be present and confused with the main venous trunk being examined. It is often helpful to move to the most distal point of the vein and scan proximally. For example, the GSV often has large tributaries just below the knee that may be confused with the main trunk of the GSV. It is helpful to move to the anterior-medial malleolar area (ankle) to identify the GSV and map the vein proximally from that point to the knee.
- Comment on the continuity of all venous segments studied and measure the length of suitable vein in centimeters (cm).
- Mark the course of the vein with an indelible marker if indicated. Marking may help in cases of unusual anatomy or to mark major tributaries and double systems.

When marking the vein on the skin, a transducer cover may be used to minimize damage by the waterproof markers to the transducer membrane.

» Keep the transducer perpendicular to the surface of the skin.
» Keep the visualized vein in the middle of the ultrasound screen in transverse view and place a small mark in the middle and just above the transducer with the marker. Continue with this method along the extremity.
» At the end of the exam, "connect-the-dots" to represent the course of the visualized vein

---

Another technique to mark the vein uses a straw placed vertically on the skin over the site of the vein, which can be rotated back and forth to create a round mark on the skin. After the gel and the transducer are removed, the circular marks on the skin can be connected, using an indelible marker, indicating the course of the vein. [1]

PRINCIPLES OF INTERPRETATION

Interpretation as to the suitable nature of a vein is left to the surgeon's discretion. In general, patent veins 3mm in diameter can usually dilate to >4mm diameter under arterial pressure for use as dialysis conduit or a bypass graft. [3]

- Criteria for suitable venous diameter differs among surgeons and according to the procedure planned. The basic interpretation of a venous mapping exam analyzes:
  » Diameter ranges
  » Health of the vein
  » Continuity of the vein

B-mode Imaging

- Determine whether echogenic material is observed within the lumen of the vein.
- Determine if the vein collapses completely with light transducer pressure.

Color Doppler

- Use color Doppler to determine if color flow is present wall-to-wall or if there is a filling defect.

Spectral Doppler Waveforms

- Observe venous flow for:
  » Spontaneity: Signal automatically heard with Doppler
  » Phasicity: Flow increases and decreases with respiration
  » Augmentation: Flow increases with distal compression

Normal

B-mode Imaging
- **Compressibility:** The vein is free of thrombus if it compresses completely and is free of echogenic material within its lumen. [8]

Check each vein of a duplicated or bifed system.

Color Doppler
- Color flow will fill the vein completely from wall-to-wall upon distal limb compression. [5,6]

Spectral Doppler Waveforms
- **Spontaneity and phasicity:** *Note:* In the superficial veins, the absence of spontaneous and phasic flow can be a normal finding.
- **Augmentation:** Compression of the limb distal to the transducer augments venous flow. [6,8]

Abnormal [5]

B-mode Imaging
- **Varicosed segments:** tortuous, dilated veins are not suitable for operative use and should be reported. [1]
- **Compressibility:** Echogenic material is visualized within the vein and full coaptation of the vein on manual compression is absent or limited due to thrombus. [6,8]
  - » It is possible for only one vein of a pair to be thrombosed. For this reason, it is important to make sure all veins are studied carefully.
  - » If the vein is sclerosed, its walls will appear very thickened, although the lumen may be collapsible. [1]
- **Thrombus:** If thrombus is present, determine whether the thrombus is partial or totally occlusive, its location, as well as the extent and the characteristics of the thrombus.

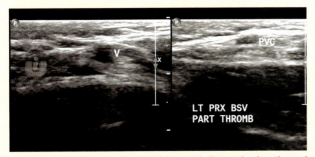

Fig. 34-9: *Partially incompressible/partially occlusive thrombus*

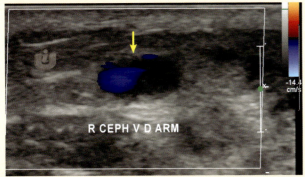

Fig. 34-10: *Acute, partially occlusive thrombus does not fill the entire lumen in transverse view*

» **Acute thrombus:** Characteristics include lightly echogenic or anechoic clot, spongy texture and thrombus which is poorly attached to the venous wall or "free floating" within the lumen. A moving tail may be seen at the end of the thrombus. The vein is often dilated in diameter. [5,7]

In cases of DVT, the superficial system can act as the primary pathway for venous return. Documentation of the deep veins can also be part of a venous mapping exam. The surgeon may want to confirm there is no evidence of DVT before removing superficial veins.

» **Chronic thrombus:** Characteristics include brightly echogenic or heterogeneous echoes, irregular surface texture and thrombus which is attached to the venous wall. The vein often contracts in diameter over time. There may be chronic thickening (sclerosis) of the vein walls observed, accompanied by calcific shadowing in cases where the vein has recanalized after a thrombus. Collateral veins may be observed adjacent to the affected vein(s). [5,7]

The term, chronic postthrombotic change has been suggested as a replacement for "chronic thrombus". The SRU has suggested that only acute events should be referred to as " acute thrombus". When it is technically difficult to determine whether findings are acute/chronic, use the term "indeterminate". [10]

» **Indeterminate age:** Characteristics of both acute and chronic stages may be present, making age difficult to determine. (*Fig. 34-13*).
  - *Subacute* is another term used by labs. Reports have suggested using this term only to describe thrombus that appears to have changed appearance on B-mode compared to a previous study where the diagnosis of acute DVT was made some weeks earlier. [10]
- There is no need to note the location of valve sinuses unless they are stenotic or otherwise abnormal. If valve leaflets are visualized, they should appear thin and freely moving within the lumen. If the valve leaflet is rigid, brightly echoic and fixed in the lumen, report this as an abnormality.

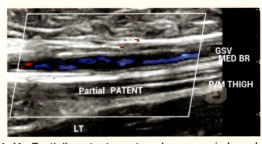

Fig. 34-11: *Partially patent great saphenous vein by color flow*

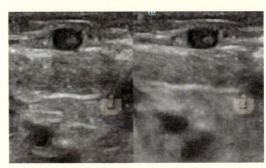

Fig. 34-12: *Dual screen image illustrating indeterminate age thrombus; the vein is neither dilated or contracted with anechoic and some bright intralumenal echoes.*

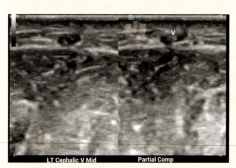

Fig. 34-13: Dual screen image illustrating chronic thrombus in a cephalic vein

Table 34-2: Thrombosis Descriptions and Characteristics

Acute	Chronic
• Light to medium echogenic/anechoic	• Bright/heterogeneous echoes
• Spongy texture on compression (homogeneous)	• Irregular texture (heterogeneous)
• Poorly attached or free floating	• Attached
• Dilated vein (if totally occluded)	• Same size as artery or vein is contracted
	• Collateral veins may be noted

- Veins can be partially or totally incompressible in both acute and chronic stages.
- Combination of events can occur (e.g., acute on top of chronic thrombus).
- Chronic thrombus with partial recanalization is seen as small color flow channels within thrombus. In some cases, the veins walls will appear chronically thickened with bright echoes or calcific shadowing only along the walls.
- Age of thrombus is sometimes indeterminate.

Color Doppler

- Color flow can be observed moving around echogenic material within the vein upon distal limb compression if partially occlusive thrombus is present. [8]
- Color flow cannot be observed upon distal limb compression if totally occlusive thrombus is present using appropriate low-flow machine settings. [6,8]

Spectral Doppler Waveforms

- **Spontaneity:** Absence of flow indicates venous obstruction. [8]
- **Phasicity:** Continuous venous flow suggests either obstruction in a proximal venous segment or extrinsic compression on the vein. [7]
- **Augmentation:** If distal compression does not produce augmentation of the venous signal, an obstruction distal to the transducer is suspected. A weak or dampened augmentation suggests a partial or total occlusion distal to the transducer and may be caused by poor filling of the vein. [7]

Table 34-3: Diagnostic Criteria for Venous Duplex Mapping

Normal	Abnormal
Complete coaptation of vein walls with light transducer pressure	Lack of complete vein compression
Absent intralumenal thrombus	Intralumenal echoes present (acute thrombus can be echolucent)
Color flow fills the lumen completely	Decrease or absence of color flow
Normal spontaneity, phasicity and augmentation	Decreased or absent spontaneity, phasicity or augmentation
No venous dilatation	Dilated or contracted veins noted

Correlation

- Venogram

REFERENCES

1. Gibson KD, Ebert A. (2010). Preoperative vein mapping. In Zierler RE (Ed.). Strandess's duplex scanning disorders in vascular diagnosis 4th ed. (231-234).Philadelphia Wolters Kluwer Lippincott Williams & Wilkins.
2. Patel, ST, Mills JL. (2005). The preoperative, intraoperative, and post-operative non-invasive evaluation of infrainguinal vein bypass grafts. In Mansour MA, Labropoulos N. (Eds.), *Vascular Diagnosis*, (277-292). Philadelphia. Elsevier Saunders.
3. Mills, JL. (2005). Infrainguinal bypass. In *Rutherford Vascular Surgery 6th edition*. (1154-1174). Philadelphia. Elsevier Saunders.
4. Dawson DL, Beals H. (2010). Acute lower extremity deep venous thrombosis. In Zierler RE (Ed.), *Strandesss's duplex scanning disorders in vascular diagnosis 4th ed.* (179-198).Philadelphia Wolters Kluwer Lippincott Williams & Wilkins.
5. Myers K, Clough A. (2004). Venous thrombosis in the lower limbs. In *Making sense of vascular ultrasound: A hands on guide*. (181-197). London: Hodder Arnold.
6. Myers K, Clough A. (2004). Diseases of vessels to the upper limb. In *Making sense of vascular ultrasound: A hands on guide*. (227-254). London: Hodder Arnold.
7. Zwiebel, WJ (2005). Ultrasound Diagnosis of Venous Thrombosis. In Zwiebel WJ, Pellerito JS (Eds.), *Introduction to Vascular Ultrasonography 5th ed*. (449-465). Philadelphia: Elsevier Saunders.
8. Meissner MH. (2005). Venous duplex scanning. In *Rutherford Vascular Surgery 6th edition*. (254-270). Philadelphia. Elsevier Saunders.
9. Robbin ML, Lockhart ME. (2005). Ultrasound evaluation before and after hemodialysis access. In Zwiebel WJ, Pellerito JS (Eds.), *Introduction to Vascular Ultrasonography 5th ed*. (325-340). Philadelphia: Elsevier Saunders.
10. Needleman, L., Cronan, J. J., Lilly, M. P., Merli, G. J., Adhikari, S., Hertzberg, B. S., DeJong, M. R., Streiff, M. B., & Meissner, M. H. (2018). Ultrasound for Lower Extremity Deep Venous Thrombosis: Multidisciplinary Recommendations From the Society of Radiologists in Ultrasound Consensus Conference. Circulation, 137(14), 1505–1515. https://doi.org/10.1161/CIRCULATIONAHA.117.030687

Definition

The use of real time B-mode imaging with spectral and color flow Doppler to assess the abdominal aorta and iliac arteries for stenosis, occlusion or the presence, location and size of any aneurysm. This examination is also used to monitor any change in aneurysm size from previous exams and assess the patency of aortoiliac bypass grafts or iliac artery stents.

Etiology

- Atherosclerosis
- Infectious aortitis (e.g., mycotic, syphilis)
- Vasculitis
- Congenital abnormalities
- Connective tissue disorders (e.g., Marfan's syndrome or Ehler-Danlos syndrome)
- Trauma

Risk Factors

- Age (increases with age)
- Smoking
- Hypertension
- Atherosclerosis
- Male gender
- Caucasian
- Immediate relative with an abdominal aortic aneurysm (AAA) history
- Trauma

A family history of AAA increases AAA development risk four-fold.[23] The risk can increase twelve-fold if an immediate family member was an AAA patient.[5]

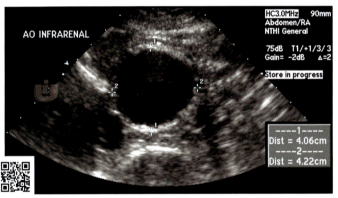

Fig. 35-1: Abdominal aortic aneurysm by B-mode imaging

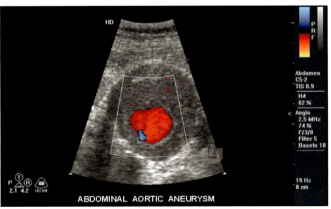

Fig. 35-2: Abdominal aortic aneurysm by B-mode imaging with mural thrombus
Courtesy of Philips Healthcare

Indications for Exam

- Surveillance of known AAA or iliac artery aneurysm
- Abdominal bruit (abnormal sound heard through auscultation caused by vibrations from turbulent flow)
- Abdominal pain
- Pulsatile aorta or mass on physical examination
- Immediate family member with a history of AAA
- History of hypertension, age >50 years with a family history of AAA
- Presence of an aneurysm at another location (e.g., iliac, femoral, popliteal)
- Aortic coarctation
- Evidence of lower extremity arterial inflow disease
- Evidence of distal emboli in the absence of a femoral-popliteal artery or cardiac source

The Deficit Reduction Act (DRA) of 2005 calls for Medicare coverage for a one-time abdominal aortic aneurysm ultrasound screening test for men ages 65-75 with a history of smoking, as well as men and women ages 65-75 with a family history of AAA. Reimbursement began Jan. 1, 2007.[26]

Contraindications/Limitations

- Obesity may cause poor visualization due to vessel depth.
- Abdominal gas may prohibit visualization of any or all vessels.

Abdominal Aortic Aneurysm Types

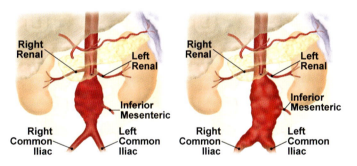

Fig. 35-3: Fusiform type aneurysm

Fig. 35-4: Fusiform type aneurysm with iliac artery involvement

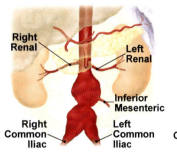
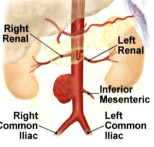

Fig. 35-5: Bi-lobed fusiform type aneurysm

Fig. 35-6: Saccular type aneurysm

Stent Location

Stents can be located within any vessel. Stents are often placed in the common or external iliac arteries.

Graft Location

The aortoiliac segment can be involved in multiple types of grafts/stents. See the chapter on "Arterial Bypass and Stent" for more detail on peripheral bypass/stents. The "Abdominal Aortic Stent" chapter focuses exclusively on endografts.

Bypass grafts connect two arteries to direct flow around an obstruction or an aneurysm in the aorta and/or iliac arteries. The bypass grafts can be placed between any two vessels. The infrarenal aorta is typically used for the proximal anastomosis if the aorta is the inflow artery. Examples of typical aortoiliac-arterial grafts encountered in the vascular lab for surveillance include:

- Aortobifemoral (abdominal aorta to bilateral femoral arteries)
- Aortoiliac (abdominal aorta to one or both iliac arteries)
- Iliofemoral-Renal artery
- Iliac artery-Femoral artery
- Femoral-Femoral (cross-femoral or "x-fem" bypass)
- Axillo-femoral (axillary artery to a femoral artery)
- A bypass may be anastomosed to another bypass (e.g., aorto-femoral-popliteal bypass)

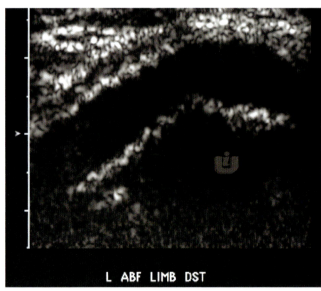

Fig. 35-7: *Aortobifemoral Bypass Graft by B-mode*

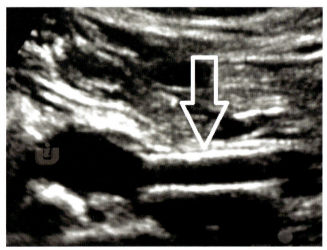

Fig. 35-8: *Common Iliac Artery Stent by B-mode*

Mechanism of Disease

- **Atherosclerosis** is the most common arterial disease. Atherosclerotic plaque forms in the artery to block flow by either narrowing the arterial lumen *(arterial stenosis)* or totally blocking the artery *(arterial occlusion)*. The term "hemodynamically significant obstruction" refers to either a stenosis or an occlusion that results in a decrease in blood pressure or flow distal to the obstruction. Typically, a stenosis must narrow the diameter of the artery by at least 50% to decrease pressure and flow distally. An arterial occlusion is typically seen from one major branch to the next. [1]
- **Emboli** may occur as contents of a plaque or fragments of an organized thrombus from the heart or aneurysm loosen and flow downstream. Emboli become lodged in a distant blood vessel, causing arterial occlusion and reduction of flow. [2] A patient presenting with "blue toe syndrome" should be worked up for AAA. [5]
- **Extrinsic compression** from tumors, musculo-skeletal configuration, hematoma, etc. can result in stenosis or occlusion by placing enough pressure on arterial walls to compromise blood flow. [1]

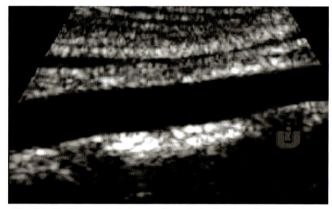

Fig. 35-9: *Normal abdominal aorta in the longitudinal plane*

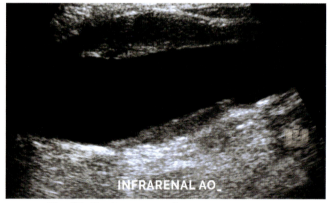

Fig. 35-10: *Aneurysm of the abdominal aorta in the longitudinal plane with mural thrombus*

- **Aneurysmal disease**

Studies estimate the prevalence of AAA discovered through ultrasound screening ranges from 4.2–8.8% for men, and 0.6–1.4% in women. [22]

> » Aneurysms are most commonly caused by atherosclerotic or inflammatory processes. Aneurysms are caused by the breakdown of the vessel wall by a multifactorial process involving: connective tissue metabolism, nutrient and oxygen levels, chronic inflammation and biomechanical wall stress.
>
> » There is increased degradation of elastin and collagen in aneurysmal arteries.

- » Elastin degradation plays a key role in aneurysmal dilatation whereas the degradation of collagen leads to rupture.
- » It has been suggested that the infrarenal abdominal aorta is at greater risk for aneurysm compared to the thoracic aorta because the infrarenal abdominal aorta has fewer vasa vasorum per medial lamellar unit. Vasa vasorum are the primary source of nutrients and oxygen for media smooth muscle cells. [5, 27]
- » Localized destruction of the arterial wall may also be caused by an infectious agent which infiltrates the adventitial layer through the vasa vasorum (mycotic aneurysm). [6]
- **Arterial thrombosis** forms as an abdominal aortic aneurysm expands. Stagnant blood in areas of the aneurysm (stasis) permits coagulation within the artery causing mural thrombosis.
- **Aortic dissection** begins with a tear in the intimal layer of the artery, allowing blood flow to access the medial layer. A dissection between the intimal and medial layers results in true and false lumens. [7] Pulsatile flow and high blood pressure may cause propagation of a dissection into multiple arteries. Blood flows through the tear in the intimal layer and may clot, flow in and out of the tear, or flow further downstream to enter the true lumen through a second tear distally.

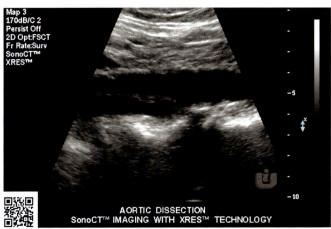

Fig. 35-11: *Dissection of the abdominal aorta by B-mode*
Courtesy of Philips Healthcare

- A **pseudoaneurysm** (PA) or "false aneurysm" forms due to trauma to all three layers of the arterial wall. A PA is a hematoma receiving its blood supply via communication with an artery through a patent "neck."
  - » One cause of PA is trauma to the aortoiliac segment (e.g., puncture for catheterization, gunshot wound, etc.).[8]
  - » PA can develop at the femoral anastomosis of an aortobifemoral graft due to degeneration of the native artery. [9]

Graft Complications
- **Technical errors** can result in failure of a bypass or stent. Kinking or twisting of the graft limb is one possible cause.[9] Early failure of either can occur even without an identifiable mechanical defect or cause.
- **Graft thrombosis** is the most frequent complication of aortofemoral bypass, usually affecting one of the limbs. [9]
  - » Failure resulting from atherosclerotic progression in the inflow/outflow beds often occurs in grafts. [9]
  - » Some patients have an undiagnosed hypercoaguable disorder which causes thrombosis or occlusion of the graft. [9]
- Additional mechanisms of complication include graft infections and trauma to the graft. [9]

Location of Disease
- Location of disease can be focal or diffuse and affect any level or multiple levels.
- For aneurysm:
  - » Infrarenal abdominal aorta (most common site)
  - » Abdominal aorta plus iliac
  - » Thoracoabdominal
  - » Isolated iliac

Over 50% of patients with a femoral artery aneurysm also have an AAA. Concurrent iliac artery aneurysms are much less frequent. [25]

- For dissection:
  - » Left subclavian artery (most common site for origin of aortic dissection)
  - » Ascending aorta or arch (2nd most common site for origin of aortic dissection)
- Common location of graft obstruction:
  - » Graft anastomotic sites
  - » Inflow arterial tract
  - » Outflow arterial tract
  - » Graft kink
- The iliac arteries are often involved in arterial stenting.

Patient History
- Many aneurysm cases are asymptomatic.
- Aneurysm may be found unexpectedly during physical exam, radiological or CT exams that were performed for unrelated reasons.
- Sense of fullness in the epigastrium
- Previous therapeutic procedure (e.g., bypass, stenting)

Physical Examination
- Pulsatile abdominal mass
- Lower back pain
- Systolic murmur in the region of the aneurysm
- Bruit in aorto-iliac region
- Pulselessness
- Cyanosis

Abdominal Aorto-Iliac Duplex Ultrasound Protocol
- Patients should be fasting for 6-12 hours to minimize the presence of air in the abdomen. A limited volume of clear liquids may be ingested prior to the examination (e.g., to swallow medications). Patients may be given Simethicone (e.g., Gas-X, Mylanta, etc.) before the exam to reduce abdominal gas.
- Obtain a patient history to include symptoms, risk factors and past vascular interventions and general dates if available. Explain the procedure to the patient.
- Patient is supine with their arms and legs adequately supported. The patient may bend their knees up to aid in relaxation of the abdominal wall and decrease lumbar pain.
- Acoustic windows used to image the abdominal aorta include: midline of the upper abdomen, left flank with patient supine or right lateral decubitus.
- Most patients require a low frequency (1-4 MHz) transducer to image these deeper abdominal structures, though some patients may require the use of a range of transducers, including a higher-frequency (5-7 MHz) transducer.

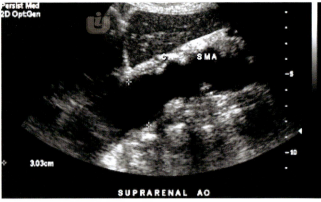

Fig. 35-12: *Suprarenal aorta diameter measured from the longitudinal plane*

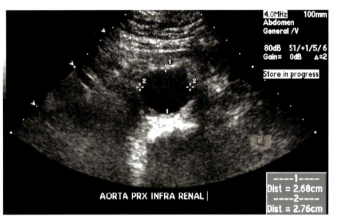

Fig. 35-13: *Infrarenal aorta diameter measured in transverse*

- The aortic lumen is measured from outer wall to outer wall in both the longitudinal (sagittal) and transverse (short-axis) planes.

Transverse (Short-Axis) Scan

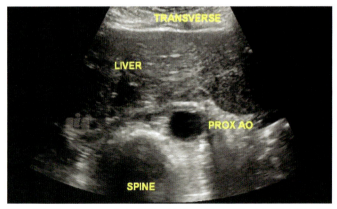

Fig. 35-14: *Transverse abdominal aorta artery and landmarks*

- Place the transducer at the midline below the xyphoid process in the transverse plane (the liver should be on the left of the display screen). Slowly move the transducer inferiorly towards the umbilicus. Use color flow as needed as a guide. Evaluate the aorta for atherosclerotic plaque, aneurysm, calcification, thrombus, dissection and tortuosity during the scan.
- At the aortic bifurcation (near the umbilicus), the right and left common iliac arteries should be clearly demonstrated.

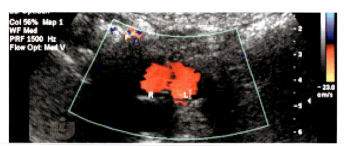

Fig. 35-15: *Transverse iliac artery bifurcation*

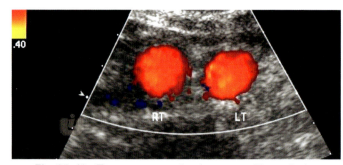

Fig. 35-16: *Transverse proximal common iliac arteries*

- The maximum anterior-posterior and medial-lateral (transverse) diameters of the aorta should be measured at the following levels:
  » Suprarenal aorta, at or above the celiac trunk
  » Juxtarenal aorta, at the level the renal arteries
  » Infrarenal aorta, below the renals, but above the iliac bifurcation
  » Proximal common iliac arteries

Place calipers parallel to the axis of flow when measuring diameters.

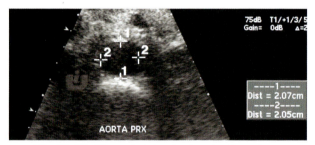

Fig. 35-17: *Normal abdominal aorta diameters (caliper #1-anterior-posterior and caliper #2- transverse measurements)*

Since it is perpendicular to the flow channel, the anterior-posterior arterial diameter measurement is more reliable than the transverse arterial diameter.[5,17]

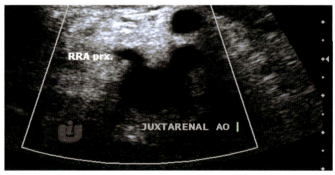

Fig. 35-18: *Juxtarenal transverse*

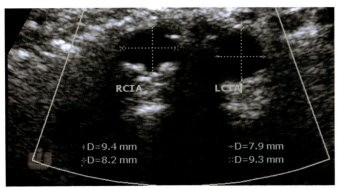

Fig. 35-19: *Proximal common iliac artery transverse diameters*

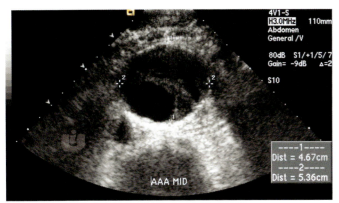

Fig. 35-20: *Abnormal abdominal aorta diameters-aneurysm*

- A transverse aortic aneurysm evaluation should include:
  » Maximum anterior-posterior and transverse diameters of the true lumen
  » Location of the aneurysm (level)
  » Documentation regarding presence and location of thrombus and attempt to classify the type of aneurysm (e.g., fusiform, saccular)
  » Use of B-mode and color flow Doppler to identify the residual vessel lumen if present

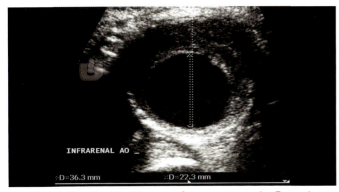

Fig. 35-21: *Residual lumen of an aneurysm by B-mode*

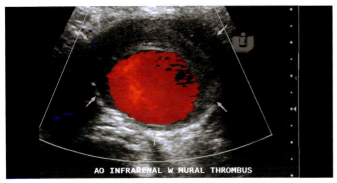

Fig. 35-22: *Residual lumen of an aneurysm with color flow*

Longitudinal (Sagittal) Scan and Images

- Place the transducer at the midline below the xyphoid process and turn the transducer longitudinally. The B-mode image of the abdominal aorta from the diaphragm to the aorta-common iliac bifurcation is evaluated for the presence of atherosclerotic plaque, aneurysm, calcification, thrombus, dissection or tortuosity.

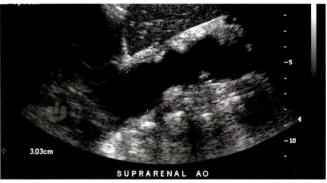

Fig. 35-23: *Longitudinal abdominal aorta on B-mode (Note: diffuse plaque)*

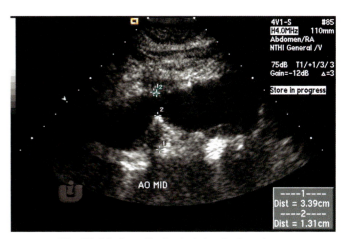

Fig. 35-24: *Longitudinal abdominal aorta on B-mode with lumenal reduction calculation*

- Document the maximum longitudinal diameter from outer wall to outer wall on axis at the following levels:
  » Suprarenal aorta, at or above the celiac trunk
  » Juxtarenal aorta, at the level the renal arteries
  » Infrarenal aorta, below the level the renal arteries, but above the iliac bifurcation
- Longitudinal aortic aneurysm evaluation should include:
  » Maximum longitudinal diameters
  » Location of the aneurysm (level)
  » Length of aneurysm
  » Use of color flow Doppler to identify true vessel lumen
  » Documentation regarding presence and location of thrombus, atherosclerotic plaque and/or calcification

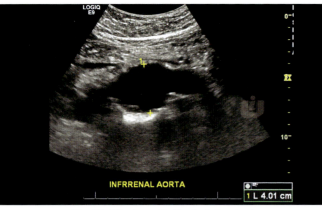

Fig. 35-25: *Longitudinal abdominal aorta diameter measurement*

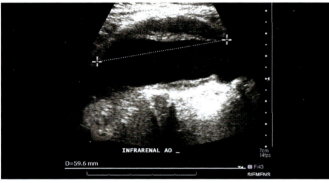

Fig. 35-26: *Length of the aneurysm measured*

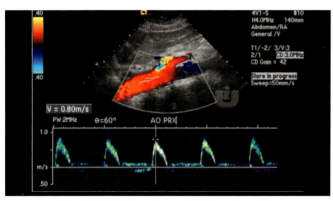

Fig. 35-27: *Normal spectral Doppler within the suprarenal abdominal aorta*

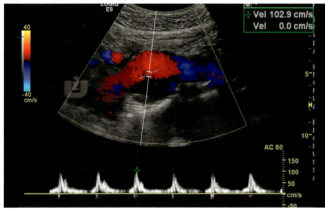

Fig. 35-28: *Spectral Doppler within an abdominal aortic aneurysm*

- Determine the peak systolic velocities (PSV), and end-diastolic velocities (EDV) using spectral Doppler (≤60° Doppler angle with the angle cursor parallel to the vessel walls and sample volume within the flow stream) at the following levels:
  - » Suprarenal aorta, at or above the celiac trunk
  - » Juxtarenal aorta, at the level the renal arteries
  - » Infrarenal aorta, below the renal arteries but above the iliac bifurcation
  - » Right common iliac artery and left common iliac artery
  - » Document the highest obtainable velocity through any stenotic area(s) by moving the sample gate through the area of stenosis and obtain representative waveforms. Record velocities and waveforms just proximal to the stenosis and just distal to the stenosis. Document post-stenotic turbulence and color bruit when present.
  - » Extremely low flow states are possible both above and below occlusions. Color Doppler parameters must be adjusted to detect low velocities. If this is not done, the length of the occlusion could be overestimated.

Table 35-1: Abdominal Aortoiliac Duplex Protocol Summary

Transverse (Short-Axis) Scan

- Measure the anterior-posterior (AP) and transverse diameters of the abdominal aorta in B-mode from outer wall-outer wall at the following levels:
  - » Suprarenal aorta, at or above the celiac artery
  - » Juxtarenal aorta, at the level of the renal arteries
  - » Infrarenal aorta, below the renal arteries, but above the iliac bifurcation
  - » Right and left common iliac arteries

Longitudinal (Sagittal) Scan

- Measure peak systolic and end diastolic velocities with spectral Doppler and measure the longitudinal diameters of the abdominal aorta in B-mode at the following levels:
  - » Suprarenal aorta, at or above the celiac artery
  - » Juxtarenal aorta, at the level of the renal arteries
  - » Infrarenal aorta, below the renal arteries, but above the iliac bifurcation
  - » Right and left common iliac arteries
- When an area of stenosis is identified, "walk" the sample gate through the area of stenosis and obtain representative waveforms at the point of highest velocity within the stenosis, as well as just proximal and distal to the stenosis.

Aortoiliac Bypass Graft/Stent Surveillance Protocol

- Obtain a patient history to include symptoms and risk factors.
- Obtain past surgical reports and records including type of bypass graft or stent placement and general date of surgery.
- Patient is typically examined in the supine position for grafts and stents.
- Obtain bilateral ABIs. (Never put a blood pressure cuff over a bypass graft or stent without first consulting the Medical Director of the lab or lab protocol.)
- Some patients may require the use of a range of transducers; including high-frequency (5-7 MHz) transducer and a lower frequency (1-4 MHz) transducer.
- Evaluate for graft or stent abnormalities while scanning (e.g., anastomotic pseudoaneurysm, thrombosis, stenosis, intimal hyperplasia, perigraft fluid).

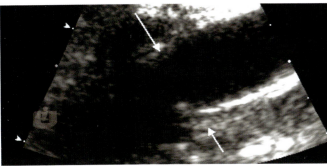

Fig. 35-29: *Proximal anastomosis of aortobifemoral bypass graft (AFB)*

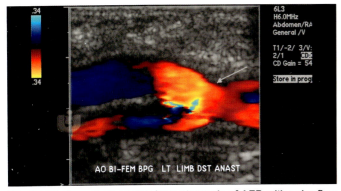

Fig. 35-30: *Longitudinal distal anastomosis of AFB with color flow*

- Record transverse and longitudinal images with and without color flow of the:
  » Inflow/proximal native artery
  » Proximal anastomosis or stent origin
  » Proximal graft or stent
  » Mid graft or stent
  » Distal graft or stent
  » Distal anastomosis or end of stent
  » Outflow/distal native artery
  » Any areas where a lumenal reduction or color bruit are noted

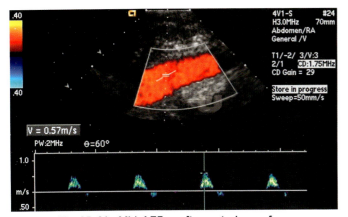

Fig. 35-31: *Mid-AFB graft spectral waveform*

- Record and measure the peak systolic velocity (PSV) in the longitudinal plane using spectral Doppler (≤60° Doppler angle with the angle cursor parallel to the vessel walls and sample volume within the center of the flow stream) at the following levels:
  » Inflow/proximal native artery
  » Proximal anastomosis or stent origin
  » Proximal graft or stent
  » Mid graft or stent
  » Distal graft or stent
  » Distal anastomosis or end of stent
  » Outflow/distal native artery

Early post-operative flow patterns (within the 1st month) in a bypass graft may have increased diastolic flow (post-operative reactive hyperemia) and may not have a triphasic waveform.

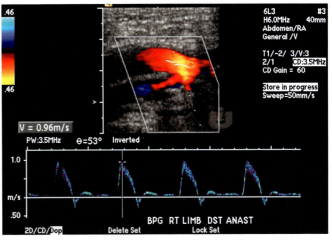

Fig. 35-32: *Normal distal AFB anastomosis by spectral Doppler*

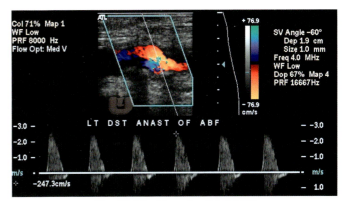

Fig. 35-33: *Stenotic distal AFB anastomosis by spectral Doppler*

- When an area of stenosis is identified, "walk" the sample gate through the area of stenosis and obtain representative waveforms proximal, at and distal to the stenosis. Post-stenotic turbulence and color bruit should be documented when present.
- Determine classification of stenosis according to laboratory diagnostic criteria.
- Repeat protocol for other grafts as necessary.

Native Aorto-Iliac Duplex

PRINCIPLES OF INTERPRETATION

B-mode Imaging

Assess all arteries for intraluminal echoes. Determine plaque location and plaque characteristics:

- **Diffuse plaque:** Long segment of the artery lined with plaque, but <50% diameter reduction at any point.
- **Stenotic:** Lumen is narrowed and velocity increases. A hemodynamically significant stenosis typically occurs when narrowing results in a >50% diameter reduction (75% area reduction). A stenosis can be focal or involve a long segment.
- **Calcific:** Highly reflective plaque(s) with acoustic shadowing
- **Occluded:** Complete occlusion of the vessel
- **"Moving"/"Mobile":** Debris within the lumen is poorly adhered to the vessel wall, e.g., moving thrombus.
- **Arterial diameters:** Measure arterial diameters to assess for aneurysmal dilatation.

Color Doppler

Color flow is used to show patency of the arterial lumen, the degree of narrowing when there is disease and flow direction.

Arterial Waveform Terminology

The terminology used to describe arterial waveforms is not consistent across laboratories. A consensus document was published in 2020 by the Society of Vascular Ultrasound and the Society for Vascular Medicine regarding the terminology and interpretation of peripheral arterial and venous waveforms. See the Arterial Hemodynamics chapter for more detail on arterial waveforms.

Spectral Doppler Waveforms

Any change in spectral waveform analysis depends on the terminology used by the lab; from triphasic to monophasic or changes in resistance may be significant.

Flow Velocities

- Determine peak systolic velocity (PSV) and flow direction
- Calculate the velocity ratio:

$$Vr = V_2 \div V_1$$

V_2 = the maximum PSV of a stenosis
V_1 = PSV of the proximal normal segment.

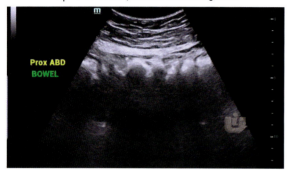

Fig. 35-34: Bowel gas can limit visualization in the abdomen

- Abdominal gas is similar to calcific shadowing in that gas/shadowing can prohibit Doppler and color flow analysis of a specific arterial segment. Use indirect signs to evaluate hemodynamically significant lesions:
  » If post-stenotic turbulence is present distal to the shadowing, there could be a stenosis through the area not visualized. Conversely, if there is no change in the waveform pattern, it is unlikely that a significant obstruction exists.
  » Comparing the Doppler waveform proximal and distal to the non-visualized segment can point to a hemodynamically significant obstruction under the shadowing.

Interpretation/Diagnostic Criteria

Normal

B-mode Imaging
- The artery is free of intralumenal echoes.
- **Arterial diameters:** The mean diameter of a normal infrarenal aorta is approximately 2.0cm.[5]

Color Doppler
- When utilized, color Doppler fills the entire arterial lumen.

Spectral Doppler Waveforms
- A *high resistance waveform* pattern is normal in the aortoiliac arteries with a quick downstroke that ends with a short period of reversed flow direction (below the baseline) at end systole/early diastole. This reversed flow segment in the waveform may or may not be followed by a third segment with a low, short segment of forward flow. This waveform can also be referred to as *triphasic*.

The third phase of the high resistant waveform may be missing in the suprarenal aortic segment, especially in patients with less vessel compliance.

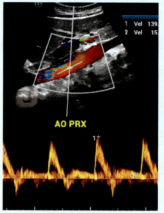 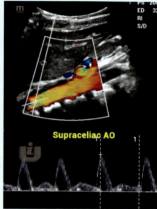

Fig. 35-35: Most labs would consider these waveforms normal from a proximal (suprarenal) abdominal aorta.

Flow Velocities
- **Flow velocities:** Normal flow velocities should be >40cm/s.[10] PSV and Vr are essentially uniform throughout the sampled arterial segment. Velocity ratios <2.0 are expected between segments.

Table 35-2: Normal Arterial Diameters and Peak Systolic Velocities

Arterial Vessel	Average Diameter ± SD*	Velocity + SD*
Infrarenal aorta	2.0 ± 0.3cm	65 ± 15cm/s
Common iliac artery	1.6 ± 2cm	95 ± 20cm/s
External iliac artery	0.79 ± 0.13cm	119 ± 22cm/s
Common femoral artery	0.82 ± 0.14cm	114 ± 25cm/s

*SD, standard deviation

Source: Armstrong PA, Bandyk DF. (2007). Duplex scanning for lower extremity arterial disease. In AbuRahma AF, Bergan JJ (Eds.). Non-invasive Vascular Diagnosis: A Practical Guide to Therapy 2nd ed. (253-261). London:Springer Verlag.

Abnormal

B-mode Imaging

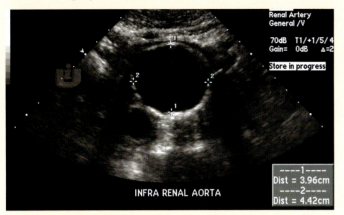

Fig. 35-36: *Abnormal transverse diameters of the abdominal aorta*

- Intralumenal echoes are visualized in cases of atherosclerotic disease within the artery resulting in a measurable lumenal reduction.
- Visualization of mural thrombus is possible within an aneurysm. Observed echoes are often heterogeneous in nature and create a residual lumen.[3]

Diameter reduction measurements should only be used in conjunction with peak systolic velocity measurements.

- **Arterial diameters:**
  » Mild dilatation of the aorta >2.0 and <3.0cm is describe as *ectatic*.[3]
  » A moderate aortic aneurysm is 3-5cm in diameter.[5]
  » Severe aneurysmal disease is present when diameters are >5.0cm.[12]

Color Doppler

- When utilized, color Doppler does not fill the entire arterial lumen. A color bruit may be observed, suggesting a hemodynamically significant lesion.[13]

Color is never diagnostic without spectral Doppler confirmation.

Spectral Doppler Waveforms

- As the obstruction becomes more severe, changes in the spectral waveform are expected before a stenosis or occlusion, at the point of greatest stenosis and after a stenosis/occlusion as described in the *Arterial Physiology* chapter.
- *Spectral broadening* represents the wide range of velocities usually present when there is disturbed, non-laminar flow. This waveform change occurs in the early stages of arterial disease. The normally clear window below the systolic peak begins to fill in.
- *Monophasic* arterial Doppler waveforms reflect low resistance and are characterized by a slow upstroke, low amplitude, and broad peak with continuous forward flow in diastole that does not cross the zero baseline. The upstroke has a general direction of being tipped to the right. Monophasic waveforms are typically present distal to an occlusion or a very high-grade stenosis.[17]

- A *high-resistance waveform* with a sharp upstroke and brisk downstroke may be noted in a stenotic region. There may or may not be flow reversal in diastole.[17] When there is a diastolic component, it may be elevated or absent depending on the degree of downstream resistance.
- *Turbulent waveforms* or "post-stenotic turbulence" are indicative of chaotic flow reflecting how blood moves in many directions just past the stenosis.
- *Parvus tardus* is an alternative term for "monophasic" used by some laboratories to describe a waveform with continuous forward flow and a slow, blunted systolic component.
- **Staccato:** A "spiked" high-resistant waveform with a short upstroke/downstroke and little to no diastolic component is often a signal of impending occlusion.
- Flow through an aneurysm can exhibit systolic dampening and a prominent diastolic reversal associated with the swirling of blood within the dilated lumen.[5,12]

Flow Velocities

- A hemodynamically significant lesion (>50%) will result in a focal velocity increase (at least double the velocity in the proximal arterial segment).[13] There will be a velocity ratio ≥2.0 between segments.

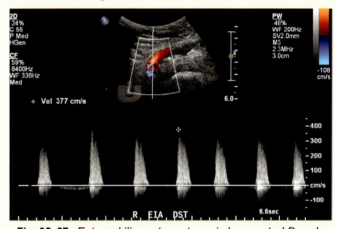

Fig. 35-37: *External iliac artery stenosis by spectral Doppler*

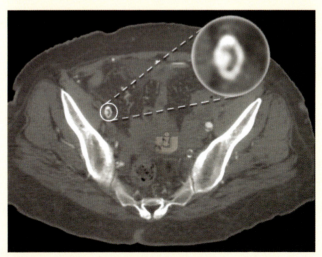

Fig. 35-38: *Same external iliac artery stenosis by CT scan*

- **Occlusion:** An occlusion is recognized in a native artery or stent/bypass graft by the absence of both color saturation and confirmed by the lack of an audible Doppler signal in the artery with appropriate low-flow settings.[13]

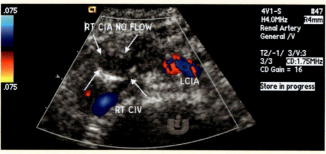

Fig. 35-39: *Right common iliac artery occlusion is suspected by color flow in the transverse plane*

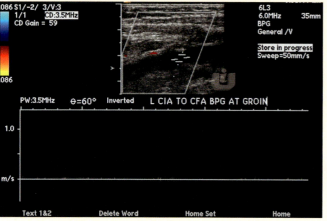

Fig. 35-40: *Absent Doppler signal in the common iliac artery explains common femoral bypass graft-occlusion*

Other Pathology

- **Arteriomegaly** is the term used to describe uniform arterial dilatation throughout an artery greater than 50% the typical diameter.[15] The artery can also be described as "ectatic" in some vascular laboratories.
- **Pseudoaneurysm** A pseudoaneurysm is diagnosed in the aortoiliac segment when a pulsatile mass is identified by color and Doppler flow communicating with the native artery or an anastomotic site through a patent "neck."[16] The neck must demonstrate to and fro (pendulum) Doppler flow patterns to indicate a pseudoaneurysm.
- **Dissection**: A dissection of the arterial lumen is recognized as two distinct flow channels by B-mode and/or color Doppler. One lumen is known as the "true lumen" while the other is referred to as the "false lumen." Waveform patterns in the false lumen will be turbulent, irregular and/or bidirectional compared to the more "normal" or expected waveform in the true lumen. An intimal flap may be seen within the arterial lumen by B-mode image.[7]

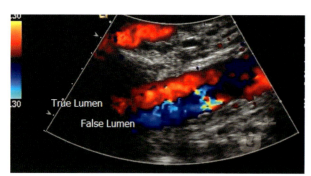

Fig. 35-41: *Arterial dissection (Note two distinct flow channels)*

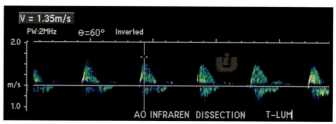

Fig. 35-42: *Spectral Doppler within true lumen*

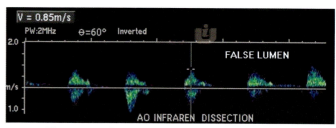

Fig. 35-43: *Spectral Doppler within false lumen*

Table 35-3: Diagnostic Criteria Summary for Abdominal Aortic Aneurysm and Dissection

Condition	Diameter (cm)
Ectasia	2.0-3.0
Aneurysm	>3.0
– Moderate	3.0-5.0
– Severe	>5.0
Dissection	True and false lumen present

Aortoiliac Bypass Graft/Iliac Stent Interpretation

PRINCIPLES OF INTERPRETATION

Analyze all of the following data from the physiologic and duplex exams. Use the exam data collected to determine if the graft or stent is normal or abnormal. Explain reasons why image and velocity data may not agree (e.g., size mismatch between stent/graft and native artery).

B-mode Imaging

- Assess the inflow/outflow vessels of the bypass or stent using B-mode for the presence of intralumenal echoes, vessel diameter changes or other unusual pathology.
- Stents can typically be seen within the lumen of clearly visualized arteries. Deeper stents may be difficult to identify with certainty.

Color Doppler

- Assess the inflow/outflow vessels of the bypass or stent using color flow and document flow at the point of intralumenal echoes, vessel diameter changes or other unusual pathology.

Segmental Pressures

- Compare duplex exam findings to the ankle-brachial indices (ABI).

Spectral Doppler Waveforms

- Observe for changes in the Doppler waveform proximal and distal to any segment with increased velocity which can point to a hemodynamically significant obstruction.

Flow Velocities
- Determine peak systolic velocity (PSV) and flow direction
- Calculate the velocity ratio:

$$Vr = V_2 \div V_1$$

V_2 = the maximum PSV of a stenosis

V_1 = PSV of the proximal normal segment.

Interpretation/Diagnostic Criteria

Normal

(absence of a hemodynamically significant stenosis, <50%)

B-mode Imaging
- Synthetic aortic bypass grafts have a characteristic "textured" appearance on B-mode image. [17]
- Normally, there is no echogenic material within the arterial lumen of an aortic bypass.

Color Doppler
- Color fills the lumen from wall-to-wall in transverse and longitudinal views with appropriate settings. [17]
- Turbulent color flow at an anastomotic site is expected. Correlate with flow velocities and spectral Doppler waveforms to determine if any color disturbances are significant.

Segmental Pressures
- If the ABI is ≥1.0, the presence of a hemodynamically significant stenosis or occlusion is unlikely in the graft/stent.

Spectral Doppler Waveforms
For details on waveform terminology, see the interpretation section in this chapter for native aortoiliac duplex. Additional considerations for aortoiliac bypass graft/iliac stent include:
- **Inflow artery:** A normal arterial inflow waveform is triphasic.
- **Proximal anastomosis:** Waveforms may demonstrate the typical disturbed flow patterns seen at bifurcations/branches or areas of angulation. These changes are focal at the anastomosis and normalize distally. [17,18]
- **Body of graft/stent:** Waveform configurations remain essentially the same as in the inflow artery throughout a non-obstructed conduit.

Flow Velocities
- **Inflow artery:** Velocity ratios (Vr) are <2.0 in the inflow tract.[17,18]
- **Anastomotic sites (proximal):** Normal Vr are <2.0. A large inflow artery feeding a small diameter graft may result in a higher velocity ratio due to the size change. The image should be scrutinized for the presence of intralumenal echoes. [17,18]
- **Body of graft/stent:** Velocity ratios are <2.0 throughout the graft/stent body. [17,18]
- **Distal anastomosis:** There is often a size change between the wider bypass graft and smaller diameter native artery resulting in a velocity increase. A normal distal anastomosis demonstrates a Vr <3.4. The image should be scrutinized for the presence of intralumenal echoes. Waveform configuration may be disturbed due to vessel angulation and size change.
- **Outflow artery:** Velocities remain fairly constant with Vr <2.0. Outflow arterial waveforms are similar to those in the graft body.[17,18] Flow direction may be retrograde in the native artery proximal to the distal anastomosis.

Abnormal

Definitive criterion for abdominal aortoiliac bypass/stent stenosis have not been widely addressed in the literature so it varies across institutions. Some labs use the same criterion used for the lower extremities.

B-mode Imaging
- There is echogenic material within the arterial lumen of the aortoiliac bypass/stent typically at the point of highest velocity.

Color Doppler
- Correlate turbulent color flow within the graft/stent or at an anastomotic site with flow velocities and spectral Doppler waveforms to determine if any color disturbances are significant.

Segmental Pressures
- If the ABI is < 1.0, the presence of a hemodynamically significant stenosis or occlusion is possible in the graft/stent.
- Generally, in any arterial intervention, findings of a decrease in ABI >0.15 on serial exam is indicative of significant disease progression in the inflow, graft or outflow arteries. [19]

Spectral Doppler Waveforms
For details on waveform terminology, see the interpretation section in this chapter for native aortoiliac duplex. Additional considerations for aortoiliac bypass graft/iliac stent include:
- **Inflow artery:** Post-stenotic turbulence and waveform changes (depending on the terminology used in your lab: triphasic to biphasic or monophasic) indicate a hemodynamically significant stenosis (≥50%). [14,17,20, 28]
- Low resistance waveform patterns at least 2cm proximal to the anastomosis indicate a significant inflow artery obstruction.
- **Anastomotic sites (proximal/distal):** Stenotic waveform patterns, spectral broadening and post-stenotic turbulence indicate a hemodynamically significant stenosis (≥50%).
- **Body of graft/stent:** Monophasic waveforms throughout the graft can indicate an obstruction in the inflow tract. Graft waveforms that demonstrate high-resistance, with no end diastolic velocity or a staccato pattern, indicate a distal anastomotic or outflow tract obstruction.

It is important to look at the images for intralumenal defects at the anastomosis or marked diameter changes that may account for velocity increases.

- **Outflow artery:** There is a change in the waveform configuration (triphasic to biphasic or monophasic) proximal and distal to any segment with increased velocity which can point to a hemodynamically significant obstruction.

Flow Velocities
- **Inflow artery:** Velocity ratios >2.0 within the native artery associated with post-stenotic turbulence and waveform changes (depending on the terminology used in your indicate a hemodynamically significant stenosis (≥50%). [14,17,20, 28]
- **Body of graft/stent:** Velocity >300cm/s and a Vr >2.0 within an iliac stent indicate a hemodynamically significant stenosis (≥50%). [21]
- **Distal anastomosis:** A PSV >275cm/s and velocity ratio >3.5 is indicative of a hemodynamically significant stenosis (≥80%) [28]
- **Outflow artery:** Vr >2.0 suggest a hemodynamically significant stenosis.

Other Pathology

- **Graft occlusion**: An occlusion of the graft or stent is present when echogenic material is observed within the graft/stent lumen **and** no flow is detected by spectral Doppler, and color in transverse and longitudinal views with appropriate low-flow settings. [17]

An occlusion suspected by color is never diagnostic without spectral Doppler confirmation

- A **pseudoaneurysm** is diagnosed when a pulsatile mass is identified by color and Doppler flow (often near an anastomotic site) which is observed communicating with the bypass or native artery through a patent "neck." The neck must demonstrate to and fro (pendulum) Doppler flow patterns to indicate a pseudoaneurysm. [17]
- **Perigraft fluid** is suspected when anechoic, fluid-filled structures surround the bypass conduit. Ultrasound cannot determine the exact fluid substance which may be related to infection, hematoma, etc. [17]

Differential Diagnosis

- Acute appendicitis
- Myocardial infarction
- Chronic diseases of the digestive tract
- Urinary tract infections
- Pancreatitis
- Renal calculi (kidney stones)

Correlation

- Spiral CT scan
- MRI
- Aortography

The predicted expansion rate of AAA is 0.2-0.5cm per year.[5]

Medical Treatment

- Treat underlying cause (e.g., systemic hypertension)
- Serial imaging exams to monitor changes in diameter or disease progression

Surgical Treatment

- Open repair for aneurysm diameter >5.0cm and/or for aneurysms rapidly increasing in size (>1.0cm per year)
- Aortic rupture is a surgical emergency
- The primary complication of AAA is rupture (in excess of 80% mortality rate). [24] Symptoms of impending rupture or rupture include:[5]
  » Severe abdominal pain radiating through to the back
  » Temporary loss of consciousness
  » Hypotension
  » Shock
  » Sudden death (rupture)

Endovascular Treatment

- Endolumenal graft
- Stent (e.g., iliac artery stenosis)
- Angioplasty

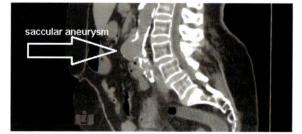

Fig. 35-44: *Saccular abdominal aortic aneurysm by CT scan*

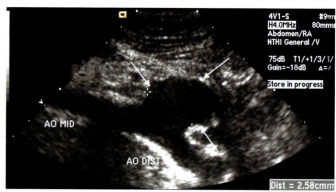

Fig. 35-45: *Saccular aneurysm off the abdominal aorta by B-mode imaging*

REFERENCES

1. Sumner DS, Zierler RE. (2005). Vascular physiology: essential hemodynamic principles. In *Rutherford Vascular Surgery 6th edition*. (75-123). Philadelphia. Elsevier Saunders.
2. Fecteau SR, Darling III RC, Roddy SP. (2005). Arterial thomboembolism. In *Rutherford Vascular Surgery 6th edition*. (971-986). Philadelphia. Elsevier Saunders.
3. Dawson DL, Lee ES, Lindholm K. (2010). Aortic and peripheral aneurysms. In Zierler RE (Ed.), Strandess's duplex scanning disorders in vascular diagnosis 4th ed. (157-168). Philadelphia Wolters Kluwer Lippincott Williams & Wilkins
4. Stary HC, Chandler AB, Dinsmore RE, Fuster V, Glagov S, Insull W, Rosenfeld ME, Schwartz CJ, Wagner WD, Wissler RW. A definition of advanced types of atherosclerotic lesions and histological classification of atherosclerosis. *Atherosclerosis, Thrombosis and Vascular Biology*. 1995; 15; 1521-1531.
5. Schermerhorn ML, Cronenwett JL. (2005). Abdominal aortic and iliac aneurysms. In *Rutherford Vascular Surgery 6th edition*. (1408-1452). Philadelphia. Elsevier Saunders.
6. Reddy DJ, Weaver MR. (2005). Infected aneurysms. In *Rutherford Vascular Surgery 6th edition*. (1581-1596). Philadelphia. Elsevier Saunders.
7. Black III JH, Cambria RP. (2005). Aortic dissection: perspectives for the vascular/endovascular surgeon. In *Rutherford Vascular Surgery 6th edition*. (1512-1533). Philadelphia. Elsevier Saunders.
8. Coimbra R, Hoyt DB. (2005). Epidemiology and natural history of vascular trauma. In *Rutherford Vascular Surgery 6th edition*. (1001-1006). Philadelphia. Elsevier Saunders.
9. Brewster DC. (2005). Direct reconstruction for aortoiliac occlusive disease. In *Rutherford Vascular Surgery 6th edition*. (1106-1136). Philadelphia. Elsevier Saunders.
10. Myers K, Clogh A. (2004) Renovascular diseases. In *Making Sense of Vascular Ultrasound*. (255-282). London: Hodder Arnold.
11. Zierler RE, Olmstead KA. (2010). Renal duplex scanning. In Zierler RE (Ed.), *Strandess's duplex scanning disorders in vascular diagnosis 4th ed.* (283-310).Philadelphia Wolters Kluwer Lippincott Williams & Wilkins.
12. Hallett JW, Brewster DC, Rasmussen TE. (2001). Aneurysms and aortic dissection. In: *Handbook of Patient Care in Vascular Diseases*. (204-221). Philadelphia Lippincott Williams & Wilkins
13. Burns PN. (1993). Principles of deep Doppler ultrasonography. In Bernstein EF (Ed.). *Vascular Diagnosis 4th ed.* (249-268). St. Louis: Mosby Yearbook Inc.
14. Rzucidlo EM, Zwolak RM. (2005). Arterial duplex scanning. In *Rutherford Vascular Surgery 6th edition*. (233-253). Philadelphia. Elsevier Saunders.
15. Cronenwett JL. (2005). Arterial aneurysms. In *Rutherford Vascular Surgery 6th edition*. (1403-1408). Philadelphia. Elsevier Saunders.
16. Brewster DC. (2005). Direct reconstruction for aortoiliac occlusive disease. In *Rutherford Vascular Surgery 6th edition*. (1106-1136). Philadelphia. Elsevier Saunders.
17. Zwiebel, WJ (2005). Ultrasound assessment of the aorta, iliac arteries and inferior vena cava. In Zwiebel WJ, Pellerito JS (Eds.), Introduction to Vascular Ultrasonography 5th ed, (530-552). Philadelphia: Elsevier Saunders.
18. Zierler RE. (2005). Ultrasound assessment of lower extremity arteries. In Zwiebel WJ, Pellerito JS (Eds.), Introduction to Vascular Ultrasonography 5th ed. (341-356). Philadelphia: Elsevier Saunders.
19. Bandyk, DF. (2005). Ultrasound assessment during and after peripheral intervention. In Zwiebel WJ, Pellerito JS (Eds.), *Introduction to Vascular Ultrasonography 5th ed*, (357-379). Philadelphia: Elsevier Saunders.
20. Hallett, JW, Brewster DC, Rasmussen TE, (2001) Non-invasive Vascular Testing, In Handbook of Patient Care in Vascular Diseases, (29-49), Philadelphia: Lippincott Williams & Wilkins
21. Back MR, Novotney M, Roth SM, Elkins D, Farber S, Cuthbertson D, Johnson BL, Bandyk DF. (2001). Utility of duplex surveillance following iliac artery angioplasty and primary stenting *J Endovasc Ther*. Dec;8(6):629-37.
22. Primary care screening for abdominal aortic aneurysm (2/2005). U.S. Preventive Services Task Force Evidence Syntheses, formerly Systematic Evidence Reviews. *Retrieved from*: http://www.ncbi.nlm.nih. gov/bookshelf/br.fcgi?book=es35&part=A30099.
23. Gerhard-Herman M, Gardin JM, Jaff M, Mohler E, Roman M, Naqvi TZ. (2006). Guidelines for non-invasive vascular laboratory testing: a report from the american society of echocardiography and the society of vascular medicine and biology. J Am Soc Echocardiogr 19:955-972.
24. Nordon IM, Hinchliffe RJ, Loftus IM, Thompson MM. (2010). Pathophysiology and epidemiology of abdominal aortic aneurysms *Nat Rev Cardiol*. Nov 16.
25. Van Bockel JH, Hamming JF. (2005). Lower extremity aneurysms. In Rutherford Vascular Surgery 6th edition. (1534-1551). Philadelphia. El Sevier Saunders.
26. Centers for medicare and medicaid services. (09/20/2010 1:09:09 PM). *Retrieved from* https://www.cms. gov/deficitreductionact.
27. Curci JA, Baxter TB, Thompson RW. (2005). Artery aneurysms. In *Rutherford Vascular Surgery 6th edition*. (475-492). Philadelphia. Elsevier Saunders.
28. Baril, D. T., Rhee, R. Y., Kim, J., Makaroun, M. S., Chaer, R. A., & Marone, L. K. (2009). Duplex criteria for determination of in-stent stenosis after angioplasty and stenting of the superficial femoral artery. Journal of vascular surgery, 49(1), 133–139. https://doi.org/10.1016/j.jvs.2008.09.046

ABDOMINAL ARTERIAL TESTING
36. Aortic Stent Graft (Endograft) Duplex Ultrasound

Definition
The combination of real time B-mode ultrasonography with spectral and color flow Doppler to assess an aortic endograft for the presence of possible endoleak, stenosis or occlusion and to monitor any changes in size of a previously documented aneurysm sac.

Etiology *(of endograft complications)*
- Endoleak
- Graft migration
- Graft infection
- Graft-limb external compression or kinking
- Embolization
- Thrombosis
- Technical error (graft misplacement)
- Limb separation
- Graft material complications (tears)
- Atherosclerosis

Risk Factors *(for endograft complications)*
- Age (increases with age)
- Smoking
- Hypertension
- Atherosclerosis
- Male gender
- Caucasian
- Immediate relative with an abdominal aortic aneurysm (AAA) history
- Trauma

Indications for Exam
- Post-operative surveillance of endovascular repair

Post-operative surveillance is generally performed at 1, 6, 12 and 18 months. Annual surveillance is recommended thereafter.

- Hip/buttock claudication or impotence in patients post-operative for endovascular repair.

Contraindications/Limitations
- Obesity may cause poor visualization due to vessel depth
- Abdominal gas may prohibit visualization of any or all vessels

Endograft Configurations
- Bifurcated aortoiliac
- Aorto uni-iliac
- Straight aortic tube graft
- Fenestrated (FEVAR): graft with openings for stents that can be placed into the arteries coming off the aorta, Fenestrated grafts can be bifurcated.
- ChEVAR: technique involving "chimney" like stent/grafts which run along the sides of the EVAR graft body to help maintain branch patency (e.g., renal branches). There are also combo grafts called FEVARCh.
- "Scalloped:" type of fenestrated graft with a U-shaped cutout proximally that goes around an arterial branch, preventing impingement

Mechanism of Endograft Complications
- **Embolization** can occur when introducing an endograft into the sac of an AAA, especially when there is intramural thrombus.[1] Renal failure (from renal obstruction) and distal embolization to the legs are concerns.

Anytime the aneurysm sac is still receiving flow, pre-operative concerns of aneurysm enlargement and rupture remain.

- **Endoleaks** may occur for the following reasons: [2]
  - » **Type I**: Poor attachment of the graft to the vessel wall
  - » **Type II**: Patent arterial branches communicate with the aneurysm sac. Multiple patent branches can supply an inflow/outflow channel to the sac. Sources include the lumbar, inferior mesenteric, accessory renal arteries, etc.
  - » **Type III**: A separation between the graft-limb modules
  - » **Type IV**: Abnormal porosity of the graft material
  - » **Type V**: sometimes called endotension is not a true endoleak but there is still expansion of the aneurysm sac. One theory suggests that increased graft permeability allows pressure to be transmitted through the aneurysm sac which affects the native aortic wall.
- **Stent migration** occurs when displacement forces exceed the strength of fixation at the proximal/distal attachment site. Movement of the endograft can cause an endoleak, kink or graft-limb thrombosis.

Patient History
- Endovascular repair of an abdominal aortic aneurysm
- Complication found unexpectedly during physical exam, radiological or CT exams
- Many complications of endovascular repair present without symptoms

Physical Examination
- Pulsatile abdominal mass
- Lower back pain
- Systolic murmur in the region of the aneurysm
- Peripheral edema due to obstruction of the inferior vena cava

Abdominal Aortic Stent Graft Examination
- Patients should be fasting for 6-12 hours to minimize the presence of air in the abdomen. A limited volume of clear liquids may be ingested prior to the examination (e.g., to swallow medications).
- Patient is supine with arms and legs adequately supported. The patient may bend their knees up to aid in relaxation of the abdominal wall and decrease lumbar pain. Explain the procedure to the patient.
- Acoustic windows for imaging the abdominal aorta include: midline of the upper abdomen, left flank with patient supine or right lateral decubitus.
- A low frequency (1-4 MHz) transducer should be used for imaging these deep structures.
- To detect flow within the aneurysm sac, use program settings sensitive for low-color flow and Doppler velocities.

Transverse (Short-Axis) Scan
- The transducer is placed at the midline, below the xyphoid process and moved slowly, inferior toward the umbilicus during exam. Image the abdominal aorta in B-mode from the diaphragm to the aortic bifurcation with intermittent color flow Doppler. Scan the iliac arteries to the inguinal ligament. Document any areas of graft compression, lumenal defect, separation of modular junctions or areas of color flow or echolucency within the sac.

- The aneurysm sac is measured from outer wall to outer wall in both the anterior-posterior and transverse planes, perpendicular to the flow axis. Document the maximum cross sectional diameter to assess for enlargement. Note the anatomic level of the image.

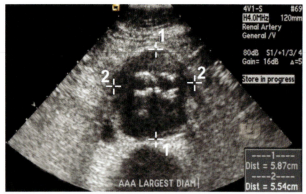

Fig. 36-1: *Duplex measurements of an aneurysm sac (Caliper #1 is the anterior-posterior measurement, Caliper #2 is the transverse measurement)*

- During serial examination, labs may measure and document the circumference of the aneurysm sac at its greatest diameter using the "area calculation" function of the duplex scanner. Document any noticeable changes regarding clot formation within the aneurysm sac.
- Determine the proximal fixation site between the stent and vessel wall. B-mode imaging without color is recommended in most cases. In transverse, record the aortic diameter at this site.

Longitudinal (Sagittal) Scan

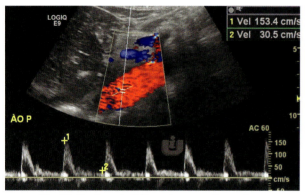

Fig. 36-2: *Spectral Doppler waveforms from abdominal aorta above stent*

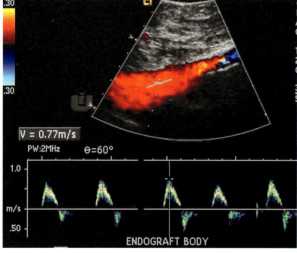

Fig. 36-3: *Spectral Doppler waveforms from body of the endograft*

- Turn the transducer longitudinally. Using spectral Doppler (≤60° Doppler angle, with the angle cursor parallel to the vessel walls in the center of the flow stream) record a spectral waveform in the abdominal aorta above the stent (typically suprarenal aortic segment). Observe for dissection or evidence of intimal flap at this level.
- Document a B-mode image of the proximal fixation site. Record peak systolic velocity (PSV) and end diastolic velocity (EDV) at this point. Turn color flow on and observe for evidence of endoleak within the aneurysm sac at this level.

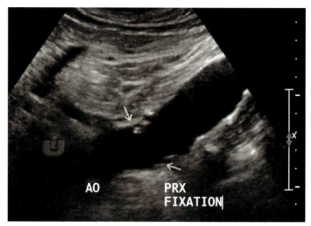

Fig. 36-4: *Proximal fixation site of stent- longitudinal B-mode view*

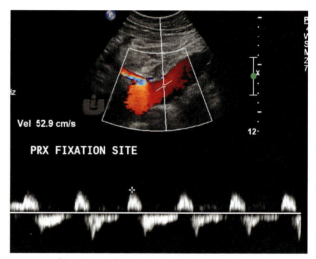

Fig. 36-5: *Spectral Doppler waveforms at the proximal fixation site*

- Analyze the body of the endovascular graft using color flow and spectral Doppler to look for any flow abnormalities or intralumenal defects. Record PSV and EDV from the body of the graft. Special attention should be given to any areas of kinking within the graft that may display increased velocities or stenosis and a decrease in distal flow. Record additional velocities pre and post any stenotic areas.
- The aneurysm sac is measured from outer wall to outer wall in the longitudinal plane. Remember to keep the transducer perpendicular to the axis of the aorta. Document the maximum diameter to assess for enlargement. Note anatomic level of image taken for accurate comparison to previous exams.
- Using color Doppler as a guide, sweep the Doppler cursor through the aneurysm sac to detect any areas of extrastent flow. An area of leak will generate uniform, reproducible color flow which should persist through diastole.

Care should be taken to differentiate between color-bleeding and artifact (due to low scales) versus a true endoleak.

- Confirm the absence or presence of flow outside the stent in multiple scan planes. Document waveform, velocity and flow direction in any areas of extrastent flow. Note anatomic location.

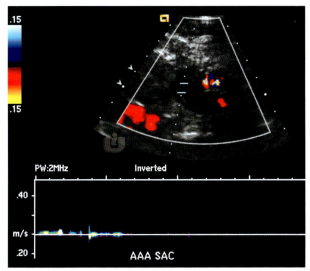

Fig. 36-6: *Spectral Doppler recorded in the transverse plane; no evidence of endoleak in the AAA sac.*

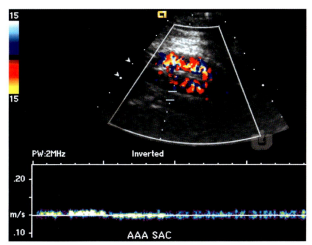

Fig. 36-7: *Spectral Doppler recorded in the longitudinal plane; no evidence of endoleak.*

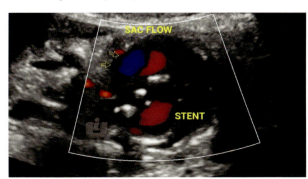

Fig. 36-8: *Color Doppler recorded in the transverse plane indicates evidence of endoleak*

Post-operatively, the movement of non-clotted blood within the aneurysm sac may be seen moving due to pulsatility from the adjacent endovascular graft.

Wall calcification and patient movement may produce flashes of color within the aneurysm sac.

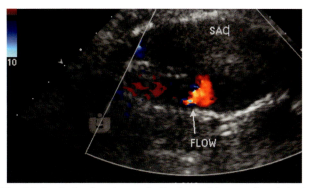

Fig. 36-9: *Color flow image indicates evidence of endoleak*

- If no color is noted within the sac with the patient supine, have the patient turn on their side (right lateral decubitus position) and scan again (from the side or back of the patient), as this position may uncover a leak not previously seen.

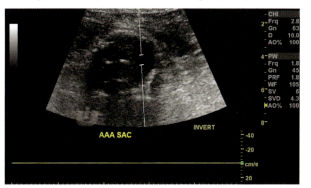

Fig. 36-10: *No leak evident by spectral Doppler when patient is in supine position.*

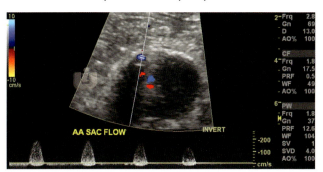

Fig. 36-11: *Evidence of leak in the same patient when scanned in the lateral decubitus position.*

- If an endoleak is present, determine the source (e.g., at a fixation site, from a branch or at junction between graft modules). Typical spectral waveform patterns will be "to-and-fro." Observe for small jets of flow in real time, filling the aneurysm sac.

When the source of a true endoleak cannot be determined, reporting should indicate that the inflow/outflow source is indeterminate.

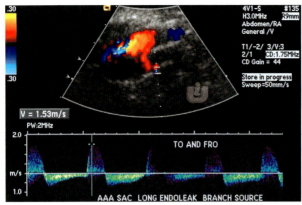

Fig. 36-12: *To-and-fro Doppler waveforms due to an endoleak.*

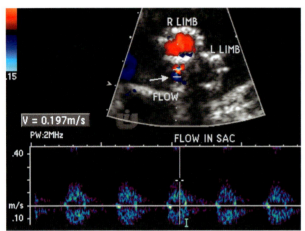

Fig. 36-13: *Transverse view of an endograft with an occlusion of the left graft limb and evidence of an endoleak.*

- Assess velocity and waveforms from each graft-limb to detect stenosis due to graft compression or occlusion. Calculate the velocity ratios (Vr), where the highest peak systolic velocity at stenosis (V_2) is divided by the PSV of the proximal normal segment (V_1).

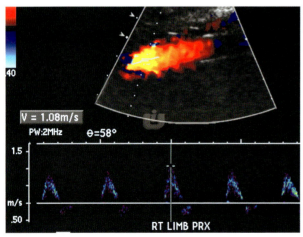

Fig. 36-14: *Spectral Doppler waveforms from the right graft limb*

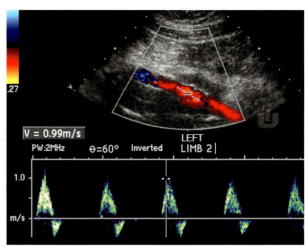

Fig. 36-15: *Spectral Doppler waveforms from the left graft limb*

- Determine the distal fixation site between the stent and vessel wall. Note the anatomic location. Turn color flow on and observe for evidence of endoleak at this level.
- Assess velocity and waveforms from the outflow artery, inferior to the distal attachment site. Calculate the velocity ratio in any areas of increased velocity.
- Analyze the bilateral common femoral waveforms to document aortoiliac inflow to the legs.
- During follow-up exams, the location of the graft is compared to previous studies for evidence of graft migration.

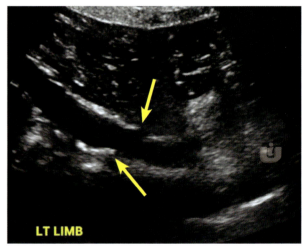

Fig. 36-16: *Distal fixation site on B-mode image*

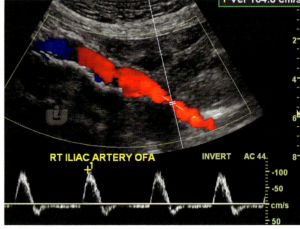

Fig. 36-17: *Arterial waveforms distal to the endograft*

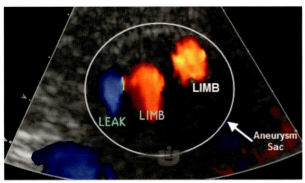

Fig. 36-18: *Transverse view of endoleak with color flow*

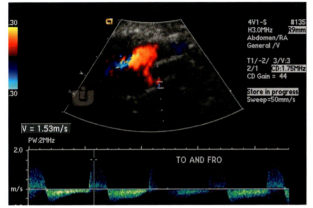

Fig. 36-19: *Endoleak spectral Doppler waveforms (to-and-fro waveform pattern)*

Table 36-1: Abdominal Aortic Stent Graft Protocol Summary

Scan in longitudinal (sagittal) and transverse (short-axis) planes with B-mode, low color and spectral Doppler velocity scales.

- Measure aneurysm sac from outer wall to outer wall in both anterior-posterior and transverse planes in both transverse and long views. Keep perpendicular to the vessel axis when measuring. Document maximum cross sectional diameter.
- Determine the proximal fixation site.
- Record peak systolic velocity (PSV), end diastolic velocity (EDV) and waveforms in the abdominal aorta above the stent.
- Observe body of the endograft in transverse and long views using low scale color flow and spectral Doppler to look for any flow abnormalities/intralumenal defects.* Record PSV, EDV and waveform from the body of the stent.
- Sweep the Doppler cursor throughout the aneurysm sac to detect any areas of extrastent flow and document any waveforms.
- Determine source of any endoleaks present.
- Record PSV, EDV and waveforms from each graft-limb.
- Determine the distal fixation site.
- Record outflow PSV, EDV and waveforms.
- Record bilateral common femoral PSV, EDV and waveforms.

* Observe for and document any areas of graft compression, luminal defect or separation of modular junctions.

PRINCIPLES OF INTERPRETATION

Analyze all of the following data from the physiologic and duplex exams. Use the exam data collected to determine if the endograft is normal or abnormal. Explain reasons why image and velocity data may not agree (e.g., size mismatch between stent/graft and native artery)

B-mode Imaging

- Assess the inflow/outflow vessels and the stent graft using B-mode image and document flow at the point of intralumenal echoes, vessel diameter changes or other unusual pathology. Diameter reduction measurements should only be used in conjunction with peak velocities. Diameter reduction measurements should only be used in conjunction with peak velocities.
- Arterial diameters: Measure diameters of the residual aneurysm sac and compare to previous exams when available.

Color Doppler

- Assess the inflow/outflow vessels and the stent graft using color flow especially at the point of any intralumenal echoes, vessel diameter changes or other unusual pathology.
- Assess for aneurysm sac with color for extra stent flow.

Spectral Doppler Waveforms

- Assess for waveform changes between the inflow, endograft and outflow arteries.
- Typically, the inferior mesenteric and lumbar arteries occlude after endovascular repair.[4] If they remain patent, determine flow direction in these side vessels and analyze carefully for possible endoleak.[7]

Flow Velocities

- Determine peak systolic velocity (PSV) and flow direction
- Calculate the velocity ratio:

$$Vr = V_2 \div V_1$$

V_2 = the maximum PSV of a stenosis
V_1 = PSV of the proximal normal segment.

- Abdominal gas is similar to calcific shadowing in that gas/shadowing can prohibit Doppler and color flow analysis of a specific arterial segment. Use indirect signs to evaluate hemodynamically significant lesions:
  » If post-stenotic turbulence is present distal to the shadowing, there could be a stenosis through the area not visualized. Conversely, if there is no change in the waveform pattern, it is unlikely that a significant obstruction exists.

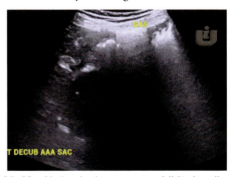

Fig. 36-20: *Abdominal gas can prohibit visualization.*

  » Comparing the Doppler waveform proximal and distal to the non-visualized segment can point to a hemodynamically significant obstruction under the shadowing.

Interpretation/Diagnostic Criteria

Normal

B-mode Imaging
- There are no intralumenal echoes within the native arteries or stent.
- There are no areas of echolucency within the aneurysm sac by B-mode image.
- **Aneurysm size:** Expect the sac/aneurysm size to decrease or remain stable post-operatively after exclusion from circulation.

Color Doppler
- The body and limbs of the endograft should be widely patent by color. There should be wall-to-wall color filling in the appropriate direction for each segment of the graft and native artery.
- There is no evidence of color flow within the aneurysm sac with appropriate low-flow settings. [3,4]

Spectral Doppler Waveforms
- A *high resistance waveform* pattern is normal in the aortoiliac arteries with a quick downstroke that ends with a short period of reversed flow direction (below the baseline) at end systole/early diastole. This reversed flow segment in the waveform may or may not be followed by a third segment with a low, short segment of forward flow. This waveform can also be referred to as *triphasic*.

The third phase of the triphasic waveform may be missing in the suprarenal aortic segment, especially in patients with less vessel compliance.

- There should be no waveform changes between the inflow, endograft and outflow arteries.

Flow Velocities
- No evidence of significant velocity increase (e.g., Vr <2.0).

Color is never diagnostic without spectral Doppler confirmation.

Abnormal

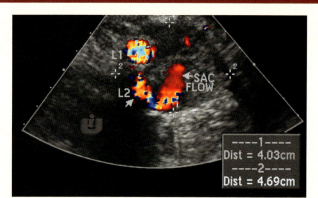

Fig. 36-21: *Duplex measurement of aneurysm sac-endoleak*

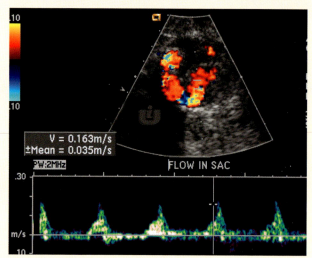

Fig. 36-22: *Spectral Doppler from aneurysm sac-endoleak*

B-mode Imaging
- An area of endoleak is recognized on the B-mode image by echolucency or pulsation within the aneurysm sac and confirmed by color and spectral Doppler waveforms. [3-5] Always attempt to reproduce evidence of an endoleak to reduce false-positive reports. [4]

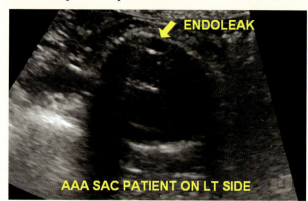

Fig. 36-23: *Endoleak suspected by an area of echolucency on B-mode image*

- **Aneurysm size:** A >0.5cm increase in the diameter of the aneurysm sac on B-mode image is suggestive of endoleak. [2,4] Further imaging (e.g., CT scan) may be needed to confirm such findings. [3,4]
- **Endotension** is indicated when an increase in the aneurysm's size is measured, without any endoleak detected by duplex. [2]

Color Doppler
- Color Doppler does not fill the entire arterial lumen, instead a color jet can be visualized through the narrowed lumen of the native artery/stent.
- There is evidence of color flow within the aneurysm sac with appropriate low-flow settings. [3,4]
- **Endoleak:** True endoleaks create reproducible uniform color Doppler data, including waveforms in sync with the patient's cardiac cycle. [4] Doppler waveforms of the endoleak should differ from the waveform characteristics in the endograft. [6]

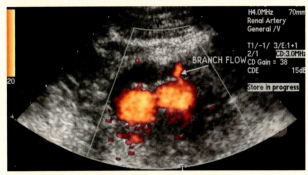

Fig. 36-24: *Endoleak documented with power Doppler*

Spectral Doppler Waveforms

- As the obstruction becomes more severe, changes in the spectral waveform are expected before a stenosis or occlusion, at the point of greatest stenosis and after a stenosis/occlusion as described in the *Arterial Physiology* chapter.
- *Spectral broadening* represents the wide range of velocities usually present when disturbed, non-laminar flow occurs. This waveform change occurs in the early stages of arterial disease. The normally clear window below the systolic peak begins to fill in.
- *Monophasic* arterial Doppler waveforms reflect low resistance and are characterized by a slow upstroke, low amplitude, and broad peak with continuous forward flow in diastole that does not cross the zero baseline. The upstroke has a general direction of being tipped to the right. Monophasic waveforms are typically present distal to an occlusion or a very high-grade stenosis. [17]
- A *high-resistance waveform* with a sharp upstroke and brisk downstroke will be noted in a stenotic region. There may or may not be flow reversal in diastole. [17] When there is a diastolic component, it may be elevated or absent depending on the degree of downstream resistance.
- *Turbulent waveforms* or "post-stenotic turbulence" are indicative of chaotic flow reflecting how blood moves in many directions just past the stenosis.
- *Parvus tardus* is an alternative term for "monophasic" used by some laboratories to describe a waveform with continuous forward flow and a slow, blunted systolic component.
- **Staccato:** A "spiked" high-resistant waveform with a short upstroke/downstroke and little to no diastolic component is often a signal of impending occlusion.
- Flow through an aneurysm can exhibit systolic dampening and a prominent diastolic reversal associated with the swirling of blood within the dilated lumen. [5,12]
- **Endoleak:** The direction of flow will be used to determine the afferent (inflow) and afferent (outflow) sources communicating with the aneurysm. [4] Depending on the source of the endoleak, describe waveforms according to the terminology used in your lab. [3,4,6]
  - » In a small research series, biphasic waveforms suggested that the endoleak had an inflow and outflow source. Endoleaks with monophasic and bidirectional waveforms are more likely to spontaneously thrombose. [6]

Flow Velocities

- **Stenosis:** A limb stenosis is recognized by color aliasing and confirmed by increased velocities. [4,7] Compare velocities at the level of the stenosis to the velocities in the proximal normal segment. A velocity ratio >2.0 and the presence of post-stenotic turbulence indicate a hemodynamically significant stenosis. Diameter reduction measurements should only be used in conjunction with peak systolic velocity measurements.
- **Occlusion:** An occlusion is recognized by the absence of color saturation confirmed by the lack of an audible spectral Doppler signal in the endograft or native artery with appropriate settings.

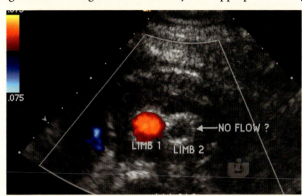

Fig. 36-25: *Occlusion of a graft limb suspected in transverse view by color flow*

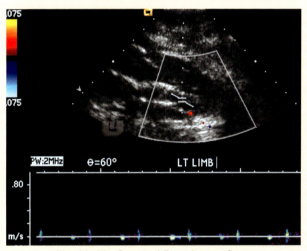

Fig. 36-26: *Spectral Doppler confirms occlusion of the graft limb*

Table 36-2: Endoleak Classification

Type	Source of Endoleak
Type I	Attachment site (either proximal or distal)
Type II	Branch site (such as; lumbar, inferior mesenteric, intercostal, internal iliac, hypogastric or accessory renal arteries)
Type III	Modular disconnection, fabric tear
Type IV	Porosity
Type V	Endotension, expansion of the aneurysm sac without a true endoleak source identified

Correlation
- CT scan
- MRI
- Aortography

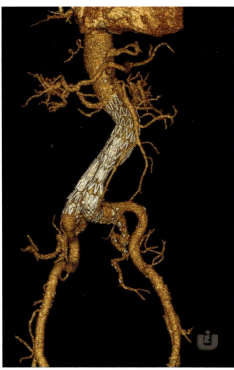

Fig. 36-27: *CTA revealing abdominal and iliac stents*

Surgical Treatment
- Open repair of aortic aneurysm

Endovascular Treatment
- Balloon dilatation of the involved graft component (to treat a leak or stenosis)
- Placement of supportive stenting or endograft extension pieces

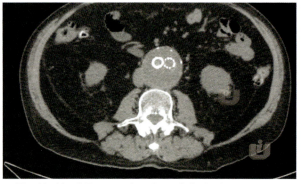

Fig. 36-28: *CT scan of endograft limbs in transverse*

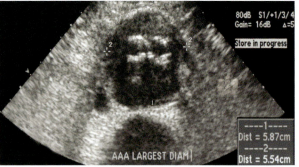

Fig. 36-29: *Duplex of endograft limbs in transverse*

REFERENCE

1. Sumner DS, Zierler RE. (2005). Vascular physiology: essential hemodynamic principles. In Rutherford Vascular Surgery 6th edition. (75-123). Philadelphia. Elsevier Saunders.
2. Fecteau SR, Darling III RC, Roddy SP. (2005). Arterial thomboembolism. In Rutherford Vascular Surgery 6th edition. (971-986). Philadelphia. Elsevier Saunders.
3. Dawson DL, Lee ES, Lindholm K. (2010). Aortic and peripheral aneurysms. In Zierler RE (Ed.), Strandess's duplex scanning disorders in vascular diagnosis 4th ed. (157-168). Philadelphia Wolters Kluwer Lippincott Williams & Wilkins
4. Stary HC, Chandler AB, Dinsmore RE, Fuster V, Glagov S, Insull W, Rosenfeld ME, Schwartz CJ, Wagner WD, Wissler RW. A definition of advanced types of atherosclerotic lesions and histological classification of atherosclerosis. Atherosclerosis, Thrombosis and Vascular Biology. 1995; 15; 1521-1531.
5. Schermerhorn ML, Cronenwett JL. (2005). Abdominal aortic and iliac aneurysms. In Rutherford Vascular Surgery 6th edition. (1408-1452). Philadelphia. Elsevier Saunders.
6. Reddy DJ, Weaver MR. (2005). Infected aneurysms. In Rutherford Vascular Surgery 6th edition. (1581-1596). Philadelphia. Elsevier Saunders.
7. Black III JH, Cambria RP. (2005). Aortic dissection: perspectives for the vascular/endovascular surgeon. In Rutherford Vascular Surgery 6th edition. (1512-1533). Philadelphia. Elsevier Saunders.
8. Coimbra R, Hoyt DB. (2005). Epidemiology and natural history of vascular trauma. In Rutherford Vascular Surgery 6th edition. (1001-1006). Philadelphia. Elsevier Saunders.
9. Brewster DC. (2005). Direct reconstruction for aortoiliac occlusive disease. In Rutherford Vascular Surgery 6th edition. (1106-1136). Philadelphia. Elsevier Saunders.
10. Myers K, Clogh A. (2004) Renovascular diseases. In Making Sense of Vascular Ultrasound. (255-282). London: Hodder Arnold.
11. Zierler RE, Olmstead KA. (2010). Renal duplex scanning. In Zierler RE (Ed.), Strandess's duplex scanning disorders in vascular diagnosis 4th ed. (283-310).Philadelphia Wolters Kluwer Lippincott Williams & Wilkins.
12. Hallett JW, Brewster DC, Rasmussen TE. (2001). Aneurysms and aortic dissection. In: Handbook of Patient Care in Vascular Diseases. (204-221). Philadelphia Lippincott Williams & Wilkins
13. Burns PN. (1993). Principles of deep Doppler ultrasonography. In Bernstein EF (Ed.). Vascular Diagnosis 4th ed. (249-268). St. Louis: Mosby Yearbook Inc.
14. Rzucidlo EM, Zwolak RM. (2005). Arterial duplex scanning. In Rutherford Vascular Surgery 6th edition. (233-253). Philadelphia. Elsevier Saunders.
15. Cronenwett JL. (2005). Arterial aneurysms. In Rutherford Vascular Surgery 6th edition. (1403-1408). Philadelphia. Elsevier Saunders.
16. Brewster DC. (2005). Direct reconstruction for aortoiliac occlusive disease. In Rutherford Vascular Surgery 6th edition. (1106-1136). Philadelphia. Elsevier Saunders.
17. Zwiebel, WJ (2005). Ultrasound assessment of the aorta, iliac arteries and inferior vena cava. In Zwiebel WJ, Pellerito JS (Eds.), Introduction to Vascular Ultrasonography 5th ed, (530-552). Philadelphia: Elsevier Saunders.
18. Zierler RE. (2005). Ultrasound assessment of lower extremity arteries. In Zwiebel WJ, Pellerito JS (Eds.), Introduction to Vascular Ultrasonography 5th ed, (341-356). Philadelphia: Elsevier Saunders.
19. Bandyk, DF, (2005). Ultrasound assessment during and after peripheral intervention. In Zwiebel WJ, Pellerito JS (Eds.), Introduction to Vascular Ultrasonography 5th ed, (357-379). Philadelphia: Elsevier Saunders.
20. Hallett, JW, Brewster DC, Rasmussen TE, (2001) Non-invasive Vascular Testing, In Handbook of Patient Care in Vascular Diseases, (29-49), Philadelphia: Lippincott Williams & Wilkins
21. 21 Back MR, Novotney M, Roth SM, Elkins D, Farber S, Cuthbertson D, Johnson BL, Bandyk DF. (2001). Utility of duplex surveillance following iliac artery angioplasty and primary stenting
22. J Endovasc Ther. Dec;8(6):629-37.
23. Primary care screening for abdominal aortic aneurysm (2/2005). U.S. Preventive Services Task Force Evidence Syntheses, formerly Systematic Evidence Reviews. Retrieved from: http://www.ncbi.nlm.nih.gov/bookshelf/br.fcgi?book=es35&part=A30099.
24. Gerhard-Herman M, Gardin JM, Jaff M, Mohler E, Roman M, Naqvi TZ. (2006). Guidelines for non-invasive vascular laboratory testing: a report from the american society of echocardiography and the society of vascular medicine and biology. J Am Soc Echocardiogr 19:955-972.
25. Nordon IM, Hinchliffe RJ, Loftus IM, Thompson MM. (2010). Pathophysiology and epidemiology of abdominal aortic aneurysms Nat Rev Cardiol. Nov 16.
26. 25 Van Bockel JH, Hamming JF. (2005). Lower extremity aneurysms. In Rutherford Vascular Surgery 6th edition. (1534-1551). Philadelphia. El Sevier Saunders.
27. Centers for medicare and medicaid services. (09/20/2010 1:09:09 PM). Retrieved from https://www.cms.gov/deficitreductionact.

ABDOMINAL ARTERIAL TESTING
37. Renal Duplex Ultrasound

Definition
The combination of real time B-mode ultrasonography with spectral and color flow Doppler to assess the renal arteries for the presence of stenosis/occlusion or other disease states such as fibromuscular dysplasia. Doppler and color flow are also used to evaluate the renal veins for evidence of thrombus.

Etiology of Renal Vessel Disease
- Atherosclerosis, resulting in stenosis or occlusion
- Fibromuscular dysplasia (FMD)
- Embolus
- Vasculitis
- External compression
- Thrombosis
- Aneurysm
- Arteriovenous fistula
- Trauma
- Occlusion

Risk Factors
- Age (increased risk with age)
- Hypertension
- Race (African-Americans have the highest risk)
- Diabetes
- Kidney disease
- Family history of kidney disease
- Smoking
- Hyperlipidemia
- Obesity
- Coronary artery disease
- Young, middle-aged Caucasian women (highest risk for fibromuscular dysplasia)

Indications for Exam
- Hypertension (HTN)
  » of unknown origin (essential hypertension)
  » malignant, benign or secondary types of types of HTN
  » changes in previously controlled HTN
- Elevated blood-urea-nitrogen (BUN) levels (*azotemia*)
- Known atherosclerosis of the aortoiliac segment, especially accompanied by HTN
- Unilateral, small (atrophic) kidney
- Cystic kidney disease
- Aneurysm/pseudoaneurysm
- Pre and post-operative surgical intervention, revascularization, endovascular procedure or percutaneous translumenal dilatation of the renal arteries

Atherosclerosis is the most common cause of renovascular hypertension (RVH).[17] FMD accounts for a smaller percentage of all RVH cases.

Contraindications/Limitations
- Obesity may cause poor visualization due to vessel depth.
- Abdominal gas may prohibit visualization of any or all vessels.
- Patient inability to hold their breath or suspend breathing for short periods of time may make it difficult to obtain accurate Doppler recordings.

Renal artery scanning is a difficult exam which requires time, patience and a long learning curve.

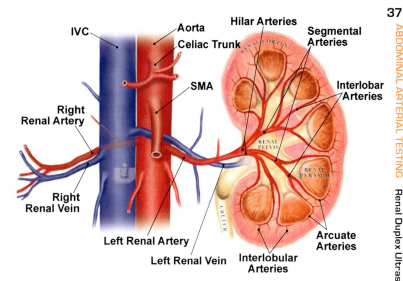

Fig. 37-1: *Renal Vessel Anatomy*

Anatomic Variations of the Kidney and Renal Arteries
- A "horseshoe kidney" is a congenital abnormality which results in the fusion of both kidneys. Beginning the scan with a midline abdominal approach is suggested for this situation.
- In 20-30% of patients, one to three accessory renal arteries may be present, especially on the left side. They usually originate from the aorta below the main renal artery and often enter the kidney directly.
- A renal artery may also branch anywhere before entering the kidney.

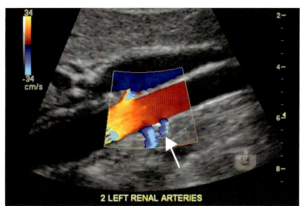

Fig. 37-2: *Left accessory renal artery (Note second left-sided branch off the aorta)*
Image courtesy of GE Healthcare-Ultrasound Division

Mechanism of Disease
- Renal arterial stenotic or occlusive disease results in decreased renal blood flow to the kidney.[1]
  » When baroreceptors detect a decrease in blood flow, the enzyme, renin is released.

The kidney maintains blood pressure by regulating the balance of sodium and water retention.[1]

» The renin-angiotensin system is activated, which increases angiotensin II levels. Sodium and water retention ensues. If the contralateral kidney is healthy, it can compensate by increasing its urine output to prevent volume expansion.

» Angiotensin II increases blood pressure and causes peripheral vasoconstriction.

» A sustained increase in hypertension results.

» When there is only single kidney function, if that renal artery is obstructed, the kidney cannot rely on increased urine output from the contralateral kidney to prevent sodium and water retention. The volume expansion which results causes elevated blood pressure and suppresses renin production by the stenotic kidney.

- **Atherosclerosis** is the most common arterial disease. Atherosclerotic plaque forms in the artery to block flow by either narrowing the arterial lumen (arterial stenosis) or totally blocking the artery (arterial occlusion). The term "hemodynamically significant obstruction" refers to either a stenosis or an occlusion that results in a decrease in blood pressure or flow distal to the obstruction. Typically, a stenosis must narrow the diameter of the artery by at least 50% to decrease pressure and flow distally. An arterial occlusion is typically seen from one major branch to the next.[2]

- **Emboli** may occur as contents of a plaque or fragments of an organized thrombus from the left-side of the heart, suprarenal aneurysm or ulcerative aortic plaque loosen and flow downstream.[3] Emboli become lodged in a distant blood vessel, causing an arterial obstruction which reduces flow.[4] Sources for renal emboli include renal artery dissection, traumatic renal artery occlusion or cardiac sources.[1]

- **Fibromuscular dysplagia (FMD)** is a non-atherosclerotic arterial disease which affects the mid/distal renal arteries. Typically, focal or "multifocal" stenoses are present, resembling a "string of beads" on imaging studies. "Focal" FMD involves the renal artery origin and is less common. The exact mechanism of disease is unclear.

- **Renal artery thrombosis** can occur when there is advanced atherosclerosis of the aorta and its branches.[3]

- **Renal vein thrombosis** can occur in adults in one or both renal veins due to cancer (especially renal cell carcinoma), hypercoaguable states, pregnancy, use of contraceptive medications, trauma or sickle cell anemia. Neonates are also at risk for renal vein thrombosis.[3]

- **Renal vein compression syndrome:** Compression of the renal vein between the aorta and superior mesenteric artery can occur in rare cases. "Nutcracker syndrome" was a previous term used to describe this type of compression which often involves the left renal vein (also known as "renal vein entrapment syndrome.")[5]

- **Aneurysmal disease** results from atherosclerosis or congenital defect.[6]

- **Arterial dissection** of the renal artery can occur spontaneously with atherosclerosis, trauma or dysplastic renovascular disease as the underlying cause.[6]

Location of Disease

- In atherosclerosis, the ostial or proximal renal arterial segment is affected.

- In cases of multifocal FMD, the mid-distal renal arterial segments are affected. Focal FMD can just affect the renal artery origin.

- In renal vein compression syndrome, venous dilatation occurs distal (upstream) to the compression.

Patient History

- Systemic hypertension
- Unexplained hypokalemia
- Renal failure
- Abnormal urinalysis (e.g., serum potassium, creatinine)
- Unexplained episodes of congestive heart failure (CHF)
- Flash pulmonary edema
- Left flank abdominal pain radiating to the buttocks (renal vein compression syndrome)
- Hematuria
- Anemia

Physical Examination

- Abdominal bruit-abnormal sound heard through auscultation caused by turbulent flow.

Duplex Examination of the Renal Arteries

- To minimize technical difficulties due to bowel gas, renal exams are best performed in the morning after the patient has fasted overnight. Encourage the patient not to smoke or chew gum before the exam.

- Patient should be fasting for 6-12 hours to minimize the presence of air and fluids in the abdomen. A limited volume of clear liquids may be ingested prior to the examination to swallow medications. Patient may be given Simethicone (Gas-X, Mylanta, etc.) before the exam to reduce abdominal gas.

- Obtain any past surgical reports or records of bypass graft or stent placement and general date of surgery if available. Explain the procedure to the patient.

- Patient should be supine with their arms and legs adequately supported. The patient may bend their knees up to aid in relaxation of the abdominal wall and decrease lumbar pain. The patient may also lie on their side to be scanned from the right and left flank (*lateral decubitus* position).

- A low frequency transducer (2.0-4.0MHz) should be used for imaging deep renal structures.

- Spectral Doppler should be at a ≤60° angle in the renal arteries. The sample volume should be parallel to the vessel walls and within the center of the flow stream. In the kidney parenchyma, the Doppler angle should be set to 0° (zero).

A 0-degree angle is used in the kidney parenchyma since waveform morphology is the only concern, not velocities.

Imaging of the renal arteries can be accomplished using the following approaches:

Transverse/short-axis View (most common approach)

» The origin and proximal portion of the renal arteries can be visualized with the patient in the supine position and the transducer oriented to obtain a transverse view. The right RA arises from the lateral aspect of the abdominal aorta at approximately 10-o'clock. The right renal vein is anterior to the right RA. The left RA, originating from the aorta at approximately the 3- 4-o'clock position, lies inferior to the left renal vein and can be more difficult to image than the right RA.

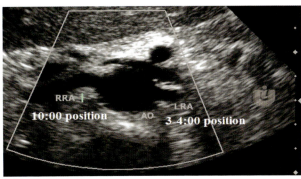

Fig. 37-3: Renal artery origins off the abdominal aorta (transverse B-mode view)

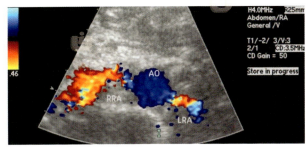

Fig. 37-4: Right and left renal artery origins off the abdominal aorta

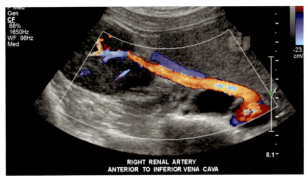

Fig. 37-5: Right renal artery coursing from the abdominal aorta to the kidney

Image courtesy of Philips Healthcare

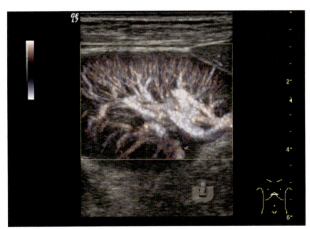

Fig. 37-6: Kidney parenchyma with color flow

Image courtesy of GE Healthcare-Ultrasound Division

"Banana Peel" View

- With the patient placed in a left lateral decubitus position, the right RA can be seen "peeling" off the aorta upward and the left RA can be seen peeling away from the aorta.
- Views of the liver, inferior vena cava and abdominal aorta can be accessed from this window.

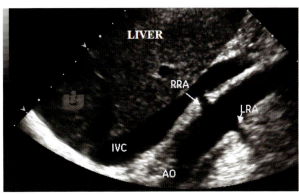

Fig. 37-7: The liver and renal arteries can be visualized using the "banana peel" view.

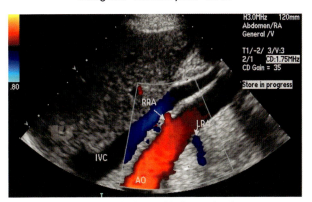

Fig. 37-8: Right and left renal artery origins off the aorta with color flow

Intercostal views may be necessary to visualize the kidneys.

Using the liver as a window

The patient is turned to a right-side-up-decubitus position and the liver is used as a window to visualize the origin of the right RA.

Spleen as a window

With the patient placed in a left lateral decubitus position, the spleen and the left kidney are used as acoustic windows to visualize the left renal artery.

Renal Artery Scanning Protocol

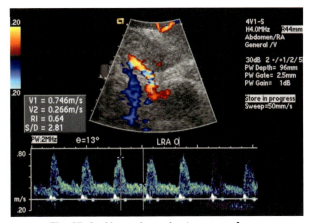

Fig. 37-9: Normal renal artery waveforms

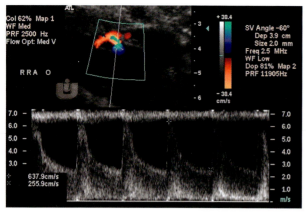

Fig. 37-10: *Abnormal (stenotic) renal artery waveforms*

Abdominal Aorta

- Examine the abdominal aorta for aneurysm, plaque, thrombus, dissection, tortuosity and/or other abnormalities.
- Record a spectral Doppler peak systolic velocity (PSV) in the suprarenal abdominal aorta, at or above the superior mesenteric artery, to be used in the renal artery/aortic ratio (RAR) calculation.
- Observe for important variants of the renal arteries (e.g., renal artery duplication).

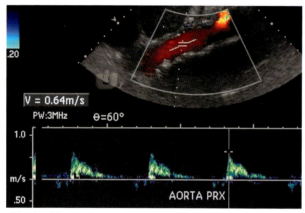

Fig. 37-11: *Abdominal aorta normal spectral waveforms*

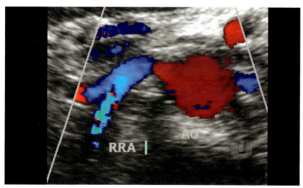

Fig. 37-12: *Branching of the right renal artery. Note: This is a "branch" and not an accessory renal since it does not originate off the actual aorta.*

Renal Artery

- Locate the superior mesenteric artery in a transverse view and then move the transducer slightly distal to image the right RA.
- Measure the PSV and EDV at the origin, proximal, mid and distal portions of the right RA. A transverse transducer orientation is often best when recording from the ostia and proximal segments, while a longitudinal (sagittal) orientation

works for the mid and distal segments. Scroll or "walk" the Doppler sample volume through the renal artery checking for focal changes in velocity and waveform configuration.
- Include additional recordings of any visualized accessory renal arteries when present.
- Document the highest PSV and EDV through any stenotic area(s) and document post-stenotic turbulence.
- Examine the renal artery for aneurysm, plaque, thrombus, dissection and/or other abnormalities.

Color flow Doppler and power Doppler may aid in locating the arteries and areas of interest.

- Image the right kidney, with and without color flow, and examine the kidney for anomalies such as cysts, dilated collection systems and/or tumors.
- Obtain a long-axis image of the right kidney and measure kidney length, pole-to-pole. A difference between both kidneys of >2cm calls for re-measurement of the smaller kidney to confirm the discrepancy.

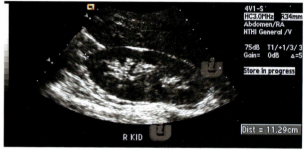

Fig. 37-13: *Pole-to-pole diameter measurement of the kidney*

- Document PSV/EDV in the parenchymal/hilar arteries (when appropriate).
- Calculate the RAR by dividing the highest PSV of the renal artery by the highest PSV in the suprarenal abdominal aortic segment.

Renal Vein

- Place the transducer in the right lower quadrant over the kidney and angle medially. Use color flow as a guide to locate the right renal vein.

Even with RV occlusion, you may observe venous flow within the kidney from hilar collaterals.[7]

- Document patency of the right RV using color flow and spectral Doppler.

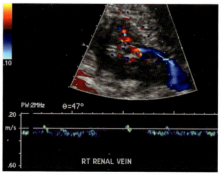

Fig. 37-14: *Normal spontaneous, phasic renal vein spectral Doppler waveform.*

The left renal vein can be a useful landmark when it crosses over the aorta near the origin of the right RA.

Renal Parenchyma

- Record PSV, EDV and Doppler spectral waveforms from the upper and/or lower poles of the kidney in the medullary and cortical regions of the organ from the arcuate and interlobar arteries. Use a 1.5-2mm sample volume and a 0⁰ (zero) Doppler angle for these measurements. Since parenchymal vessels are not easily imaged, color flow is a useful tool to guide placement of the Doppler sample volume. Waveforms with the highest amplitude and velocity should be documented from the parenchyma.

It may improve the kidney visualization by asking the patient to take a deep breath in and hold it.

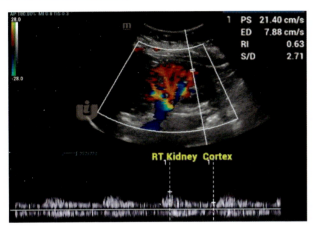

Fig. 37-15: *Cortical flown in the kidney measured near the outer border of the kidney*

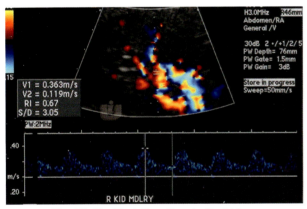

Fig. 37-16: *Medullary flow in the kidney*

Stenosis of the renal artery may be unilateral, although bilateral renal stenoses are possible, especially when atherosclerotic disease is the cause.

- Calculate the resistive index (RI) using the arcuate and interlobar arteries in the medulla and cortical regions of the kidney. The formula for RI is (1 - [EDV/maximum systolic velocity] x 100) or (PSV-EDV)/PSV. Many duplex scanners will automatically calculate RI from the spectral tracings during the exam.
- Determine classification of stenosis according to laboratory diagnostic criteria.
- Repeat for the left RA, RV and parenchyma.

When fibromuscular dysplasia (FMD) is detected in the renal arteries, you may be asked to scan the carotid and mesenteric arteries since the disease commonly coexists in these vessels. FMD can be either unilateral or bilateral.

Renal Bypass Graft/Stent Surveillance Protocol

- Evaluate for graft or stent abnormalities while scanning (e.g., thrombosis, stenosis, residual valves, aneurysm, kinks, intimal hyperplasia, perigraft fluid, arteriovenous fistula).
- Record images in a longitudinal view with and without color flow of the:
  » Inflow/proximal native artery
  » Proximal anastomosis
  » Proximal graft or stent
  » Mid graft or stent
  » Distal graft or stent
  » Distal anastomosis
  » Outflow/distal native artery
- Scroll or "walk" the Doppler sample volume through the bypass graft/stent checking for focal changes in velocity and waveform configuration.
- Record and measure the peak systolic velocity (PSV) in longitudinal using spectral Doppler (≤60⁰ Doppler angle with the angle cursor parallel to the vessel walls and sample volume within the center of the flow stream) at the following levels:
  » Inflow/proximal native artery, at least 2cm proximal to the anastomosis
  » Proximal anastomosis
  » Proximal graft or stent
  » Mid graft or stent
  » Distal graft or stent
  » Distal anastomosis
  » Outflow/distal native artery
- Determine classification of stenosis according to laboratory diagnostic criteria.
- Report any incidental findings so additional diagnostic studies may be obtained if necessary.[14]

Table 37-1: Renal Duplex Protocol Summary

Abdominal Aorta
- Evaluate the abdominal aorta for aneurysm, plaque, thrombus, dissection, and/or tortuosity.
- Obtain a spectral Doppler peak systolic velocity (PSV) in the abdominal aorta, at or above the superior mesenteric artery, for use in the renal artery/aortic ratio (RAR).

Renal Arteries
- Record PSV and EDV at the origin, proximal, mid and distal portions of the right and left renal arteries.

Kidneys
- Image the right and left kidneys in the long-axis. Measure its diameter.
- Identify arterial flow in the cortical and medullary segments of the kidney using color flow. Record PSV and EDV in the upper and/or lower poles of the kidney according to lab criteria.

Renal Veins
- Identify the right and left RV using color flow and record spectral waveforms of these veins.

Calculations
- Calculate the renal artery/aortic ratio (RAR) (bilaterally) and determine the classification of disease.

$$\frac{\text{The highest renal artery PSV}}{\text{The highest PSV in the suprarenal abdominal aortic segment}}$$

- Calculate the resistive indices (RI) bilaterally using cortical and medullary flow to determine the presence of intrinsic disease.

Resistive index = 1 - [EDV/PSV] x 100
or (PSV - EDV) ÷ PSV x 100

PRINCIPLES OF INTERPRETATION

B-mode Imaging
- Determine whether echogenic material such as plaque or thrombus results in a luminal reduction in the arteries and describe the location (proximal or distal).
- Observe the appearance of the renal parenchymal and the echogenicity of the kidney.
- Measure kidney size/diameter

Color Doppler
- Observe the renal arteries and veins for patency using color flow.

Spectral Doppler Waveforms
- Observe for changes in the Doppler waveform proximal and distal to any segment with increased velocity which can point to a hemodynamically significant obstruction.
- Observe the renal veins for spontaneity and phasicity.

Flow Velocities
- Measure peak systolic (PSV) and end diastolic velocity (EDV)
- V_2/V_1 peak systolic velocity ratio (Vr); where V_2 represents the maximum PSV of a stenosis and V_1 is the PSV of the proximal normal segment
- Renal-aortic ratio: Calculate the renal artery/aortic ratio (RAR) bilaterally and determine the classification of disease.

The highest renal artery PSV
highest PSV in the suprarenal abdominal aorta

- Kidney parenchyma: Calculate the resistive indices (RI) bilaterally using cortical and medullary flow to determine the presence of intrinsic disease.

Resistive index = 1 - (EDV ÷ PSV) x 100
or (PSV - EDV) ÷ PSV x 100

The RAR is only reliable when abdominal aortic velocities are normal. Base interpretation on absolute velocities instead of RAR when the aortic PSV is <45cm/s or >100cm/s.[12,13]

- Abdominal gas is similar to calcific shadowing in that gas/shadowing can prohibit Doppler and color flow analysis of a specific arterial segment. Use indirect signs to evaluate hemodynamically significant lesions:
  » If post-stenotic turbulence is present distal to the shadowing, there could be a stenosis through the area not visualized. Conversely, if there is no change in the waveform pattern, it is unlikely that a significant obstruction exists.
  » Comparing the Doppler waveform proximal and distal to the non-visualized segment can point to a hemodynamically significant obstruction under the shadowing.

Interpretation/Diagnostic Criteria

Normal

B-mode Imaging
- No echogenic material should be observed within the lumen of the native artery, vein, graft or stent by B-mode and color flow.
- Two separate areas of the kidney parenchyma around the renal sinus should be evident by B-mode image: the medulla and cortex. The echogenic characteristics of a normal cortex are similar to the liver or spleen at a similar depth. The cortex should have a "scalloped" or "notched" appearance.[14]
- **Kidney diameter**: A normal kidney length is 10-12cm with a 4.5-6cm width.[13,14] There should be <2cm difference in the diameter between both kidneys.

Color Doppler
- Color flow fills the lumen of the renal artery/vein completely from wall-to-wall.

Spectral Doppler Waveforms
- The normal low resistance waveform of the renal artery has a rapid upstroke in systole followed by a downstroke that decelerates into continuous forward flow throughout the cardiac cycle with no reversed flow phase or notch.[8,9]
- **Kidney parenchyma**: Normal parenchymal arterial flow will appear similar to the distal renal artery; a low resistance waveform (forward flow in diastole).[14]
- **Venous flow**: The renal veins are normally pulsatile near their origins by spectral Doppler. Venous signals recorded near the renal hilum will be more phasic with respiration.[14]

Flow Velocities
- Normal peak systolic arterial velocities are <180-200cm/s.[8,10]
- **Renal-aortic ratio**: A normal renal-aortic ratio (RAR) is <3.5.[10,11]
- **Kidney parenchyma**: The average peak systolic velocity should be between 20-30cm/s in the cortex and 30-40cm/s in the medullary region at a 0° angle.[14]
- Normal RI values are <0.70.[13]

Table 37-2: Normal Renal-Aortic PSV

Arterial Vessel	Peak Systolic Velocity
Aorta	80-100cm/s
Renal artery	<180cm/s
Medullary artery	30-40cm/s (at 0° angle)
Cortical artery	20-30cm/s (at 0° angle)

Source: Zierler RE, Olmstead KA. (2004). Renal Duplex Scanning: in Strandess's Duplex Scanning of Vascular Disorders, (283-310). Philadelphia: Lippincott Williams and Wilkins.

Abnormal

B-mode Imaging
- Echogenic material is observed within the lumen of the native artery, graft or stent by B-mode.
- Incidental findings on B-mode imaging include renal calculi (kidney stones), tumors, etc. Renal cysts are a common finding. Single or multiple cysts may be observed in any part of the kidney. These cysts are typically round or oval, anaechoic and smooth in appearance.[14]

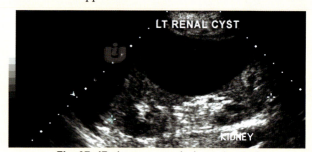

Fig. 37-17: *Large, anechoic cyst noted in the kidney on B-mode image*

- **Kidney diameter**: A kidney length under 9cm is highly suspicious for decreased blood flow.[9,15] Bilateral kidney diameters should be within 2cm of each other.[14]

Color Doppler
- Color flow does not fill the arterial lumen completely especially at the point of any intralumenal echoes, vessel diameter changes or other unusual pathology.

- A hemodynamically significant arterial stenosis is recognized by color aliasing, and confirmed by increased PSV. [8,10]
- The presence of post-stenotic turbulence and color bruit support the diagnosis of an arterial stenosis. [9,10]

Spectral Doppler Waveforms

- As the obstruction becomes more severe, changes in the spectral waveform are expected before a stenosis or occlusion, at the point of greatest stenosis and after a stenosis/occlusion as described in the *Arterial Physiology chapter*. These changes are important to note in the interpretation of the vascular exam.
- *Spectral broadening* represents the wide range of velocities usually present when there is disturbed, non-laminar flow. This waveform change occurs in the early stages of arterial disease. The normally clear window below the systolic peak begins to fill in.
- Abnormal renal arterial Doppler waveforms are characterized by a slow upstroke, low amplitude, and broad peak with no evidence of the reversed flow component in late systole. Diastolic flow may be absent if there is distal resistance from an additional high-grade distal obstruction, for example. [9,10,15]
  » The term "parvus tardus" meaning "low and slow" was previously used to describe the dampened waveform. Diameter reduction measurements should only be used in conjunction with peak systolic velocity measurements. [17]
- **Venous flow**: Pulsatile flow through the entire renal vein from the origin to the renal hilum suggests increased central venous pressure due to congestive heart failure, pulmonary edema, etc. [14]
  » Slow-moving venous flow in the renal vein suggests proximal obstruction in the absence of observed thrombus. [7]

Renal vein thrombosis may be secondary to a tumor or other source of extrinsic compression. [13]

Flow Velocities

- A hemodynamically significant arterial stenosis is recognized by color aliasing, and confirmed by increased PSV >180-200cm/s. [8,10]
- **Renal-aortic ratio**: An abnormal renal-aortic ratio (RAR) is >3.5. [8,10,11]
- **Kidney parenchyma**: Abnormal parenchymal arterial flow will exhibit increased pulsatility and decreased diastolic flow. [8,9]
  » An RI >0.80 is abnormal. [8-10,15]

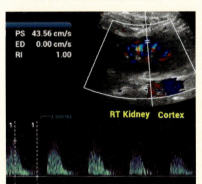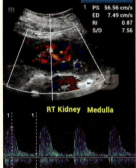

Fig. 37-18: *Abnormal resistive indices measured in the cortical (RI=1.0) and medullary (RI=0.87) regions of the kidney.*

Other Pathology

- **Renal vein thrombosis**:[13,14] Echogenic material may or may not be observed with the lumen of the RV by B-mode image depending on the age of the thrombus. Color flow will be observed flowing around echogenic material or may be absent, depending on whether the clot is partially or totally occlusive. Confirm any suspected thrombosis by spectral Doppler.
  » Dilatation of the vein proximal to the occlusion and an enlarged kidney may be observed in an acute event. The thrombus may be echolucent in acute cases.
  » Echogenic material within the lumen of the vein suggests a chronic event. Continuous venous flow signals may be observed if the vein has recanalized. [14]

Blood in the urine (hematuria) and abdominal pain are signs of acute renal vein thrombosis. In cases of acute renal vein occlusion, an enlarged kidney and atypical echogenicity of the renal parenchyma may be noted including: [7]

- Hypoechoic cortex, with or without usual separation of the cortical/medullary regions.
- Loss of typical intrarenal echogenicity and observation of linear "streaks" through the parenchyma.

- **Occlusion**: An arterial occlusion is present when no flow is detected by spectral Doppler and color. [9,10,13,15]

An occlusion should never be based on color alone. Always confirm flow by placing the Doppler sample volume in the vessel lumen.

- **Fibromuscular Dysplasia**: When a series of hemodynamically significant velocity increases are noted in the mid/distal segment of the renal artery along with significant turbulence, FMD is suspected. [9] A "string of beads" is the classic appearance on B-mode and color Doppler images (where segments of the artery can be seen narrowing and then widening in series). [6,16]

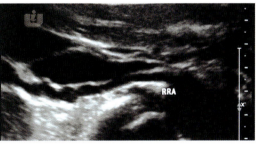

Fig. 37-19: *Fibromuscular dysplasia of the renal artery: "string of beads" appearance noted on B-mode image*

- **Renal vein compression syndrome (venous compression)**: Increased venous velocities (up to 5 times greater than the velocities at the hilum of the kidney) are observed at the point of entrapment. The renal vein is typically enlarged about five times the measured diameter at the point of entrapment. [5] Doppler waveforms will exhibit either decreased spontaneity, phasicity and continuous renal vein flow or an absent Doppler signal in renal vein compression syndrome. [5]

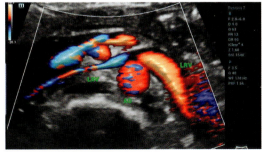

Fig. 37-20: *A venous compression syndrome ("nutcracker syndrome") is suggested by increased renal vein diameter distal to an area of compression on the vein.*

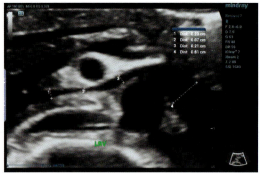

Fig. 37-21: *LRV diameters measured were 0.2cm (proximal), 0.07cm (at compression) and 0.8cm (distal); 11 x's larger past the point of entrapment*

- **Aneurysmal disease**: Renal artery aneurysms usually occur before the artery reaches the parenchyma and are often saccular. Aneurysm diameters between 5-9cm have been reported. [6] Fusiform aneurysms are less common with diameters <2cm. [6] PSV may decrease proximal to the dilatation and normalize distally. [9]
- **Arterial dissection**: A dissection of the arterial lumen is recognized by two distinct flow channels by B-mode and/or color Doppler separated by an intimal echo. One lumen is known as the "true lumen" while the other is referred to as the "false lumen." One of the lumens may demonstrate increased velocities and stenotic waveforms. [9]

Table 37-3: Diagnostic Criteria for Renal Artery Stenosis

Normal: no detectable renal artery stenosis
- Low resistance waveform
- No focal velocity increase
- RAR <3.5
- Peak systolic velocity <180-200cm/s

<60% diameter reduction: mild narrowing; no hemodynamic significance
- Low resistance waveform
- Focal velocity increase with possible post-stenotic turbulence
- RAR >2.0 but <3.5
- Peak systolic velocity <180-200cm/s

>60% diameter reduction: hemodynamically significant stenosis
- Post-stenotic turbulence (mosaic flow pattern by color flow Doppler) with focal velocity increases
- RAR >3.5
- Peak systolic velocity >180-200cm/s

Occlusion: complete obstruction of renal artery
- No detectable renal artery signal by color or spectral Doppler
- Kidney length <9cm (when occlusion is chronic)

The same diagnostic criteria used for native renal arteries has shown to be accurate in the diagnosis of post-intervention (e.g., renal bypass) duplex data. [8,10]

Table 37-4: Diagnostic Criteria for Significant Renovascular Resistance Within the Kidney

- Normal low renovascular resistance: RI <0.70
- Borderline increased renovascular resistance: RI between 0.70-0.80
- Increased renovascular resistance: RI >0.80

Source: Tublin, M. E., Bude, R. O., & Platt, J. F. (2003). Review. The resistive index in renal Doppler sonography: where do we stand? AJR. American journal of roentgenology, 180(4), 885–892.

Differential Diagnosis
- Hypotension, due to ACE inhibitors

Correlation
- Spiral CT scan
- MRA
- Renal arteriography

Medical Treatment
- Vasodilator therapy (e.g., ACE inhibitors)

Surgical Treatment
- Endarterectomy
- Bypass grafting (aorto-renal, splachno-renal)
- Renal artery reimplantation
- Ex-vivo reconstruction

Endovascular Treatment
- Balloon angioplasty, with or without stenting

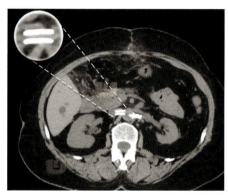

Fig. 37-22: *Bilateral renal artery stents by CT scan*

REFERENCES

1. Hansen KJ, Pearce JD. (2005). Renal complication. In *Rutherford Vascular Surgery 6th edition*. (863-874). Philadelphia. Elsevier Saunders.
2. Sumner DS, Zierler RE. (2005). Vascular physiology: essential hemodynamic principles. In *Rutherford Vascular Surgery 6th edition*. (75-123). Philadelphia. Elsevier Saunders.
3. Desai TR, Gupta N, Gewertz BL. (2005). Acute renovascular occlusive events. In *Rutherford Vascular Surgery 6th edition*. (1871-1877). Philadelphia. Elsevier Saunders.
4. Fecteau SR, Darling III RC, Roddy SP. (2005). Arterial thromboembolism. In *Rutherford Vascular Surgery 6th edition*. (971-986). Philadelphia. Elsevier Saunders.
5. Alimi YS, Hartung O. (2010). Iliocaval venous obstruction. In Cronenwett JL. Johnston KW (Eds.), *Rutherford Vascular Surgery 7th edition*. (Chapter 59) Philadelphia: Saunders Elsevier.
6. Calligaro KD, Dougherty MJ. (2005). Renal artery aneurysms and arteriovenous fistulae. In *Rutherford Vascular Surgery 6th edition*. (1861-1870). Philadelphia. Elsevier Saunders
7. Pellerito JS, Zwiebel, WJ (2005). Ultrasound assessment of native renal vessels and renal allografts. In Zwiebel WJ, Pellerito JS (Eds.), *Introduction to Vascular Ultrasonography 5th ed*. (611-636). Philadelphia: Elsevier Saunders.
8. Zierler RE. (2005). Vascular diagnosis of renovascular disease. In Mansour MA, Labropoulos N. (Eds.), *Vascular Diagnosis*, (333-340). Philadelphia: Elsevier Saunders.
9. Neumyer MM, Isaacson J. (1995). Direct and indirect renal arterial duplex and Doppler color flow evaluations. *J Vasc Technol*, 19(5-6):309-316.
10. Rzucidlo EM, Zwolak RM. (2005). Arterial duplex scanning. In *Rutherford Vascular Surgery 6th edition*. (233-253). Philadelphia. Elsevier Saunders.
11. Kohler TR, Zierler RE, Martin RL, et al. (1986). Non-invasive diagnosis of renal artery stenosis by ultrasonic duplex scanning. *J Vasc Surg* 4:450-456.
12. Armstrong PA, Bandyk DF. (2010). Arterial duplex scanning. In Cronenwett JL. Johnston KW (Eds.), *Rutherford Vascular Surgery 7th edition*. (Chapter 15). Philadelphia: Elsevier Saunders.
13. Myers K, Clogh A (2004). Renovascular diseases. In *Making Sense of Vascular Ultrasound*. (255-282). London: Hodder Arnold.
14. Zierler RE, Olmstead KA. (2004). Renal Duplex Scanning: in *Strandess's Duplex Scanning of Vascular Disorders*, (283-310). Philadelphia: Lippincott Williams and Wilkins.
15. Cairols M. (2005). Renal artery color-flow scanning: technique and applications. In Mansour MA, Labropoulos N. (Eds.), *Vascular Diagnosis*, (341-349). Philadelphia: Elsevier Saunders.
16. Stanley JC, Wakefield TW. (2005). Arterial fibrodysplasia. In *Rutherford Vascular Surgery 6th edition*. (431-452). Philadelphia. Elsevier Saunders.
17. DeLoach SS, Mohler III F. Atherosclerotic risk factors. In Cronenwett JL. Johnston KW (Eds.), *Rutherford Vascular Surgery 7th edition*. (Chapter 29). Philadelphia: Saunders Elsevier.
18. Kim, E. S., Sharma, A. M., Scissons, R., Dawson, D., Eberhardt, R. T., Gerhard-Herman, M., Hughes, J. P., Knight, S., Marie Kupinski, A., Mahe, G., Neumyer, M., Poe, P., Shugart, R., Wennberg, P., Williams, D. M., & Zierler, R. E. (2020). Interpretation of peripheral arterial and venous Doppler waveforms: A consensus statement from the Society for Vascular Medicine and Society for Vascular Ultrasound. Vascular medicine (London, England), 25(5), 484–506. https://doi.org/10.1177/1358863X20937665

Definition

Combination of real time B-mode imaging with spectral and color Doppler to provide monitoring for both early post-operative evaluation and long term follow up of renal transplants. The terms graft/allograft will be used in this chapter to refer to the transplant. An *allograft* is defined as a tissue graft from a donor of the same species as the recipient which may not always be genetically identical.[3]

Etiology *(of allograft complications)*

- Vascular complications
- Parenchymal complications
- Perinephric fluid collections
- Urological complications
- Post biopsy complications

Risk Factors

- Surgical trauma or incorrect surgical technique
- Donor hypotension and prolonged warm ischemic time (acute tubular necrosis (ATN))
- After an episode of acute transient rejection, patients have higher risk for chronic rejection.
- Renal vein thrombosis: hypercoagulable states, acute rejection, and venous compression by fluid collections
- Renal biopsy (increased risk of hemorrhage and arteriovenous fistula (AVF))
- Kinked or tortuous renal arteries
- Atherosclerosis in the donor or recipient's renal or iliac arteries

Indications for Exam

- Routine follow up of post-operative transplant kidney
- Investigation and follow-up of transplant dysfunction or complications
- Suspected renal artery stenosis
  » Hypertension: severe hypertension refractory (resistant) to medical therapy.
  » Renal artery graft bruit
  » Reduction in renal function following ACE inhibitor treatment.
- Guide for interventional procedures including biopsy, nephrostomy and drainages.

Contraindications/Limitations

- Exam can be time consuming and requires patience.
- Surgical dressings over the suture site immediately post-transplant
- Multiple renal arteries may increase the difficulty of the examination, and the examination time.
- Transplant renal artery may be difficult to assess completely because of its tortuosity.
- To minimize the risk of radiation exposure to the technologist, avoid examining the patient immediately post-nuclear medicine examination.

Technique of Renal Transplantation

Renal transplantation has become the treatment of choice for end-stage renal disease, offering significantly decreased mortality and increased quality of life. Grafts are obtained from cadavers or donated from living donors.

- The transplanted kidney is commonly placed in the extraperitoneal space, into the right or left iliac fossa, anterior to the psoas muscle.
- The donor renal artery and renal vein are anastomosed with an end-to-side configuration to the external iliac artery and vein respectively (less commonly to the internal iliac vessels).
- Renal transplants are typically harvested with an attached portion of the aorta (**Carrel patch**) which is anastomosed end-to-side to the recipient's external iliac artery. When there are multiple renal arteries of the donor kidney, either a long Carrel patch containing both renal artery origins or separate patches are obtained. In the living donor with multiple renal origins, the arteries may be reconstructed to have a common stem.

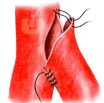

Fig. 38-1: *End-to-side anastomosis*

- The anastomosis is formed by attaching the donor ureter to the dome of the bladder. The ureter is tunneled through the bladder wall to create a pseudo sphincter, and as the bladder fills, the increasing pressure compresses the ureter preventing reflux.

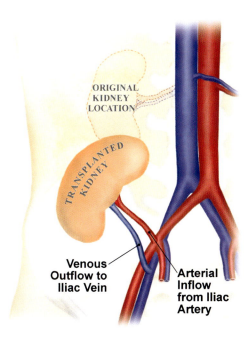

Fig. 38-2: *Renal transplant anatomy*

Mechanisms of Disease

Vascular Complications

- **Renal artery stenosis (RAS)** is the most common vascular complication of renal transplantation.
  - » Early presentation occurs within the first three months. Most stenoses occur at the anastomosis or proximal renal artery and are directly related to surgical technique or kinking of the vessel.
  - » Late presentation is generally due to intimal hyperplasia of the artery. Stenosis of the anastomotic site is more common, although mid/distal renal artery stenoses may be due to intimal hyperplasia in response to turbulent flow.
- **Renal artery thrombosis**: occurs within the first week of the post-operative period, and almost invariably leads to graft loss.
  - » **Complete occlusion**: usually results from errors in surgical technique, such as kinking or torsion of the artery, or dissection of the arterial wall. Other causes include acute rejection, ATN, and a hypercoagulable state.
  - » **Segmental infarction**: results from thrombosis of the intrarenal arterial branches or accessory arteries, or may occur as a result of rejection.
- **Renal vein thrombosis or stenosis** is a rare cause of transplant dysfunction, usually occurring within the first week post-transplant. Causes include surgical technique, renal vein compression by fluid collections, hypercoaguable states and acute rejection.
- **Arteriovenous fistula (AVF)** is usually secondary to vascular trauma during a percutaneous biopsy. AVF forms when a needle penetrates both the artery and vein, creating a communication between them.
  - » Small AVFs are usually asymptomatic and resolve spontaneously.
  - » Large AVFs may result in renal ischemia due to a "steal" phenomenon or a high cardiac output failure, and this may require urgent treatment.
- **Pseudoaneurysms** may also result from renal biopsy, although only the artery is injured. A communication via a neck is formed between the artery and the pseudoaneurysm. Most are asymptomatic and resolve spontaneously.
- **Extrarenal arteriovenous fistula and pseudoaneurysm** are extremely uncommon, and are usually a consequence of surgical technique rather than percutaneous biopsy. Extrarenal pseudoaneurysms have a high incidence of spontaneous rupture and are potentially catastrophic.

Parenchymal Complications

- **Acute rejection** occurs in the first few weeks post-transplant.
- **Chronic rejection** results in a gradual deterioration in graft function beginning at least three months after transplant.

Chronic rejection is irreversible and cannot be treated effectively

---

- **Drug nephrotoxicity:** Immunosuppressive agents that are required post-transplant have nephrotoxic potential, which may result in direct damage to the tubules.
- **Acute tubular necrosis (ATN)** is common in the early post-transplant period and usually resolves during the first two weeks. ATN is a result of ischemia of the donor kidney during the process of transplantation (greater risk with cadaveric donors).
- **Post-transplant neoplasm:** the prevalence of cancers is significantly higher in transplant recipients. Risk for primary renal carcinoma may be increased in transplant recipients, with approximately 90% occurring in the native kidneys and approximately 10% in the renal transplant.

Perinephric Fluid Collections

Peritransplant fluid collections are very common. Many are asymptomatic and are noted during routine sonographic evaluation of the kidney post-operatively.

- **Hematomas** are common immediately post-operative as the result of trauma or biopsy. They are usually small and resolve spontaneously. Large hematomas can displace the allograft and may produce a mass effect.
- **Lymphoceles** are very common. They are a result of intra-operative trauma to lymphatic vessels and they have the potential to produce a mass effect and obstruct the ureter.
- **Urinomas** are relatively rare, occurring within the first 2 months post-transplant. Urinomas are formed by urine leaks, which are secondary to ureteral necrosis from inadequate vascular supply of the distal ureter or from surgical technique.
- **Peritransplant abscesses** are an uncommon complication and may occur secondary to development of pyelonephritis or infection of a perinephric fluid collection.

Urological Complications

- **Obstructive hydronephrosis**: early obstruction may be attributable to a blood clot within the ureter or bladder or suboptimal surgical technique. Late obstruction can be due to ureteral stricture of the distal ureter occurring as a result of ischemia, compression by fluid collections, ureteral kinking or renal calculi.
- Transient dilatation of the collecting system as a result of ureteral anastomotic edema frequently occurs immediately after renal transplantation and usually resolves spontaneously.

Patient History

Patient symptoms are often non-specific and may not be helpful in identifying the cause of the dysfunction.

- Fever (may be masked by immunosuppressants)
- Pain over the graft site
- Impaired or delayed renal function
- Oliguria or anuria (decreased or absent urine output)
- Rising creatine levels
- Hematuria
- Proteinuria
- Hypertension: severe hypertension refractory to medical therapy

Physical Examination

- Swelling and tenderness over the graft
- Swelling or "puffiness;" a sign of fluid retention
- Bruit (abnormal sound heard through ausculation caused by turbulent flow)

Renal Transplant Duplex Protocol

- Obtain patient history to include symptoms and risk factors. Explain the procedure to the patient.
- Obtain past surgical reports/records including a general date of surgery.
- Some patients may require the use of a range of transducers depending on body habitus, for example a 5-7MHz may be used to image anatomical detail along with a 1.0-4.0MHz low frequency, curved linear array transducer.

Transplant Kidney Imaging

A post-operative ultrasound examination should be obtained within the first 24-48 hours to establish a baseline for further monitoring. Follow-up examinations are then performed as needed, based on the patient's clinical status.

B-mode Imaging

Renal transplant biopsy is generally accepted as the gold standard for clarifying the cause of renal dysfunction.

- B-mode imaging of the transplant, urinary bladder, and perinephric area should be performed first with the patient in a supine or oblique position, utilizing an anterolateral approach. In the case of immediate post-operative ultrasound, sterile gel should be used. Record B-mode images of the bladder in both longitudinal and transverse planes.
- In the longitudinal (sagittal) plane, B-mode images and measurements of the kidney length should be documented. Evaluation should also include:
  » Cortical thickness
  » Renal echogenicity
  » Calyceal dilatation
  » Measurement of any perinephric collections
- Any evidence of distension of the renal pelvis should be documented by measuring the pelvic diameter in the transverse (short axis) plane.
- If the collecting system is dilated, attempt to follow the ureter to the bladder.
- Transverse images of the transplant kidney are also recorded in the upper, mid and lower poles.
- If there is an indication of ureteric obstruction, color Doppler can be used to look for evidence of a ureteric jet at the transplant vesicoureteral junction.

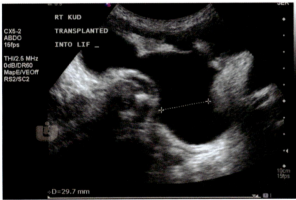

Fig. 38-3: *Transplant hydronephrosis. The diameter of the renal pelvis is measured in the longitudinal plane.*

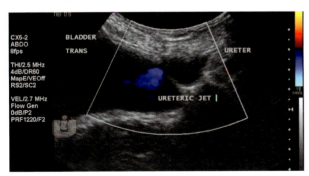

Fig. 38-4: *Ureteric jet: Using color Doppler, a ureteric jet is demonstrated at the vesicoureteral junction.*

Color and Spectral Doppler Waveforms

- A baseline Doppler examination is performed to evaluate transplant renal perfusion, as well as vascular flow in the renal and iliac vessels. This will identify any complications that need to be addressed.

Doppler of the transplant renal artery can be technically difficult. It may be difficult to obtain a Doppler angle ≤60° at the anastomosis site, or in a tortuous artery. Angles >60° may result in elevated velocities and turbulent flow and mimic a renal artery stenosis, which would be a false positive result.

- Color, power and spectral Doppler are applied observing for vessel patency, flow direction, waveform characteristics and velocity of blood flow. A Doppler angle of <60° is required for accurate velocity measurement sampled at the following locations:
  » Interlobar arterial branches: upper, mid and lower poles
  » Main renal artery (and accessory arteries): anastomosis, proximal, mid and distal renal arterial segments
  » Main renal vein
  » Ipsilateral external iliac artery: proximal, at, and distal to the anastomosis

Resistive Index (RI) measures the resistance to arterial flow within the renal vascular bed. This is a non-specific marker of renal transplant dysfunction.

- The spectral parameters most commonly assessed include:
  » Peak systolic velocity (PSV)
  » End-diastolic velocity (EDV)
  » Acceleration time (AT)
  » Acceleration index (AI)
  » Resistive index (RI)
  » Main transplant artery to iliac artery PSV ratio

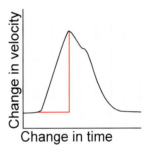

Fig. 38-5: *The formula for Acceleration Time (AT) is $a = \Delta v/\Delta t$. Most duplex machines will calculate the value from the spectral Doppler trace.*

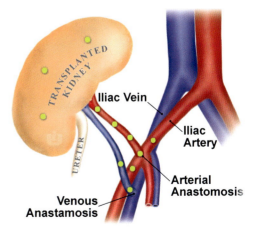

Fig. 38-6: *Renal transplant Doppler sample sites*

Intrarenal Transplant Vessels

- Using a longitudinal or transverse plane, interrogate and document the intrarenal vessels using color or power Doppler to assess renal transplant perfusion, in particular cortical perfusion. Using a high frequency linear transducer, a normal transplant should demonstrate flow extending all the way to the renal capsule.
- Use spectral Doppler to study the distal interlobar or arcuate arteries in the upper, mid and lower portions of the kidney. A resistive index of each of these sections is recorded.

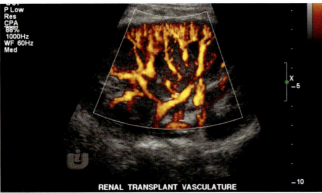

Fig. 38-7: Power Doppler demonstrates renal transplant perfusion, with flow extending to the renal capsule

Image courtesy of Philips Healthcare

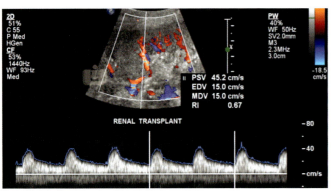

Fig. 38-8: PSV, EDV and resistive index measurements of an intrarenal artery

Extrarenal transplant vessels

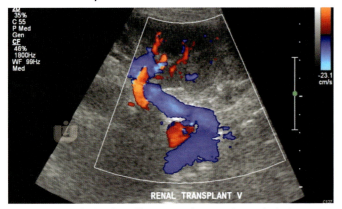

Fig. 38-9: Color flow illustrates the anastomosis between the transplant renal vein and external iliac vein

Table 38-1: Renal Transplant Duplex Protocol Summary

B-mode imaging
- Transplant kidney
    - » Sagittal plane: measurements of renal length
    - » Transverse planes: upper, mid & lower poles
- Bladder– sagittal and transverse planes
- Perinephric region
- Document calyceal or renal pelvis dilatation
- Measure and document evidence of perinephric collections

Color, power, and spectral Doppler
- Assess transplant renal perfusion
- Observe vessel patency, direction, velocity and characteristics of blood flow at the following locations:
    - » Interlobar arterial branches
    - » Upper, mid & lower poles
    - » Main renal artery (and accessory arteries)
    - » Anastomosis: proximal, mid & distal
    - » Main renal vein
    - » Ipsilateral external iliac artery: proximal to anastomosis, at the anastomosis, and distal to anastomosis
- Measure RI (resistive index) at each site

- In the longitudinal or transverse plane, record a spectral waveform in the main renal vein, assessing it along the entire length to the anastomotic site with the iliac vein. Note the direction of flow and any regions of high velocities.
- Assess the main renal artery along the entire length for any indication of stenosis with color Doppler. Measure the PSV and EDV in the distal, mid and proximal portions of the main renal artery, or at regions of high velocities. Careful attention should be given to the anastomosis with the iliac artery. In the presence of renal artery stenosis, document any post-stenotic turbulence.

It is often difficult to optimize the angle of insonation relative to the vessel at the arterial anastomosis. The patient may need to be rolled, or alternatively a "heel-toe" technique with the transducer may be necessary.

Iliac Vessels

- Orient the transducer in an oblique plane using the bladder as a window to locate the external and internal iliac vessels. Determine the anastomotic site of the main renal artery and vein.
- Measure the PSV and EDV of the iliac artery (external or internal) proximal to the anastomosis, at the anastomosis, and distal to the anastomosis. Assess the iliac arteries for evidence of stenosis.

PRINCIPLES OF INTERPRETATION

B-mode Imaging and Color Doppler

- Renal parenchymal appearance: Observe the appearance of the renal parenchymal and the echogenicity of the cortex and renal pyramids. Consider the spacing between the pyramids for irregularity.
- Determine whether echogenic material is observed within the lumen of the vein.
- Measure kidney size/diameter
- Assess patency and flow direction using color flow especially in areas of abnormality.

Spectral Doppler Waveforms and Flow Velocities
- Determine peak systolic velocity (PSV) and flow direction
- Calculate the velocity ratio:

$$V_r = V_2 \div V_1$$

V_2 = the maximum PSV of a stenosis

V_1 = PSV of the proximal normal segment.

- Resistive Index (RI): Calculate the resistive indices (RI) (bilaterally) using cortical and medullary flow to determine the presence of intrinsic disease.

$$\text{Resistive index} = 1 - [EDV \div PSV] \times 100$$

$$\text{or } (PSV - EDV) \div PSV \times 100$$

- Observe for phasicity of venous flow in the iliac veins.

Interpretation/Diagnostic Criteria

Normal

B-mode Imaging and Color Doppler
- **Kidney parenchyma:** The transplant kidney appears similar to a native kidney, although anatomical detail is better appreciated due to the superficial nature of the transplant, and the opportunity to use a higher frequency transducer.
  » The cortex should be homogeneous, with mid to low level echoes and a uniform cortical thickness. The central renal sinus is relatively hyperechoic.
  » The renal pyramids are mildly hypoechoic relative to the parenchyma and are regularly spaced with no communication between them (differentiating feature from dilated calyces).
  » The renal pelvis may be identified but should not be distended or dilated; typically, the calyces are collapsed. Over time a mild degree of distension is common presumably because the ureter is denervated (loses nerve function) and becomes "baggy."
  » Make sure image settings do not remove all echoes. Sometimes the echoes are "real" and indicate pus, blood or debris. Seeing some echoes is preferred to assure that real echoes have not been removed.
- **Kidney diameter:** The kidney size is usually enlarged, with the volume increasing by up to 30% within the first 3 weeks.

Mild hydronephrosis immediately following surgery may reflect ureteral anastomotic edema or denervation of the kidney. This hydronephrosis is transient, resolving over time, and can be reassessed by follow-up examinations.

- Color fills the vessel lumen wall-to-wall in transverse and longitudinal views with appropriate settings and flows in the appropriate direction. Intrarenal arteries demonstrate cortical perfusion that extends to the renal capsule.

Spectral Doppler Waveforms and Flow Velocities
- Normal transplants can display a wide variation of velocities, and it is important to compare the patient's previous results to identify a significant change in velocities.

Velocities immediately post-transplant are often elevated with turbulent flow (including at the anastomosis), and revert back to normal at 1 - 3 months post-transplant. This suggests a physiological adaptation rather than a true stenosis.

- **Resistive Index (RI):** Normal intra and extra renal arterial flow is represented by a low resistive waveform as these arteries feed a low resistance vascular bed. Normal RI is <0.7.
- Iliac arteries display lower resistance (bi or monophasic) flow proximal to the anastomosis, and triphasic flow distal to the anastomosis. Alternate terms may be used in some labs to describe biphasic and monophasic waveforms.
- **Venous flow:** The main renal vein is represented by continuous, low-velocity, phasic flow, typically between 40-60cm/s.
- Iliac veins display continuous phasic flow.

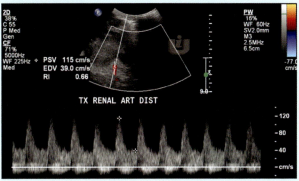

Fig. 38-10: *Normal transplant renal artery demonstrating a low resistance waveform pattern*

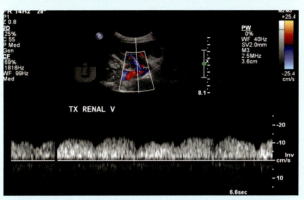

Fig. 38-11: *Normal transplant renal vein waveform*

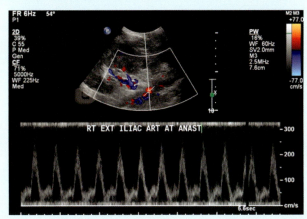

Fig. 38-12: *The external iliac artery displays biphasic/intermediate resistive flow proximal to the anastomosis*

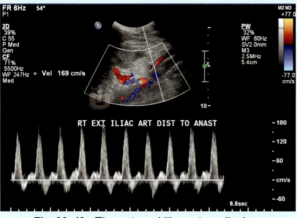

Fig. 38-13: *The external iliac artery displays triphasic flow distal to the anastomosis*

Table 38-2: Resistive Index (RI) Severity for Renal Transplant

RI	Severity
<0.70	Normal
0.70-0.80	Indeterminate
>0.80-0.90	Abnormal

Source: Langer JE, Jones LP. (2007). Sonographic evaluation of the renal transplant. Ultrasound Clinics; 2:73-88.

Abnormal

It is important to note that a wide range of parameters for stenosis criteria are used by different laboratories.

B-mode Imaging and Color Doppler

For abnormal B-mode and color Doppler findings relevant to renal transplants, see "Other Pathology" in this chapter.

Flow Velocities

Resistive Index (RI): An elevated RI may be seen in all forms of graft dysfunction and, although it cannot differentiate the causes, it is a good predictor of immediate graft function. The severity of an abnormal RI is:

- Indeterminate RI 0.7-0.8
- Abnormal RI >0.8-0.9
- Serial measurements may determine if there are changes from the patient's baseline values.

Vascular Complications

Renal artery stenosis (RAS) (≥50% diameter reduction)

- Elevated arterial and venous velocities may be seen immediately post-transplantation and return to normal at one to three months post-transplant. This finding suggests physiologic adaptation rather than true stenosis.
- Direct signs (most sensitive Doppler criteria)
  » Color aliasing at a focal velocity increase with appropriate Doppler settings.
  » Increased velocities: PSV >200cm/s with marked spectral broadening, and post-stenotic turbulence
  » Transplant renal artery to iliac artery systolic ratio >2, considering the velocities of stenotic regions compared with the pre-stenotic segments in the iliac artery (2cm upstream from the anastomosis in the iliac artery).

A velocity cutoff <250cm/s improves specificity, but may decrease sensitivity. Using this criterion reduces the number of patients referred for an unnecessary angiogram.

Transplant Renal Artery Stenosis

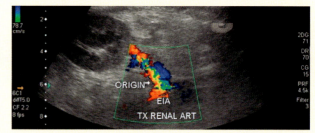

Fig. 38-14: *Color aliasing of the transplant renal artery at the anastomosis*

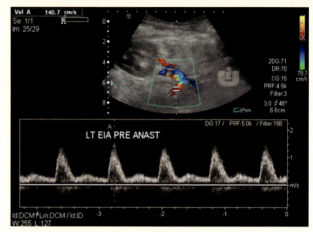

Fig. 38-15: *External iliac arterial velocities are 141 cm/s proximal to the stenosis.*

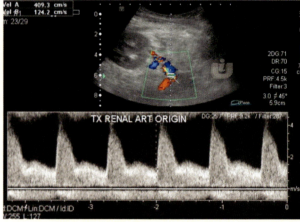

Fig. 38-16: *Renal transplant artery demonstrating elevated velocities at the anastomosis. The transplant renal artery to iliac artery systolic ratio would be abnormal at 2.9 (409cm/s divided by 141cm/s).*

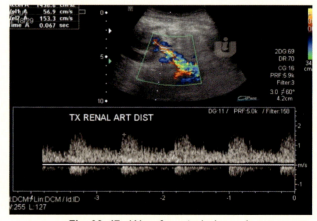

Fig. 38-17: *Waveform turbulence is noted distal to the stenosis*

- Indirect signs (should be used in conjunction with the direct criteria) include:
  » Dampened waveforms of the intrarenal arteries or distal to a stenosis will exhibit "low and slow" flow, with lower peak systole and delayed upstroke (previous terminology was "parvus tardus").
  » Acceleration Time (AT) >100msec in the renal or intrarenal arteries and decreased acceleration index <300cm/s².

Mimics of renal artery stenosis include tortuosity or transient kinking of the renal artery, which may cause increased velocities and spectral broadening in normal vessels.

Renal vein stenosis

- Visible as an area of narrowing and color aliasing with a three-four fold increase in velocity through the region of stenosis relative to the pre-stenotic region.

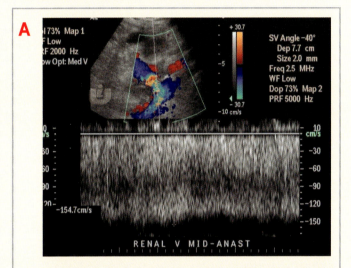
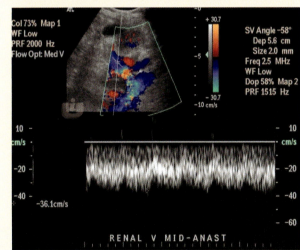

Fig. 38-18: *Renal Vein Stenosis: A) The renal vein proximal to the anastomosis demonstrates high velocities, which are >4 times higher in comparison to velocities proximal to the stenosis in B.*

Renal artery thrombosis

- **Complete occlusion:** Absence of arterial flow with appropriate settings is seen in the renal arteries and intrarenal vessels on color Doppler examination. Depending on the position of the thrombus, duplex sampling may demonstrate a highly resistive damped waveform, with absent diastolic flow at the proximal renal artery ("thump at the stump" pattern). B-mode imaging may demonstrate an enlarged and hypoechoic kidney.

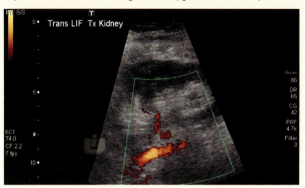

Fig. 38-19: *Power Doppler demonstrates occlusion of the intrarenal arteries*

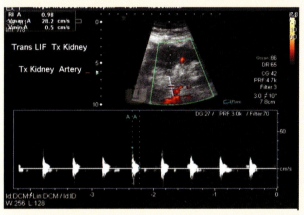

Fig. 38-20: *"Thump at the stump" type waveform is seen at the renal hilum, indicating intrarenal artery occlusion*

It is critical to adjust technical parameters appropriately to avoid a false-positive result. The use of power Doppler may help to demonstrate flow in a technically difficult patient.

- **Segmental occlusion/infarct:** This may appear as focal hypoechoic wedge-shaped regions in the cortex without any demonstrable flow. Eventually the infarcted segment reduces in volume and forms an echogenic wedge, and finally a linear echogenic focus with a cortical scar.

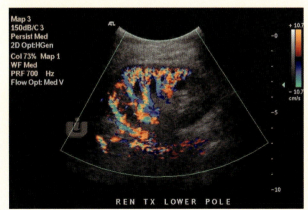

Fig. 38-21: *Segmental infarct demonstrated as a loss of flow on color Doppler in the lower pole of the transplant kidney*

Renal vein thrombosis

- The main renal vein can be dilated on B-mode image due to thrombus. Acute thrombus can appear hypoechoic and is difficult to demonstrate, although echogenicity may increase over time. Absent or diminished venous flow is demonstrated on color or spectral Doppler. Non-occlusive thrombus may be seen with partial flow around the thrombus.
- B-mode imaging may demonstrate an enlarged and hypoechoic kidney with increased cortical thickness.
- Elevated resistive index: flow in the renal artery is reduced, with absent or reversed diastolic flow, depending on the extent of the thrombus.

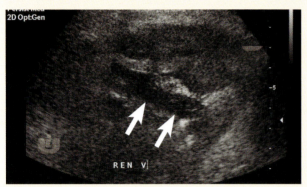

Fig. 38-22: *Transplant renal vein thrombosis seen with hypoechoic thrombus distending the main renal vein*

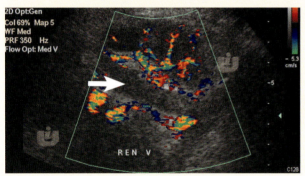

Fig. 38-23: *Color Doppler confirming renal vein thrombosis*

Other Pathology

Arteriovenous Fistula (AVF)
- Color Doppler shows aliasing (mosaic appearance) at focal areas of turbulent flow.
- Spectral Doppler demonstrates turbulent flow with high velocities and a low resistance waveform at the AVF and in the inflow artery.
- The draining vein demonstrates pulsatile flow due to arterialization.

Pseudoaneurysm
- Pseudoaneurysms resemble simple or complex cystic masses on B-mode image.
- Color Doppler will demonstrate a turbulent, swirling flow pattern.
- Spectral Doppler reveals a waveform with forward and reverse flow pattern (referred to as the "yin-yang" sign).

Arteriovenous Fistula

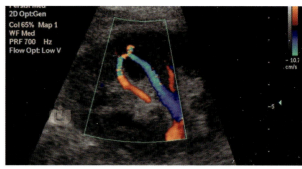

Fig. 38-24: *Color Doppler reveals an AVF between a feeding artery and draining vein*

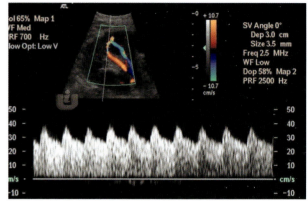

Fig. 38-25: *Spectral Doppler demonstrates a low resistive feeding artery*

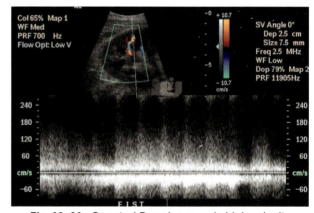

Fig. 38-26: *Spectral Doppler reveals high velocity and turbulent flow within the AVF*

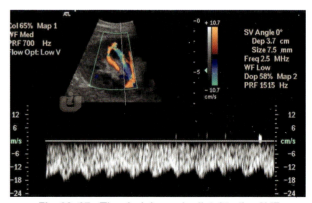

Fig. 38-27: *The draining vein distal to the AVF appears pulsatile due to arterialization*

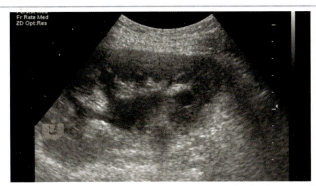

Fig. 38-28: *B-mode imaging shows an area in the lower pole that has the appearances of a simple cyst*

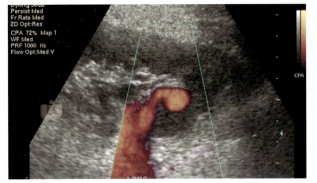

Fig. 38-29: *Power Doppler indicates how this region actually contains flow and is suggestive of a pseudoaneurysm.*

Parenchymal complications

ATN, rejection and drug nephrotoxicity are difficult to differentiate on imaging and a renal biopsy is required to establish the diagnosis. Several non-specific sonographic findings are demonstrated in patients who have graft dysfunction due to these complications, although these findings may only be apparent in the late stages. Sonographic findings may include:

- Renal enlargement
- Decreased cortical and renal medullary echogenicity (loss of corticomedullary differentiation)
- Effacement of the renal sinus
- Thickening of uroepithelium
- Absence of diastolic flow or flow reversal (acute rejection)
- Elevated intrarenal RI (ATN, acute rejection)
- Decreased venous flow with severe acute rejection
- Chronic rejection displays decreased renal size, with a thinned echogenic cortex.

Ultrasound appearances of ATN, rejection and drug nephrotoxicity are non-specific as they often have similar sonographic and Doppler features. This can cause a diagnostic dilemma for the interpreting physician. Interpretation of dysfunction should be made based on the time of onset, the patient's clinical status, as well as results of biochemical testing.

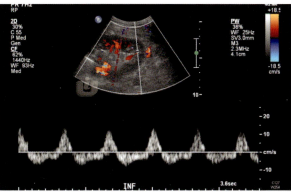

Fig. 38-30: *Reverse end-diastolic flow seen in the intrarenal artery of a patient with graft dysfunction*

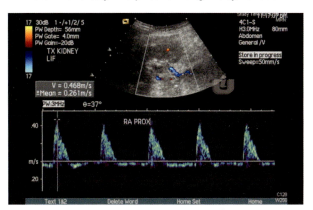

Fig. 38-31: *Reverse end-diastolic flow seen in the main renal transplant artery.*

Perinephric fluid collections

- Hematomas are usually hyperechoic and complex in the acute phase, and resolving hematomas are typically hypoechoic.
- Lymphoceles are seen as loculated anechoic collections that may have thin septations and internal echoes.
- Urinomas are observed as well-defined anechoic fluid collections with occasional septations, usually visualized between the kidney and the bladder. These may rapidly increase in size.
- Abscesses are demonstrated as a complex perirenal cystic mass, which may contain air or fluid.

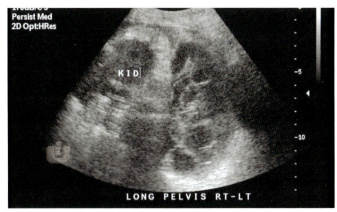

Fig. 38-32: *B-mode imaging shows a complicated cystic mass adjacent to the transplant kidney representative of an urinoma*

Urological complications

- **Obstructive hydronephrosis** is demonstrated by dilated renal pelvis and calyces. The graft can become distended and edematous, and an increased RI may be apparent.
- **Pyelonephritis**: the kidney may be enlarged with regions of increased or decreased echogenicity and areas of altered parenchymal flow. Internal echoes within the collecting system may be noted.

Peritransplant Collections

- **Lymphoceles**: most are small and asymptomatic, and intervention is not necessary. Lymphoceles that cause compression of the ureter or vascular pedicle require percutaneous drainage.

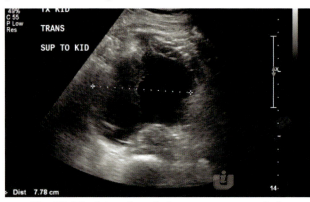

Fig. 38-33: *A lymphocele is seen as an anechoic collection with internal septations*

- **Urinoma**: large urinomas may rupture, producing urinary ascites, or compress vascular or ureteral structures. These urinomas should be drained percutaneously to relieve extrinsic compression and reduce the risk of infection.
- **Abscess**: prompt surgical or percutaneous drainage, combined with antibiotics is mandatory due to the immunosuppressed state of transplant patients.

Urological Complications

- **Urinary leaks**: percutaneous nephrostomy and stent placement can divert urinary flow to allow ureteral healing. Surgical revision is required in some cases.
- **Hydronephrosis** is often managed by percutaneous nephrostomy. Ureteral stenting or balloon dilatation can be utilized if obstruction persists.

Differential Diagnosis
None

Correlation
- Renal transplant biopsy
- Laboratory studies
- Radionuclide imaging (Tc-99 MAG3)
- CTA (iodinated contrast avoided due to nephrotoxic effects)
- MRA
- Angiography for vascular intervention

Medical Treatment

Acute rejection
- High-dose steroids or antibody therapy
- Plasma exchange (plasmapheresis) is used to treat steroid resistant transplant rejection

Chronic rejection (irreversible with no effective treatment)
- Temporary measures include controlling blood pressure and avoiding nephrotoxins.
- Reduce episodes of acute rejection to decrease the risk of chronic rejection.

Surgical Treatment

The decision to intervene on a renal artery stenosis diagnosed by Doppler is often based on the combination of a high clinical suspicion, the patient's clinical status and biochemical testing.

- Surgical resection and revision of the anastomosis is indicated for recurrent stenoses and lesions that cannot be treated by or recur after PTA.
- Surgical thrombectomy with arterial/venous repair (for cases of early graft thrombosis)
- Nephrectomy (for graft thrombosis that cannot be salvaged)

Endovascular Treatment
- Angioplasty, with or without stenting (for renal artery and venous stenosis)
- Intra-arterial directed thrombolysis (early graft thrombosis)
- Coil embolization (post-biopsy bleeds, arteriovenous fistulas, and pseudoaneurysm)

REFERENCES
1. Baxter, GM, Imaging in Renal Transplantation, (September 2003). US Quarterly, 19 (3), 123-127.
2. Irshad, A, Ackerman SJ, Campbell AS, & Anis, M (August 2009). An Overview of Renal Transplantation: Current Practice and Use of Ultrasound. US CT and MRI, 30 (4), 298-314.
3. Oxford Languages. Google. (2023).

ABDOMINAL ARTERIAL TESTING
39. Celiac and Mesenteric Artery Duplex Ultrasound

Definition
The combination of real time B-mode ultrasonography with spectral and color flow Doppler to evaluate the celiac and mesenteric arteries for the presence and severity of stenosis or occlusion, as well as other disease states and to assess hemodynamics after vascular reconstruction.

Etiology
- Atherosclerosis
- Median arcuate ligament syndrome
- Fibromuscular dysplagia
- Embolus (acute ischemia)
- Thrombosis (acute ischemia)
- Occlusion
- Aneurysm
- Arteriovenous fistula
- Trauma
- Status post-angioplasty/stent
- Aortic dissections (male>female)
- Neurofibromatosis
- Takayasu's arteritis
- Radiation injury
- Systemic lupus
- Drug use

Risk Factors
- Hypertension
- Diabetes
- Obesity
- Hypercholesterolemia
- Smoking
- Female
- Age
  » Patients with median arcuate ligament syndrome are typically young.
  » Patients with chronic mesenteric ischemia are typically elderly.

Indications for Exam
- Abdominal pain and cramping, associated with eating
- Significant unexplained weight loss
- Abdominal bruit
- Suspected visceral artery aneurysm
- Unexplained gastrointestinal symptoms
- Post-operative evaluation of a mesenteric vascular reconstruction

Contraindications/Limitations
- Obesity may cause poor visualization due to vessel depth.
- Abdominal gas may prohibit visualization of any or all vessels.
- Recent abdominal surgery (tenderness and staples may limit visualization).
- Breathing difficulties may limit evaluation (e.g., shortness of breath, rapid breathing, etc.).

Mechanism of Disease
- Mesenteric blood flow is regulated by several mechanisms: intrinsic (metabolic) and extrinsic (neural and hormonal).[1]

  » A lack of oxygen to the mesenteric organs causes cellular injury and mucosal ischemia within the intestines. Tissue necrosis and metabolic acidosis are significant consequences.[1,2]

  » The renin-angiotensin system regulates blood volume, pressure and vascular resistance. When extracellular volume decreases the renin-angiotensin system is activated, releasing renin which will increase angiotensin II levels, causing vasoconstriction.[1]

  » Blood volume is lost and an abnormal increase in the concentration of fluids results in the release of vasopressin (antidiuretic hormone) from the pituitary gland, causing mesenteric vasoconstriction and venorelaxation.[1]

- **Atherosclerosis** can significantly narrow the arterial supply to the intestinal organs. Atherosclerotic plaque forms in the artery which blocks flow by either narrowing the arterial lumen (arterial stenosis) or totally blocking the artery (arterial occlusion). The term "hemodynamically significant obstruction" refers to either a stenosis or an occlusion that results in a decrease in blood pressure or flow distal to the obstruction. Typically, a stenosis must narrow the diameter of the artery by at least 50% to decrease pressure and flow distally.[3]

- **Vasospasm**, usually affecting the SMA, occurs as a result of neurohormonal triggers. Mesenteric vasospasms occur while the body releases vasopressin and angiotensin to help correct hypervolemic states or cardiogenic shock.[2]

- **Compression syndromes** occur when there is enough abnormal pressure on a blood vessel to limit the amount of blood that can flow through the artery causing mesenteric ischemia.[1] Arteries can either cause compression of other structures or can be compressed themselves. There are numerous compression syndromes that can occur in the body. The most common abdominal compression syndromes include:

  » Compression of the celiac trunk by the median arcuate ligament of the diaphragm. Lumenal stenosis is thought to be caused by intimal fibrosis from the compression. Compression increases during expiration.[4]

  » Superior Mesenteric Artery Syndrome: A section of the duodenum (small intestines) can be compressed between the abdominal aorta and the SMA.

- **Thrombosis** may result from low-flow states.[5]

- **Mesenteric ischemia** is categorized as acute or chronic:

  » Chronic Mesenteric Ischemia[6]
    - Most commonly caused by progression of atherosclerotic disease (stenosis or occlusion) in the aorta, celiac or proximal mesenteric arteries.
    - Less common causes include arteritis, aneurysm, mesenteric artery dissection or hypercoaguable conditions.

  » Acute Mesenteric Ischemia[5]
    - Caused by arterial occlusion due to thrombosis of the SMA.
    - The condition of acute mesenteric ischemia has a high mortality rate, (70%).
    - Caused by arterial occlusion usually due to a cardiac embolism, occurring most frequently in the SMA due to its smaller size.
    - Caused by small vessel insufficiency (e.g., poor collateral circulation).

- **Aneurysm:** Aneurysmal disease results from atherosclerosis, infectious disease, trauma or congenital defect. Arterial dissection of the *splanchnic arteries* (visceral or gut) can occur spontaneously with hypertension, atherosclerosis, and weakening of the arterial walls during pregnancy as the underlying causes.[14]

Location of Disease
- Typical at the ostia (opening) of proximal celiac or mesenteric arterial segments.

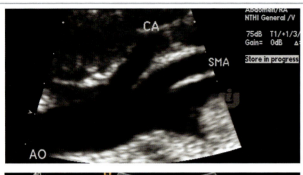

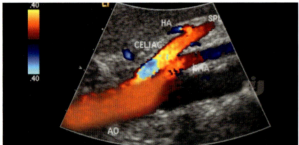

Fig. 39-1: *Celiac and superior mesenteric arteries-origin off the proximal aorta with B-mode and color*

See the Abdominal Arterial Vasculature chapter for more anatomy.

Graft Location
Typical arterial grafts encountered for surveillance include:
- Abdominal aorta-Celiac artery
- Abdominal aorta-Superior mesenteric artery (SMA)
- Abdominal aorta-Celiac and SMA

Graft Type
- PTFE (Polytetrafluoroethylene)

Patient History
- Significant weight loss
- Abdominal pain 30-60 minutes after eating
- Complaints of bloating, nausea, vomiting, or diarrhea

Patients usually describe pain about 30 minutes after eating that can last for several hours. This experience can result in a patient's "fear of food" and they may skip meals to avoid the pain, resulting in weight loss.

Physical Examination
- Abdominal bruit (abnormal sound heard through auscultation caused by turbulent flow)
- Abdominal tenderness
- Ischemic symptoms include: fever, abdominal distention, dehydration, shock, gastrointestinal bleeding and peritoneal signs (rebound tenderness, guarding).

Celiac/mesenteric artery scanning is a difficult exam which requires time, patience and a long learning curve. Patients may be given Simethicone (Gas-X, Mylanta, etc.) before the exam to reduce abdominal gas.

Celiac and Mesenteric Artery Duplex Protocol
- Fasting 6-12 hours before examination minimizes air in the abdomen. A limited volume of clear liquids may be ingested prior to the examination (e.g., to swallow medications). Studies are usually performed in the morning.
- Patient is studied while supine with the head slightly elevated and the arms and legs adequately supported. The patient may bend their knees up to aid in relaxation of the abdominal wall and decrease lumbar pain.
- Obtain a patient history, including symptoms and risk factors and explain the procedure to the patient.
- The celiac and superior mesenteric arteries may be stented.
- Some patients may require the use of a range of transducers; including high-frequency (5-7 MHz) and low frequency transducers (2.0-4.0 MHz for imaging deeper structures).
- Spectral Doppler angle should be ≤60° with the angle cursor parallel to the vessel walls and the sample volume within the center of the flow stream.

Doppler angles >60° result in falsely elevated velocities.

Evaluation of Abdominal Aorta
- Place the transducer just beneath the xyphoid process. Orient the transducer to obtain a transverse view of the abdominal aorta. Examine the abdominal aorta for aneurysm, plaque, thrombus, dissection, tortuosity and other abnormalities.
- Record B-mode images in longitudinal (sagittal) view of the supraceliac abdominal aorta. Document additional images using color flow as needed.
- Record a spectral Doppler peak systolic velocity (PSV) and end diastolic velocity (EDV) of the supraceliac aorta in the longitudinal plane.
- Document B-mode and color images in areas of suspected stenosis. Measure diameter reduction, especially in hemodynamically significant lesions. Document any post stenotic turbulence or color bruit.

Patient's inability to hold his/her breath for short periods of time, shortness of breath or rapid breathing may make it difficult to obtain accurate Doppler recordings.

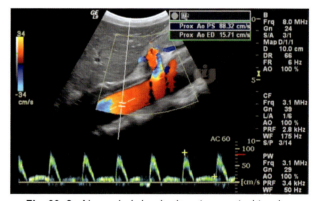

Fig. 39-2: *Normal abdominal aorta spectral tracing*

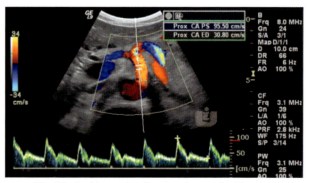

Fig. 39-3: *Normal celiac trunk spectral tracing*

Images courtesy of GE Healthcare Ultrasound Division

Evaluation of Celiac Artery

- Orient the transducer to obtain a longitudinal view of the celiac trunk and its ostia. Record B-mode images in a longitudinal view. Document additional images using color flow as needed. Examine for tortuosity or abnormalities such as plaque, aneurysm or thrombus. In some cases, a transverse orientation will provide a better axis for evaluation.

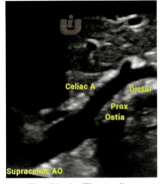

Fig. 39-4: The celiac artery is a branch off the proximal aorta.

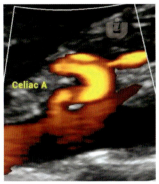

Fig. 39-5: Tortuosity of the CA noted by power Doppler

- Measure the PSV and EDV from the origin, proximal, and distal portions of the celiac trunk/artery. Note direction of flow.
- Measure PSV and EDV in the branches of the celiac trunk: the common hepatic (HA) and the splenic (SA) arteries. Note direction of flow.

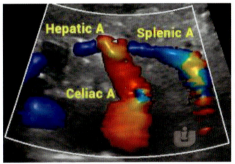

Fig. 39-6: The hepatic and splenic artery branches off the celiac trunk

Typically, at least two of the three mesenteric arteries (CA, SMA, IMA) have significant disease before symptoms of severe or chronic mesenteric ischemia are noted. The SMA is almost always one of the arteries involved.[1,6,12]

- Document PSV and EDV with spectral Doppler through any area(s) of stenoses. Document post stenotic turbulence.
- Determine the classification of disease according to laboratory diagnostic criteria.

Color flow Doppler and power Doppler may aid in locating arteries.

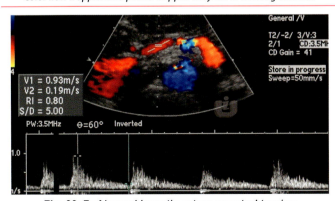

Fig. 39-7: Normal hepatic artery spectral tracing

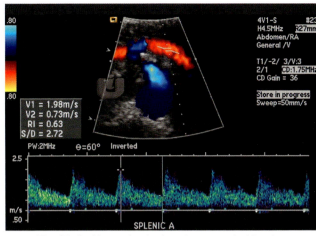

Fig. 39-8: Normal splenic artery spectral tracing

When instructed to "image arteries in transverse," because of the angulation of visceral arteries it may look like you are holding the transducer longitudinally while the arteries appear transverse on the monitor. Image abdominal arteries transverse to the axis of the vessel and not transverse to the body.

Evaluation for Median Arcuate Ligament Syndrome (MALS)

- In each and every patient that has an increased PSV in the celiac artery, ask the patient to take a deep breath in and hold while recording the PSV again. If the celiac artery PSV normalizes, there is evidence of the CA being compressed by the median arcuate ligament.

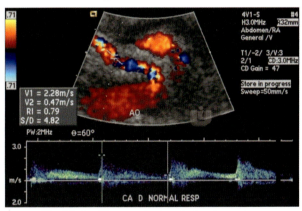

Fig. 39-9: Abnormal, elevated celiac artery PSV during quiet respiration

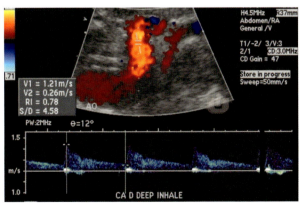

Fig. 39-10: Normal celiac artery PSV while patient takes a deep breath

Evaluation of Superior Mesenteric Artery
- Slide the transducer distally 1-2cm down the aorta from the celiac origin. Orient the transducer to obtain a longitudinal view of the superior mesenteric artery at its ostia. Examine for tortuosity or abnormalities such as plaque, aneurysm or thrombus.
- Record PSV and EDV with spectral Doppler from the origin, proximal, mid and distal portions of the SMA. Note direction of flow.
- Record B-mode images in a longitudinal view of the SMA, especially near its origin. Document additional images using color flow as needed.
- Document the highest PSV and EDV through any area(s) of stenoses. Document post-stenotic turbulence.
- Document B-mode and color images in areas of suspected stenosis. Measure diameter reduction, especially in hemodynamically significant lesions.
- Determine the classification of disease according to laboratory diagnostic criteria.
- Research suggests that there is no significant benefit from post-prandial evaluation (rescanning after ingestion of a meal) for the diagnosis of ≥70% stenosis. PSV will be significantly elevated either fasting or nonfasting.[9]

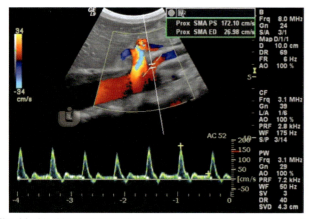

Fig. 39-11: *Normal superior mesenteric artery spectral tracing*
Image courtesy of GE Healthcare-Ultrasound Division

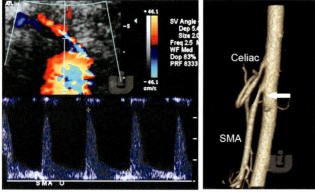

Fig. 39-12: *Abnormal (stenotic) SMA spectral tracing correlates to the abnormal CT image shown.*

Evaluation of Inferior Mesenteric Artery
- The inferior mesenteric artery originates off the aorta and lies superior to the common iliac arteries, 3-5cm above the iliac bifurcation. In transverse, the artery comes off at approximately the 1–2 o'clock position. This artery is sometimes difficult to visualize due to abdominal gas at this level.

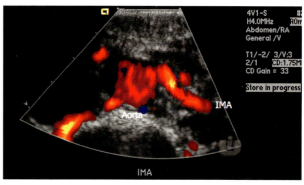

Fig. 39-13: *Transverse inferior mesenteric artery*

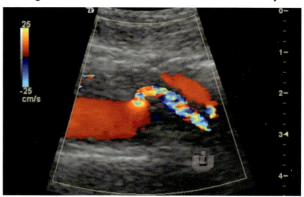

Fig. 39-14: *Inferior mesenteric artery (longitudinal)*
Image courtesy of GE Healthcare-Ultrasound Division

- Orient the transducer to obtain a longitudinal view of the inferior mesenteric artery at its ostia. Examine for tortuosity or abnormalities such as plaque, aneurysm or thrombus.
- Record B-mode images of the IMA in longitudinal view. Document additional images using color flow as needed. In some cases, a transverse orientation will provide a better axis for documentation.
- Record PSV and EDV from the origin and proximal segment of the IMA. Note direction of flow. Record additional velocities from the mid/distal artery as necessary.

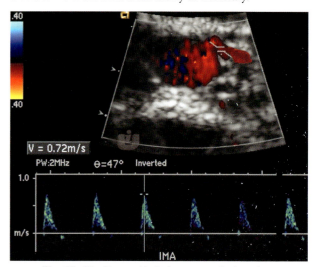

Fig. 39-15: *Normal inferior mesenteric artery*

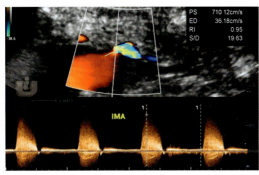

Fig. 39-16: *Abnormal (stenotic) inferior mesenteric artery*

- Document the highest PSV and EDV through any area(s) of stenoses. Document post-stenotic turbulence.
- Document B-mode and color images in areas of suspected stenosis. Measure diameter reduction, especially in hemodynamically significant lesions.
- Determine the classification of disease according to laboratory diagnostic criteria.

Table 39-1: Celiac and Mesenteric Artery Duplex Protocol Summary

Abdominal Aorta
- Evaluate the abdominal aorta for aneurysm, plaque, thrombus, dissection and/or tortuosity. Document a longitudinal (sagittal) B-mode image of the artery.
- Obtain a spectral Doppler peak systolic velocity (PSV) and end diastolic velocity (EDV) of the abdominal aorta, superior to the celiac (CA) and superior mesenteric (SMA) arteries.

Celiac Trunk
- Document a B-mode image of the proximal CA, either in longitudinal (sagittal) or transverse view, depending on the course of the vessel.
- Record the highest PSV and EDV of the celiac trunk at the following levels:
  » Celiac trunk ostia
  » Proximal celiac artery
  » Distal celiac artery

Hepatic and Splenic Arteries
- Document a transverse image of the proximal hepatic and splenic arteries.
- Record the highest PSV and EDV in each artery.

Superior Mesenteric Artery
- Document a longitudinal (sagittal) B-mode image of the superior mesenteric artery.
- Record the highest PSV and EDV of the SMA at the following levels:
  » SMA ostia   » Mid SMA
  » Proximal SMA   » Distal SMA

Inferior Mesenteric Artery
- Document a longitudinal (sagittal) or transverse B-mode image of the inferior mesenteric artery, depending on the course of the vessel.
- Record PSV and EDV of the ostial and proximal portion of the IMA.

- Document B-mode and color images in areas of suspected stenosis. Measure diameter reduction, especially in hemodynamically significant lesions.
- Determine the classification of disease according to laboratory diagnostic criteria.

Post-operative Duplex Evaluation of Splanchnic Bypass or Stent

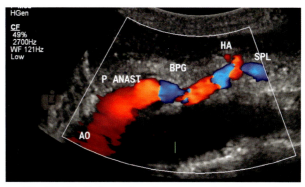

Fig. 39-17: *Celiac artery bypass graft off the aorta*

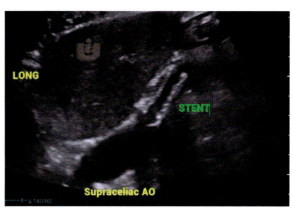

Fig. 39-18: *Stented celiac artery*

- Record images in a longitudinal view with and without color flow Doppler of the:
  » Inflow/proximal native artery
  » Proximal anastomosis
  » Proximal graft or stent
  » Mid graft or stent
  » Distal graft or stent
  » Distal anastomosis
  » Outflow/distal native artery.

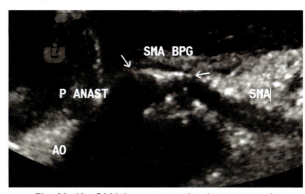

Fig. 39-19: *SMA bypass-proximal anastomosis*

- Record the PSV in longitudinal using spectral Doppler (≤60° Doppler angle with the angle cursor parallel to the vessel walls and sample volume within the center of the flow stream) at the following levels:
  » Inflow/proximal native artery
  » Proximal anastomosis
  » Proximal graft or stent
  » Mid graft or stent
  » Distal graft or stent
  » Distal anastomosis
  » Outflow/distal native artery

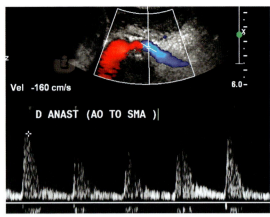

Fig. 39-20: *SMA bypass: distal anastomosis spectral waveforms*

PRINCIPLES OF INTERPRETATION

B-mode Imaging
- Determine whether echogenic material such as plaque or luminal reduction is observed within the lumen of the arteries and describe the location.
- Measure arterial diameters (when indicated)

Color Doppler
- Observe the with color flow for patency and appropriate flow direction.

Spectral Doppler Waveforms
- Observe for changes in the Doppler waveform proximal and distal to any segment with increased velocity which can point to a hemodynamically significant obstruction.
- Observe waveform patterns at rest and with any provocative maneuvers and report changes in the Doppler waveform (high to low resistive, for example) proximal and distal to any segment with increased velocity which can point to a hemodynamically significant obstruction.

Flow Velocities
- Determine peak systolic velocity (PSV) and flow direction
- Calculate the velocity ratio:

$$V_r = V_2 \div V_1$$

V_2 = the maximum PSV of a stenosis
V_1 = PSV of the proximal normal segment.

- Abdominal gas is similar to calcific shadowing in that gas/shadowing can prohibit Doppler and color flow analysis of a specific arterial segment. Use indirect signs to evaluate hemodynamically significant lesions:
  » If post-stenotic turbulence is present distal to the shadowing, there could be a stenosis through the area not visualized. Conversely, if there is no change in the waveform pattern, it is unlikely that a significant obstruction exists.
  » Comparing the Doppler waveform proximal and distal to the non-visualized segment can point to a hemodynamically significant obstruction under the shadowing.

Interpretation/Diagnostic Criteria

Normal

Duplex may not demonstrate elevated flow velocities in elderly patients or those with low cardiac output even when hemodynamically significant disease is present.[8]

B-mode Imaging
- The artery is free of intralumenal echoes.

Color Doppler
- When utilized, color Doppler fills the entire arterial lumen.

Spectral Doppler Waveforms

Supraceliac aorta
- A *high resistance waveform* pattern is normal in the aortoiliac arteries with a quick downstroke that ends with a short period of reversed flow direction (below the baseline) at end systole/early diastole. This reversed flow segment in the waveform may or may not be followed by a third segment with a low, short segment of forward flow This waveform can also be referred to as *triphasic*.

The third phase of the triphasic waveform may be missing in the suprarenal aortic segment, especially in patients with less vessel compliance.

Celiac, hepatic and splenic arteries
- The normal *low resistance waveform* of the CA, HA and SA arteries has a rapid upstroke in systole followed by a downstroke that decelerates into continuous forward flow throughout the cardiac cycle with no reversed flow phase or notch in the downslope or reversed flow phase that crosses the zero baseline.[17]

SMA/IMA
- Normal fasting superior and inferior mesenteric arterial flow is represented by a *high resistance waveform*. There is a quick downstroke that ends with a short period of reversed flow direction (below the baseline) at end systole/early diastole. This reversed flow segment in the waveform may or may not be followed by a third segment with a low, short segment of forward flow.
- Consider whether the patient fasted before the exam. SMA/IMA waveforms normally change post-prandially (after eating) because the intestines require more blood flow during digestion. In order to meet the extra demand for blood flow, post-prandial SMA and IMA waveforms will be low resistant, similar to the celiac arteries.[16]

Flow Velocities
- The normal peak systolic velocity for the CA, HA and SA should be <200cm/s.[7]

SMA/IMA fasting
- The peak systolic velocity will be <275cm/s.[7]
- Normal IMA PSV range from 93-189cm/s.[8] When aortic or mesenteric disease is present, the PSV is thought to be closer to the higher end of this range depending on how much collateral flow is present through the IMA.[13]

Table 39-2: **Normal Celiac and Mesenteric Waveforms**

- Normal celiac (CA), Hepatic (HA) and splenic (SA) artery waveforms are typically low-resistant in nature as they feed low resistance outflow beds.
- Normal SMA waveforms are high-resistant in the fasting state. This high resistance waveform will change to a low resistance waveform after ingestion of a meal.

Table 39-3: **Normal Celiac and Mesenteric Peak Systolic Velocities (PSV)**

Artery	PSV
Celiac artery	98-105cm/s
Superior mesenteric artery	97-142cm/s
Inferior mesenteric artery	93-189cm/s

Source: Pellerito JS. (2005). Ultrasound assessment of the splachnic (mesenteric) arteries. In Zwiebel WJ, Pellerito JS (Eds.), In *Introduction to Vascular Ultrasonography* 5th ed, (571-583). Philadelphia: Elsevier Saunders.

Abnormal

B-mode Imaging
- Lumenal reduction or wall irregularities may be observed by B-mode image.[8] Diameter reduction measurements should only be used in conjunction with peak systolic velocity measurements.

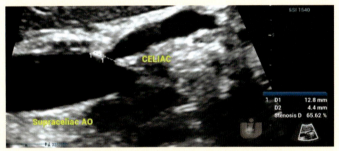

Fig. 39-21: *Diameter reduction measurement of any artery should be used in conjunction with velocity data.*

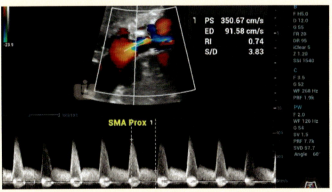

Fig. 39-22: *Significant SMA stenosis at the same point diameter reduction was documented.*

Color Doppler
- Color Doppler does not fill the entire arterial lumen, instead a color jet can be visualized through the narrowed lumen.[8]
- An occlusion of the artery is present when no flow is detected by color flow with the appropriate settings to detect low flow.[8]

> *Always confirm lack of flow by using spectral Doppler, placing the Doppler sample gate in the artery.*

Spectral Doppler Waveforms
- As the obstruction becomes more severe, changes in the spectral waveform are expected before a stenosis or occlusion, at the point of greatest stenosis and after a stenosis/occlusion as described in the *Arterial Physiology* chapter.
- **Stenosis**: A hemodynamically significant stenosis is initially recognized by color aliasing and confirmed by increased peak systolic velocities. The presence of post-stenotic turbulence supports the presence of a stenosis.[8]
  » Retrograde color flow in a mesenteric artery suggests hemodynamically significant stenosis or occlusion (e.g., retrograde SMA flow can be present with an occlusion at the origin of the SMA).[8]
  » Retrograde common hepatic artery flow suggests a hemodynamically significant stenosis or occlusion of the celiac artery.[10]
- *Spectral broadening* represents the wide range of velocities usually present when there is disturbed, non-laminar flow. This waveform change occurs in the early stages of arterial disease. The normally clear window below the systolic peak begins to fill in.
- A *high-resistance waveform* with a sharp upstroke and brisk downstroke will be noted in a stenotic region. There may or may not be flow reversal in diastole.[17] When there is a diastolic component, it may be elevated or absent depending on the degree of downstream resistance.
- *Turbulent waveforms* or "post-stenotic turbulence" are indicative of chaotic flow reflecting how blood moves in many directions just past the stenosis.

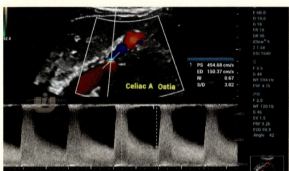

Fig. 39-23: *Significant celiac artery stenosis*

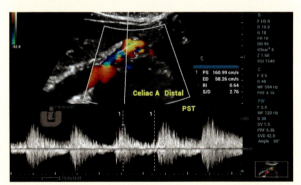

Fig. 39-24: *Post-stenotic turbulence in the distal CA*

Flow Velocities
- **Celiac artery**: PSV >200cm/s in the celiac artery suggests a stenosis >70%.[7]
  » An EDV ≥55cm/s in the celiac artery suggests a stenosis >50%.[9]
- **Superior or inferior mesenteric arteries**: PSV >275cm/s in the SMA or IMA suggests a stenosis >70%.[7]

» An end diastolic velocity of >45cm/s is used to diagnose a hemodynamically significant stenosis >50% in the SMA.[11]

- **Post-intervention restenosis**: The same criterion is often used to categorize initial stenosis and post-intervention restenosis. Comparison of PSV recorded during a baseline duplex evaluation soon after the procedure and follow-up studies is another method to diagnose disease progression.

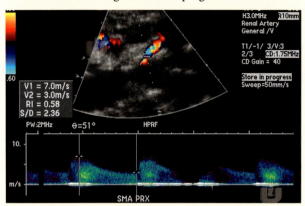

Fig. 39-25: *Significant SMA stenosis*

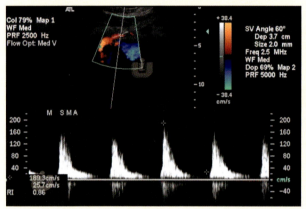

Fig. 39-26: *Post-stenotic turbulence in a mid SMA*

- **Occlusion**: An occlusion of the artery is present when no flow is detected by spectral Doppler with appropriate settings. The extent of the occlusion can often be determined by identifying a large collateral at the proximal and distal end of the occlusion.[8] These collaterals often exit or enter the artery at 90° to the vessel.
  » Retrograde flow may be observed in the hepatic/splenic arteries in cases of occlusion.

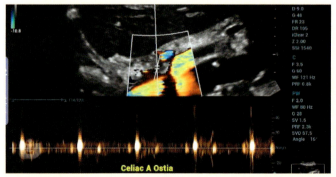

Fig. 39-27: *Celiac artery occlusion suspected on color duplex.*

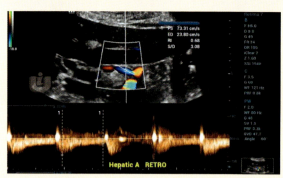

Fig. 39-28: *Reverse flow is noted in the hepatic artery as a result of the CA occlusion.*

Intestinal collaterals are able to compensate for ischemia to some extent for up to about 12 hours before substantial injury occurs.

Table 39-4: Diagnostic Criteria of Celiac for Mesenteric Artery Stenosis

<70% diameter reduction

- Low resistance waveform celiac (CA), Hepatic (HA) and splenic (SA) arteries
- An end diastolic velocity >45cm/s in the SMA suggests a >50% stenosis.
- An end diastolic velocity >55cm/s in the CA suggests a >50% stenosis.

≥70% diameter reduction: Hemodynamically significant stenosis

- Peak systolic velocity >200cm/s in the celiac arteries
- Retrograde common hepatic artery flow suggests significant celiac disease.
- Peak systolic velocity >275cm/s in the mesenteric arteries
- Mosaic color flow pattern and a focal velocity increase and evidence of post-stenotic turbulence by spectral Doppler distal to the increase

Occlusion: Complete obstruction of celiac/mesenteric arteries

- No detectable CA, SMA and/or IMA color flow and spectral Doppler signal.

Sources: Moneta GL, Lee RW, Yeager RA et al. (1991). Duplex ultrasound criteria for diagnosis of splachnic artery stenosis or occlusion. *J Vasc Surg* 14:511: 520.
Moneta GL, Lee RW, Yeager RA et al. (1993). Mesenteric duplex scanning: A blinded prospective study. *J Vasc Surg* 17:79: 86

Other Pathology

- **Median arcuate ligament compression:** If the celiac artery PSV increases with expiration and normalizes with inspiration, this suggests that the CA is being compressed by the median arcuate ligament.[8]

A "syndrome" refers to a group of physical symptoms that consistently occur together but can often be a part of other diagnoses. MALS (median arcuate ligament syndrome) is the appropriate term to use only when the patient has evidence of compression of the celiac artery on imaging AND has symptoms.[8]

- **Aneurysm:**[15] Although celiac and mesenteric artery aneurysms are rare, there is a high risk of death in cases of rupture. Almost 10% of these aneurysms accompany an abdominal aortic aneurysm.

- » Diameters of 15-22mm are considered abnormal with an approximate 5% chance of rupture. Diameters >30mm have a 50-70% chance of rupture.

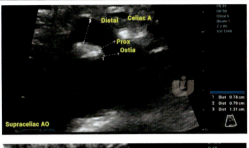
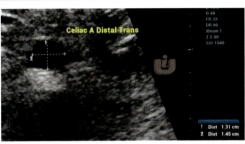

Fig. 39-29: Dilated segment of the CA measuring near 1.5cm on duplex scan.

- **Arterial dissection:** A dissection of the arterial lumen is recognized by two distinct flow channels by B-mode and/or color Doppler separated by an intimal echo. One lumen is known as the "true lumen" while the other is referred to as the "false lumen." One of the lumens may demonstrate increased velocities and stenotic waveforms.

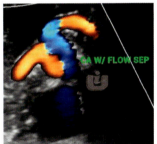
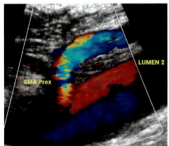

Fig. 39-30: Note two distinct flow channels of the distal CA by color flow.

Fig. 39-31: The SMA originates off the true lumen of a dissected artery.

Flow velocities may be elevated in younger patients without mesenteric disease being present. [8]

Differential Diagnosis
- Cholecystitis
- Diverticulitis
- Appendicitis
- Intestinal obstruction
- Cancer
- Peptic ulcer disease
- Pancreatitis
- Inflammatory bowel disease

Correlation
- Spiral CT scan
- Barium study of the upper/lower GI tract
- Endoscopy
- Arteriography

Medical Treatment
- Vasodilator therapy (e.g., papaverine)

Surgical Treatment
- Endarterectomy
- Bypass grafting (supraceliac or infrarenal aorto-mesenteric)
- Vein patch

- Arteriotomy/thromboembolectomy
- Decompression of the median arcuate ligament and diaphragmatic crura with/without bypass grafting
  - » Laparoscopic surgery
  - » Celiac endarterectomy/patch angioplasty
  - » Aneurysmal resection and revascularization

Emergent surgical/interventional treatment is often required for acute mesenteric ischemia.

Endovascular Treatment
- Angioplasty (with or without stenting)

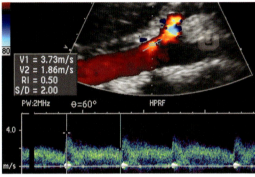

Celiac artery peak systolic velocities; pre and post- surgical decompression of the median arcuate ligament (shown in two photos below)

Fig. 39-32: Celiac artery pre-operative spectral waveforms

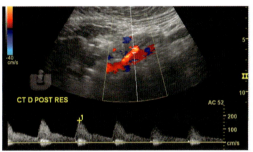

Fig. 39-33: Celiac artery intra-operative spectral waveforms

REFERENCES
1. Wyers MC, Zwolak RM. (2005). Physiology and diagnosis of splanchnic arterial occlusion. In *Rutherford Vascular Surgery 6th edition*. (1707-1717). Philadelphia. Elsevier Saunders.
2. Desai TR, Bassiouny HS. (2005). Diagnosis and treatment of nonocclusive mesenteric ischemia. In Rutherford Vascular Surgery 6th edition. (1728-1731). Philadelphia. Elsevier Saunders.
3. Sumner DS, Zierler RE. (2005). Vascular physiology: essential hemodynamic principles. In Rutherford Vascular Surgery 6th edition. (75-123). Philadelphia. Elsevier Saunders.
4. Aziz F, Comerota AJ. (12-3-2009). Abdominal Angina. eMedicine. Retrieved from http://emedicine.medscape.com/article/188618-overview. (12-11-2010).
5. Moore EM, Endean ED. (2005). Treatment of acute intestinal ischemia caused by arterial occlusions. In Rutherford Vascular Surgery 6th edition. (1718-1728). Philadelphia. Elsevier Saunders.
6. Huber TS, Lee WA, Seeger JM. (2005). Chronic mesenteric ischemia. In Rutherford Vascular Surgery 6th edition. (1732-1747). Philadelphia. Elsevier Saunders.
7. Moneta GL, Lee RW, Yeager RA et al. (1991). Duplex ultrasound criteria for diagnosis of splanchnic artery stenosis or occlusion. J Vasc Surg 14:511-520.
8. Pellerito JS. (2005). Ultrasound assessment of the splanchnic (mesenteric) arteries. In Zwiebel WJ, Pellerito JS (Eds.), In *Introduction to Vascular Ultrasonography 5th ed,* (571-583). Philadelphia: Elsevier Saunders
9. Bowersox JC, Zwolak RM, Walsh DB et al. (1991). Duplex ultrasonography in the diagnosis of celiac and mesenteric artery occlusive disease. *J Vasc Surg* 14:780-788.
10. Rzucidlo EM, Zwolak RM. (2005). Arterial duplex scanning. In *Rutherford Vascular Surgery 6th edition*. (233-253). Philadelphia. Elsevier Saunders.
11. Moneta GL, Lee RW, Yeager RA et al. (1993). Mesenteric duplex scanning: A blinded prospective study. *J Vasc Surg* 17:79-86.
12. Hallett, JW, Brewster DC, Rasmussen TE, (2001) Intestinal ischemia. In *Handbook of Patient Care in Vascular Diseases,* (231-237), Philadelphia: Lippincott Williams & Wilkins .
13. Erden A, Yurdakul M, Cumhur T.(1998).Doppler waveforms of the normal and collateralized inferior mesenteric artery. *Am J Roentgenol* 171:619-627.
14. Vaidya, S., & Dighe, M. (2010). Spontaneous celiac artery dissection and its management. Journal of radiology case reports, 4(4), 30–33. https://doi.org/10.3941/jrcr.v4i4.408
15. Takeuchi, N., Soneda, J., Naito, H., Iida, A., Yumoto, T., Tsukahara, K., & Nakao, A. (2017). Successfully-treated asymptomatic celiac artery aneurysm: A case report. International journal of surgery case reports, 33, 115–118. https://doi.org/10.1016/j.ijscr.2017.02.018
16. Danczyk RC, Moneta GL, 2013 Clinical Evaluation and Treatment of Mesenteric Vascular Disease, in Vascular Medicine: A Companion to Braunwald's Heart Disease Second Edition (Creager MA, Beckman JA, Loscalzo J (Eds), W.B. Saunders, Pages 328-339, ISBN 9781437729306, https://doi.org/10.1016/B978-1-4377-2930-6.00027-6. (https://www.sciencedirect.com/science/article/pii/B9781437729306000276)

ABDOMINAL ARTERIAL TESTING
40. Hepatoportal Duplex Ultrasound

Definition

The use of real time B-mode imaging with spectral and color flow Doppler to evaluate the portal and hepatic veins for evidence of portal hypertension (PHT). *Portal hypertension* is the elevation of pressures within the portal circulation.

Etiology

Portal hypertension and its causes can be divided into 3 categories: pre-hepatic, intrahepatic and post hepatic.

- Pre-hepatic causes
  - » Portal or splenic vein thrombosis
  - » Portal or splenic vein invasion or extrinsic compression by tumor
  - » Arteriovenous fistula
- Intrahepatic causes (most common cause of PHT)
  - » Pre-sinusoidal (e.g., schistosomiasis)
  - » Post-sinusoidal (e.g., cirrhosis, acute hepatitis, congenital hepatic fibrosis)
- Post-hepatic causes
  - » Right sided heart disease
  - » Budd Chiari Syndrome
    - Hepatic vein thrombosis (may be associated with hypercoaguable risk factors, including oral contraception)
    - Right atrial tumors
    - IVC webs or obstruction
    - Hepatic veno-occlusive disease

Risk Factors

> *Cirrhosis is the most common cause of PHT.*

- Chronic liver disease that precedes fibrosis or cirrhosis such as:
  - » Viral hepatitis: chronic hepatitis B or C
  - » Alcoholic liver disease
  - » Autoimmune disorders: primary biliary cirrhosis, primary sclerosing cholangitis
  - » Metabolic & genetic disorders
    - Hemachromatosis
    - Wilson's disease
  - » Schistosomiasis
  - » Sarcoidosis
  - » Non-alcoholic steatohepatitis (NASH)
- Heart disease resulting in increased right sided heart pressures including:
  - » Tricuspid regurgitation
  - » Congestive heart failure
  - » Constrictive pericarditis

Indications for Exam

- Suspected or known chronic liver disease
- Acute liver failure
- Unexplained ascites
- Unexplained gastrointestinal bleeding
- Documented gastroesophageal varices or portal hypertensive gastropathy
- Follow-up post trans-jugular intrahepatic portosystemic stent (TIPS)
- Post-liver transplant

Contraindications/Limitations

- Small, contracted liver with abundant ascites
- Bowel gas and floating bowel in ascites
- Poor patient cooperation (caused by hepatic encephalopathy or otherwise)
- Severe fatty livers often result in poor image quality

Mechanisms of Disease

- Portal hypertension refers to the elevation of portal pressure within the portal circulation caused by an increased resistance to flow, usually within the hepatic parenchyma.
- The portohepatic system naturally attempts to reduce increased pressure by diverting blood away from the liver directly into the systemic system, via portosystemic collaterals (e.g., gastroesophageal varices).
- Rupture of these varices can result in life-threatening hemorrhage.
- Other consequences of portal hypertension are ascites, hepatic encephalopathy, and splenomegaly (in about 50% of patients), which can lead to low platelet counts.

Location of Disease

- Hepatic veins
  - » Right hepatic veins
  - » Middle hepatic veins
  - » Left hepatic veins
- Portal veins
  - » Main portal veins
  - » Right portal veins
  - » Left portal veins

Patient History

- Some patients are asymptomatic
- Abdominal distension from ascites
- Manifestations of liver disease, and conditions associated with its cause (e.g., pancreatitis, if alcohol related)
- Variceal hemorrhage (hematemesis and melena)
- Bacterial peritonitis

Physical Examination

- Jaundice (if liver is sufficiently impaired)
- Splenomegaly
- Dilated abdominal wall veins (including caput medusa around the umbilicus)
- Hepatic encephalopathy (confusion due to poor liver function)

Hepatoportal Duplex Protocol

- Patients should fast 6-12 hours before examination to minimize the presence of air and fluids. A limited volume of clear liquids may be ingested prior to the examination (e.g., to swallow medications).
- Review any past imaging or surgical reports if available. Explain the procedure to the patient.
- Some patients may require the use of a range of transducers; including high-frequency (5-7 MHz) transducer and lower frequency (1-4 MHz) curved linear, phased sector or vector array transducers.

- Multiple patient positions may be used during examination, including:
  » Supine
  » Left lateral decubitus
  » Oblique
- Multiple scanning windows are utilized:
  » Subcostal
  » Substernal
  » Intercostal
- Spectral Doppler angles should be at ≤60º with the angle cursor parallel to the vessel walls and the sample volume within the center of the flow stream. Doppler samples are taken at several locations and should include the following observations:
  » Presence and direction of flow
  » Flow velocity and characteristics
  » Vessel diameter measurements

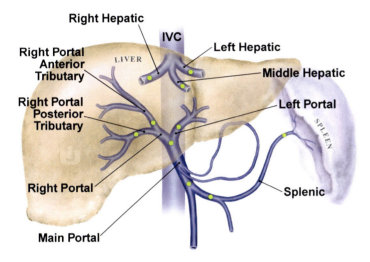

Fig. 40-1: *Color and spectral Doppler sample locations*

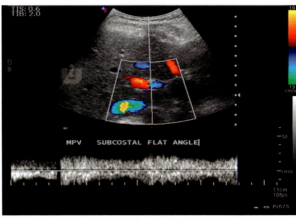

Fig. 40-2: *MPV: Using a subcostal approach often results in a 90° Doppler angle*

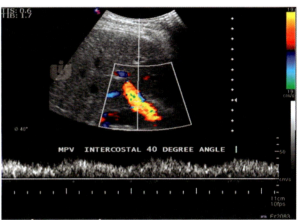

Fig. 40-3: *MPV: Intercostal approach is more favorable for an optimal Doppler angle*

Doppler Sample Locations and Typical Probe Orientation

- **Main portal vein (MPV):** With the patient in a 45º left posterior oblique position, a subcostal approach with the transducer angled superiorly can be used to image the MPV. If the MPV has a flat orientation, a right lateral intercostal approach, angling medially is more favorable for an optimal Doppler angle. *(See Fig. 40-2 and 3 for examples)*
- **Right portal vein (RPV):** A subcostal or intercostal window can be used to image the RPV in the transverse plane.

Interrogation of both the right anterior and right posterior branches is necessary, as reverse flow or thrombus may occur in either of these branches.

- **Left portal vein (LPV):** With the patient supine, a substernal approach is utilized to document the LPV.
- **Splenic vein (SV):** A spectral Doppler trace is obtained from the anterior abdominal wall in midline, with the patient supine. Documentation is also taken at the splenic hilum with the patient in a right lateral decubitus position.
- **Right hepatic vein (RHV):** The RHV is best interrogated with a right lateral intercostal window for an optimal Doppler angle and visualization of the vessel.
- **Middle hepatic vein (MHV):** A substernal or subcostal approach is the best position to document the MHV.
- **Left hepatic vein (LHV):** With the patient in the supine position, the LHV is examined from a substernal approach, angling superiorly.

Hepatic veins should ideally be interrogated during expiration, as deep inspiration can dampen the normal hepatic vein pulsatility.

- **Inferior vena cava (IVC):** Assessment for thrombus and direction of flow in the IVC can be documented in a longitudinal plane.
- **Paraumbilical vein:** This vessel traverses the ligamentum teres within the falciform ligament. It extends anteriorly and inferiorly from the LPV. Assessment for recanalization should be made with color, power and spectral Doppler. Evaluation for a patent paraumbilical vein is possible using a retrograde approach from the umbilicus.
  » The falciform ligament can be seen on ultrasound as an echogenic band with a hypoechoic channel. It extends superficially and inferiorly from the anterior aspect of the LPV, exits the liver, and travels along the anterior abdominal wall to the umbilical region. If a hypoechoic channel is seen, its diameter is measured.

Use a higher frequency transducer for the paraumbilical vein.

- **Collaterals:** Evidence of venous collaterals should be documented, e.g., at the splenic hilum, between the spleen and left kidney, midline around the pancreas, gallbladder fossa, anterior abdominal wall towards umbilicus, and along the liver surface.

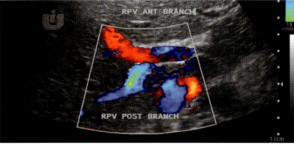

Fig. 40-4: *Doppler interrogation of the anterior and posterior branches of the right portal vein (performed to assess for hepatofugal flow or thrombus)*

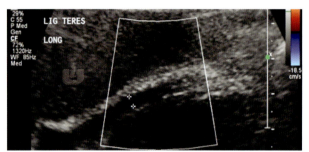

Fig. 40-5: *Measurement of hypoechoic lumen within the ligamentum teres*

Other Diagnostic Parameters

- **Measure the main portal vein** diameters anterior to the IVC on inspiration.
- **Measure splenic length:** A preferred technique is to measure the splenic length in the coronal plane, from the top at the diaphragm to the inferior border of the spleen.
- **Assess for presence of ascites**

Use a higher frequency transducer for liver surface assessment.

- **Liver texture and liver surface:** Examine the liver for coarse echo texture and irregular liver surface which accompanies cirrhosis. Fibrosis and cirrhosis do not attenuate the ultrasound beam as much as a fatty liver.
- **Hepatic vein surface:** Assess for waviness of the hepatic vein wall, which results from the nodularity of cirrhosis.

Carefully examine the entire liver with the focal zone in the near field, and repeat examination with the focal zone in the far field, searching for possible focal liver lesions.

- **Assess for focal liver lesions:** Cirrhosis is associated with an increased risk of hepatocellular carcinoma (HCC).

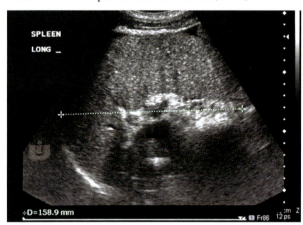

Fig. 40-6: *Splenic length measured in the coronal plane*

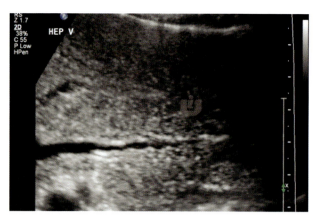

Fig. 40-7: *Irregular (wavy) hepatic vein in a cirrhotic liver*

- Consider using multiple scan planes in difficult patients. Do not persist with a gas filled window.
- Attempt all respiratory states, roll the patient, utilize the erect position in a difficult patient.
- Utilize an intercostal approach, especially with small contracted livers.
- Try different transducers:
  » Deep attenuating structures or a cirrhotic liver require a lower frequency (e.g., phased array).
  » Surface detail requires a higher frequency transducer.

Table 40-1: Hepatoportal Duplex Protocol Summary

Obtain a spectral Doppler peak systolic velocity (PSV) at the following locations:
- Main portal vein (MPV)
- Right portal vein (RPV)
- Left portal vein (LPV)
- Splenic vein (SV)
- Right hepatic vein (RHV)
- Middle hepatic vein (MHV)
- Left hepatic vein (LHV)

IVC
- Assess the inferior vena cava (IVC) for thrombus and document flow direction.

Paraumbilical Vein
- Assess for recanalization with color, power and spectral Doppler. Measure the diameter of the hypoechoic channel of the falciform ligament if seen.

Collaterals
- Document any venous collaterals noted (such as between the spleen and left kidney, midline around the pancreas, gallbladder fossa, etc.).

Hepatic Vein
- Assess for waviness of the vein wall.

Liver
- Examine the liver for coarse echo texture and irregular liver surfaces.
- Assess for focal liver lesions.

Measurements
- Main portal vein
- Splenic length

* Include assessment for ascites

PRINCIPLES OF INTERPRETATION

B-mode Imaging
- Determine whether echogenic material such as plaque or luminal reduction is observed within the lumen of the arteries and describe the location.
- Assess for echogenic material within the lumen of the veins that would suggest venous thrombosis.
- Assess liver texture and report any lesions or wall irregularities in the hepatic vein, for example.
- Report other abnormal pathology (e.g., presence of ascites).
- Measure the main portal vein diameters
- Determine splenic length

Spectral Doppler Waveforms and Color Doppler
- Determine whether there is antegrade/retrograde or hepatofugal/hepatoportal flow direction in the IVC, hepatoportal arteries and veins.
- Observe waveform patterns and report changes in the Doppler waveform proximal and distal to any segment with increased velocity which can point to a hemodynamically significant obstruction.
- Assess the arteries and veins for patency and document flow direction using color flow.

Flow Velocities
- Analyze the spectral Doppler and calculate:
  » Peak systolic (PSV) and end diastolic velocity (EDV)
  » Calculate the velocity ratio:

$$Vr = V_2 \div V_1$$

V_2 = the maximum PSV of a stenosis
V_1 = PSV of the proximal normal segment

Interpretation/Diagnostic Criteria

Normal

Spectral Doppler Waveforms and Color Doppler

Table 40-2: Normal Hepatoportal Doppler Waveform Analysis

Vessel	Wave Characteristics
Main portal vein	Hepatopetal, and continuous
Right portal vein	Hepatopetal and continuous
Left portal vein	Hepatopetal and continuous
Hepatic artery	Hepatopetal and pulsatile (low resistance)
Splenic vein	Continuous
Superior mesenteric vein	Continuous
Right hepatic vein	Multiphasic
Middle hepatic vein	Multiphasic
Left hepatic vein	Multiphasic

- Portal veins demonstrate mild respiratory and cardiac phasicity.

Hepatopetal refers to flow direction towards the liver.
Hepatofugal refers to flowing direction away from the liver.

- **Hepatic veins waveforms:** The pulsations from the right heart are reflected in the waveform of the hepatic veins, with a multiphasic flow pattern consisting of two periods of forward flow corresponding to atrial diastole and ventricular systole. The period of transient flow reversal corresponds to the right heart contraction of atrial systole.

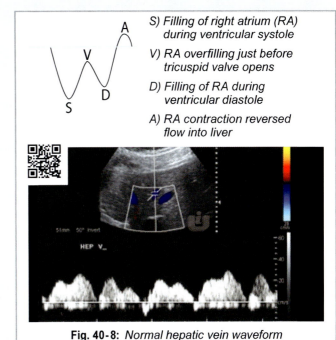

S) Filling of right atrium (RA) during ventricular systole
V) RA overfilling just before tricuspid valve opens
D) Filling of RA during ventricular diastole
A) RA contraction reversed flow into liver

Fig. 40-8: Normal hepatic vein waveform

Flow Velocities

Table 40-3: Normal Hepatoportal Velocity Ranges Reported in the Literature

Results from various studies have shown a great variation in normal maximum portal vein velocity ranges:

Velocity Range	Source
8-18cm/s (fasting)	Patriquin. et al
26.5cm/s (± 5.5)	Haag et al
16-31cm/s	Abu-Yousef et al
11-39cm/s	Kok et al
20-33cm/s	Cioni et al

- The large variation in ranges can be a result of intraobserver variability, diversity in fasting and respiratory states, differing cardiac outputs, and the presence of varied collateral pathways (especially the recanalized paraumbilical vein).
- This variation makes it difficult to rely on velocities as an indicator of portal hypertension. In general, unusually low velocities in the portal vein indicate portal hypertension, although velocities in the normal range do not exclude this diagnosis.

Source: Robinson, KA, Middleton WD, AL-Sukaiti R, Teefey SA & Dahiya N. (March 2009). Doppler sonography of portal hypertension, *Ultrasound Quarterly.* 25(1), 3-13..

Table 40-4: Normal Hepatoportal Interpretation Summary

No detectable hepatoportal disease
- Portal vein
  » Low velocity hepatopetal flow with respiratory variation
  » Maximum velocities vary within 15-30cm/s
- Hepatic artery
  » Low resistance flow
  » PSV range 70-150cm/s
- Hepatic Vein
  » Multiphasic flow pattern

Source: Robinson, KA, Middleton WD, AL-Sukaiti R, Teefey SA & Dahiya N. (March 2009). Doppler sonography of portal hypertension, *Ultrasound Quarterly*. 25(1), 3-13.

Abnormal

In this chapter, abnormal hepatoportal interpretation will be grouped by condition instead of separating each duplex finding.

A spleen diameter >13cm measured in the coronal plane is a sign of splenomegaly.

Portal Hypertension

- Hepatofugal flow in the main portal vein or its branches is only seen in advanced PHT cases.

Both right and left portal veins may show reversed flow, but if there is a large patent paraumbilical vein, the right portal vein may be reversed, while the left and main portal veins are flowing in the normal direction.

- Hepatofugal flow in the splenic vein is abnormal.
- Hepatofugal flow in the SMV (uncommon)
- Enlarged diameter of portal veins (MPV >13mm) may be observed, although is not a sensitive sign of disease (found only in about 40% of patients with PHT).
- A patent umbilical vein demonstrating hepatofugal venous flow on spectral Doppler is the most reliable and sensitive ultrasound sign, seen in up to 85% of patients with PHT. An umbilical vein diameter >2.5mm, also indicates portal hypertension.

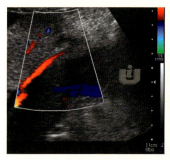
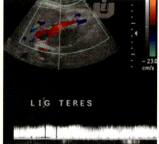

Fig. 40-9: *Patent umbilical vein seen on color and spectral Doppler*

- Dilated mesenteric or splenic veins diameters >10mm.

Acute Thrombus

- Acute thrombus may result in little to no expansion of the vessel lumen and consist of hypoechoic to echogenic intraluminal echoes identified within the hepatic, portal veins or IVC. No flow will be observed by color or spectral Doppler especially in cases of complete thrombosis.

Acute thrombus occurs in up to 5% of patients with PHT due to cirrhosis.

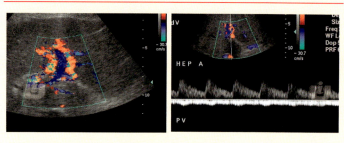

Fig. 40-10: *Hepatofugal flow in the left portal vein seen by color and spectral Doppler (below the baseline).*

Chronic Thrombosis

- Chronic thrombosis with cavernous transformation appears as a small echogenic lumen with multiple, tortuous collateral channels seen within the porta hepatis. *(Fig. 40-12)* These form a bypass route from the splanchnic veins to the intrahepatic portal veins around the thrombosed portal vein. (This may take up to a year to develop.)
- Echogenic material may be visualized expanding the lumen of the portal vein in cases of malignant thrombus from vascular invasion of hepatocellular carcinoma (HCC). Pulsatile arterial flow may be present within the thrombus. The main portal vein diameter is usually >2cm in this context, so a large occluded portal vein (or branches) should suggest the presence of HCC.

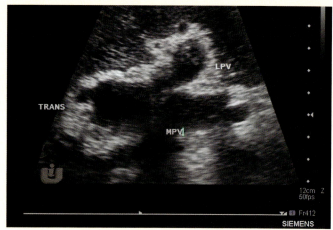

Fig. 40-11: *Hepatocellular carcinoma, malignant thrombus increasing portal vein diameters*

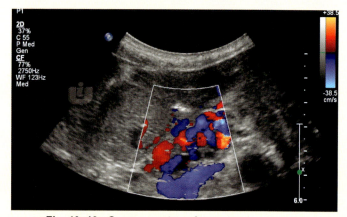

Fig. 40-12: *Cavernous transformation in a patient with chronic thrombosis of the portal vein*

Be aware of transmitted arterial wall thump. This is not umbilical venous flow.

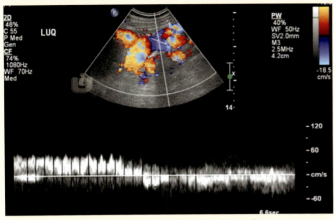

Fig. 40-13: *Splenorenal collaterals demonstrated with spectral Doppler.*

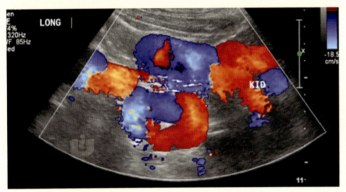

Fig. 40-14: *Splenorenal collaterals demonstrated with color Doppler*

- A mass of tortuous, worm-like vessels, with no accompanying artery and a low-mid velocity, turbulent Doppler signal suggests gastro-esophageal, splenorenal and/or retroperitoneal collaterals.

Budd-Chiari Syndrome
- Decreased, absent, or reversed flow in any of the hepatic veins
- Decreased venous flow, or narrowing of the IVC
- Intrahepatic venovenous collaterals
- Echogenic intralumenal echoes in the hepatic veins or IVC
- Dampened spectral tracing in the hepatic vein if there is an obstructing lesion in the hepatic vein or IVC
- Caudate lobe hypertrophy

Right-sided Heart Failure/Tricuspid Valve Regurgitation
- Increased hepatic vein pulsatility
- Pulsatile portal vein

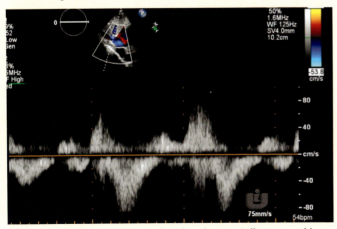

Fig. 40-15: *Spectral Doppler showing systolic reversal in the hepatic vein from severe tricuspid regurgitation.*

Table 40-5: Diagnostic Criteria for Abnormal Hepatoportal Disease

Portal Hypertension
- Hepatofugal (reverse) flow in the main portal vein or its branches, splenic vein, or SMV
- Slow portal vein flow
- Portal flow alternating between retrograde and antegrade flow
- Main portal vein diameter >13mm
- Splenic vein diameter >10mm
- Portal vein thrombosis +/- cavernous transformation
- Patent paraumbilical vein
- Paraumbilical vein diameter >2.5mm
- Presence of other portal systemic collaterals
- Spleen coronal length >13mm
- Presence of ascites

Budd-Chiari Syndrome
- Decreased, absent, or reversed flow in any of the hepatic veins
- Narrowing of the IVC
- Intrahepatic venovenous collaterals
- Echogenic thrombus in hepatic veins or IVC
- Dampened spectral tracing in hepatic veins
- Caudate lobe hypertrophy

Right-sided Heart Failure/Tricuspid Valve Regurgitation
- Increased hepatic vein pulsatility
- Pulsatile portal vein

Source: Robinson, KA, Middleton WD, AL-Sukaiti R, Teefey SA & Dahiya N. (March 2009). Doppler sonography of portal hypertension, *Ultrasound Quarterly.* 25(1), 3-13.

TIPS (Transjugular Intrahepatic Portosystemic Shunt)

Under angiographic guidance, a stent is inserted via the right internal jugular vein to connect the hepatic vein with the portal vein (usually RPV to RHV).

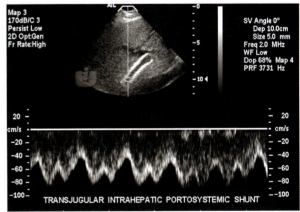

Fig. 40-16: *Spectral Doppler of TIPS*

TIPS is used to treat life threatening varices.

Normal

B-mode Imaging
- A normal stent on ultrasound appears with echogenic walls and an anechoic lumen. The ends of the stent should be located right in the hepatic (proximal end) and portal (distal end) veins (not in the liver parenchyma).

Color Doppler
- Color flow is uniform and fills the stent wall to wall.

Spectral Doppler Waveforms
- Portal vein (PV) branch flow changes normal direction and is instead shunted into/towards the stent (hepatofugal) after creation of the TIPS.
- Normally venous waveforms are phasic and pulsatile. Mild to moderate spectral broadening is not uncommon.

Flow Velocities
- Normal PV velocity should be about 30 cm/s proximal to the stent, with a typical range between 37-47 cm/s.
- Flow velocities should be relatively uniform through the shunt. Normal PSV for a TIPS ranges between 90-190cm/s. [12,13]

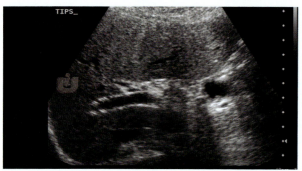

Fig. 40-17: *TIPS demonstrated with echogenic corrugated walls on B-mode image.*

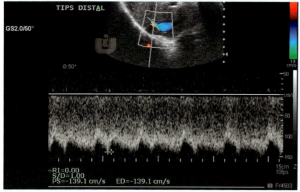

Fig. 40-18: *Distal end of a TIPS draining into the R-hepatic vein.*

Abnormal

B-mode Imaging
- A shunt stenosis on ultrasound appears with visible echogenic material and narrowing within the lumen.

Color Doppler
- Localized high-velocity color flow and post-stenotic turbulence is suggestive of a stenosis.
- An occlusion of the shunt is present when no flow is detected by color flow with the appropriate settings to detect low flow.

Spectral Doppler Waveforms
- Post-stenotic turbulence is often observed when there is a stenosis.
- Venous waveforms are continuous (non-pulsatile).
- Portal or splenic venous flow is hepatofugal or bidirectional (to-fro).
- An occlusion of the shunt is present when no flow is detected by spectral Doppler. Hepatopetal flow (away from the stent) is an indirect sign of stent malfunction which supports occlusion.

Flow Velocities
- Elevated PSV >190 cm/s in the stent suggest a hemodynamically significant for a TIPS. [13]
- PSV <90cm/s suggests possible stenosis of about 50%. PSV <50-60cm/s suggests a stenosis with impending failure. [8,10]
- A decrease in velocity >100cm/s anywhere in the shunt especially when accompanied by a luminal reduction is thought to be suggestive of shunt stenosis.
- Decreased PSV in the MPV post-operatively, especially <30cm/s suggests shunt malfunction.

Correlation
- Upper GI series
- CT scan
- MRI
- Endoscopic examination
- Angiography

Medical Treatment
- Managing the cause of portal hypertension (e.g., anticoagulation for hepatic vein thrombosis, treating any identified cause of liver disease).
- Beta-blockers can reduce portal pressure
- Management of complications:
    » Varices
        - Endoscopic banding
        - Sclerotherapy
    » Ascites
        - Diuretics
        - Salt restriction
        - Paracentesis
        - Treat any supervening bacterial peritonitis

Surgical Management
- Esophageal devascularization
- Liver transplant– considered if liver function is poor
- Portosystemic vascular shunts
    » Distal splenorenal shunt (DSRS)
    » Portocaval shunt (main portal blood flow shunted to the IVC)
    » Mesocaval shunt (blood from the superior mesenteric vein shunted to the IVC)

REFERENCES

1. Baxter GM, (2003). Imaging in renal transplantation. Ultrasound quarterly. 19(3) 123-137.
2. Ditchfield MR, Gibson RN, Donlan JD, Gibson PR. (1992). Duplex Doppler ultrasound signs of portal hypertension: relative diagnostic value of examination of paraumbilical vein, portal vein and spleen. Australasian Radiology, 36: 102-105
3. Gibson RN, Gibson PR, Donlan JD, Padmanabhan R. (1993). Modified Doppler flowmetry in the splanchnic circulation. Gastroentererology; 105:1029-1034.
4. Gibson RN, Gibson PR, Donlan JD, Clunie DA. (1989). Identification of a patent paraumbilical vein using Doppler sonography: importance in the diagnosis of portal hypertension. AJR, 153: 513-516.
5. Irshad A, Ackerman SJ, Campbell AS, A. (2009). An overview of renal transplantation: current practice and use of ultrasound. Seminars in Ultrasound, CT and MRI. 30 (4) 298-314.
6. Robinson, KA, Middleton WD, AL-Sukaiti R, Teefey SA & Dahiya N. (March 2009). Doppler sonography of portal hypertension, Ultrasound Quarterly. 25(1), 3-13.
7. Vessal S, Naidoo S, Hodson J, Stella D, Bibson RN. (2009). Hepatic vein morphology- a new sonographic diagnostic parameter in the investigation of cirrhosis. J Ultrasound Med. 28:1219-1227.
8. Zwiebel, WJ (2005). Ultrasound assessment of the hepatic vasculature. In Zwiebel WJ, Pellerito JS (Eds.), Introduction to Vascular Ultrasonography 5th ed, (586-609). Philadelphia: Elsevier Saunders.
9. Saxon RS, Barton RE, Keller FS, Rösch J: Prevention, detection, and treatment of TIPS stenosis and occlusion. Semin Intervent Radiol 1995;12(4):3
10. Franklin VR, Simmons LQ, Baker AL. Transjugular Intrahepatic Portosystemic Shunt: A Literature Review. Journal of Diagnostic Medical Sonography. 2018;34(2):114-122. doi:10.1177/8756479317746338
11. Saxon RS, Barton RE, Keller FS, Rösch J: Prevention, detection, and treatment of TIPS stenosis and occlusion. Semin Intervent Radiol 1995;12(4):375–383
12. Kliewer, M. A., Hertzberg, B. S., Heneghan, J. P., Suhocki, P. V., Sheafor, D. H., Gannon, P. A., Jr, & Paulson, E. K. (2000). Transjugular intrahepatic portosystemic shunts (TIPS): effects of respiratory state and patient position on the measurement of Doppler velocities. AJR. *American journal of roentgenology*, 175(1), 149–152.
13. Darcy M. (2012). Evaluation and management of transjugular intrahepatic portosystemic shunts. AJR. *American journal of roentgenology*, 199(4), 730–736.

ADDITIONAL TESTING
41. Hemodialysis Access Duplex Evaluation

Definition
The use of a combination of real time B-mode imaging with spectral and color flow Doppler (duplex scan) to evaluate maturity of arteriovenous fistulas (AVF) prior to hemodialysis and to assess patency of dialysis fistulas or grafts (AVG) already in use.

Rationale
Hemodialysis requires high flow in a vessel that is easily accessible and can withstand multiple punctures with the dialysis catheters. To accomplish this, an arteriovenous fistula is often created surgically by connecting an artery and a vein together, so that a high flow situation is created as blood flows directly from a large high pressure artery to the vein. When an AVF is not an option, an AVG may be surgically inserted, which also connects an artery to a vein for hemodialysis access using a prosthetic graft or transposing a vein as conduit.

Etiology (for complications of hemodialysis access)
- Intimal hyperplasia
- Atherosclerosis
- Thrombosis
- Aneurysm
- Pseudoaneurysm
- Embolization
- Trauma (e.g., punctures)
- Extrinsic compression
- External radiation

Risk Factors for Renal Disease
- Age (increased risk with age)
- Hypertension
- Race (African Americans having the highest risk)
- Diabetes
- Kidney disease
- Family history of kidney disease
- Smoking
- Hyperlipidemia
- Obesity
- Coronary artery disease

Indications for Exam
- Abnormal measurements during a dialysis session including: elevated recirculation, elevated venous pressures or low urea reduction rates
- Onset of extremity symptoms post-intervention
- Decreased bruit or thrill in the access conduit
- Evaluation of AVF maturity
- Pulsatile mass

Contraindications/Limitations
- Obesity or severe edema/swelling may cause poor visualization due to vessel depth.
- Extensive bandaging or any open wounds limiting access by the ultrasound transducer
- IV lines
- Severe hypotension affecting velocities/volume flow
- Extreme angles at anastomotic sites may limit visualization.

Common Connections of AVF/AVG
- Brescia-Cimino (radial artery-cephalic vein)
- "Snuffbox" fistula (thenar branch of the radial artery-cephalic vein)
- Radial artery-basilic vein forearm transposition
- Brachial artery-upper arm basilic vein transposition
- Brachial artery-cephalic vein (antecubital area)
- Brachial artery-cephalic vein (upper arm)
- Thigh graft connections involve:
  » Great saphenous, common femoral or femoral vein
  » Common femoral artery or superficial femoral artery
- Axillary artery-axillary vein
- Axillary artery-ipsilateral or contralateral jugular vein
- Subclavian artery-contralateral subclavian vein "necklace graft"

"Transposition" refers to removal and tunneling of a vein to a more superficial level.

Graft Types *Configurations*
- Straight graft in the forearm or upper arm
- Loop graft in the forearm or upper arm
- Thigh grafts (typically loop)
- Access anastomoses configurations include: End-to-side, End-to-end, and Side-to-side

Graft Types *Materials Used*
- Prosthetic
  » **Biological**: bovine heterografts, cryopreserved veins
  » **Synthetic**: Dacron or PTFE (Polytetrafluoroethylene)
- Autogenous
  » **In-situ vein**: using native veins as conduit
    - Basilic vein
    - Cephalic vein
    - Great saphenous vein
    - Endo AVF is a non-surgical technique which uses magnets to line up and connect the artery and vein via a perforator to create an AVF
    - Femoral veins

Studies indicate that the overall patency rate is higher for an AVF than it is for a prosthetic graft. [2-5,19]

Inflow Sites
- Radial artery at the wrist
- Brachial artery at the antecubital fossa
- Proximal brachial artery
- Axillary artery
- Common femoral artery
- Superficial femoral artery
- Subclavian artery

Outflow Sites
- Cephalic vein
- Median antecubital vein
- Basilic vein
- Great saphenous vein
- Femoral vein
- Subclavian vein

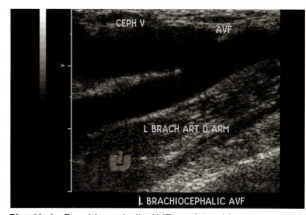

Fig. 41-1: *Brachiocephalic AVF: end-to-side anastomosis*

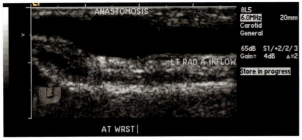

Fig. 41-2: *Radiocephalic AVF: end-to-end anastomosis*

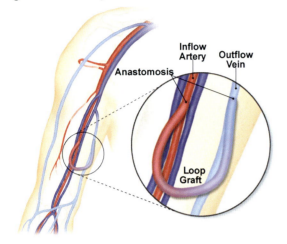

Fig. 41-3: *Arteriovenous graft (AVG) loop graft configuration*

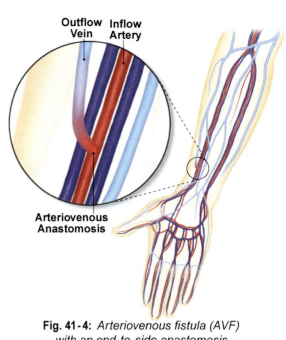

Fig. 41-4: *Arteriovenous fistula (AVF) with an end-to-side anastomosis*

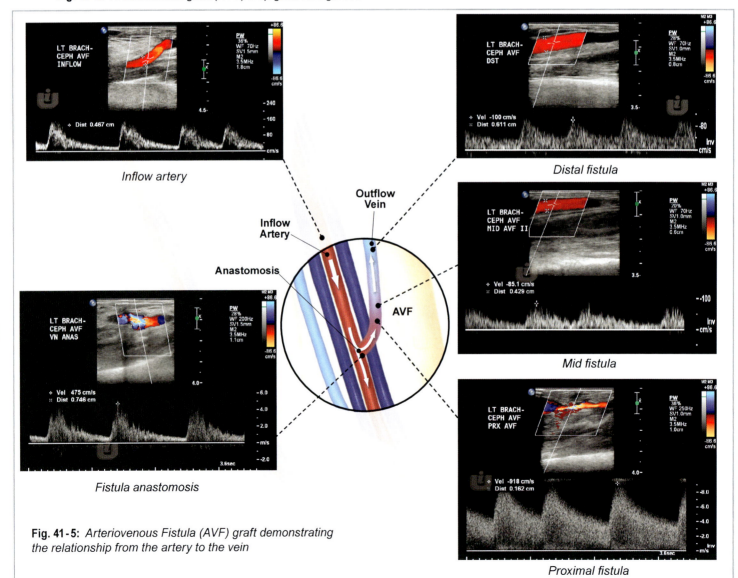

Fig. 41-5: *Arteriovenous Fistula (AVF) graft demonstrating the relationship from the artery to the vein*

Normal Flow Within Arteriovenous Fistula/Grafts

- Flow is increased in the proximal portion of the artery feeding the AVF.
- Low resistance waveforms are found in the proximal artery before the AVF.
- Increased flow velocity and volume is dependent on the size of the AVF, venous out-flow resistance, collaterals and the overall resistance of the distal peripheral bed.
- In distal arteries, the flow pattern is dependent on the fistula's resistance, proximal artery, collaterals and the distal vascular bed.
- Flow into the proximal venous segment is from an artery with high pressure which jets into the low pressure vein.
- High pressure gradients increase flow volume and velocities in the vein.
- Venous pressure at and beyond the AVF site is low and has a more pulsatile waveform.

AVF generally have a greater long term success rate when the pre-operative assessment has documented the absence of arterial disease (including a complete palmar arch) and superficial venous diameters >4.0mm in the chosen extremity. [9]

Mechanism of Access Complication/Failure

- A hemodynamically significant stenosis at the anastomosis or in the venous outflow track of an AVF can occur due to intimal hyperplasia and the inherent turbulent flow conditions of the access.[1-3] Hyperplasia typically occurs within 1 month to 2 years of access placement. Prosthetic dialysis grafts can also develop stenoses from intimal hyperplasia, typically at the venous anastomosis.[4]
- Hemodynamic abnormalities can arise in a vein after being arterialized. Besides venous intimal hyperplasia, abnormalities may be caused by valve position, venous wall thickening or a central venous stenosis.

Infection can occur at needle insertion sites. [5]

- Thrombosis can occur early in the post-operative period due to technical errors in the construction of the access (e.g., poor choice of inflow/outflow, anastomotic configuration) undiagnosed hypercoaguable states or poor cardiac output (hypotension).[4]

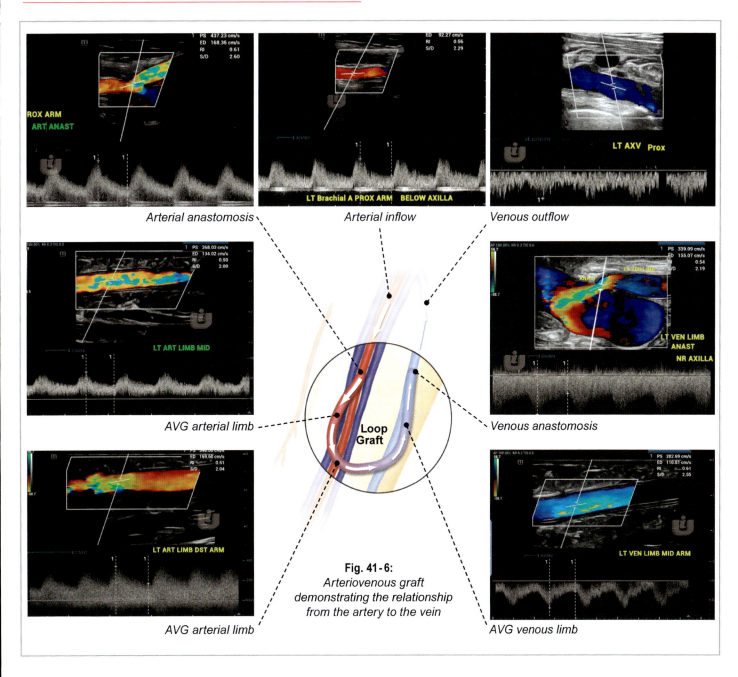

Fig. 41-6: Arteriovenous graft demonstrating the relationship from the artery to the vein

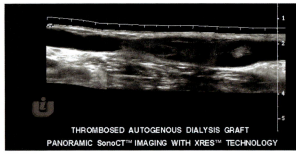

Fig. 41-7: *Graft thrombosis by B-mode image*
Courtesy of Philips Healthcare

- **AVF immaturity:** Venous branches which are significantly larger than the outflow vein of a fistula, can be the reason for AVF immaturity. When the branches are surgically ligated, oftentimes the AVF can mature. [2,3]

- **Steal syndrome:** Blood flow in the tissues distal to the AVF may be "stolen" by the fistula when the AVF offers lower resistance to flow than the distal arteries. In this case, the flow in the artery distal to the AVF is reversed, flowing away from the hand and "stealing" flow from the hand and digits. In the presence of a steal in the upper extremity, flow to the digits may be compromised, unless adequate collateral circulation is present. Note: AV grafts can also develop a steal. [2,4]

Some arterial steals can be asymptomatic. [2]

- **Pseudoaneurysm:** Insertion of a needle during a dialysis session creates "trauma" to the fistula or prosthetic graft. Over time, the access wall can weaken and a pseudoaneurysm or aneurysmal degeneration can develop in mature access conduits. [5,6]

Pseudoaneurysms are linked with increased risk of graft thrombosis. They can also cause difficulty for the dialysis technician when accessing the graft. [4]

Early graft failure can occur even without an identifiable mechanical defect or cause. [6]

Patient History
- End-stage renal disease (ESRD)
- Previous dialysis access conduits
- Chronic arterial disease
- Extremity pain
- Claudication

The outflow tract may appear "lumpy" on physical exam due to the presence of multiple aneurysmal dilatations

Physical Examination
- Steal phenomenon symptoms include hand coolness or pain and tingling of the digits, which may worsen during dialysis.
- Absent "thrill" within the fistula or graft
- Pulsatile mass
- Signs of infection, (e.g., fever of unknown origin)
- Presence of an indwelling catheter being used for dialysis, (e.g., in the jugular or subclavian veins)

Duplex Protocol of Arteriovenous Fistulas and Grafts for Hemodialysis

- Obtain a patient history to include any symptoms experienced during a dialysis session and past vascular interventions with general dates. Explain the procedure to the patient.

Obtain as much patient history as possible. This will make it easier locating the graft and is very helpful when multiple grafts are present. Many dialysis patients are good historians and they can usually tell you what conduit is currently being used during their dialysis session.

- Obtain past surgical reports/records if available, especially concerning creation of any dialysis access conduits. Dialysis patients can usually point out which access is currently being used when questioned. Look for incision scars on the extremity to give you a hint what type of access there is or where the anastomosis might be if a report of the operation is unavailable.

- The patient is typically examined in the supine position with the arm resting at the side. The patient can also sit in a chair with the arm extended on a pillow if unable to lie down for the exam, as long as the graft/fistula can be adequately assessed.

- Some patients may require the use of a range of transducers; including high-frequency (5-7 MHz) (8-15 MHz) transducers and a lower frequency (1-4 MHz) transducer.

- Use your hand to feel for the "thrill" or pulsatility of the graft or fistula. This information can help with transducer placement when trying to locate the fistula or graft.

Venous hypertension can result if an access is placed in the same arm as a venous thrombosis, resulting in severe arm edema. [5]

- Identify any abnormalities during scanning (e.g., thrombosis, occlusion, stenosis, perigraft fluid, pseudoaneurysm, aneurysm).

Duplex protocols vary depending on the configuration and type of hemodialysis access in place. Protocols for three typical access types (prosthetic-loop graft, prosthetic-straight graft and arteriovenous fistula) are as follows:

Prosthetic Dialysis: Loop Graft Protocol

Duplex scanning of prosthetic grafts may be technically difficult 24-48 hours immediately post-op due to the presence of air within the walls of the graft, which ultrasound cannot penetrate.

Transverse Scan and Images
- Follow the dialysis graft in transverse to determine its course. Locate the arterial and venous anastomoses in the transverse (short-axis) plane.
- Record transverse images of the: inflow artery, arterial anastomosis, arterial limb of the graft, venous limb of the graft, venous anastomosis and venous outflow using duplex, with color flow Doppler on and off.

Longitudinal Scan and Images
- Scan the entire inflow artery in long view in color, looking for any flow or lumenal abnormalities.
- Record longitudinal (sagittal) images of the inflow artery, arterial anastomosis, arterial limb of the graft, venous limb of the graft, venous anastomosis and venous outflow using duplex, with color flow on and off.
- Return the transducer back to the arterial anastomosis and concentrate on the inflow. Rotate your transducer onto the inflow artery above the anastomosis in the longitudinal plane. Record a longitudinal image with color flow Doppler on and off, using small transducer manipulations to capture the inflow artery and arterial anastomosis in the same image. Observe for any lumenal reduction or other abnormality.

> Color Doppler can overestimate plaque and diameter reductions due to bleeding of the color flow. For increased accuracy, measure lumenal reduction in B-mode whenever possible.

- When recording PSV in the longitudinal plane with spectral Doppler, use a ≤60° Doppler angle with the angle cursor parallel to the vessel walls and a sample volume that is in the center of the flow stream.
  » Record the PSV of the inflow (afferent) artery, at least 2cm proximal to the arterial anastomosis.
  » Record the PSV of the inflow artery 2cm distal to the arterial anastomosis. Determine flow direction to check for steal syndrome.
  » Record the highest PSV at the arterial anastomosis. Observe for any lumenal reduction or other abnormality.
  » Move the transducer longitudinally through the arterial limb of the graft. Record the highest PSV in the arterial limb. Observe for any lumenal reduction or other abnormality.
  » As the graft curves around, the venous limb of the graft will be observed. Record the highest PSV in the venous limb. Observe for any lumenal reduction or other abnormality.

> Since there is typically a high-flow state, set scales high to avoid aliasing color or waveforms.

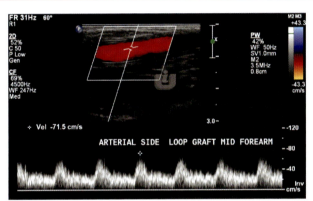

Fig. 41-8: Spectral tracing-arterial limb of graft

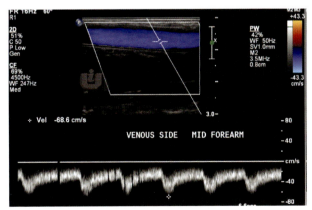

Fig. 41-9: Spectral tracing-venous limb of graft

  » Using small transducer manipulations, insonate the venous limb of the graft as it connects to the venous anastomosis. Record the highest PSV at the venous anastomosis. Observe for any lumenal reduction or other abnormality.

> The most common sites for stenosis in a prosthetic graft are at the venous anastomosis [2-4] (>50%) or in the venous outflow tract (approximately 25%). Stenosis of the graft limbs, arterial anastomosis and central veins are less common. Multiple stenoses are possible.

- Record images with color flow on and off at the venous anastomosis. Use either a longitudinal or transverse approach depending on the angulation at the anastomosis. Observe for any lumenal reduction or other abnormality.
- Record the PSV of the venous outflow (efferent vein) in longitudinal using spectral Doppler and a ≤60° Doppler angle with the angle cursor parallel to the vessel walls and a sample volume that is in the center of the flow stream.
  » If the cephalic vein is the outflow, evaluate the cephalic-subclavian venous confluence. Record images of the confluence with color flow on and off. Record sample waveforms from this site and assess for spontaneity, phasicity and augmentation. Measure a PSV if possible.
  » If the basilic is the outflow vein, record images and assess spectral Doppler waveforms from the basilic-brachial vein confluence and the axillary vein.
  » Record spectral Doppler waveforms from the subclavian and internal jugular veins.
- Record additional velocities proximal, at and distal to any stenosis.
- Measure diameter of any aneurysmal dilatations or lumenal reductions at points of stenosis or thrombus.
- Determine classification of stenosis according to laboratory diagnostic criteria.

Prosthetic Dialysis: Straight Graft Protocol

Transverse Scan and Images

- Locate the arterial anastomosis in the transverse (short-axis) plane. Follow the dialysis graft in transverse to determine its course.
- Record transverse views of the inflow artery, arterial anastomosis, body of the graft, venous anastomosis and venous outflow using duplex, with and without color flow.

Longitudinal Scan and Images

- Return the transducer back to the arterial anastomosis and concentrate on the inflow. Rotate your transducer onto the inflow artery above the anastomosis in the longitudinal plane. Record a longitudinal image with color flow on and off, using small transducer manipulations to capture the inflow artery and arterial anastomosis in the same image. Observe for any lumenal reduction or other abnormality.
- When recording peak systolic velocities (PSV) in the longitudinal plane with spectral Doppler, use a ≤60° Doppler angle with the angle cursor parallel to the vessel walls and a sample volume that is in the center of the flow stream.
  » Record the PSV of the inflow (afferent) artery, at least 2cm proximal to the arterial anastomosis.
  » Record the PSV of the inflow artery, 2cm distal to the arterial anastomosis. Determine flow direction to check for steal syndrome.
  » Record the highest PSV at the arterial anastomosis.

- » The access created should run in a straight line. Record several representative samples of flow within the body of the graft and measure the highest PSV.
- » Using small transducer manipulations, capture an image of the body of the graft as it connects to the venous anastomosis. Record the highest PSV at the venous anastomosis. Observe for any lumenal reduction or other abnormality.
- Record images with color flow on and off at the venous anastomosis. Use either a longitudinal or transverse approach depending on the angulation at the anastomosis. Observe for any lumenal reduction or other abnormality.
- Record the PSV of the venous outflow (efferent vein) in the longitudinal plane.
  - » If the cephalic vein is the outflow, evaluate the cephalic-subclavian venous confluence. Record images of the confluence with color flow on and off. Record sample waveforms from this site and assess for spontaneity, phasicity and augmentation. Measure a PSV if possible.
  - » If the basilic is the outflow vein, record images and assess spectral Doppler waveforms from the basilic-brachial vein confluence and the axillary vein.
  - » Record spectral Doppler waveforms from the subclavian and internal jugular veins.
  - » Record additional velocities proximal, at and distal to any stenosis.
- Measure the diameter of any aneurysmal dilatations or lumenal reductions at points of stenosis, thrombus.
- Determine classification of stenosis according to laboratory diagnostic criteria.

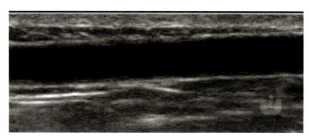

Fig. 41-10: *Normal graft with clear vessel lumen*

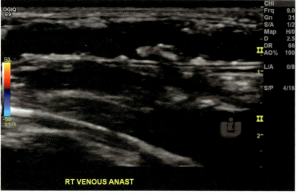

Fig. 41-11: *Abnormal access with intraluminal echoes*

Arteriovenous Fistula Protocol
Transverse Scan and Images

There is a single connection between the arterial and venous system in these access types, the AVF anastomosis.

- Locate the anastomosis of the AVF in the transverse (short-axis) plane. Follow the fistula in transverse to determine its course.
- Record transverse views of the inflow artery, anastomosis and several representations of the outflow vein using duplex, with and without color flow.

Longitudinal Scan and Images

- Record longitudinal (sagittal) views of the: inflow artery, anastomosis and several representations of the outflow vein using duplex, with and without color flow Doppler. Flow is sometimes increased in the proximal portion of the artery feeding the AVF.
- Return the transducer back to the anastomosis and concentrate on the inflow. Rotate your transducer onto the inflow artery above the anastomosis in the longitudinal plane. Record a longitudinal image with color flow Doppler on and off, using small transducer manipulations to capture the inflow artery and arterial-venous anastomosis in the same image. Observe for any lumenal reduction or other abnormality.

Be careful not to "create" a stenosis by putting too much compression on the outflow vein since these vessels are very superficial.

- When recording PSV in the longitudinal plane with spectral Doppler, use a ≤60° Doppler angle with the angle cursor parallel to the vessel walls and a sample volume that is in the center of the flow stream.
  - » Record the PSV of the inflow (afferent) artery in the longitudinal plane, at least 2cm proximal to the arterial anastomosis.
  - » Record the PSV of the inflow artery in the longitudinal plane, 2cm distal to the arterial anastomosis. Determine flow direction to check for steal syndrome.
  - » Record the highest PSV at the arterial-venous anastomosis.

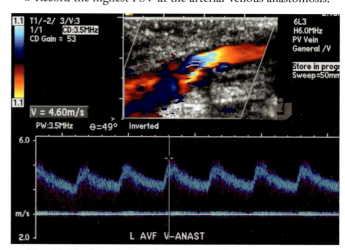

Fig. 41-12: *Spectral tracing at an AV fistula anastomosis*

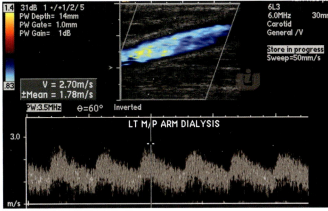

Fig. 41-13: *Normal efferent vein spectral waveforms*

» Record several representative samples of flow within the outflow (efferent) vein or body of the access and measure the highest PSV. Take several samples and annotate according to the anatomical level, e.g., "outflow-mid arm."
  • Assess for spontaneity, phasicity and augmentation. Measure a PSV if possible.
  • If the cephalic is the outflow vein, evaluate the cephalic-subclavian venous confluence.
  • If the basilic is the outflow vein, evaluate the basilic-brachial vein confluence and the axillary vein.
  • Subclavian and internal jugular veins
» Record additional velocities proximal, at and distal to a stenosis

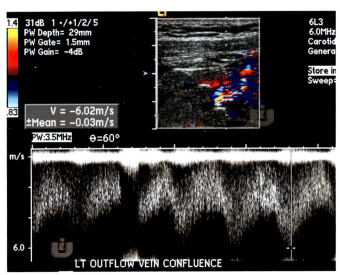

Fig. 41-14: *Significant stenosis at an AVF anastomosis*

• Measure the diameter of any lumenal reductions from stenosis or thrombus and any aneurysmal dilatations.
• Velocity increases can also occur in AVF conduits due to valve cusps. Determine the significance of the velocity increase by calculating the PSV ratio (Vr) in the vicinity of the valve.

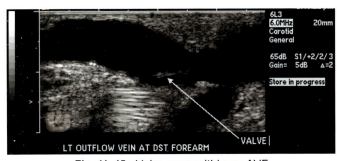

Fig. 41-15: *Valve cusp within an AVF*

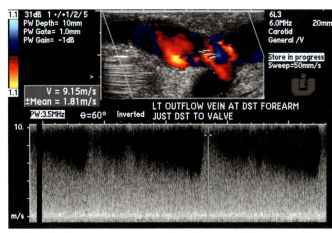

Fig. 41-16: *Increased velocity within an AVF at valve site*

• Determine classification of stenosis according to laboratory diagnostic criteria.

• Measure several outflow vein diameters to assess for fistula maturity (e.g., distal, mid and proximal arm).

• Measure the distance from the skin to the anterior wall of the outflow vein. This can be reported to the dialysis center and may assist dialysis technicians when cannulating the conduit.

There is a maturation period of approximately 1-3 months before an access can be used for dialysis. [2,5,11,15]

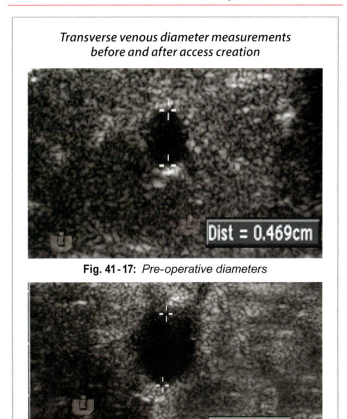

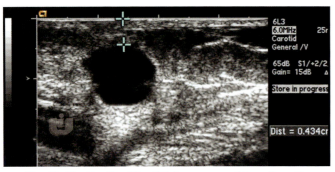

Fig. 41-19: *Depth of the fistula measured from the skin*

Evaluation of Volume Flow

The calculation of volume flow assumes laminar flow was used. Significant error in calculation will occur if the segments used for measurement were aneurysmal, stenotic or exhibited turbulent flow patterns.

- Volume flow measurements indicate the volume of fluid passing through a cross sectional area of the access per unit time.

Studies indicate that there is a high success rate in AVF patency when the volume flow >500 mL/min and the outflow venous diameters >4mm. [2,12]

- Calculate volume flow using a straight, non-tapering segment of the access. Activate the "time average maximum" calculation or its equivalent on the duplex scanner.
  » Measure the diameter of the segment, placing the calipers perpendicular to the vessel wall.
  » At the same location, open the Doppler gate to include the entire width of the vessel. Measure at least 1-3 cycles (PSV to PSV or EDV to EDV) on the spectral tracing to obtain volume flow (mL/min). Use complete cycles if measuring more than one.
- Repeat these steps in one or two additional areas of the dialysis access. Use an average volume flow or choose the highest value if all flow calculations are similar.

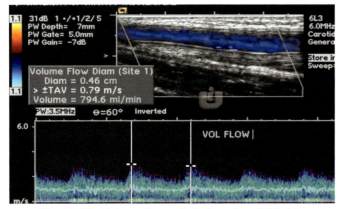

Fig. 41-20: *Volume flow calculation of an AV fistula*

Measurement of Volume Flow (VF)

VF (mL/min) = Cross-sectional area x mean velocity x 60
where Cross-sectional area (cm^2) = π d^2/4
d = diameter

Evaluation for Steal Syndrome

- Obtain baseline photoplethysmography (PPG) waveforms and digital pressures in the affected digits. Additional evaluation of non-affected digits can be used for comparison. *For detailed instructions, see chapter on PPG testing.*

- Repeat PPG waveforms and digital pressures while compressing the fistula or graft just beyond the anastomosis until you can no longer feel a "thrill" within the dialysis conduit.
- Compare pre-compression digital pressures and PPG waveforms to those taken during compression of the fistula or graft.
- Duplex imaging can also be used to illustrate steal syndrome.
  » Assess for retrograde flow in the inflow artery distal to the anastomosis.
  » Observe for large outflow venous branches. Measure PSV before the branch, in the branch, and after the branch to see how it affects flow in the fistula.

Be careful not to compress the inflow artery, only the graft or fistula just beyond the anastomosis.

Evaluation of Incidental Findings

- Document potential fluid collections or "masses" around the access. Document pulsatility/non-pulsatility using color flow and spectral Doppler with low scales.
- Measure anterior-posterior and transverse diameters of any structures and describe location and echogenicity (e.g., homogeneous, anechoic, etc.).
- No flow should be observed in a contained fluid collection. Noninfectious fluid collections include: hematoma, perigraft seroma or lymphocele. A typical location for a seroma is near the arterial anastomosis. [5]

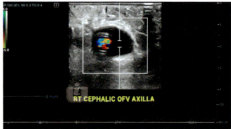

Fig. 41-21: *Perigraft fluid was noted around this dialysis conduit. Document lack of pulsatility/ color flow.*

Table 41-1: Protocol Summary for Dialysis Arteriovenous Fistula/Prosthetic Dialysis-Loop Graft

Scan transverse (short-axis) in B-mode and color and longitudinal (sagittal) with B-mode, color and spectral Doppler

- Inflow/proximal to arterial anastomosis *
- Inflow artery distal to arterial anastomosis **
- Arterial anastomosis *
- Document the following segments depending of the type of access:

AVF	AVG
Body of access at several levels **	• Mid arterial limb ** • Mid venous limb ** • Venous anastomosis **

- Continue by documenting venous outflow
  » Cephalic-subclavian confluence (if cephalic is outflow) *
  » Basilic-brachial confluence (if basilic is outflow)
- Subclavian and internal jugular veins *
- Document velocities proximal, at and distal to a stenosis*
- Evaluate for graft abnormalities. Measure diameter of any lumenal reductions and any aneurysmal dilatations.
- Determine classification of stenosis according to laboratory diagnostic criteria.

* Record peak systolic velocity (PSV).
** Record PSV and check for flow direction.

PRINCIPLES OF INTERPRETATION

B-mode Imaging and Color Doppler
- Assess all arteries for intralumenal echoes. Determine location and characteristics of any thrombus, plaque, retained valve cusps, etc.
- Report measured diameters and the depth of the access from the skin's surface.
- Color flow is used to show patency of the arterial lumen, the degree of narrowing when there is disease and flow direction.

Spectral Doppler Waveforms
- Characterize the waveform characteristics within the dialysis access as well as before/after any anastomotic site.
- Any change in spectral waveform may be significant.

Flow Velocities
- Peak systolic velocity ratios (V_2/V_1) are used more than absolute velocities in most cases to determine the severity of stenosis.

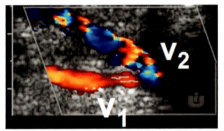

Fig. 41-22: Example of velocity ratio points for V_r calculation

- Report the volume flow calculated in mL/min.

AVF/AVG waveforms
Normal hemodialysis conduit waveforms reflect high-flow states (a low resistance waveform with elevated peak systolic and end diastolic velocities).[7]

Interpretation/Diagnostic Criteria

Normal

B-mode Imaging and Color Doppler
- No lumenal reduction by B-mode image [7]

Depth: A depth of less than 5-6mm from the skin surface is needed for successful access of a fistula for hemodialysis.[2,8,20]

Diameter
- ≥4-6mm is the optimal vessel diameter for a mature AVF.[20,21]
- There should be wall-to-wall color filling in the appropriate direction for each segment of the dialysis access, inflow and outflow arteries.[7]

Spectral Doppler Waveforms
Arterial inflow
- Arterial waveform patterns should normally be low resistant above the anastomosis of the AVF/AVG and high resistant below the AVG anastomosis or AVF connection.[7]

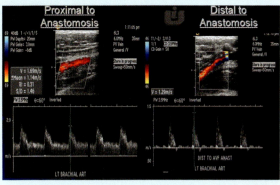

Fig. 41-23: Typical waveform resistance proximal (low-resistance) and distal to the anastomosis (high-resistance)
Note: The patient's head is to the right in these images since the patient was reversed on the cart during scanning for ergonomic issues.

Flow Velocities
- PSV <400cm/s is considered normal for both dialysis grafts and fistulas.
- Dialysis grafts:
  » Normal PSV are 100-400cm/s with EDV between 60-200cm/s.[7]
  » A normal peak systolic velocity ratio (V_2/V_1) is <2.0.[9]
  » Normal PSV in the outflow vein is expected to be 30-100cm/s.[7]
- Dialysis fistulas: A normal peak systolic velocity ratio is <2.0. A ratio <3.0 is considered normal at the fistula anastomosis.[9,10]

Volume flow: A volume flow >800mL/min is suggested for optimal dialysis graft performance.[11] A volume flow greater than 500mL/min is suggested for optimal fistula performance.[12]

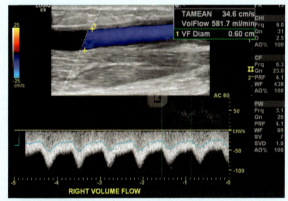

Fig. 41-24: Normal volume flow >600 mL/min is suggested for optimal fistula performance.[20]

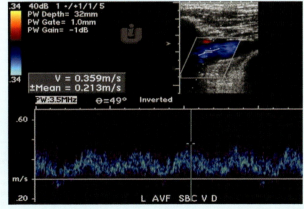

Fig. 41-25: Normal SCV waveforms in a patient with an AVF

Abnormal

B-mode Imaging and Color Doppler

- Lumenal reduction by B-mode image (e.g., intimal hyperplasia).[7]
- **Depth:** A depth of >5-6mm from the skin surface is not likely to be successful. The fistula may need to be "elevated" surgically.
- **Diameter:** Vessel diameters measuring <4-6mm suggest that the AVF will not "mature" enough for a successful access. [20,21]
- High velocity color jets together with increased velocities and post-stenotic turbulence support the presence of a significant stenosis. Take care to note a diameter change in the vessel with lumenal debris that may explain an increased velocity in the smaller diameter section of the vessel. [7] Alternately, a dilated area will have lower velocities that increase as the sample volume is moved to a normal diameter segment of the vessel.

Spectral Doppler Waveforms

- Decreased venous spontaneity and respirophasicty suggests the presence of obstruction (thrombus, stenosis, etc.) in the outflow vein. [7] *See venous chapters for a detailed description of spontaneity and phasicity.*
- Evaluate the spontaneity, phasicity and pulsatility of the subclavian and internal jugular veins. Abnormal pulsatility, lack of spontaneity or decreased phasicity suggests central venous obstruction. [7]

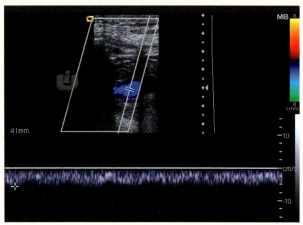

Fig. 41-26: *Abnormal SCV waveform with non-phasic, non-pulsatile flow in an AVF patient*

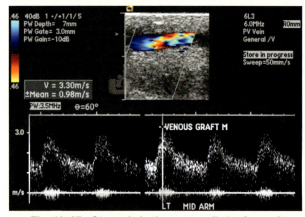

Fig. 41-27: *Stenosis in the venous limb of a graft*

Flow Velocities

- A peak systolic velocity ratio (V_2/V_1) >3.0 indicates a hemodynamically significant stenosis (≥50%) at the anastomotic site of an AVF. [7]

- PSV ratio between 2-2.9 in an AVG correlates with a 50-79% stenosis on angiography while a ratio >3.0 suggested a stenosis >75%. [7]
- >2.0 indicates a hemodynamically significant stenosis (≥50%) in the draining vein of AVF or AVG. [7,10]
- A peak systolic velocity ratio (V_2/V_1) >3.0 indicates a hemodynamically significant stenosis (≥75%) in the dialysis access. [7,10]

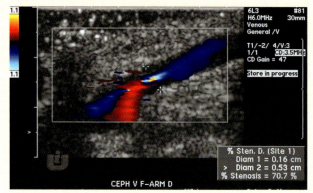

Fig. 41-28: *Significant lumenal reduction by color in an AVF*

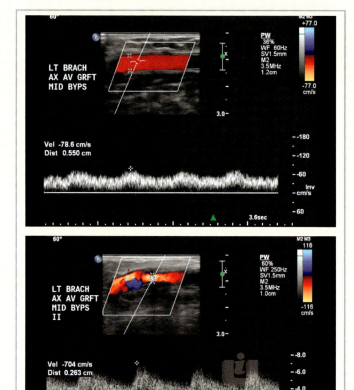

Fig. 41-29: *Significant stenosis by spectral Doppler in an AVF (pre and at stenosis). Calculating the Vratio: 704/79=8.9, categorizes this stenosis as hemodynamically significant.*

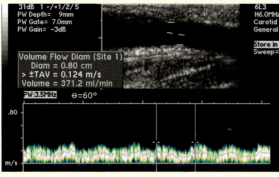

Fig. 41-30: *Abnormal volume flow*

Volume flow: A volume flow less than 800 mL/min [11] may result in suboptimal dialysis graft performance. A volume flow <500-600mL/min may result in suboptimal fistula performance. [7,12,20]

Access occlusion: The absence of spectral Doppler waveforms and measurable flow velocity with appropriate settings suggests occlusion of a fistula/graft. Intralumenal echoes visualized on B-mode image and/or the lack of color flow must be documented to support access occlusion.

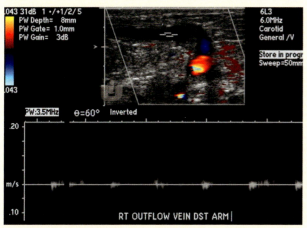

Fig. 41-31: *Occluded AVF by color and Doppler waveform*

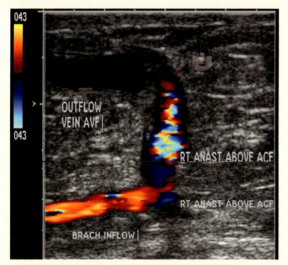

Fig. 41-32: *Occluded AVF by color*

Steal Syndrome

- When using PPG and digital pressures to evaluate the hand for steal syndrome, if there is a significant difference between the baseline digital *pressure* and amplitude of the PPG waveform compared to the post-compression pressure and PPG waveforms, there is an indication that the access is stealing flow from the hand. [15] Some labs use a pressure difference >30mmHg.

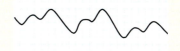
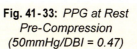
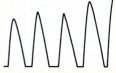

Fig. 41-33: *PPG at Rest Pre-Compression (50mmHg/DBI = 0.47)*

Fig. 41-34: *Repeat PPG after AVF compression (100mmHg/DBI = 0.94)*

- Flow reversal in the inflow artery distal to the anastomosis suggests the presence of arterial steal.
- A "side branch steal" is possible when an accessory branch of the outflow vein is at least one-third the diameter of the fistula. A significant reduction in velocity through the fistula after the branch and abnormal volume flows support the presence of a steal. [16] A large side branch may also prevent a fistula from maturating. [2]

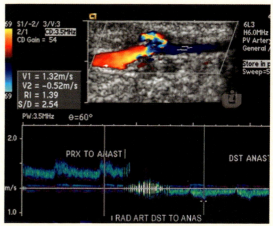

Fig. 41-35: *Steal by duplex: flow reversal noted in the native artery distal to AVF anastomosis*

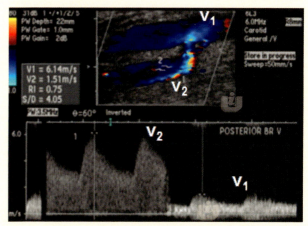

Fig. 41-36: *Elevated velocities in a venous branch of the outflow tract*

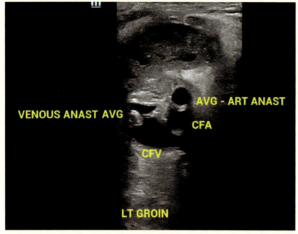

Fig. 41-37: *Compression of the venous anastomosis*

Other Pathology

Pseudoaneurysm: A pseudoaneurysm is diagnosed when a pulsatile mass is identified by color and Doppler flow which is observed communicating with the access through a patent "neck." The neck/mass demonstrates a "to and fro" (pendulum) Doppler flow patterns to indicate a pseudoaneurysm. This may be difficult to assess due to the high flow states present in an arteriovenous fistula or graft. [17]

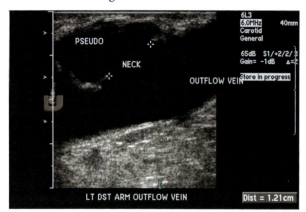

Fig. 41-38: *Pseudoaneurysmal dilatation of a dialysis graft*

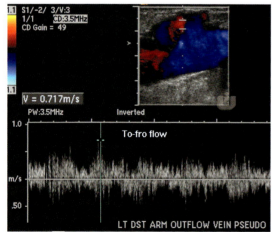

Fig. 41-39: *Spectral waveforms within the pseudoaneurysm of the graft*

Aneurysm: A focal enlargement with a diameter measurement that is at least twice the diameter of the proximal vessel indicates an aneurysmal dilatation. Aneurysms involving the arterial anastomosis of a fistula are a significant complication to be reported, as a surgical revision may be necessary. [8]

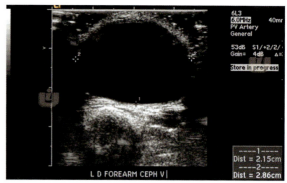

Fig. 41-40: *Aneurysmal dilatation of an AVF*

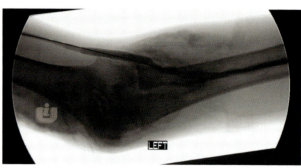

Fig. 41-41: *AVF fistulogram*

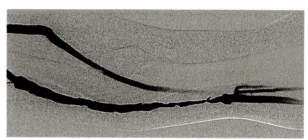

Fig. 41-42: *AVG shuntogram*

Table 41-2: **University of Chicago Diagnostic Criteria for ≥50% Stenosis in a Hemodialysis AVF**

Location of stenosis	PSV (V2) distal/PSV (V1) proximal ratio*
Arterial inflow or venous outflow	>2.0
At anastomosis	>3.0

- **Occlusion:** Absent signal, No color saturation identifiable in an occlusion
- **Abnormal volume flow:** <500 mL/min

Source: Grogan J, Castilla M, Lozanski L, Griffin A, Loth F, Bassiouny, H. (2005). Frequency of critical stenosis in primary arteriovenous fistulae prior to hemodialysis access: should duplex ultrasound surveillance be the standard of care? *The Journal of Vascular Surgery*, June 41(6), 1000-1006

Differential Diagnosis for Steal Syndrome
- Neuropathy

Correlation
- Fistulogram/Shuntogram

Medical Treatment
- Modify risk factors (e.g., smoking cessation)
- Antiplatelet medication (e.g., aspirin)
- Anticoagulation (warfarin)
- Thrombolysis (acute blockage)
- Limb elevation

Table 41-3: Diagnostic Criteria for Prosthetic Hemodialysis Grafts

	Peak Systolic Velocity (PSV)	PSV (V_2) distal/ PSV (V_1) proximal ratio	Diameter Reduction
Within normal limits (0-49%)	NA	<50% increase	0-49%
Hemodynamically significant (50-74%)		>2.0	50-74%
Hemodynamically significant at venous anastomosis	>400cm/s	1.9	
Hemodynamically ≥ 75%		>3.0	≥75%
Occlusion	absent signal		

• No color saturation identifiable in an occlusion

Source: Lockhart, ME, Robbin, ML. (2001). Hemodialysis Access Ultrasound. Ultrasound Quarterly Vol. 17, No. 3, pp. 157-167 Lippincott Williams & Wilkins, Inc., Philadelphia.

Surgical Treatment
- Open surgical thrombectomy
- Open surgical thrombectomy with patch angioplasty
- Pseudoaneurysm resection with interposition graft
- Bypass around a section of pseudoaneurysm
- Access revision (banding)
- Distal revascularization interval ligation (DRIL) procedure for vascular steal

Endovascular Treatment
- Intra-arterial directed thrombolysis
- High pressure balloon angioplasty
- Mechanical clot-removing endolumenal devices
- Stenting
- Patch angioplasty

The National Kidney Foundation has published the Kidney Disease Outcomes Quality Initiatives (KDOQI). These guidelines recommend that all dialysis patients receive regular monitoring and surveillance which can include duplex scanning to assess the anatomy and blood flow of the access.

REFERENCES

1. Pierre-Paul D, Gahtan V, Conte MS. (2005). Molecular biology and gene therapy in vascular disease. In Rutherford Vascular Surgery 6th edition. (172-192). Philadelphia. Elsevier Saunders.
2. Robbin ML, Lockhart ME. (2005). Ultrasound evaluation before and after hemodialysis access. In Zwiebel WJ, Pellerito JS (Eds.), Introduction to Vascular Ultrasonography 5th ed, (326-340). Philadelphia: Elsevier Saunders.
3. Lumsden AB, Bush RL, Lin PH, Peden EK. (2005). Management of thrombosed dialysis access. In Rutherford Vascular Surgery 6th edition. (1684-1692). Philadelphia. Elsevier Saunders.
4. Sidawy AN. (2005). Strategies of arteriovenous dialysis access. In Rutherford Vascular Surgery 6th edition. (1669-1676). Philadelphia. Elsevier Saunders.
5. Adams ED, Sidawy AN. (2005). Nonthrombotic complication of arteriovenous access for hemodialysis. In Rutherford Vascular Surgery 6th edition. (1692-1706). Philadelphia. Elsevier Saunders.
6. Hallett, JW, Brewster DC, Rasmussen TE (2001). Hemodialysis access. In Handbook of Patient Care in Vascular Diseases, 4th ed. (279-285). Philadelphia. Lippincott Williams and Wilkins.
7. Lockhart ME, Robbin ML. (2001). Hemodialysis access ultrasound. Ultrasound Quarterly. 17(3), 157-167.
8. NKF KDOQI Guidelines "Clinical Practice Guidelines and Clinical Practice Recommendations 2006 Updates Hemodialysis Adequacy, Peritoneal Dialysis Adequacy, Vascular Access." National Kidney Foundation. Retrieved from http://www.kidney.org/professionals/Kdoqi/guideline_upHD_PD_VA/va_guide1.htm. (12-7-2010).
9. Robbin ML, Oser RF, Allon M, Clements MW, Dockery J, Weber TM, Hamrick-Waller KM, Smith JK, Jones BC, Morgan DE, Saddekni S. (1998). Hemodialysis access graft stenosis: US detection. Radiology Sep 208(3), 655-661.
10. Grogan J, Castilla M, Lozanski L, Griffin A, Loth F, Bassiouny, H. (2005). Frequency of critical stenosis in primary arteriovenous fistulae prior to hemodialysis access: should duplex ultrasound surveillance be the standard of care? The Journal of Vascular Surgery. June 41(6), 1000-1006.
11. Back MR, Maynard M, Winkler A, Bandyk DF. (2008). Expected flow parameters within hemodialysis access and detection for remedial intervention of nonmaturing conduits. Vascular and Endovascular Surgery. 42(2), 150-158.
12. Robbin ML, Chamberlin NE, Lockhart ME, et al: Hemodialysis arteriovenous fistula maturity: US evaluation. Radiology 225(1):59-64,2002
13. Older RA, Gizienski TA, Wilkowski MJ, Angle JF, Cote DA. (1998). Hemodialysis access stenosis: early detection with color Doppler ultrasound. Radiology 207, 161-164.
14. Dumars MC, Thompson WE, Bluth EI, Lindberg JS, Yoselevitz M, Merritt CR. (2002). Management of suspected hemodialysis graft dysfunction: usefullness of diagnostic ultrasound. Radiology 222, 103-107.
15. White JG, Kim A, Josephs LG, Menzoian JO. (1999). The hemodynamics of steal syndrome and its treatment. Ann Vasc Surg. May;13(3):308-12.
16. Beathard GA: (2003). Aggressive treatment of early fistula failure in hemodialysis patients. Kidney Int 63(1):346-352.
17. Arshad FH, Sutijono D, Moore CL. (2010). Emergency ultrasound diagnosis of a pseudoaneurysm associated with an arteriovenous fistula. Acad Emerg Med. Jun;17(6):e43-5. Epub 2010 May 14
18. Bohannon WT, Silva MB. (2005). Venous transposition in the creation of arteriovenous access. In Rutherford Vascular Surgery 6th edition. (1677-1683). Philadelphia. Elsevier Saunders.
19. Voormolen EH, Jahrome AK, Bartels LW, Moll FL, Mali WP, Blankestijn PJ (2009.) Nonmaturation of arm arteriovenous fistulas for hemodialysis access: A systematic review of risk factors and results of early treatment. Vasc Surg. May;49(5):1325-36.
20. Oliver M. J. (2018). The Science of Fistula Maturation. Journal of the American Society of Nephrology: JASN, 29(11), 2607–2609. https://doi.org/10.1681/ASN.2018090922
21. Wavelinq EndoAVF System. (2023), Post-Creation Ultrasound Assessment Sheet. wavelinq.bd.com/resources.

ADDITIONAL TESTING
42. Pseudoaneurysm Duplex Ultrasound

Definition
The use of a combination of real time B-mode imaging with spectral and color flow Doppler to evaluate peripheral arterial vessels, dialysis conduits or arterial grafts for pseudoaneurysm.

A pseudoaneurysm (PA) or "false aneurysm" forms due to trauma to all three layers of the arterial wall. The "false aneurysm" is actually a pulsating hematoma, receiving its blood supply via communication with an artery through a patent "neck." These "necks" vary in size and length.

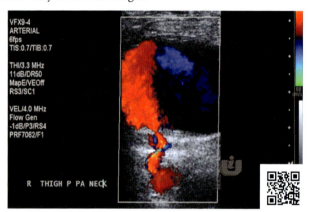

Fig. 42-1: Pseudoaneurysm of the superficial femoral artery-transverse image

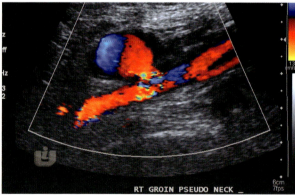

Fig. 42-2: Pseudoaneurysm of the common femoral artery-longitudinal image

Etiology of Pseudoaneurysm Development
- Iatrogenic arterial puncture
- Trauma

Risk Factors
- Post-cardiac catheterization
- Post-angiography
- Post-endarterectomy
- Patients on renal dialysis (It is common to develop PA in synthetic grafts)

Indications for Exam
- Presence of pulsatile mass at anastomotic, catheterization or puncture sites
- Bruit (abnormal sound heard through auscultation caused by vibration of tissue from turbulent flow)

Contraindications/Limitations
- Allergy to thrombin or bovine products prohibits PA injection as a repair option.
- Patients on medication for anticoagulation make thrombosis of PA technically difficult.
- Size and width of PA neck can influence treatment options
- Ischemia of the distal limb being treated
- Skin infection at PA site
- Contraindications for ultrasound guided pseudoaneurysm injection repair include:
  » Patients currently on anticoagulation (thrombus will not form in the PA)
  » The size and width of the PA neck (there may be less success when larger necks are present)
  » Known allergy to thrombin or bovine products

Mechanism of Disease
- Insertion of a needle for diagnostic or therapeutic purposes is still a trauma to the arterial wall.
- Repeated puncture of hemodialysis grafts leads to formation of subcutaneous hematomas and pseudoaneurysms.

In dialysis conduits, there are risks of graft thrombosis, infection and bleeding associated with pseudoaneurysms. [4]

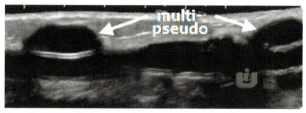

Fig. 42-3: Multiple pseudoaneurysms of a dialysis access

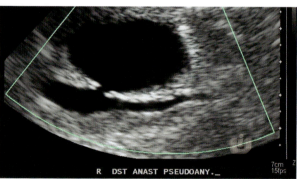

Fig. 42-4: Pseudoaneurysm of a bypass graft at the distal anastomosis

Pseudoaneurysm formation is less common in autogenous AV fistulas compared to prosthetic grafts. [4]

- Reasons for pseudoaneurysm at an anastomotic site include, infection, tension at the anastomosis, thin-walled arteries, suture deterioration or improper suture technique.
- A reduction in tensile strength, post-endarterectomy may weaken arterial walls, increasing the risk of pseudoaneurysm.

Location of Disease
- Common femoral artery
- Superficial femoral artery
- External iliac artery
- Deep femoral artery
- Brachial artery
- Axillary artery
- Radial artery
- Carotid artery
- Anastomotic sites
- Hemodialysis grafts or AV fistulas

Patient History
- Recent percutaneous arterial catheterization/puncture
- History of arteriovenous graft (AVG)
- Recent surgery
- Trauma

Physical Examination
- Tenderness/swelling at puncture site
- Pain in vicinity of puncture
- Pulsatile mass
- Bruit near puncture site
- Palpable thrill (vibration caused by turbulent blood flow)

Duplex Examination for Suspected Pseudoaneurysm
- Obtain a patient history to include approximate location where catheter/needles were injected. If catheterization of the artery was recent, an entry point can usually be identified by physical exam on the skin. A pseudoaneurysm is likely to be located at or proximal to the entry point.
- Patient is examined in the supine position. Explain the procedure to the patient. Note: Since patients are often very tender post-procedure at the site of suspected PA, use extra gel to help obtain images comfortably.
- Some patients may require the use of a range of transducers, including high-frequency (5-7 MHz) (8-15 MHz) transducers and lower frequency (1-4 MHz) transducers.

Transverse Scan and Images
- Document B-mode and color images in areas of suspected pseudoaneurysm (PA). Begin imaging in the transverse plane so more than one vessel can be visualized at one time.
- Moving the transducer through the suspected area in every direction: cephalad, caudad, lateral; and medial: observe the regional arteries and veins.
- Survey for evidence of pulsatile mass, hematoma or fluid collection.
  » If a mass is detected, color Doppler is useful to distinguish between a pulsatile and non-pulsatile mass. Areas of flow disturbance or flow absence prompt close observation by color Doppler. Adjust the color scale sensitivity (low-sensitivity versus high-sensitivity) depending on the flow states encountered.
  » Obtain a color flow image of the mass. A pseudoaneurysm typically displays a half red-half blue appearance in at least one view, denoting flow into the mass and circling around it. An occluded pseudoaneurysm will show echogenic material and little to no color flow or may be a mass caused by another etiology.
  » Measure the anterior-posterior and transverse diameters of any mass noted.

There is often a pulsatile mass on the physical exam which can guide your transducer placement to locate the PA.

The size of a pseudoaneurysm varies in diameter, but is typically between 1-5cm.

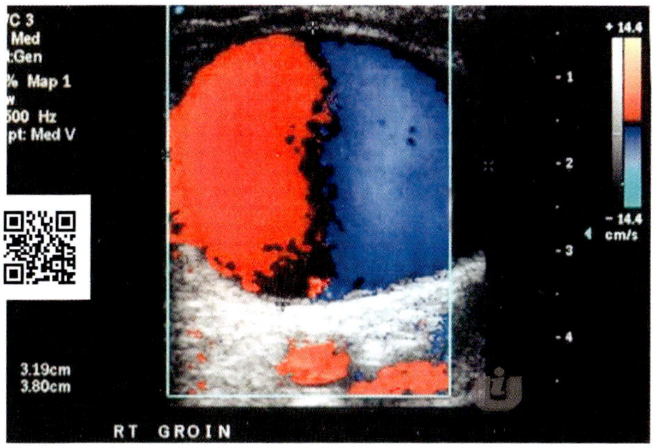

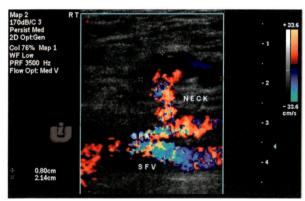

Fig. 42-5: *Typical color flow within a pseudoaneurysm*

- Determine the communication point between any pulsatile mass (pseudoaneurysm) and a native artery by locating the "neck" using color Doppler. Place the sample volume in the neck and obtain a Doppler spectral display. A to-and-fro Doppler flow pattern is characteristic of a pseudoaneurysm whereby pulsatile flow escapes the native artery or graft, enters the mass, circles around the mass, and then returns to the artery.

Use dual screen to measure a larger PA.

- Document the presence of any intramural thrombus present by B-mode image within the pseudoaneurysm.

The groin is a common location for pseudoaneurysm.

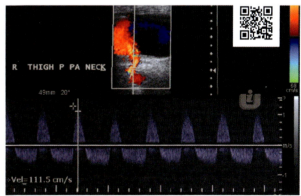

Fig. 42-6: *Color flow observed in a PA neck*

Fig. 42-7: *Characteristic "to and fro" flow pattern in a PA neck. Attempt to measure the length and diameter of the neck using equipment calipers.*

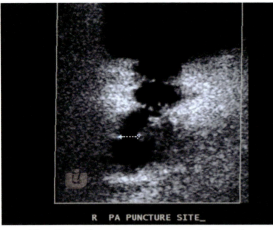

Fig. 42-8: *Pseudoaneurysm neck diameter*

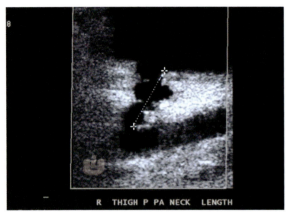

Fig. 42-9: *Pseudoaneurysm neck length*

- Estimate the distance between the top of the pseudoaneurysm cavity and skin to help choose an appropriate length needle for possible PA repair procedure.
- Document Doppler flow within the pseudoaneurysm. Use color flow imaging as a guide to place the sample volume for this recording. Measure peak systolic velocity (PSV) when directed.

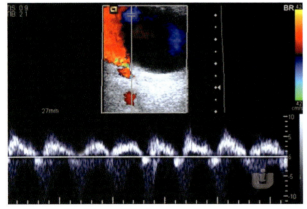

Fig. 42-10: *Flow within the pseudoaneurysm cavity*

Longitudinal Scan and Images

- **Scan arteries:** Perform spectral Doppler waveform analysis in the adjacent arteries above and below the PA and its neck. Measure PSV. When recording PSV in the longitudinal plane with spectral Doppler, use a ≤60° Doppler angle with a sample volume that is in the center of the flow stream.

    Example: *For a groin PA, assess common femoral, proximal superficial femoral and deep femoral arteries.*

- **Scan veins:** Perform spectral Doppler waveform analysis in the adjacent veins as well as above and below the PA and its neck. Assess for spontaneity, phasicity and augmentation of these venous signals. Record velocity when appropriate.

    Example: *For a groin PA, assess common femoral, proximal great saphenous, femoral and deep femoral veins.*

- Occasionally, there may be multiple lobes or multiple pseudoaneurysms present. Evaluate all lobes or pseudoaneurysms in the same manner described above.

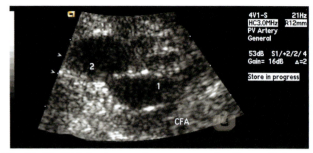

Fig. 42-11: *Bi-lobed pseudoaneurysm by B-mode image*

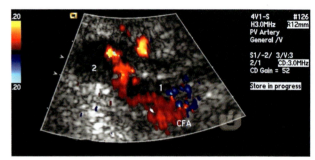

Fig. 42-12: *Bi-lobed pseudoaneurysm with color flow*

Table 42-1: Pseudoaneurysm Duplex Protocol Summary

- Document suspected area of PA using B-mode and color Doppler.
- Measure AP and transverse diameters of any pulsatile or non-pulsatile masses noted.
- Document depth of PA from skin.
- Identify communication site (or neck) between arterial source and PA. Measure diameter and length of neck.
- Document Doppler waveforms within the neck of the PA.
- Document flow within the PA using color and spectral Doppler.
- Document PSV and waveform patterns in the arterial and venous segments above and below the level of the PA.

Ultrasound-Guided Pseudoaneurysm Repair Using Thrombin Injection [1]

- Document pre-injection pedal pulses and/or ABIs.
- Create a sterile field for the injection procedure. Probe covers and sterile gel may be used.

Pre and post-procedural ABI measurements can detect embolic complications resulting from repair procedures.

- Pain medication or local anesthetic is administered to the patient before injection at the physician's discretion.
- Place the transducer over the PA so it can be visualized by B-mode image, while leaving sufficient access for injection needles.

- The physician will typically insert a 21-22 gauge endoscopic needle with an echogenic tip containing thrombin at 1000 U/mL. A biopsy guide may be used.
- After confirming with duplex that the echogenic needle tip is within the PA cavity, turn on color Doppler.
- The physician will slowly inject the thrombin into the cavity. Observe for immediate thrombosis of the PA upon injection.

Observe patients for complaints of local or distal symptoms (e.g., sudden lower extremity numbness or pain, toe discoloration) which may result from thrombosis of local arteries or micro thrombotic embolization during any repair.

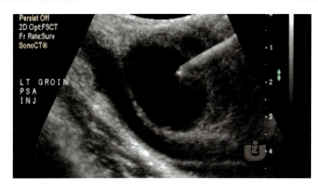

Fig. 42-13: *Confirm needle is within PA by B-mode.*

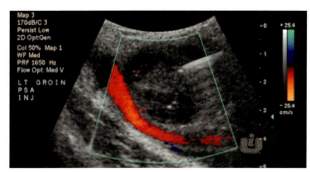

Fig. 42-14: *Once thrombin is injected into PA, thrombosis is noted.*

- Additional thrombin may need to be redirected to other areas within the PA cavity should partial color flow remain. Avoid injecting too close to the native artery as this may introduce thrombin into the native vessel.
- Reassess for flow within the PA cavity using color and spectral Doppler. (use low-sensitivity settings to detect any possible flow)
- Document post-injection pedal pulses and/or ABIs.
- Re-image the PA and surrounding area 20 minutes post-injection to confirm total thrombosis.

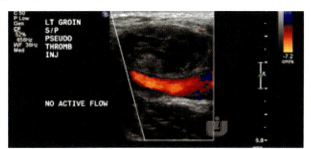

Fig. 42-15: *No color flow in pseudoaneurysm cavity post-injection.*

Table 42-2: Ultrasound-Guided Pseudoaneurysm Injection Protocol Summary

- Document pre-injection pedal pulses and/or ABIs.
- Image PA using B-mode while physician inserts a needle into the PA cavity.
- Using color duplex, monitor flow within the PA cavity as physician injects thrombin.
- Confirm complete thrombosis of PA using color flow and spectral Doppler.
- Document post-injection ABIs and arterial Doppler waveforms in peri-PA arteries.

PRINCIPLES OF INTERPRETATION

B-mode Imaging and Color Doppler

- Measure AP and transverse diameters of any pulsatile or non-pulsatile masses noted and measure depth from the skin.
- Measure diameter and length of neck.
- Document flow within the PA using color Doppler.

Spectral Doppler Waveforms

Please see the UE/LE Arterial Duplex chapter for a detailed description of arterial waveform terminology.

- Analyze communication site (or neck) between arterial source and PA.
- Document Doppler waveforms within the neck of the PA.
- Document flow within the PA using spectral Doppler.
- Measure PSV and document waveform patterns in the native arterial and venous segments.

Interpretation/Diagnostic Criteria

Pre-Intervention

B-mode Imaging

- A pulsatile mass observed communicating with a native artery or arterial graft is indicative of a pseudoaneurysm. To-and-fro Doppler flow patterns will be apparent within the "neck" of the PA.
- Intramural thrombus may or may not be observed by duplex within the pseudoaneurysm.

Spectral Doppler Waveforms

- Changes in spectral waveform (depending on the terminology used by the lab), post stenotic turbulence and color bruit may be observed in the arterial segments above and below the pseudoaneurysm, but are more likely to be unchanged except for a focal area at the exit site.

Post-Thrombin Injection

B-mode Imaging and Color Doppler

- Expect thrombus to form immediately while imaging after thrombin injection and color flow to cease as a result.
- Use color flow to confirm complete thrombosis of the PA and patency of the artery/vein post injection.
- There is a change in the echogenicity within the pseudoaneurysm cavity from pre-injection (echolucent) to post injection (echogenic).

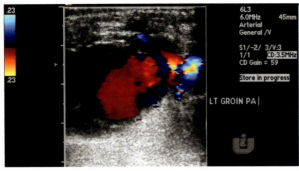

Fig. 42-16: *Pseudoaneurysm pre-injection by color flow*

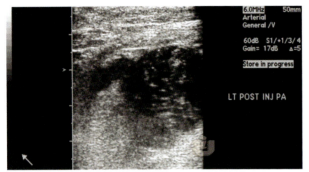

Fig. 42-17: *Same pseudoaneurysm post-injection. Note echoic thrombus in B-mode.*

Spectral Doppler Waveforms

- There should be no change between pre-injection and post-injection ABI/pedal pulses. A significant change in either is indicative of intra-arterial thrombus or embolization, post-injection.
- It is important to check the peri-mass native artery for thrombus formation following injection.

Differential Diagnosis

- Hematoma without communication to an artery
- Hyperemic lymph nodes
- Arteriovenous fistula
- Vascular mass

Correlation

- CT angiography
- Angiography

Medical Treatment

- Follow-up observation of pseudoaneurysms <2cm in diameter
- Thrombin injection under duplex ultrasound-guidance
- Duplex-guided compression repair

Surgical Treatment

- Open repair to evacuate the hematoma and repair the arterial wall
- In hemodialysis conduits: resection of the pseudoaneurysm site and surrounding graft
- Interposition graft placement or bypass around the affected segment

Pseudoaneurysms may spontaneously thrombose without treatment, so not all pseudoaneurysms require treatment. [3]

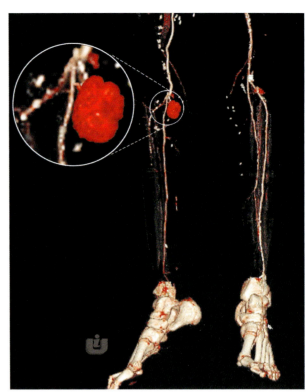

Fig. 42-18: *CT angiogram (in 3-D) of a pseudoaneurysm off a bypass graft*

Endovascular Treatment

- Covered stent

RESOURCES

1. Kang, SS, (2005). Pseudoaneurysm: diagnosis and treatment. In Mansour MA, Labropoulos N. (Eds.), Vascular Diagnosis, (319-323). Philadelphia: Elsevier Saunders.
2. Lenartova M, Tak T. (2003). Iatrogenic pseudoaneurysm of femoral artery: case report and literature review. *Clinical Medicine & Research*. 1(3): 243-247
3. Burke BJ, Friedman SG. (2005). Ultrasound in the diagnosis and management of arterial emergencies. In Zwiebel WJ, Pellerito JS (Eds.), Introduction to Vascular Ultrasonography 5th ed, (381-399). Philadelphia: Elsevier Saunders
4. Lumsden AB, Peden E, Bush RL, Lin PH. (2005). Complications of endovascular procedures. In Rutherford *Vascular Surgery 6th edition*. (809-820) Philadelphia. Elsevier Saunders.
5. Adams ED, Sidway AN. (2005). Nonthrombotic complications of arteriovenous access for hemodialysis. In Rutherford *Vascular Surgery 6th edition*. (1692-1706) Philadelphia. Elsevier Saunders.v

ADDITIONAL TESTING
43. Thoracic Outlet Testing

Definition
A non-invasive physiological test or duplex evaluation comparing upper extremity waveform patterns at rest and during provocative postural maneuvers.

Rationale
The thoracic outlet is comprised of the clavicle, first rib and the scalene muscle. Either the subclavian vessels or nerve network, known as the *brachial plexus*, can be compressed by the bones/muscles at the thoracic outlet as they leave the chest (TOS-thoracic outlet syndrome).

Arterial compression can cause flow disturbance in certain arm or shoulder positions, disruption of the intimal layer, aneurysm, thrombosis or embolism. This compression can be reflected in the arterial waveform as a marked reduction or cessation of the arterial flow signal.

The nerve and/or vein may also be compressed at the thoracic outlet but this chapter concentrates on non-invasive arterial and venous testing resulting from thoracic outlet compression.

Etiology (Symptoms from TOS)
- Extrinsic compression of artery, vein and/or nerve at the thoracic outlet
- Thrombus in the SCV
- Atherosclerosis
- Trauma to the vessel
- Embolization from the subclavian/axillary arteries
- Aneurysm

Risk Factors
- Anatomical variations of the cervical ribs
- Head or neck trauma
- Large pectoral muscles
- Hyperlipidemia
- Excessive breast tissue
- Obesity
- History of radiation
- Klipple-Fiel Syndrome

Indications for Exam
- Thoracic outlet symptoms (numbness, tingling, arm pain in certain positions)
- Claudication (exercise-related arm pain)
- Bruit (abnormal sound heard through ausculation caused by turbulent flow vibration)
- Limb pain at rest
- Digital cyanosis
- Arterial aneurysm
- Upper extremity swelling indicates venous testing

Contraindications/Limitations
- Upper extremity venous thrombosis is a contraindication to arterial testing.
- Patient's inability to perform functional maneuvers
- Direct imaging of the subclavian vessels is limited by the clavicle.
- Patients with extensive bandages or casts which cannot be removed limits direct visualization.
- Obesity or severe edema (depth of vessels)
- Open wounds can limit access with the imaging transducer.

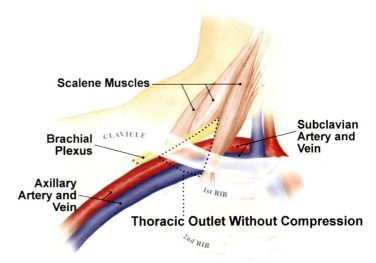

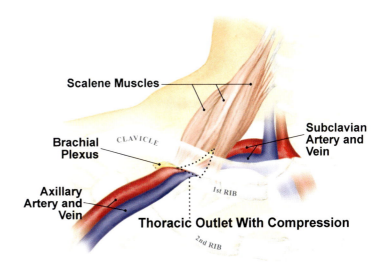

Fig. 43-1: Upper extremity arterial and venous anatomy. Illustrated with and without compression in the thoracic outlet region

Mechanism of Syndrome

Mechanical compression of the subclavian vein or artery can occur in the thoracic outlet region. Anatomical defects, such as a congenital abnormality of the first rib or fracture of the clavicle, are examples of possible sources of this compression. There are three causes for the types of thoracic outlet syndrome: neurogenic, venous and arterial.

The cause of thoracic outlet syndrome (TOS) is neurogenic in 93% of cases. A venous cause is present in 5%, while an arterial cause is present in only 1% of cases.[9] A combination of these causes is also possible.[1]

Types of thoracic outlet syndrome [1]

- **Neurogenic** (most common): compression of the brachial plexus from the cervical ribs, first rib, anterior scalene muscles, congenital myofascial bands and ligaments
- **Venous**: also known as *effort thrombosis* or *Paget-Schroetter syndrome* results from repetitive trauma to the subclavian vein (SCV).[5] Arm abduction causes the SCV to be compressed against the first rib and scalenus anticus muscle, causing the trauma. Venous thrombosis can result.
- **Arterial** (least common): The head of the humerus can cause arterial compression when the arm is abducted and externally rotated. Extrinsic compression of the SCA, post-stenotic dilatation or aneurysm develops. The typical pathogenesis then is focal compression, dilation, ulceration, and thrombus formation.[1]
- Venous or arterial compression results in:
  » **Stenosis**: Significant narrowing of the artery or vein, decreasing the vessel lumen and possibly resulting in decreased blood flow.
  » **Occlusion**: Plaque, thrombus, or external compression of the artery or vein completely blocking blood flow in that segment.
  » **Embolization**: Contents of a plaque and/or fragments of an organized thrombus become lodged in a distant blood vessel.
  » **Swelling**: Significant compression of the subclavian vein causes limb swelling.

Approximately 25% of the population have asymptomatic compression.[6]

Location of Disease

- Subclavian vein
- Subclavian artery
- Distal obstruction caused by emboli from a thoracic outlet artery

Patient History

- Cold/painful/numb extremity during certain limb positions
- Claudication
- Limb pain at rest
- Acute arterial occlusive symptoms
- Previously fractured clavicle
- History of upper extremity venous thrombosis
- Swelling
- Regular exercise of upper extremity (e.g., weight lifting)

Physical Examination

- Most of these patients will present with thromboembolic symptoms.
- Patients also present with ischemic complications secondary to repeated episodes of embolization.
- Bruit (abnormal sound heard through auscultation caused by turbulent flow vibration)
- Cyanosis
- Marked temperature difference between hand/fingers
- Pallor
- Pulselessness
- Rubor
- Palpable thrill (vibration caused by turbulent blood flow)
- Swelling

Thoracic Outlet Testing Protocol

- Obtain a patient history to include symptoms and risk factors. Explain the procedure you will perform to the patient.
- Patient is examined in a sitting position with the hands palm up, resting on a pillow in the patient's lap.

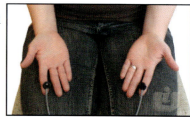

Fig. 43-2: *Resting Position*

NOTE: A baseline upper extremity arterial physiologic exam at rest is recommended prior to performing provocative maneuvers to check for underlying arterial disease.

- Perform a baseline exam at rest of either the digits using photoplethysmography (PPG), or of the upper extremity using volume pulse recording (VPR). Duplex imaging of the subclavian vessels may also be used as an additional baseline study. Any asymptomatic digits/hand can be used as a baseline or comparison to the symptomatic hand.

Continuous wave Doppler is not recommended for TOS testing since one can easily slip off the vessel and misinterpret an obstruction.

PPG

- Attach the PPG photocell to the pad of the digit using double-stick tape. Typically, the index finger is used. However, any symptomatic digit may also be tested.
- Alternative sensors used by some labs include a digital clip similar to a pulse oximeter which eliminates the need for tape or Velcro to keep the sensor in place.

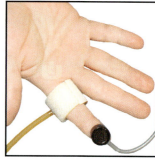

Fig. 43-3: *PPG Placement on Digit*

- The PPG device with strip chart recorder or computer monitor is set to the "arterial" or AC setting.
- Run the PPG recording at a slow speed (5mm/sec) to record the amplitude of the waveform. Center the PPG tracings on the paper or monitor. Ideally the baseline tracing consists of a series of horizontal pulses.
- Continue recording while performing the functional maneuvers listed at the end of this section. Observe for significant waveform changes.

VPR

- Apply cuffs with 10-12cm bladder (in width) on the upper arm and forearm bilaterally.
- Inflate the cuff to 65mmHg. Set the gain settings appropriately to create a waveform that is moderate in amplitude. Settings should not be changed while the positional maneuvers are being performed.

Particular VPR gain settings are not necessary for TOS testing, as long as waveforms are moderately sized.

- Record baseline VPR waveforms at each level.
- Record VPR waveforms while performing the functional maneuvers listed at the end of this section. Observe for any waveform changes.

Duplex Imaging

Venous Duplex

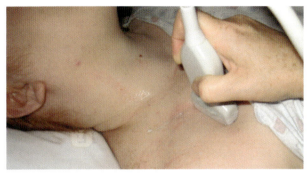

Fig. 43-4: *Probe position for visualization of the distal subclavian-proximal axillary arteries and veins.*

- Locate the subclavian vein (SCV) and axillary vein (AXV). Observe for patency and look for venous thrombosis.
- Record baseline waveforms and peak velocities in the proximal and distal SCV and AXV.
- Have the patient perform the functional maneuvers listed at the end of this section slowly while re-recording the distal SCV and AXV waveforms. Observe for any waveform changes.
- Record additional velocities and waveforms proximal, at and distal to any venous stenosis.
- Note any symptoms the patient experiences during these maneuvers. Patients may test positively without any symptoms so this is also very important to note.

Arterial Duplex

- Locate the subclavian artery (SCA) above the clavicle and the proximal axillary artery (AXA) below the clavicle and record baseline waveforms and PSV. Remember to set the Doppler angle parallel to flow in order to measure accurate arterial velocities.
- Ask the patient to slowly perform the functional maneuvers listed at the end of this section while re-recording the SCA and AXA waveforms and measuring the PSV. Observe for any waveform and velocity changes.
- Record additional waveforms proximal, at and distal to any stenosis.

Thoracic Outlet Functional Maneuvers [2,3]

Note: Some labs choose to constantly move the arm through any and all positions while recording tracings, describing what positions cause a change and symptoms. Other labs prefer to document responses to certain standard positions.

The most important positions are with the shoulder back and the arm back at 180° and any position the patient reports causing symptoms.

These positions can be performed one arm at a time, or simultaneously if equipment allows monitoring of both arms at once.

- **Adson's maneuver:** Instruct the patient to take a deep breath in, hold it, and look over the right shoulder, then over the left shoulder while recording the waveforms.
- **Costoclavicular maneuver:** The shoulders are in exaggerated "military" position (back and down). Instruct the patient to look over the right and left shoulders while recording the waveforms.
- **Hyperabduction:** The arms are extended straight out to the side (90°) with the shoulders back and while the patient looks to their right and left. Next the arms are positioned straight over-head (180°) while the shoulders are back and the patient looks to their right and left sides. Record waveforms during each maneuver.
- **Alternative positions:** Question the patient whether there is a special position they know to cause symptoms. Record waveforms during these maneuvers. Take note whether there is signal loss at the same time the patient experiences symptoms during testing.

Functional Positions for TOS Testing

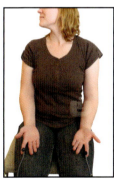
Adson's maneuver with head turned

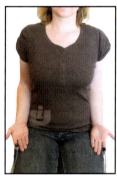
Costoclavicular maneuver with head straight

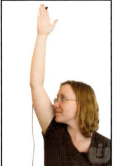
Arm abducted 180° with head turned

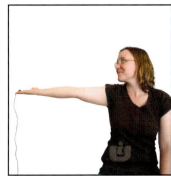
Arm abducted 90° with head turned

Fig. 43-5: *Functional positions for TOS testing.*

Table 43-1: **Thoracic Outlet Examination Protocol Summary**

- Using PPG, VPR or duplex scanning, obtain baseline arterial waveforms in the upper extremity with the patient in a neutral position (e.g., sitting). Duplex scanning is the method used to obtain baseline venous waveforms.
- Instruct the patient to perform functional maneuvers while re-recording vessel waveforms.
- Typical maneuvers include:
  - » Adson's
  - » Costoclavicular
  - » Hyperabduction
  - » Any alternative position the patient can describe which evokes symptoms
- Compare baseline waveforms to those performed during exercise.
- Ask the patient if the symptoms develop during the maneuvers and observe for the presence or absence of pulses/color flow at that time.

PRINCIPLES OF INTERPRETATION

PPG Digital Waveforms

The PPG waveform from any digit is categorized as *pulsatile, reduced or non-pulsatile* based on the upstroke (amplitude) of the waveform and downslope and compared at rest and during provocative postural maneuvers.

B-mode Imaging

- Use B-mode imaging to determine if a thrombus is present. *For a detailed description for venous thrombosis interpretation see the Upper Extremity Venous Duplex chapter.*
- Confirm the vein collapses completely with light transducer pressure.

Color Doppler

- Wall-to-wall color flow will fill the artery/vein spontaneously and upon distal compression in the veins.
- Use color Doppler to determine if color flow is present wall-to-wall or if a filling defect is present.

Spectral Doppler Waveforms and Flow Velocities

- Compare baseline arterial/venous waveforms and velocities to those performed during exercise.

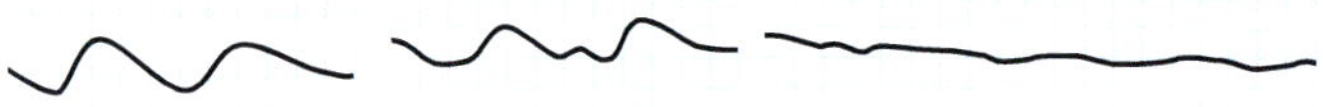

Neutral position	Hyperabduction 90° (no change)	Hyperabduction 180° (abnormal loss of signal)

Fig. 43-6: *PPG Waveforms: TOS Testing*

Interpretation of Arterial Waveforms

A flat PPG tracing or obliteration of the CW Doppler signal may occur even in normal patients when raising the arm overhead.[3] In such cases, question whether the patient is experiencing symptoms at the time. If not, such findings are suggestive of asymptomatic TOS.

Normal

PPG Digital Waveforms

- Normal waveforms exclude the presence of significant compression/disease.[8] Normal PPG waveform characteristics include:[4,6,7,9]
  - » Short onset to peak (subjective)
  - » Downslope that bows toward the baseline
  - » A dicrotic notch in the downslope
- The amplitude of any waveform tracing during maneuvers should remain unchanged or increase compared to baseline. A slight decrease (without patient complaint of symptoms) is not suggestive of significant TOS.[4-6]

B-mode Imaging

- The artery is free of echogenic material.

Color Doppler

- Wall-to-wall color flow will fill the artery.

Spectral Doppler Waveforms and Flow Velocities

- There is uniform flow and change in the baseline waveforms or velocities recorded in the SCA by duplex scan during functional maneuvers. (Vratio <2.0).

Abnormal

PPG Digital Waveforms

- Abnormal ("reduced") PPG waveform characteristics (secondary to obstruction) include:[4,6,9]
  - » Prolonged onset to peak (subjective)
  - » Rounded peak
  - » Downslope that bows away from the baseline
- An "absent" or non-pulsatile digital waveform is reported when the PPG tracing reflects a flat-line. An obstruction is suspected.[4]
- **Thoracic outlet compression** is suggested when the arterial signal demonstrates a highly significant, persistent decrease in waveform amplitude or the waveform completely disappears during functional maneuvers and the patient experiences symptoms during the loss of pulse.[4,6]

B-mode Imaging

- There is echogenic material within the arterial lumen.

Color Doppler

- Color flow does not fill the artery wall-to-wall.

Spectral Doppler Waveforms and Flow Velocities

- **Arterial stenosis:** A subclavian artery (SCA) stenosis is identified by duplex scan during functional maneuvers. A significant stenosis is at least a two-fold increase from the baseline velocity followed by post-stenotic turbulence.[5]

It is very important to ensure the Doppler sample volume remains within the artery and has not moved off during positional changes.

Interpretation of Venous Waveforms

Normal

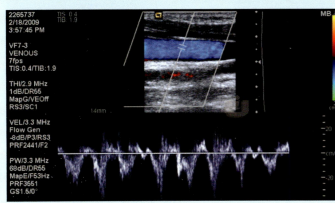

Fig. 43-7: *Normal venous Doppler waveform during TOS testing.*

B-mode Imaging
- The veins are free of echogenic material and compress completely when it is technically possible.

Color Doppler
- Wall-to-wall color flow will fill the vein spontaneously and upon distal compression.

Spectral Doppler Waveforms and Flow Velocities
- The main characteristics of the venous waveform considered in TOS testing are spontaneity and phasicity. A normal venous waveform demonstrates:
  » **Spontaneity:** The vein demonstrates spontaneous flow, especially in the central veins (jugular, brachiocephalic (innominate), subclavian) and axillary vein. In the distal arm veins, the absence of spontaneous flow can be a normal finding.
  » **Phasicity:** Venous signals are phasic and vary with respiration and the cardiac cycle. During deep exhalation, venous signals typically decrease or discontinue and increase with inhalation due to changes in intrathoracic pressures during the respiratory cycle.
- There should be no significant change in the venous flow velocity at rest and during provocative postural maneuvers. The phasic respirations expected of any venous tracing should remain unchanged or increase compared to baseline waveforms during maneuvers. A slight decrease (without patient complaint of symptoms) is not suggestive of significant TOS. [4,5]

Abnormal

B-mode Imaging
Venous thrombosis
- Intralumenal echoes are visualized within the vein and the vein is not completely compressible. Partial or totally occlusive venous thrombosis can be present in the subclavian vein/axillary segment. [5]

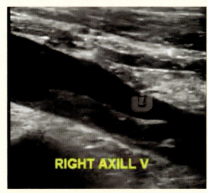

Fig. 43-8: *Acute thrombosis of the axillary vein*

- Refer to the *UE Venous Duplex* chapter for information on how to report the age of any identify venous thrombus.

Color Doppler
- If a thrombus does not completely inhibit blood flow, color flow will be seen flowing around echogenic material.
- Use color flow in the adjacent artery as a guide to identify an occluded vein. But always confirm the absence of flow by placing sample volume in the vessel while using spectral Doppler.

Spectral Doppler Waveforms and Flow Velocities
- **Spontaneity:** Reduced Doppler waveforms indicate venous compression/obstruction. The absence of spontaneous flow by spectral Doppler indicates total venous obstruction. Use color flow in the adjacent artery to confirm reduced/absent flow when an obstructed vein is suspected.
- **Phasicity:** Reduced phasicity or continuous venous flow (does not vary with respiratory and cardiac cycles) suggests compression/obstruction in the vein.
- **Venous thrombosis:** Partially occlusive thrombus can still produce spontaneous, phasic signals with augmentation.
- **Thoracic outlet compression** is suggested when the venous signal significantly loses phasic respiration or the signal completely disappears during functional maneuvers [7] and the patient experiences symptoms during loss of the signal.
- **Venous stenosis:** A hemodynamically significant venous stenosis is diagnosed when there is a velocity ratio of at least 2.5 in comparison to the adjacent venous segment. [8] An increased velocity may be demonstrated as the vein is compressed, followed by cessation of venous flow if the vein becomes totally occluded by the compression. The increased flow velocity may only be demonstrated if insonation is at or very near the point of compression. Velocity ratios (Vr):

$$\frac{\text{Highest peak systolic velocity}}{\text{PSV of the proximal normal segment } (V_1)}$$

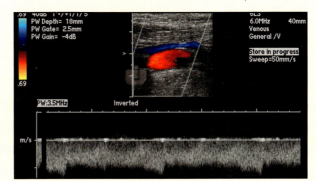

Fig. 43-9: *Compression of the vein suspected by Doppler waveform during TOS maneuvers since there is loss of phasicity. Set angle and calculate venous velocity ratios in this area to confirm.*

Table 43-2: Diagnostic Criteria for TOS Disease

Normal

- Amplitude of the arterial waveform remains unchanged or increases compared to baseline.
- Spontaneous, phasic respirations of venous tracings remain unchanged or increase compared to baseline.

Abnormal

- Amplitude of the arterial waveform decreases compared to baseline during functional maneuvers AND the patient experiences symptoms during loss of pulse.
- Spontaneous, phasic respirations of venous tracings decrease compared to baseline or is completely lost during functional maneuvers AND the patient experiences symptoms during loss of signal.
- Vr ≥2.5 suggest a venous stenosis.

Differential Diagnosis for Arterial or Venous TOS

- Nerve compression or nerve diseases
- Vascular compression by tumors
- Musculoskeletal problems
- Venous thrombosis, without venous compressions at the thoracic outlet
- Arterial obstruction or emboli proximal or distal to the thoracic outlet

Correlation

- Duplex ultrasound
- Spiral CT scan
- MRA
- Arteriography

Medical Treatment

- Modify risk factors (e.g., reduce cholesterol, manage HTN and DM, smoking cessation)
- Anti-inflammatory meds
- Muscle relaxants
- Physical therapy
- Anticoagulation (warfarin)

Surgical Treatment

- Removal of the first rib or cervical rib
- Dividing scalene muscle attachments and fibromuscular bands
- Cervical sympathectomy
- Resection (aneurysmal disease)
- Embolectomy
- Breast reduction

Endovascular Treatment

- Angioplasty
- Stent
- Intra-arterial directed thrombolysis

REFERENCES

1. Kreienberg PB, Shah, DM, Darling III, RC, Change BB, Paty SK, Roddy SP, Ozsvath KJ, Manish,, (2005). Thoracic Outlet Syndrome. In Mansour MA, Labropoulos N. (Eds.), *Vascular Diagnosis*, (517-522). Philadelphia,: Elsevier Saunders.
2. Daigle, R. (2002). Arterial evaluation of the upper extremities. In Daigle, R. (Ed.) *Techniques in non-invasive vascular diagnosis*. (187-196). Littleton: Summer Publishing..
3. Myers K, Clogh A, (2004). Disease of vessels to the upper limbs: In *Making Sense of Vascular Ultrasound*, (227-254). London: Hodder Arnold.
4. Talbot, SR, and Zwiebel, WJ. (2005). Assessment of upper extremity arterial occlusive disease. In Zwiebel, WJ (Ed). *Introduction to Vascular Ultrasonography (5th ed)* (297-323). Philadelphia: Elsevier.
5. Longo MG, Pearce WH, Sumner DS. (2005). Evaluation of upper extremity ischemia. In *Rutherford Vascular Surgery 6th edition*. (1274-1293). Philadelphia. Elsevier Saunders
6. Raines JK. (1993). The pulse volume recording in peripheral arterial disease. In Bernstein EF (Ed). Vascular Diagnosis 4th ed. (534-553). St Louis: Mosby
7. Green RM. (2005). Subclavian-axillary vein thrombosis. In *Rutherford Vascular Surgery 6th edition*. (1371-1384). Philadelphia. Elsevier Saunders.
8. Leon, LR, Labropoulos, N, Mansour MA. (2005). Hemodynamic principles as applied to diagnostic testing. In Mansour MA, Labropoulos N. (Eds.), Vascular Diagnosis, (7-21). Philadelphia: Elsevier Saunders.
9. Thompson RW, Bartoli MA. (2005). Neurogenic thoracic outlet syndrome. In *Rutherford Vascular Surgery 6th edition*. (1347-1365). Philadelphia. Elsevier Saunders.

ADDITIONAL TESTING
44. Penile Testing

Definition
The combination of real time B-mode imaging with spectral and color flow Doppler and/or systolic blood pressures to evaluate the penile arterial system.

Etiology (erectile dysfunction)
- Psychogenic
- Neurogenic/neurologic
- Arterial insufficiency
- Hormonal imbalance
- Cavernosal venous leak/venous insufficiency/impaired venous occlusion
- Scarring/fibrosis of the sinusoidal tissue

Risk Factors
- Hypertension
- Hypercholesteremia
- Diabetes
- Peripheral arterial occlusive disease
- Smoking
- Prostatectomy
- Hypogonadism
- Peyronie's disease (calcified plaque or fibrosis affecting the tunica albuginea)
- Coronary artery disease
- Vascular surgery (e.g., aortoiliac bypass, etc.)
- Spinal surgery
- Pelvic surgery

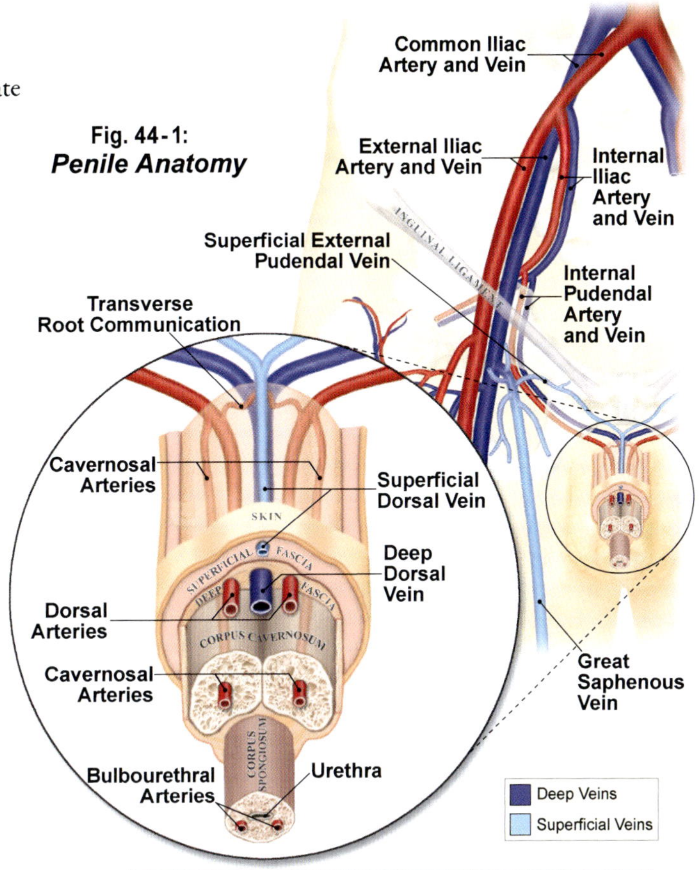

Indications for Exam
- Impotence
- Peyronie's disease
- Penile ischemia/pain
- Penile fracture/trauma

Contraindications/Limitations
- Due to the small arteries involved, duplex imaging is often difficult for a single technologist to perform without assistance, especially when working with machine controls.
- Calipers for measurement must be placed quickly. Even slight movements of the transducer can skew measurements during the process.
- Injection of a vasodilator is not recommended for all patients (e.g., patients with a penile prosthesis, history of priapism, etc.).[10]

Penile Anatomy
- The penis is composed of three chambers of spongy tissue, two corpus cavernosum, and one corpus spongiosum. A thick fascia called the *tunica albuginea* surrounds these corpora.
  » The paired corpus cavernosum (a.k.a. corpora cavernosa) contain sinusoidal chambers comprised of smooth muscle which are partially responsible for changes in resistance within the penis. The spongy tissue in these chambers fills with blood during an erection. A septum divides both corpora cavernosa.
  » A single corpus spongiosum surrounds the urethra and is located on the dorsal plantar side of the penis.
- The urethra travels through the center of the corpus spongiosum.

Penile Arteries and Inflow
- The internal iliac artery (a.k.a. hypogastric artery) and internal pudendal arteries supply blood flow to the groin.

Fig. 44-1: **Penile Anatomy**

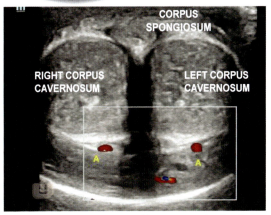

Fig. 44-2: *Penile anatomy: Transverse duplex image illustrates the three chambers of the penis*

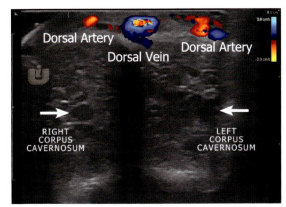

Fig. 44-3: *Dorsal artery and veins: transverse view*

- The internal pudendal artery has several branches (perineal, bulbar and urethral) before continuing as the penile artery. There are several terminal branches:
  » **Cavernosal arteries**: responsible for transporting blood to the main erectile tissues of the penis (corpora cavernosa).
    - Right cavernosal artery
    - Left cavernosal artery
    - The helicine arteries, which originate from the cavernosal arteries bring blood to the corpus cavernosa. [10]
  » **Dorsal artery (a.k.a. superficial dorsal artery)**: The two arteries responsible for supplying blood to the skin, corpus spongiosum and glans penis.
- There are multiple small connections between the cavernosal and dorsal arteries.

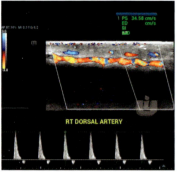

Fig. 44-4: Color duplex and waveform of the dorsal artery.

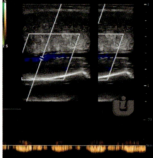

Fig. 44-5: Color duplex and waveform of the dorsal vein.

  » **Urethral artery** (a.k.a. spongiosal): responsible for transporting blood to the corpus spongiosum (urethral) and the Cowper's gland (bulbar).

Penile Veins and Outflow
- **Superficial dorsal vein**: Drains the blood from the skin
- The cavernosa is drained by the following veins:
  » Emissary veins empty into the circumflex veins and ultimately the deep dorsal veins
  » Internal pudendal vein
  » Hypogastric vein

Normal Fluid Dynamics
- Normal flow in the penis differs depending on the physiological state.
- In a non-erectile state (flaccid), there is low resistance to arterial inflow because blood flows from the arteries to the veins of the penis through a series of pre-cavernosal arterio-venous (AV) shunts. Arterioles within the cavernosa are constricted in the flaccid state.
- Increased resistance is needed to maintain an erectile state. As the penis approaches an erectile state:
  » Arterioles dilate within each cavernosum, so that resistance decreases. Blood flow in the cavernosal arteries increases, resulting in low-resistance Doppler waveforms.
  » AV shunts start to close, resulting in an increased perfusion pressure to the penis.
  » The sinusoidal chambers fill with blood causing expansion of the corpora cavernosa. Increased flow resistance in the corpora cavernosa causes occlusion of the outflow veins, so the blood flow cannot leave the sinusoidal chambers.
  » When the sinusoidal chambers fill, eventually the arterial inflow decreases, indicated by a high resistance Doppler waveform.

Successful erections have been documented with peak systolic velocities of <29cm/s, and diastolic values at zero.

Mechanism of Disease
There are several mechanisms that may contribute to erectile dysfunction (ED); anatomical, vascular, neurogenic or hormonal. [1,2]
- Failure of the AV shunts to close negatively affects flow resistance. Incompetent veins allow blood flow to leak out of the penis, reducing rigidity. [1]
- Failure to maintain adequate arterial flow results in the inability to obtain or maintain an erection. This may be due to lack of inflow by the arteries, extrinsic compression or narrowing. [1]
- Lack of psycho-erotic stimulation, heavy smoking, the use of antihypertensive drugs, etc. may fail to produce the neurochemical reaction or parasympathetic innervations needed to produce erection. [1,2]
- **Priapism** is a painful condition of sustained persistent erection unaccompanied by sexual excitement lasting for >4 hrs. [9]
  » Priapism is a potential complication post injection.
  » Priapism is also a complication in sickle cell patients.
  » Types include:
    - **Ischemic** (veno occlusive, low-flow): Ischemic is the most common type and can be caused by pelvic vascular thrombosis, dorsal penile vein thrombosis, drug therapy, or may be idiopathic.
    - **Non-ischemic** (arterial, high flow): Non-ischemic priapism is caused by unregulated arterial inflow, such as an AV fistula. This may be due to a recent trauma to the vasculature of the penis. Non-ischemic priapism does not usually present with penile pain as a symptom.
  » While both types may lead to erectile dysfunction if untreated, ischemic priapism can be painful and lead to penile necrosis or gangrene.
- **Peyronie's disease:** Scar tissue forms inside the penis causing pain in both the flaccid and erect states.

Location of Disease
- Cavernosal arteries

Patient History/Symptoms
- Impotence
- Penile pain

Physical Examination
Palpation of pulses at the groin can identify peripheral arterial disease. Poor groin pulses may indicate arterial inflow/vascular dysfunction issues.

Penile Testing Protocol
There are several techniques used to evaluate the penile vasculature. They include penile pressures, VPR tracings and duplex imaging. One or more of these techniques may be used during an evaluation and may include the injection of a vasodilator.

Duplex and penile pressures are appropriate for impotency testing and Peyronie's disease. Penile pressures are appropriate for ischemia and pain. Arterial duplex may also be used to help identify causes of priapism due to trauma.

Penile Arterial Duplex Protocol
(with and without injection)
- Obtain a patient history to include symptoms and risk factors.
- Explain the exam to the patient.
- The exam room temperature should be warm (21-24° C /70-75° F). Warm compressions applied to the penis can enhance visualization of the cavernosal artery.

- The patient is examined lying supine with the penis in a cephalad position.
- High-frequency (5-7 MHz) (8-15 MHz) linear transducers are used for imaging.

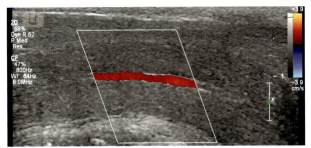

Fig. 44-6: *Pre-injection cavernosal artery by color flow*

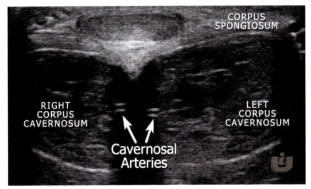

Fig. 44-7: *Pre-injection B-mode image-transverse view*

Pre-Injection Duplex

- Locate the two corpora cavernosa of the penis in the transverse (short axis) plane with B-mode imaging. The corpus spongiosum will be along the ventral side of the penis.

> To help hold the penis in place you can drape a folded towel across to maintain stability.

- Observe the echogenicity of the tissue, looking for areas of high echogenicity, as the penile tissue appears less hyperechoic than the arterial walls.
- Record B-mode images in the transverse plane of the corpora cavernosa and the corpus spongiosum. Observe for similar size between the right and left corpora cavernosa.
- Transverse diameter measurements should be taken of the cavernosal arteries at the base of the shaft. Measurements should be taken near or at systole.

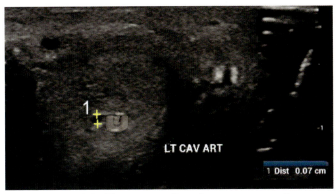

Fig. 44-8: *Transverse diameter measurement of the cavernosal artery*

- Record B-mode images in the longitudinal (sagittal) plane of the corpora cavernosa and the corpus spongiosum.

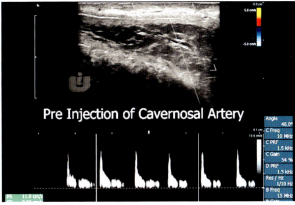

Fig. 44-9: *Cavernosal artery Doppler waveform pre-injection*

- Record and measure the peak systolic velocity (PSV) and end-diastolic velocity (EDV) at the base of the shaft using spectral Doppler (≤60° Doppler angle, with the angle cursor parallel to the vessel walls in the center of the flow stream) in the longitudinal plane of the proximal right and left cavernosal arteries.

Duplex with Injection

- The physician will inject a potent vasodilatory agent into the cavernosum (e.g., papaverine or proglastin E).[1] Only one side of the cavernosum will require injection due to communications across the intracavernosal septum.

> Normal erection time (duration) should be approximately 30 minutes.

- After intracavernosal injection of a vasodilator, the penis should be massaged by the patient to create an erection or place a 2-2.5cm penile pressure cuff or band on the penis for 2-3 minutes after injection and then remove.

> Response to the injection is enhanced if the dorsal vein at the base of the penis is compressed during the injection. If a poor erection is achieved, try placing a rubber band over the penile pressure cuff at base of penis. If improvement is noted, a venous leak is suspected.

- Record the PSV and EDV of the right and left cavernosal arteries for 20 minutes post injection in 5-minute increments (e.g., at 5 minutes, at 10 minutes, etc.). Color flow may be a useful tool to help locate these arteries.
- The inter-cavernosal arteries which balance the flows to the cavernosa are the *helicine arteries* and are seen most clearly during the immediate post-injection phase.
- Transverse diameter measurements should be taken of the cavernosal arteries at the base of the shaft. Measurements should be taken at systole and compared to pre-injection values.

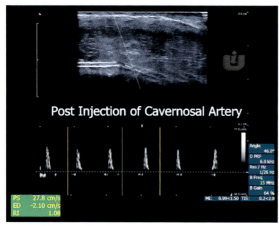

Fig. 44-10: *Cavernosal artery spectral waveforms post-injection*

Table 44-1: Penile Artery Duplex Protocol Summary

- Record baseline B-mode images of the corpus cavernosum and corpus spongiosum in transverse and longitudinal planes. Observe echogenicity of the tissues. Measure transverse diameter measurements of the cavernosal arteries.
- Record and measure the peak systolic velocity (PSV) and end diastolic velocity (EDV) in the right and left proximal cavernosal arteries.

If using intracavernosal injection:
- Inject vasodilator agent. Penis should be massaged by the patient to create an erection or wrap a tourniquet or penile pressure cuff around the base of the penis.
- Measure transverse diameter measurements of the cavernosal arteries, post injection for comparison to pre-injection values.
- Record and measure the PSV and EDV in the cavernosal arteries post-injection.
- Determine classification of disease according to laboratory diagnostic criteria.

Penile Artery Pressures Protocol

- Obtain a patient history to include symptoms and risk factors.
- Explain the procedure to the patient.
- The patient is examined in a supine position.
- Appropriately wrap a blood pressure cuff around the base of the penis. Also wrap pressure cuffs around the arm for brachial pressures. Cuffs should be placed "straight" rather than angled. All cuffs should fit snugly so that inflation of the bladder transmits the head of pressure into the tissue rather than into space between the bladder and the limb, producing falsely elevated readings.
- Locate the right and left proximal cavernosal arterial signals using a high frequency (8 MHz) CW Doppler transducer. (Use a lower frequency transducer (e.g., 4 MHz) when needed).
- Angle between 45-60°, pointing the transducer towards the heart. Manipulate the transducer slightly to obtain the strongest arterial signal. Record several representative cavernosal artery waveforms.
- The following instructions can be used when testing with an automatic cuff inflator or standard manometer:
  » Inflate the pressure cuffs 20-30mmHg above the last audible arterial signal heard using the Doppler transducer.

For patients with irregular heartbeats, decrease deflation speeds.

  » Deflate the cuff slowly (at a rate of 2-4mmHg per second). The systolic pressure is recorded as soon as the first audible arterial Doppler signal returns. The Doppler pulse must continue after hearing the first pulse to assure there is an actual pulse rather than motion artifact.
  » Obtain penile pressures using the right and left cavernosal arteries. Obtain bilateral brachial artery (BrA) pressures
  » Divide the highest cavernosal artery pressure by the highest brachial pressure to determine the penile-brachial index (PBI).
  » Determine severity of disease according to laboratory diagnostic criteria.

Table 44-2: Penile Pressures Protocol Summary

- Wrap an arterial cuff around the arm and obtain bilateral brachial artery blood pressures.
- Apply 2-2.5cm pressure cuff around the base of the penis.
- Using a high frequency 8MHz CW transducer, locate the cavernosal artery.
- Inflate the penile cuff until the Doppler signal is obliterated, about 20-30mmHg beyond the last audible arterial signal.
- Slowly decrease the pressure in the penile cuff at a rate of 2-4mmHg per second. The pressure is recorded as soon as the first audible arterial Doppler signal returns and continues.
- Calculate the penile-brachial index:

$$PBI = \frac{\text{Penile Pressure}}{\text{Higher Brachial Pressure}}$$

- Determine classification of disease according to laboratory diagnostic criteria

Penile VPR

- Patient is examined in the supine position. Explain the procedure to the patient.
- Cuffs should be placed "straight" rather than angled. Choose appropriately sized pneumatic cuffs for each section of the limb:
  » 12cm width; arm (some labs prefer a 10cm cuff)
  » 2-2.5cm width; base of penis
- Inflate the cuffs to approximately 60mmHg.
- Record VPR waveforms using the appropriate gain settings. (Consider the factory recommended settings of the VPR equipment being used).

Table 44-3: Penile VPR Protocol Summary

- Apply a 10-12cm arterial cuff around the arm and a 2-2.5cm pressure cuff around the base of the penis.
- Inflate the cuffs to approximately 60mmHg.
- Record VPR waveforms using the appropriate gain settings recommended for the VPR equipment used..

PRINCIPLES OF INTERPRETATION

VPR Tracings [7]
- The volume pulse waveform is primarily interpreted by its contour (shape) and amplitude (height).

Segmental Pressures
- Compare the arterial pressures/indices of the penis and bilateral lower extremity at the ankle.

B-mode Imaging

- Observe the echogenicity of the corpus cavernosum and corpus spongiosum tissues.
- Observe for intralumenal echoes in the arteries/veins.
- Assess transverse diameter measurements of the cavernosal arteries, pre- and post-injection.

Color Doppler

- Assess for wall-to-wall color filling in the appropriate direction for each segment.

Spectral Doppler Waveforms

See arterial chapters for a detailed description of arterial waveform terminology.

- Compare the resistance of the Doppler waveform patterns in the non-erect and erect states.
- Observe whether there is venous flow present during the erection.

Flow Velocities

- Determine PSV, EDV and flow direction, pre-and post-injection.

Interpretation/Diagnostic Criteria

Normal

VPR Tracings [7]

- Normal tracings demonstrate:
  - » Sharp upstroke
  - » Sharp systolic peak
  - » Gradual downslope bowing towards baseline
  - » Dicrotic notch, however some patients may have inward bowing on the downslope

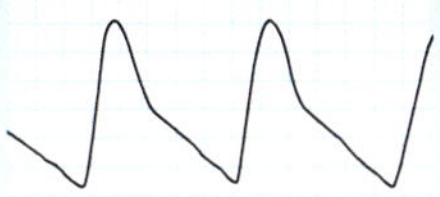

Fig. 44-11: *Normal penile VPR Tracing*

Segmental Pressures

- **PBI:** A normal penile-brachial index is >0.75. [2,8]

B-mode Imaging

Flaccid State

- General B-mode characteristics: Normal cavernosal tissue echogenicity is relatively homogeneous. The septum which divides both corpora cavernosa may normally produce acoustic shadowing. The walls of the cavernosal arteries may appear bright within the corpus cavernosa.
- The size of both corposa cavernosa should be symmetrical. The corpus spongiosum is typically smaller in comparison.

Erect State

- The injection site will be echogenic.
- The size of both corposa cavernosa should be larger than the flaccid state and small anechoic areas mixed with brightly echoic "dividers" will be noted in the spongiosum, representing the dilated sinusoids.
- The walls of the cavernosal arteries may become brightly echogenic.
- Diameters: Cavernosal arterial diameters should increase at a minimum 70-75% post-injection. [2,4]

Color Doppler [12]

Flaccid State

- Color flow fills the vessel lumen from wall-to-wall with appropriate settings. The cavernosal arteries may only be visualized at their origin in the flaccid state.

Erect State

- Color flow can normally appear to "reverse" as diastole lasts longer than systole post-injection.

Spectral Doppler Waveforms

Flaccid State

- High resistant arterial waveforms with low PSV and absent or reversed EDV are expected in the cavernosal arteries.

Erect State

- Normal response to a cavernosal injection: A low resistance waveform with high diastolic flow can be expected immediately post injection and may persist for 5 minutes. [1,4,6] As pressure increases in the intracavernosal space, the systolic peak will be sharper as the diastolic component decreases and eventually disappears.
- Waveforms may exhibit low resistant waveform characteristics if full erection is not achieved. A dicrotic notch is sometimes noted on waveforms recorded during the tumescence phase. [10]
- **Venous flow:** Venous flow in the dorsal vein is not normally observed during erection. [1,6]

Flow Velocities

Flaccid State

- Low PSV typically >12.5cm/s should be observed in the flaccid state. [6,12]
- In the flaccid state as filling occurs, PSV and EDV increase and then the EDV will decrease to zero by the full erectile state.

Erect State

- EDV when the penis is fully erect should be very low (<5cm/s) or reversed due to the increased resistance during erection. [3,4]
- *Note:* Maximum PSV usually occurs around 5 min after injection. Cavernosal artery PSV >29cm/s (post-injection) indicates normal arterial inflow adequate for an erection. [2,3,4]
- A difference in PSV of <10-15cm/s between the right and left cavernosal arteries is normal. [4]

Table 44-4: Diagnostic Criteria for Penile Brachial Index

- Normal: ≥0.75
- Marginal: 0.60-0.74
- Abnormal: <0.60

Source: Modified from Zierler RE, Sumner DS. (2005). Physiologic assessment of peripheral arterial occlusive disease. In *Rutherford Vascular Surgery 6th edition.* (197-222). Philadelphia. Elsevier Saunders.

Abnormal

VPR Tracings [7]

- Abnormal tracings demonstrate:
  - » Rounded systolic peak
  - » Loss of dicrotic notch [2]
  - » Downslope bends slightly away from the baseline
  - » Very low amplitude or flat, non-pulsatile tracing

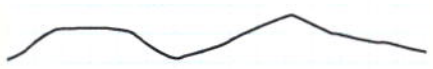

Fig. 44-12: *Abnormal Penile VPR Tracing*

Segmental Pressures

- **PBI:** Penile-brachial indices between 0.60-0.74 are considered marginally reduced.
- An abnormal penile-brachial index is <0.60. [2,8]

B-mode Imaging

- **General B-mode characteristics**: All areas of increased focal echogenicity should be noted. [4] Areas of increased focal echogenicity in the cavernosal tissue can indicate scarring or tunical plaques. [6]
- **Diameters:** An arterial diameter increase less than 70-75% post-injection in the cavernosal arteries indicates inadequate vessel compliance. [2,4]

Spectral Doppler Waveforms
- Waveform patterns remain low resistant throughout the flaccid and full erectile state.
- **Venous flow:** Continuous, rather than phasic flow in the dorsal vein may or may not be observed. [10]

Flow Velocities

Flaccid State
- Low PSV <12.5cm/s in the flaccid state would be abnormal. [12]

Erect State
- PSV <29cm/s (post-injection) indicates arterial insufficiency, especially when the PSV <25cm/s. [3,4]
- A difference in PSV of >10-15cm/s between the right and left cavernosal arteries also suggests underlying unilateral arterial disease. [4]

PSV should not be used for diagnosis in men with duplicated cavernosal arteries; the normal PSV may be <30cm/s. [6]

- **Venous flow:** Venous leakage can only be diagnosed by duplex when arterial flow is normal. When PSV are abnormal (<30cm/s), persistent EDV is less reliable. [11]
  » If arterial PSV are normal, but EDV >5cm/s, the persistent diastolic flow suggests failure of AV shunts to close and venous occlusive ED. Note: Abnormal EDV published in the literature ranges between 4.5-8cm/s. [1,4,5,6]

Other Pathology
- **Arteriovenous malformation (AVM):** An arteriovenous malformation such as an AV fistula can occur between any artery and an adjacent vein and is characterized by color bruit on duplex image along with high velocity, with pronounced end-diastolic flow, low-resistant spectral waveforms at the same site by spectral Doppler. [1,4]
- **Venous thrombosis:** Intralumenal echoes are visualized within the dorsal vein due to thrombus and the venous diameters may appear dilated in an acute event. Confirm the absence of venous flow with spectral Doppler and color flow (if possible) when suspected.

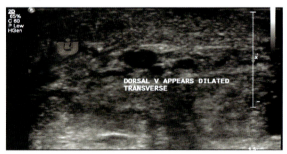

Fig. 44-13: *Acute occlusion suspected in the dorsal vein by B-mode image*

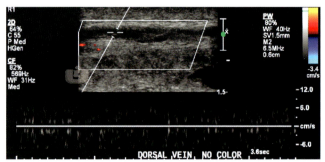

Fig. 44-14: *Acute occlusion confirmed in the dorsal vein by spectral Doppler*

- **Peyronie's disease:** Multiple, focal hyperechoic areas noted in both cavernosa are compatible with this condition. When echoes are limited to a single cavernosum, trauma may have been the cause instead. [10] Elevated flow may be noted by Doppler in early stages of Peyronie's due to inflammation.

Differential Diagnosis
- Arterial occlusive disease (ipsilateral)
- Pelvic steal
- Arterial vasospasm
- Neurological/nerve damage (e.g. spinal cord injury, CVA, diabetic neuropathy, Alzheimer's or Parkinson's disease)
- Endocrine disorders
- Hormone deficiency (e.g., hypogonadism, thyroid disease)
- Psychogenic (e.g., anxiety, depression, schizophrenia, stress)

Correlation
- Angiography
- Cavernosometry, with or without vasoreactive pharmacologic agents
- MRI
- Sonoelastography

Cavernosometry in conjunction with injection of a vasodilatory agent is the preferred method for diagnosing penile venous insufficiency. [6]

Pharmacology
- Vasodilators
  » Sildenafil (Viagra)
  » Tadalafil (Cialis)
  » Vardenafil (Levitra)
  » Alprostadil
  » Yohimbine

Medical Treatment
- In erectile dysfunction cases that do not respond to pharmaceutical therapy, a vacuum device and constriction ring may be prescribed as a medical treatment.
- For priapism: Ischemic treatment includes ice packs, walking, and decompression of the corpora via large bore needle aspiration. In more severe cases, a temporary shunt from the cavernosa to the spongiosum may be placed to reduce swelling.

Surgical Treatment
- May include an implantation of a penile prosthesis.

Corrective actions for priapism vary by type. Ischemic treatment can include ice packs, walking, and decompression of the corpora via large bore needle aspiration. In more severe cases, a temporary shunt from the cavernosa to the spongiosum may be placed to provide a reduction in swelling.

REFERENCES
1. Kornic AL, Villemarette PY, Baum N, Hower Jr. JF. (1990). Vasculogenic impotence: diagnostic application of color flow Doppler. *The Journal of Vascular Technology.* 14(4) 173-179.
2. DePalma RG. (2005). Vasculogenic erectile dysfunction. In *Rutherford Vascular Surgery 6th edition.* (1261-1270). Philadelphia. Elsevier Saunders.
3. DePalma RG, Schwab FJ, Emsellem HA, et al. (1990) Non-invasive assessment of impotence. *Surg Clinics N America.* Feb: 70(1) (119-132).
4. Hattery RR, King BF, Lewis RW, James M, McKusick MA. (1991). Vasculogenic impotence. *Contemporary Uroradiology.* 29(3). (629-645).
5. Bassiouny HB, Levine LA. (1991). Penile duplex sonography in the diagnosis of venogenic impotence. *The Journal of Vascular Surgery.* 13 (75-83).
6. Zwiebel WJ, Benson CB, Doubilet PM. Duplex ultrasound evaluation of the male genitalia. In Zwiebel WJ, Pellerito JS (Eds.), *Introduction to Vascular Ultrasonography 5th ed.* (659-684). Philadelphia: Elsevier Saunder
7. Kempczinski RF. (1982). Segmental volume plethysmography: The pulse volume recorder. In: Kempczinski RF and Yao SJS. Practical Non-invasive Vascular Diagnosis. (105--117). Chicago: Yearbook Medical.
8. Zierler RE, Sumner DS. (2005). Physiologic assessment of peripheral arterial occlusive disease. In Rutherford Vascular Surgery 6th edition. (197-222). Philadelphia. Elsevier Saunders.
9. Bassett J, Rajfer J. (2010). Diagnostic and therapeutic options for the management of ischemic and nonischemic priapism Rev Urol. 12(1): (56-63).
10. Varela, C. G., Yeguas, L. A. M., Rodríguez, I. C., & Vila, M. D. D. (2020). Penile Doppler Ultrasound for Erectile Dysfunction: Technique and Interpretation. AJR. American journal of roentgenology, 214(5), 1112–1121.
11. James, FM. (1993). Penile Ultrasound. In Vascular Diagnosis 4th edition. (754-763). St. Louis: Mosby.
12. Aversa, A, Crafa A, Greco, FA, Chiefari E, Brunetti A, La Vignera S. (2021). The penile duplex ultrasound: How and when to perform it? Andrology, Sep;9(5):1457-1466.

CARDIAC
45. Effects on Spectral Doppler

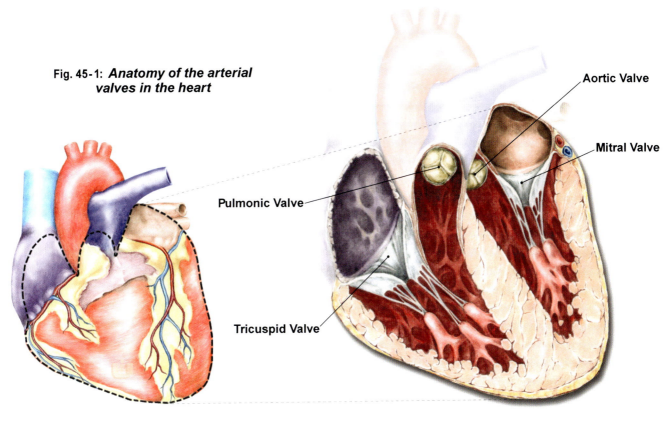

Fig. 45-1: *Anatomy of the arterial valves in the heart*

Image courtesy of Rick Duncan

Introduction

According to the American Heart Association, cardiovascular disease is still the leading cause of death for U.S. men and women and risk factors are on the rise. When performing a vascular exam in the aging population, heart disease must be considered and general knowledge of how heart disease affects the spectral Doppler waveform in the vascular examination should be understood. Abnormal Doppler waveforms may not always be associated with vascular disease. Certain conditions can either overestimate or underestimate the stenosis. Use a combination of velocities and velocity ratios, along with an algorithm, weighing the findings for each.

Any cardiac disease present may affect the vascular system. These effects can be seen in arterial and venous waveforms. Careful examination of patient history will prove useful.

Table 45-1: **Summary of Cardiac Effect on Cardiac Output**

Over Estimated Stenosis: High Cardiac Output	Under Estimated Stenosis: Low Cardiac Output
Chronic anemia	Congestive heart failure
Chronic hypercapnia	Cardiac valvular problems
Sepsis	Coronary artery disease
Beriberi heart disease	Cardiac diastolic dysfunction
Sickle cell anemia	Pericarditis
Pregnancy	Congenital heart disease
Obesity	Cardiomyopathy
Hepatic disease	Systemic hypertension
Carcinoid syndrome	Anemia
Paget's disease	Cardiac arrhythmias
Multiple myeloma	Atrial fibrillation
Cardiac arrhythmias	Cardiac tamponade

High Cardiac Output

An increase in cardiac output (normal range: 4 to 6 liters per minute (lpm)) may result in an increase in peak systolic velocities. The ICA/CCA ratio may be useful to calculate when the B-mode information does not match the increased systolic velocities. The following disease states are associated with increased cardiac output:

- Chronic anemia
- Chronic hypercapnia
- Sepsis
- Beriberi heart disease
- Pregnancy
- Obesity
- Hepatic disease
- Carcinoid syndrome
- Paget's disease
- Multiple myeloma
- Cardiac volume overload diseases
- Cardiac arrhythmias (compensatory beats)

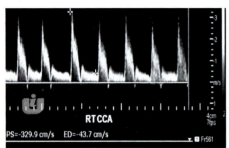

Fig. 45-2: Spectral Doppler waveform with elevated velocities of the CCA in a patient with high cardiac output. This waveform will be observed bilaterally in the CCA.

Low Cardiac Output

A reduction in cardiac output may result in a decrease in peak systolic velocities. The ICA/CCA ratio may be useful to calculate when the B-mode information does not match the decreased peak systolic velocity. Low cardiac output is defined as a cardiac output below 4 lpm. The following disease states are associated with low cardiac output:

- Congestive heart failure (CHF)
- Low ejection fraction (EF%)
- Coronary artery disease
- Cardiac diastolic dysfunction
- Pericarditis
- Congenital heart disease
- Cardiomyopathy
- Systemic hypertension
- Anemia

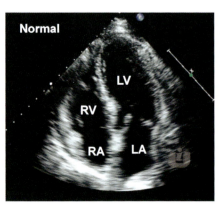

Fig. 45-3: 4-chamber with normal ejection fraction

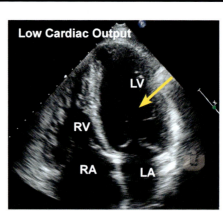

Fig. 45-4: 4-chamber low cardiac output/low ejection fraction

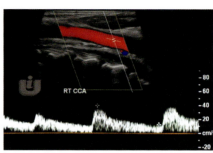

Fig. 45-5: Spectral Doppler waveform of low cardiac output with severe congestive heart failure. This waveform will be observed bilaterally in the CCA.

The low cardiac output will be seen in all the vessels examined and should not be confused with the effects of proximal high-grade stenosis.

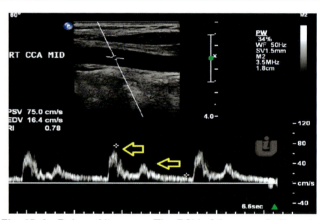

Fig. 45-6: Pulsus Alternans. The PSV of the vessel alternates between two levels on sequential beats. This rhythm can also be associated with hypocalcemia, or IVC compression. [1]

When performing vascular exams on patients with significant cardiac disease, the velocity ratio is usually more useful than the peak systolic velocity (PSV) in the exam interpretation especially when the abnormality is found throughout the cardiac cycle.

Aortic Stenosis (AS)

Aortic stenosis is the narrowing and restriction of antegrade blood flow through the aortic valve.

Left ventricular and aortic valve abnormalities mainly affect arterial hemodynamics (pulse contour and pressure).

- The most common etiologies of aortic stenosis are as follows:
  » Congenital (e.g., bicuspid aortic valve)
  » Degenerative and rheumatic. Severe aortic stenosis is defined as the narrowing of the aortic valve area <1.0cm^2.

» Doppler interrogation of the ascending aorta will usually show increased velocities.
» In cases of severe aortic stenosis, Doppler interrogation of the common carotid artery may only show a low amplitude, turbulent spectral waveform with a prolonged acceleration time. This finding may be most apparent in the proximal common carotid artery spectral Doppler tracing.
» Severe AS is associated with a body surface area (BSA) <0.06cm²

In a patient with aortic stenosis, the PSV will be underestimated; use the ratio for interpretation of disease

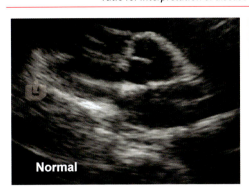

Fig. 45-7: Normal 2D aortic valve

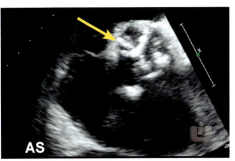

Fig. 45-8: 2D aortic valve stenosis

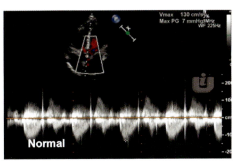

Fig. 45-9: Spectral Doppler of a normal aortic valve.

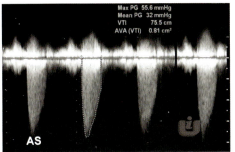

Fig. 45-10: Spectral Doppler of aortic stenosis.

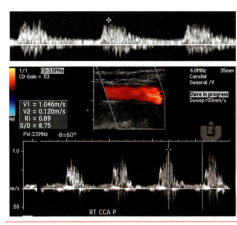

Fig. 45-11: Low amplitude and turbulent spectral Doppler waveforms of the CCA noted in cases of AS.

Abnormal waveforms due to cardiac effects may be found bilaterally in the CCA and should not be confused with a stenosis.

- The ICA/CCA ratio may be useful to calculate when the B-mode information does not match the decreased PSV.
- Overall systemic circulation will be reduced, and low amplitude signals will be present.
- Low brachial blood pressures may be seen bilaterally.
- If unilateral, you should suspect subclavian stenosis.

Cardiac valvular problems can be congenital, genetic, inflammatory, stress, or structural based.

Aortic Regurgitation (AR)

Aortic regurgitation is defined as the backflow of blood through the aortic valve during ventricular diastole into the ventricle.

Some labs may refer to aortic regurgitation as aortic insufficiency.

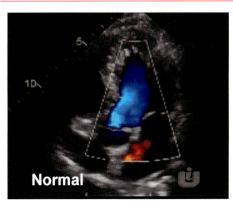

Fig. 45-12: Color Doppler of a normal aortic valve.

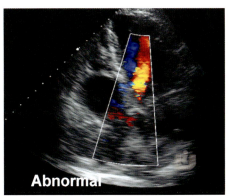

Fig. 45-13: Color Doppler of aortic regurgitation. (note reversed flow)

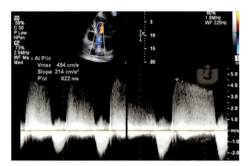

Fig. 45-14: Spectral Doppler of aortic regurgitation (Mild is >500) with an example of holo-diastolic flow measured.

Pulsus Bisferiens is seen in approximately 50% of patients with aortic valvular disease and can also be associated with hypertrophic cardiomyopathy.

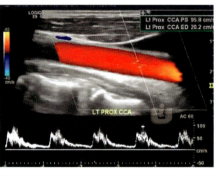

Fig. 45-15: Color and spectral Doppler waveform of pulsus bisferiens.

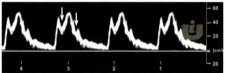

Fig. 45-16: Note the two peaks per cardiac cycle of pulsus bisferiens.

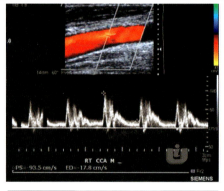

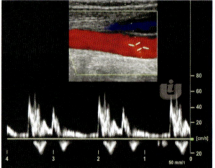

Fig. 45-17: Bisferiens waveform from two separate patients with aortic valvular disease.

High resistant arterial waveforms with a diminished or absent dicrotic notch indicate aortic valve disease may be present

- Aortic regurgitation may be acute or chronic.
- Severe aortic regurgitation results in a volume overload of the left ventricle.
- Increased pressures may inhibit pulmonary return.
- AR can result in dilation of the left ventricle.
- Doppler waveforms of the aorta and the great vessels may show holo-diastolic flow (dense backward flow noted on waveform throughout diastole).
- A "double peaked" vascular waveform may be seen when aortic regurgitation or stenosis is present.

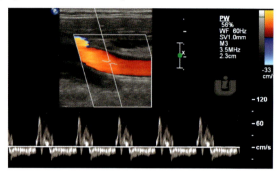

Fig. 45-18: Water-Hammer Pulse from a patient with severe aortic regurgitation. The end-diastolic flow is reversed due to severe regurgitation.

Mitral Stenosis (MS)

Mitral stenosis is the narrowing and restriction of antegrade blood flow through the mitral valve.

- Severe MS will cause a pressure overload in the left atrium and reduced filling of the left ventricle.
- Doppler waveforms of the aorta and carotid arteries may show low amplitude signals as a secondary result of MS.

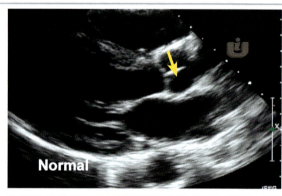

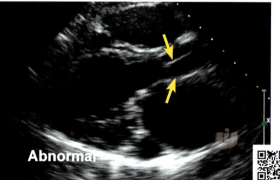

Fig. 45-19: Normal 2D of the mitral valve vs. mitral stenosis. Note dilation of the left atrium and ventricle.

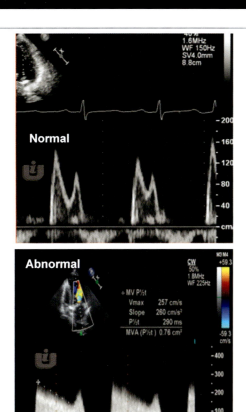

Fig. 45-20: *Normal mitral valve spectral Doppler vs. mitral stenosis*

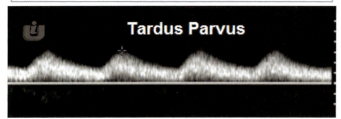

Fig. 45-21: *A low amplitude spectral Doppler waveform can result in the CCA secondary to severe mitral stenosis. Note the prolonged peak with diminished amplitude. Parvus tardus waveforms are often identified distal to severe stenosis.*

Mitral Regurgitation (MR)

Mitral regurgitation is the abnormal back flow of blood through the mitral valve.

- Severe mitral regurgitation results in a volume overload of the left atrium (LA), resulting in increased pressures in the left atrium and pulmonary capillary wedge.
- Increased pressures will inhibit pulmonary venous return.
- MR can result in dilation of pulmonic veins. (There are 4 pulmonary veins that return blood into the LA.)
- Doppler waveforms of the pulmonary veins show marked reversal characteristics during systole, particularly in the systolic pulmonary vein waveform.
- MR does not usually affect the spectral Doppler in vascular exams.

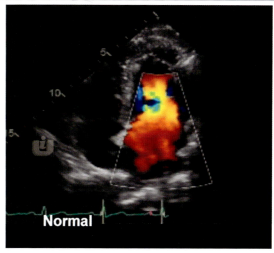
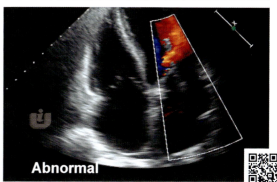

Fig. 45-22: *Normal color Doppler of the mitral valve vs. abnormal mitral regurgitation.*

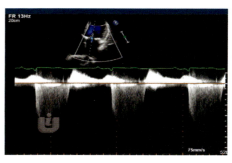

Fig. 45-23: *Mild mitral regurgitation with sparse Doppler profile and parabolic shape.*

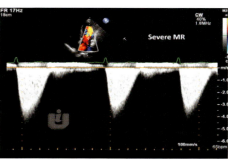

Fig. 45-24: *Severe mitral regurgitation with bright, dense spectral Doppler profile and triangular shape.*

Tricuspid Regurgitation (TR)

Tricuspid regurgitation is the abnormal back flow of blood through the tricuspid valve.

- Severe tricuspid regurgitation results in a volume overload of the right atrium.
- Increased pressures in the right atrium (RA) will restrict/inhibit venous return.
- TR can result in dilation of the RA, IVC, and hepatic veins.

- Spectral Doppler waveforms of the hepatic veins and IVC may show marked reversal characteristics during systole.
- Jugular vein distention may also be present.
- Systolic murmur may be present.
- Increased or elevated pressures within the right side of the heart may result in pulsatility of hepatic, portal, internal jugular vein, and peripheral veins.

Right ventricular and tricuspid valve abnormalities mainly affect venous hemodynamics.

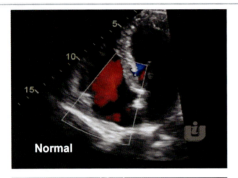
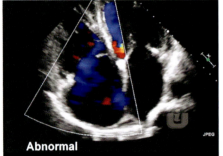

Fig. 45-25: *Normal color Doppler of the tricuspid valve vs. abnormal tricuspid regurgitation.*

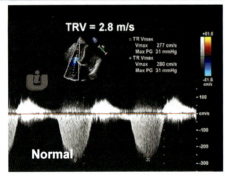

Fig. 45-26: *Spectral Doppler of tricuspid regurgitation*

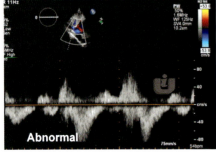

Fig. 45-27: *Spectral Doppler showing systolic reversal in the hepatic vein from severe tricuspid regurgitation.*

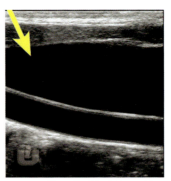
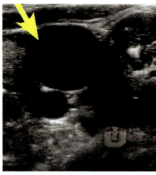

Fig. 45-28: *Dilated internal jugular vein caused from elevated pressure within the right side of the heart. (shown in long and transverse)*

Tricuspid Stenosis (TS)

Tricuspid stenosis is the narrowing and restriction of antegrade blood flow through the tricuspid valve.

- Severe tricuspid stenosis will cause a pressure overload in the right atrium and reduced filling of the right ventricle.
- Spectral Doppler waveforms of the main pulmonary artery may exhibit a turbulent waveform pattern.
- IVC and hepatic veins may become dilated.

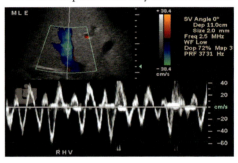

Fig. 45-29: *Increased pulsatility in the hepatic vein.*

Pulmonary Regurgitation (PR)

Pulmonary regurgitation is the abnormal back flow of blood through the pulmonic valve.

Some labs refer to pulmonary regurgitation as pulmonic insufficiency.

Severe pulmonary regurgitation results in a volume overload of the right ventricle.

- Increased pressures can inhibit venous return.
- PR can result in dilation of the right ventricle.
- Spectral Doppler waveforms of the pulmonary arteries may show marked flow reversal components during diastole.
- Increased or elevated pressures within the right side of the heart may result in pulsatility of peripheral veins.

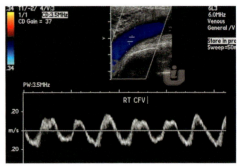

Fig. 45-30: *Increased pulsatility in a common femoral vein caused from elevated pressure within the right side of the heart.*

If pulsatile venous flow is found in the lower extremities, clinical correlation should be considered for pulmonary regurgitation (PR).

Pulmonic Stenosis (PS)

Pulmonic stenosis is the narrowing and restriction of antegrade blood flow through the pulmonic valve.
- Severe pulmonic stenosis will cause a pressure overload in the right ventricle and reduced flow to the pulmonary arteries.
- Spectral Doppler waveforms of the pulmonary arteries may show increased amplitude and turbulent waveform patterns.
- Increased or elevated pressures within the right side of the heart may result in pulsatility of peripheral veins. *(Fig. 45-30)*

Cardiac Tamponade

Cardiac tamponade is an emergency cardiac finding. There is a reduction in diastolic filling of the heart due to increased intrapericardial pressures from the accumulation of fluid or blood around the heart (pericardial effusion).
- Patients with cardiac tamponade are considered to have emergent findings which should be addressed immediately.
- The classic clinical finding for cardiac tamponade is *pulsus paradoxus*, defined as a drop in systolic blood pressure by greater than 10mmHg upon inspiration. This drop in blood pressure is due to a reduction of left ventricular filling during inspiration.
- The carotid Doppler tracing will demonstrate a decrease in PSV during inspiration and an increased PSV velocity during expiration.
- An increase in left ventricular filling with expiration results in an augmented PSV of the carotid artery during expiration. This is referred to as respiratory variation.

Constrictive Pericarditis

Constrictive pericarditis is the thickening of the pericardium due to inflammation, interfering with the diastolic filling of the heart.

IVC dilation without inspiratory collapse is a very helpful sign of constrictive pericarditis.

- Commonly seen in post-cardiac surgery.
- Distension of the internal jugular vein, IVC, and peripheral edema is usually present.
- The resultant carotid spectral Doppler tracing will demonstrate a decrease in peak systolic velocity upon inspiration.

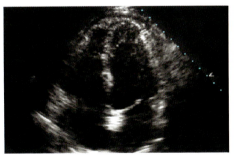

Fig. 45-31: *Constrictive pericarditis respiratory shift.*

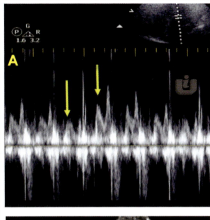
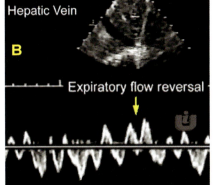

Fig. 45-32: *Constrictive pericarditis: A) Spectral Doppler of mitral valve inflow demonstrating respiratory variation B) Spectral Doppler of hepatic vein showing expiratory flow reversal.*

Cardiac Arrhythmias

Cardiac arrhythmias exhibit irregular spectral Doppler waveforms that correspond with the heart rhythm and rate.

When a cardiac arrhythmia is encountered, consider waiting for a short time period to begin or continue the exam, as these can be intermittent in some patients.

If the spectral Doppler waveform abnormality stems from cardiac issues, the waveform abnormality is usually seen throughout the vascular exam; it is important to compare waveforms bilaterally.

- Vascular labs have adopted several methods of measuring velocities when arrhythmias are present.
  » A common technique used when an irregular rhythm is present is to measure the most consistent beats. This may be a string of three or more waveforms.
  » In cases where the rhythm present is "irregularly irregular" (no pattern that can be followed), it becomes more difficult. An average of the 3-5 most consistent beats may be taken. This is more subjective, and care should be taken when reporting results using this method. Diameter and area reduction tools may prove extremely useful in cases of irregularly irregular arrhythmias.
- In cases where an intraortic balloon pump is used, it may be difficult to determine the underlying rhythm.

Some physicians will allow the balloon pump to be turned off for brief periods so underlying rhythms can be seen and measurements taken.
This should NOT be done by the sonographer!

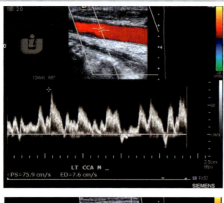
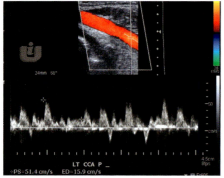

Fig. 45-33: *Spectral Doppler waveform from a patient on an intra-aortic balloon pump (IABP) with a variety of peaks making measurement difficult.*

Sinus Arrhythmia
All waveforms are normal. The heart rate increases and decreases with respiration.

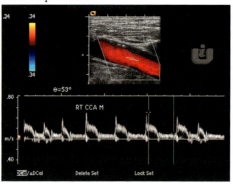

Fig. 45-34: *Spectral Doppler waveform of sinus arrhythmia*

Sinus Bradycardia
All waveforms are normal, but the heart rate is below 60bpm.

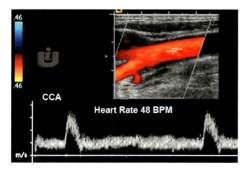

Fig. 45-35: *Spectral Doppler waveform of Sinus Bradycardia*

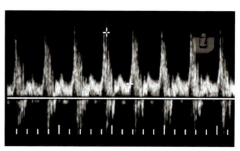

Fig. 45-36: *Spectral Doppler waveform of sinus tachycardia*

Sinus Pause (Sinus Arrest)
The SA node (natural pacemaker) fails to send out an impulse for a period of time.

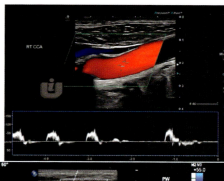

Fig. 45-37: *Spectral Doppler waveform of sinus pause from a patient with severe congestive heart failure.*

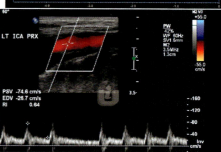

Fig. 45-38: *Measuring spectral Doppler waveform of sinus pause.*

Atrial Fibrillation/Atrial Flutter
Atrial fibrillation is a common cardiac arrhythmia. It is the fibrillation of the heart's two upper chambers (atria). The carotid spectral Doppler waveform appears to have a variety of peak systolic velocities due to the varying R-R intervals. It is recommended to measure 3 to 5 beats and average.

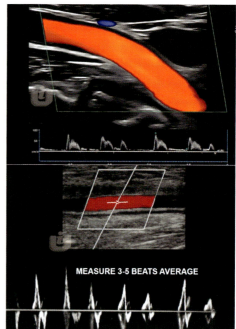

Fig. 45-39: *Spectral Doppler waveforms and color Doppler depicting atrial fibrillation*

Fig. 45-40: *Spectral Doppler waveforms of atrial fibrillation with varying PSV. Measure several waveforms and report the average velocity.*

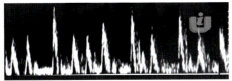

Fig. 45-41: Spectral Doppler waveforms of atrial fibrillation

Premature Ventricular Contraction (PVC)

A PVC originates from an ectopic focus (an abnormal electrical pulse) within the right or left ventricles. PVCs occur earlier than expected and are followed by a delayed beat (compensatory pause). The spectral Doppler waveform of a PVC would be lower than normal, and the following delayed beat will be higher than normal. It is recommended not to measure either beat because this is not a true representation of the velocity during normal sinus rhythm.

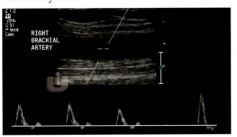

Fig. 45-42: PVC found in an artery; a repeating pattern of a PVC followed by a normal beat.

Bigeminy

A repeating pattern of two beats close together followed by a pause.

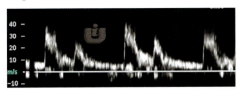

Fig. 45-43: Spectral Doppler waveforms demonstrating bigeminy of the common carotid artery

Trigeminy

A repeating pattern of a PVC following two normal beats.

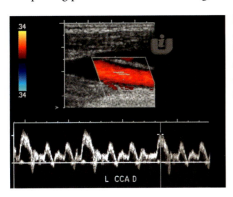

Fig. 45-44: Spectral Doppler waveforms of atrial fibrillation of trigeminy of the CCA.

Table 45-2: Effects of Cardiac Diseases on the Spectral Doppler Waveform Summarized

Disease	Effect
High cardiac output	Increased systolic velocity
Low Cardiac Output	Decreased systolic velocity
Aortic Regurgitation	Double peaked waveform and/or reversal during diastole; diminished or absent dicrotic notch
Aortic Stenosis	Low amplitude and/or turbulent waveform; parvus tardus
Mitral Stenosis	Low amplitude
Mitral Regurgitation	No effect usually noted in the vascular exam
Tricuspid Regurgitation	Increased pulsatility in the venous waveform
Pulmonic Regurgitation	Increased pulsatility of the venous waveform
Pulmonary Stenosis	Increased pulsatility of the venous waveform
Tricuspid Stenosis	Increased pulsatility of the venous waveform
Cardiac Tamponade	Decreased peak systolic velocity during inspiration and increased peak systolic velocity during expiration
Constrictive Pericarditis	Decreased peak systolic velocity during inspiration and increased peak systolic during expiration
Cardiac Arrhythmia	Varying peak systolic velocity

REFERENCES

1. Rohren E., Kliewer M., et al. (2003). A spectrum of Doppler waveforms in the carotid and vertebral arteries. *AJR, 181*, pages 1695-1704.
2. Bendick P. (2011). Cardiac effects on peripheral vascular Doppler waveforms. *Journal of Vascular Ultrasound, 35*(4), pages 237-243.
3. Palma, R. (2019). *Echocardiographers' Pocket Reference. 5th edition.* Arizona Heart School of Cardiac Ultrasound.
4. Reynolds, T. (1997). *Cardiovascular principles: A registry exam preparation guide.* Arizona Heart School of Cardiac Ultrasound.
5. Kaddoura, S. (2002). *Echo Made Easy.* Elsevier Saunders.
6. Centers for Disease Control and Prevention. (2022, October 14). *Heart Disease Facts.* CDC. gov. http://www.cdc.gov/heartdisease/facts.htm.

RESOURCES
46. Ergonomics

Purpose

Ergonomics is the study of factors that affect humans in their workplace with a focus on design and the arrangement of physical spaces so that people and objects interact efficiently and safely.

As ultrasound exams become more complex and physically demanding and volumes increase, more sonographers report experiencing workplace injury and chronic pain. As vascular testing becomes more popular and space in offices and hospitals is limited, you may be required to perform exams in tighter spaces. The demand for portable exams in intensive care units for example makes it more difficult for the technologist to use ergonomically friendly exam rooms and maintain proper posture. The percentage of sonographers experiencing musculoskeletal pain at work has increased from 84% in 1997 [1] to 90% in 2009 [2] according to published studies. Recent data published in late 2023, indicates 86% of those surveyed experience discomfort attributed to work. [12] When rest is not enough, some sonographers undergo surgery to relieve their symptoms while others are forced to leave the field of vascular sonography altogether.

The term "Work Related Musculoskeletal Disorders (WRMSDs)" is used to describe the numerous conditions that are caused by repetitive use and performing difficult activities in the workplace. Back-to-back abdominal exams or venous exams on obese patients are often part of the regular schedule in many vascular labs. WRMSDs occur over time and affect the muscles, nerves, ligaments, and tendons of those in our profession. Often, the pain and discomfort of WRMSDs will linger throughout the day well after you put the transducer down and finish scanning your patients.

Work-related injuries cost up to $20 billion/yr in medical expenses and worker's compensation benefits, with even more money being lost due to absenteeism, lost productivity, and the time needed to hire and train new staff. [3] In contrast, the approximate cost to set up an ergonomically friendly work area for the sonographer is $188,205. [6]

There is substantial physical effort needed for vascular scanning beyond the force required to compress vessels, including pushing, pulling, and gripping the transducer. Vascular exams call for the sonographer to stay in an awkward posture, sometimes for an extended amount of time to obtain the information needed to diagnose the patient's issue/disease. Wrist and shoulder flexion/extension, reaching, bending and twisting are common to vascular testing.

Congress passed the Occupational Safety and Health Act of 1970 creating the group known as OSHA (Occupational Safety and Health Administration) to ensure safe and healthy working conditions for employees. OSHA is part of the US Department of Labor and allows employees to file complaints about workplace safety and substandard conditions. If someone believes their employer is not following OSHA standards, they can file a complaint online, via fax, mail/email or in person. Call your local OSHA office for more information at 800-321-6742 (OSHA) [6]

- Sonographers share in the responsibility for complying with OSHA standards. This chapter provides guidance for practicing proper form and scanning techniques. To learn more, visit www.osha.gov/etools/hospitals/clinical-services/sonography

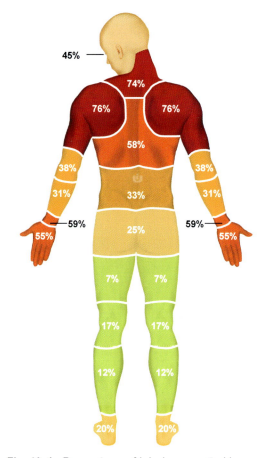

Fig. 46-1: *Percentage of injuries reported by area*

Modified from J. Baker "Musculoskeletal Injury and Sonography: The American Experience Statistical Evidence of Risk Factors" www.sonoworld.com

Common Conditions Diagnosed as a Result of a WRMSD

- Carpal tunnel syndrome
- Tendonitis/Tenosynovitis
- Bursitis (especially of the shoulder)
- Thoracic Outlet Syndrome
- Epicondylitis (tennis elbow)
- Trigger Finger- inability to extend the finger

Location of Disease

The most common WRMSD injuries involve the following areas of the body:

- Shoulder
- Hand/wrist
- Back (upper > middle and lower)
- Neck

Patient History

The physical symptoms of Musculoskeletal Disorders (MSDs) include:

- Pain
- Numbness, tingling
- Loss of control (unable to grip or feeling like you will drop the transducer, for example)
- Blurred vision, headaches
- Inflammation
- Joint stiffness and decreased range of motion

Ergonomic Advances in the Imaging Industry

Ultrasound manufacturers have made substantial improvements to equipment design over the years including some of the modifications listed here: [5]

- Central break controls (instead of one brake on every wheel)
- Height adjustable keyboards and monitors
- Footrests to encourage neutral positioning, redesigning units so technologists' knees and legs are unobstructed when sitting.
- System designs so transporting takes no more than 50 pounds of force by one technologist to push/pull equipment on bare flooring.
- Lighter weight transducers that are more slip resistant and encourage better grip
- Better cable lengths and management systems for transducers
- Optimization of control layout, options for right- and left-handed users
- Better font type and size

Height Adjustable Table

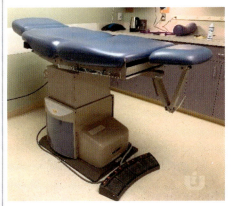

Fig. 46-2: *Motorized height adjustable exam table.*

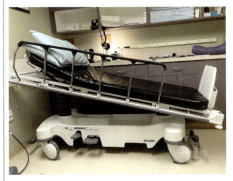

Fig. 46-3: *Manual (foot pump) height adjustable stretcher.*

Optimization Goals for Vascular Labs Pre, During, and Post Scan

Scheduling

- Scheduling templates for vascular lab exams should include time for indirect patient care (exam room set-up, time to allow the patient to change, and patient assessment), as well as direct patient care (actual scan) and the time needed afterward to clean, complete worksheets and bill.
- Some of the recommended exam times for vascular studies are listed below: [9]
  - 70 minutes for a bilateral CVI exam
  - 45 minutes for a unilateral CVI exam
  - 92 minutes for a complete renal exam
  - 67 minutes for a complete carotid exam
- Scheduling templates should allow for breaks between patients complying with local, state, and federal labor laws and workplace policies for breaks/meal periods.
- Limit the number of portable exams performed to those that are truly necessary (critically ill patients, for example) versus bedside exams just for convenience. Make sure providers know that the patient will probably receive a better-quality scan if they can travel to your department, where you have all of your equipment and additional resources.
- Try to rotate tasks between staff sonographers or try to schedule different exam types each hour if you are working alone. It is better to schedule a carotid exam in between two abdominal exams to give your body a break. Varying the type of exam(s), you perform daily allows you to use different muscle groups while you rest others. This variation will reduce the risk of repetitive use injury.

Moving Patients/Equipment

- Do not bend over when moving a patient cart.
- Raise the cart to a level that allows your arms to be at a 90° angle. This will facilitate pushing with the arms instead of the back.

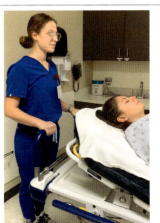
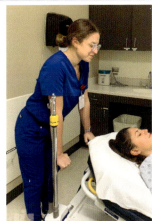

Fig. 46-4:
CORRECT POSTURE
Raise the cart so your arms are at 90°. Use your arms (not your back) to push.

Fig. 46-5:
INCORRECT POSTURE
This cart is too low and using straight arms to push will require the use of your lower back.

Moving Ultrasound Machines

- Lower the monitor so you have an unobstructed view as you move through doorways and halls.
- Do not bend over when moving equipment.

- Raise the equipment to allow your arms to be at a 90° angle. This will facilitate pushing with the arms instead of your back.
- If your machine has a "2-way steer" option, make sure it is engaged, so you will have better control when traveling long distances. If you leave the machine engaged in "all-wheel drive" it will be more difficult to control and stop.

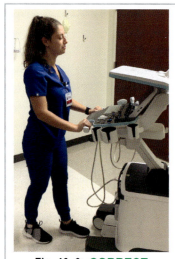

Fig. 46-6: CORRECT
The lowered screen allows for better visibility, and the machine height allows for a 90° arm angle to avoid using your back.

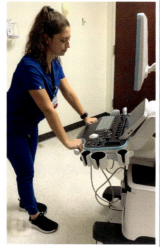

Fig. 46-7: INCORRECT
The raised screen may obstruct your view. The low height of the machine does not allow for a 90° angle of the arms, causing the use of your lower back.

Scanning

- Make sure to wear the proper sized glove for your hand to maintain a proper grip on the transducer.
  » The scanning sonographer is ultimately responsible for using proper form while scanning.
  » A proper transducer grip will be more comfortable for you and should ensure a steady image.
- Take the time to position the patient properly, as close to you as possible, and at an appropriate height. Try to minimize reaching, bending, or twisting during the scan.
- Once the patient has been safely positioned, the exam table should be raised to allow for the use of proper ergonomics.
  » Electronically controlled tables are preferred.
  » Stand in front of pedal controls used to raise the bed up/down instead of trying to make adjustments with your body at an angle.
  » If you can adjust the height of the exam table and US equipment, consider performing some exams while standing instead of sitting to vary your posture.
- Adjust window coverings and exam room lights so there is no glare on the monitor during the scan. Dimmable lighting is recommended.
- Before the start of the scan, adjust your chair, monitor, exam table, and keyboard to the best level for you.
- Your machine's monitor should be 10-15° below your eye level and an arm's length away from your eyes (about 18-30 inches). Make sure to keep the screen of your monitor clean. Refocus your eyes occasionally during the scan to give them a break.
- Keep your arm as close to your side as possible to avoid overreaching.

- Grip the transducer as lightly as possible while remaining steady.
- Hold the transducer as close to the patient's skin as possible instead of gripping closer to the transducer cable.
- Rest the side of your hand, from the tips of your pinky finger to the outside of the wrist on the patient.
- Keep your wrist as straight as possible when scanning, and try not to have too great of an angle between your wrist and forearm.
- Stop and pay attention to your body if you feel pain during the scan. Just as you would try to reposition your patient during the scan if they were uncomfortable, you should do the same for yourself. Try to keep your shoulders, arm, and wrist relaxed. Try to reposition your chair. Grab a cushion or roll up a blanket to use as a support for your arm if needed.
- Take "micro-breaks" during the scan, where you ease up on your transducer grip for a moment and then return to a tighter grip.
- Use any equipment available to you that will aid in proper positioning and result in good ergonomics.
  » Adjustable exam beds
  » Height adjustable stools/chairs
  » Support blocks and cushions
  » Raised platform or step stool.
  » Automated cuff inflation device for lower extremity venous insufficiency duplex exams.
- Work as a team on difficult patients. Ask for help from coworkers when you can. For example, one technologist can stand on the opposite side of the bed to scan the contralateral limb, while the other technologist controls the machine.

Consider regular monitoring between coworkers to support proper body mechanics as a team. Involve sonographers in the writing of safety guidelines and policies for the department.

- Ask the patient for help when you can. An example would be to ask the patient to lie on their side or in the prone position to avoid reaching and twisting to scan the back of the calf.
- Remember that there are limits to ultrasound exams. Maintain reasonable expectations about the images you can get when there are technical limitations such as body habitus, poor patient positioning, or extreme patient discomfort.

Hand and Wrist Ergonomics

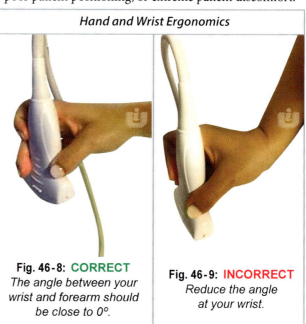

Fig. 46-8: CORRECT
The angle between your wrist and forearm should be close to 0°.

Fig. 46-9: INCORRECT
Reduce the angle at your wrist.

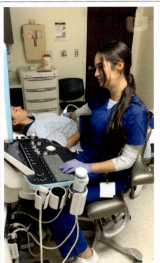
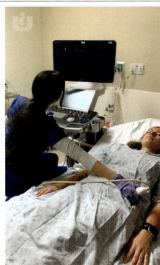

Fig. 46-10: CORRECT POSTURE Adjust the chair for support, adjust the machine height and monitor, support your arm with a cushion/rolled blanket.

Fig. 46-11: INCORRECT POSTURE Chair, machine and monitor are too high, arm and back are not supported, and the tech is not sitting in the chair properly.

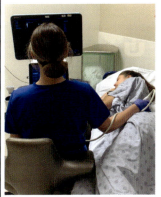
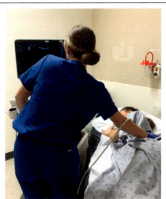

Fig. 46-12: CORRECT POSTURE Move the patient as close to you as possible. Use a chair when scanning and adjust its height. Adjust the height of the machine and monitor. The monitor should be at eye level.

Fig. 46-13: INCORRECT POSTURE Avoid neck extension/rotation, awkward trunk postures (e.g., leaning sideways) and excessive reach.

Encourage students to practice proper body mechanics early in their careers.

Standing Venous Insufficiency

Achieving good ergonomics during a standing venous insufficiency ultrasound exam requires the use of additional equipment such as a patient platform and an automatic cuff inflator.

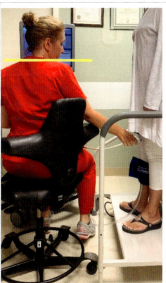
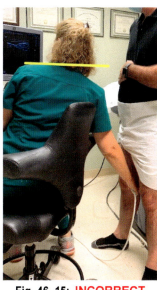

Fig. 46-14: CORRECT The shoulders should remain parallel when scanning. Use a step or platform to raise the patient to a good height.

Fig. 46-15: INCORRECT Notice how the right shoulder is much lower than the left shoulder.

Automated Cuff Augmentation Devices

Venous reflux exams rely on an augmentation of the thigh/calf muscle to propel the blood in the antegrade (normal) direction followed by a rapid release of the muscle to watch for retrograde (abnormal) flow. Automated rapid cuff augmentation devices are available to replace the need for the sonographer to manually compress the calf.

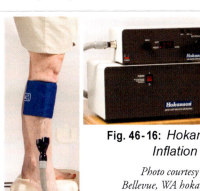

Fig. 46-16: Hokanson Rapid Cuff Inflation System

Photo courtesy of Hokanson, Bellevue, WA hokansonvascular.com

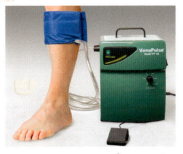

Fig. 46-17: VenaPulse Hands-Free Augmentation Device

Photo courtesy of ACI Medical San Marcos, CA. acimedical.com/products/venapulse

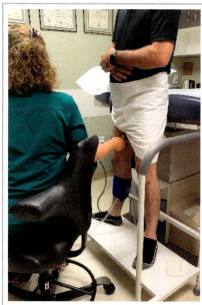

Fig. 46-18: CORRECT Using an automated cuff inflation device allows for hands-free augmentation to maintain proper posture.

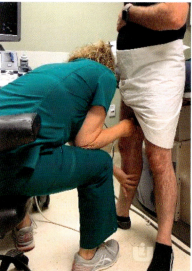

Fig. 46-19: INCORRECT Hand augmentation of the calf causes strain on multiple parts of the sonographer's body.

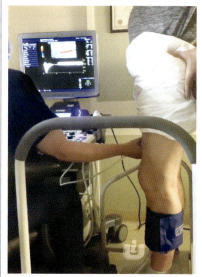

Fig. 46-20: Cine loop demonstrating the use of an automated cuff inflation device

Take the time to properly set up the room, position the patient properly and be sure to use any equipment that your employer provides such as support cushions, scanning chairs, etc. Offer input about equipment purchases so that the right equipment is selected.

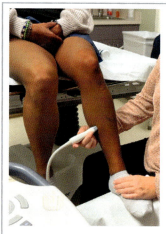 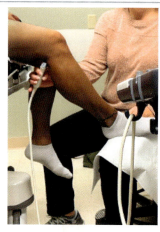

Fig. 46-21: Alternate positions for evaluation of the calf veins; seated on the side of the bed with the leg dependent and foot resting on examiner's lap or stool. When using this position, be sure the back of the leg or knee is not resting against the bed.

Scanning Chair/Stool

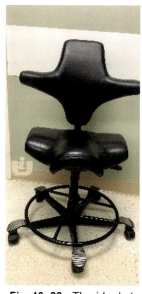 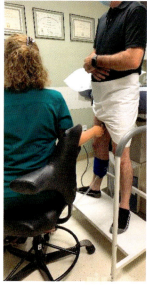

Fig. 46-22: The ideal stool for this test has a saddle-style seat which allows the user to be seated in multiple positions including the position pictured above. Note the seat and the back rest have been turned so the "wing" can support the scanning arm.

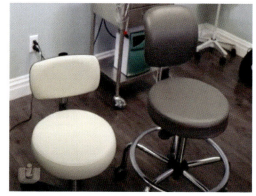

Fig. 46-23: At a minimum, the sonographer should use a stool/chair that has a pneumatic height adjustment and can easily swivel.

Sitting at Your Desk

- Use chairs that have wheels, are height adjustable and support the lumbar area (low back) with a tilt feature whenever possible. A footrest is another option. The seat should be deep enough to fit most of the thigh, up to the knee.
- Maintaining a neutral position supports the natural curves of the spine and keeps your body in proper alignment. Sustaining good posture will help you complete tasks essential to job performance. You should concentrate on trying to keep your head, neck, shoulders, elbows and hips aligned when sitting.
- Try to keep your hips higher than your knees to some extent.
- Try not to tense your shoulders, keep them relaxed.
- Keep elbows bent at >100°

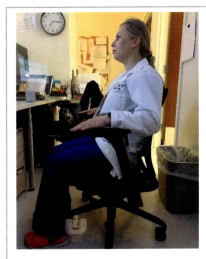

Fig. 46-24: *Neutral position when sitting; head, neck shoulders and hips are aligned, back is supported*

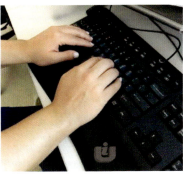

Fig. 46-25: *Keep your wrists straight when typing. Commercially available wrist supports might be helpful.*

After Scanning

- Research suggests that there are possible benefits from stretching between patients. Walking or gentle exercise increases blood flow to your joints. [4,5]
- Report symptoms early to your supervisor so you can discuss improvements and get help before it is too late
- Rest periods during the workday are believed to be essential. [4]
- Work to strengthen all of the muscle groups in the arm, hand and shoulder. Pilates or other exercises that strengthen your core have been suggested as a way to reduce the risk of WRMSDs and promote career longevity.

REFERENCES

1. Pike I, Russo A, Berkowitz J, Baker J, Lessoway V. The Prevalence of Musculoskeletal Disorders Among Diagnostic Medical Sonographers. (1997). *Journal of Diagnostic Medical Sonography 13*(5), 219-227.
2. Evans K, Roll S, Baker J. Work-Related Musculoskeletal Disorders (WRMSD) Among Registered Diagnostic Medical Sonographers and Vascular Technologists: A Representative Sample. (2009). *Journal of Diagnostic Medical Sonography, 25*(6), 287-299.
3. Murphey, S. (2017). Work related musculoskeletal disorders in sonography. *Journal of Diagnostic Medical Sonography, 33*(5), 354-369.
4. Harrison G., Harris A. (2015). Work-related musculoskeletal disorders in ultrasound: Can you reduce risk? Ultrasound, 23(4), 224-230.
5. Alaniz J, Veale B. Stretching for Sonographers: A Literature Review of Sonographer-Reported Musculoskeletal Injuries. (2013). *Journal of Diagnostic Medical Sonography, 29*(4), 188-190.
6. *How to File a Safety and Health Complaint. Occupational Safety and Health Administration* (2016). OSHA.gov. Available at: https://www.osha.gov/workers/file_complaint.html. Accessed August 23, 2021.
7. Industry Standards for the Prevention of Work-Related Musculoskeletal Disorders in Sonography. Consensus Conference on Work-Related Musculoskeletal Disorders in Sonography. (2011). *Journal of Diagnostic Medical Sonography, 27*(1), 14–18.
8. *Employer Responsibilities; Work Related Musculoskeletal Disorders in Sonography White Paper.* Society of Diagnostic Sonography. (n.d.). https://www.sdms.org/resources/careers/work-related musculoskeletaldisorders/employer-responsibilities. (Accessed Aug 30, 2021)
9. *Professional Performance Guidelines. Society for Vascular Ultrasound.* (2019.). Society of Vascular Ultrasound. https://www.svu.org/practice-resources/professional-performanceguidelines/. (Accessed Nov 24, 2023)
10. Environment Health and Safety. *Maintain a Neutral Posture.* University of California San Francisco. https://ehs.ucsf.edu/maintainneutral-posture. Accessed 8/23/21.
11. U.S. Department of Labor. (2023, November 24). Clinical Services-Sonography. Occupational Safety and Health Administration. https://www.osha.gov/etools/hospitals/clinical-services/sonography
12. Parga MR, Evans KD, Sommerich CM, Roll SC (2023), Sonographers and Vascular Technologists Offer Potential Solutions to Promote the Health and Well-being of Their Workforce, Journal of Diagnostic Medical Sonography, https://journals.sagepub.com/doi/abs/10.1177/87564793231217217

RESOURCES
47. Correlation Modalities

Definition
Correlative tests are alternative testing modalities used when there is need to further investigate disease extent and clearly define etiology identified by duplex ultrasound exam. Alternative tests are also useful when clinical correlation is suggested, the vascular exam is limited or non-diagnostic.

Differential Tests
- Computerized Tomography (CT)
- Computerized Tomography Angiography (CTA)
- Computerized Tomography Pulmonary Angiogram (CTPA)
- Magnetic Resonance Imaging (MRI)
- Magnetic Resonance Angiography (MRA)
- Magnetic Resonance Venography (MRV)
- Angiography (Arteriogram/Venogram)
- D-dimer blood test
- Ventilation/Perfusion Scan (VQ Lung Scan)

Computed Tomography (CT)

A CT is a widely used diagnostic imaging test for a multitude of specialties. Tomography is derived from the Greek word "tomo" for slice. Computed tomography is a computerized x-ray procedure that creates multiple thin cross-sectional images (stacked one on top of the other) through a narrow beam of x-rays and electronic detectors that rotate swiftly around the body in a spiral motion.

The mainly two-dimensional (2-D) image provides detailed diagnostic information of the internal organs, bones, blood vessels, other soft tissues and any abnormalities (e.g., luminal reductions, tumors, foreign bodies, etc.). Multiplanar reconstruction CT and three-dimensional (3-D) rendering techniques use computer software to provide alternative views of the information gathered. During the procedure, the patient will lie supine on a narrow, motorized table that will slide into the donut shaped device. A special dye called *contrast* may be used for certain CTs to highlight blood vessels for example. There are several types of CTs:

Spiral CT/Helical CT: traditional CT used for a broad range of diseases, abnormalities and conditions, with or without the use of contrast.

Computerized Tomography Pulmonary Angiogram (CTPA): used to specifically obtain images of the pulmonary arteries, mainly to diagnose pulmonary emboli (PE), using contrast.

Computerized Tomography Angiography (CTA): utilized to obtain images specifically of arteries, veins, associated vascular diseases and related conditions, using contrast.

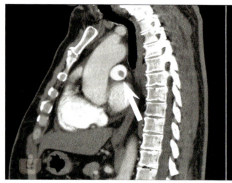
Fig. 47-1: *CTPA image of pulmonary embolus*

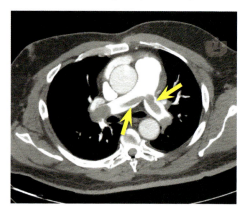

Fig. 47-2: *CPTA image of multiple areas of pulmonary embolus (saddle embolus is pictured)*

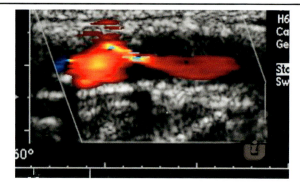
Fig. 47-3: *Duplex image of the ICA stenosis.*

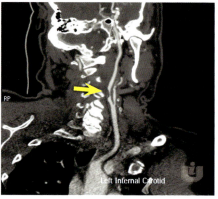
Fig. 47-4: *Multiplanar CT angio image of a left ICA stenosis*

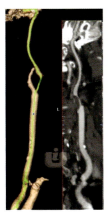 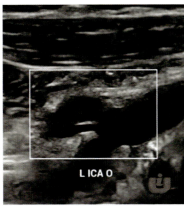

Fig. 47-5: *(Left) CTA and 3-D reconstruction of 80-99% ICA stenosis. (Right) B-mode image of 80-99% ICA stenosis resulting from an almost anechoic intraluminal source.*

Indications

- Cardiovascular related concerns
  » Initial diagnosis
  » Used to monitor disease progression and effectiveness of treatment
- Musculoskeletal related concerns
- Neurologic related concerns
- Liver & gastrointestinal related concerns
- Tumors/other diseases of the body
- Procedure guidance
- Internal injuries and bleeding

Contraindications/Limitations

- Allergy to iodinated contrast agent
- Renal impairment
- Inability to lie still/flat
- History of anaphylactic reaction
- Hyperthyroidism
- Pheochromocytoma (benign, adrenal gland tumor)
- Extreme anxiety
- Myasthenia gravis (chronic autoimmune disorder)
- Pregnancy and/or breast feeding
- Arrhythmia
- Body habitus
- Children under 2 years of age

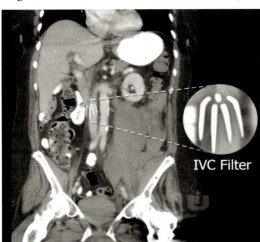

Fig. 47-6: *CT imaging of an IVC filter*

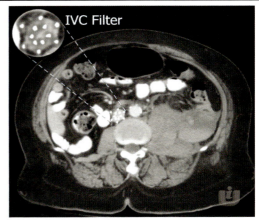

Fig. 47-7: *CT imaging of an IVC filter*

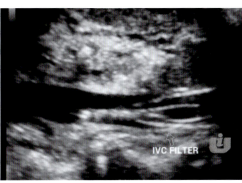

Fig. 47-8: *IVC filter on duplex scan*

Magnetic Resonance Imaging (MRI)

MRI is a diagnostic imaging test of the body's anatomy and physiological processes using magnetic components of our own natural elements. The MRI scanner is a large tube which uses a strong circular magnet, radio wave frequency and the hydrogen atoms in the body to create detailed multiple cross-sectional images (2D/3D) of internal organs, bones, blood vessels, other soft tissues and any abnormalities. When the hydrogen atoms and their protons are exposed to the magnetic field, different tissues will appear darker/lighter depending on the number of protons.

During the exam, the patient is placed on a narrow, motorized table that moves into the scanner. The scanner can be open or closed. The MRI scan itself is non-invasive, but IV or oral contrast may be used, depending on the information needed. Since MRI uses radiation in the "radiofrequency" range, there is little risk of developing cancer even with repeated exposure.

Magnetic Resonance Angiography (MRA): a study of arteries in the body including the organs, neck, chest, abdomen, pelvis and extremities. Contrast agents can be used for image enhancement.

Magnetic Resonance Venography (MRV): A study of veins in the body including the organs, neck, chest, abdomen, pelvis and extremities. Contrast agents can be used for image enhancement.

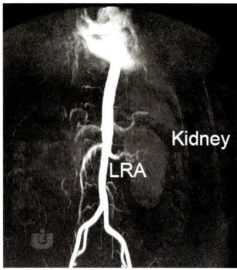

Fig. 47-9: *MRA showing a solitary left kidney and patent left renal artery*

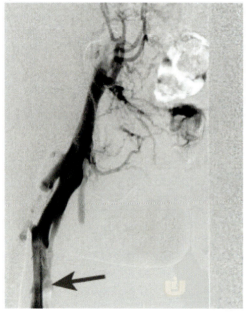

Fig. 47-10: *MRV of an iliac vein thrombosis. Note the filling defect (at arrow) and collateral network toward midline.*

Indications
- Cardiovascular related concerns
- Neurologic related concerns
- Musculoskeletal related concerns
- Liver & gastrointestinal related concerns
- Angiographic needs for diagnosis
- Tumors/diseases of the body

Contraindications/Limitations
- Metal implants in the body (total replacement joints, clips, stents, pacemaker, defibrillators, cochlear implants)
- Oxygen dependent breathing
- Extreme anxiety
- Inability to lie still/flat
- Pregnancy
- Claustrophobia
- Body habitus
- Renal impairment (non-dialysis patient)

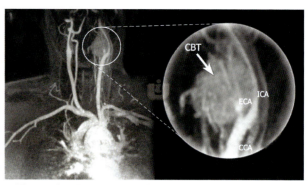

Fig. 47-11: *MRI image of a carotid body tumor (CBT)*

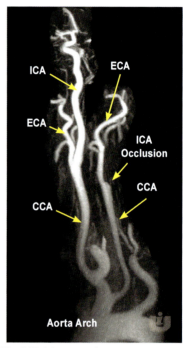

Fig. 47-12: *MRA image of an ICA occlusion (100%)*

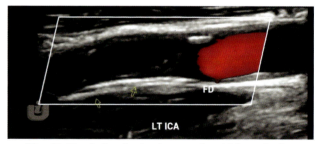

Fig. 47-13: *Color duplex image of an ICA occlusion*

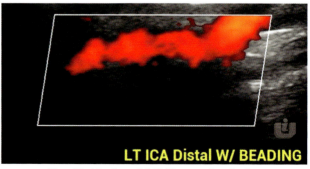

Fig. 47-14: *Carotid FMD on color duplex*

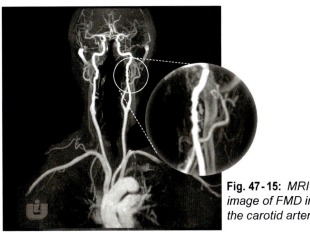

Fig. 47-15: *MRI image of FMD in the carotid artery*

Angiography (Arteriogram/Venogram)

Angiography is derived from the Greek word "angio" for vessel. An angiogram is used to image the two main kinds of blood vessels; arteries (arteriography) and veins (venography or phlebography).

Arteriogram

An arteriogram (arteriography) is an imaging test of the arteries. Angiography is an invasive imaging technique where a radio-opaque contrast material is injected into the vessels through a catheter. The contrast agent makes imaging of the arteries possible with "fluoroscopy," an x-ray imaging technology. During the procedure an x-ray beam is passed through the area of interest displaying a real-time continuous x-ray image on a computer monitor where body parts, surgical instruments and contrast agents can be visualized in detail. The images produced provide diagnostic information regarding anatomy and any vascular abnormalities. Images are taken from multiple planes when necessary for accurate evaluation of the target area.

Digital Subtraction Angiography (DSA)

DSA is a fluoroscopic technique where all overlapping tissues and radio-opaque structures are subtracted from an image to clearly define blood vessels. Prior to injection of a contrast agent, an x-ray image is obtained of the target area (mask image), which includes anatomy and radio-opaque structures. After contrast is administered, multiple images are taken as the contrast flows through the vessels. The display shows the opacified vessel overlaid on the initial mask image. The digital information from the original mask image is subtracted from the contrast images pixel by pixel, resulting in the images that only illustrate the filled vessels with greater clarity and detail.

Indication
- Peripheral vascular disease
- Renovascular disease
- Cerebrovascular disease
- Central vascular disease (aortic/visceral diseases, aneurysm, endovascular treatment)
- Subarachnoid hemorrhage
- Vascular trauma
- Aneurysmal disease
- Atypical arterial anatomy
- Arteriovenous malformation (AVM)

Contraindications/Limitations
- Pregnancy
- Allergy to iodinated contrast agent
- Renal impairment or dehydration
- Antiplatelet/blood thinning medication
- Coagulopathy
- Extreme anxiety
- Inability to lie still/flat

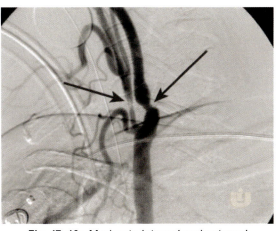

Fig. 47-16: *Moderate internal and external carotid artery stenoses by angiography*

Angiographic calculation of diameter reduction uses the distal normal vessel where walls are parallel for the true lumen because the true walls are not visible on arteriograms.

- The North American (NASCET) and Asymptomatic (ACAS) carotid surgery trials used different methods than the European (ECST) trial for measuring carotid stenosis on angiography.
  » NASCET method uses the lumen beyond the bulb where the walls are parallel.
  » NASCET derived measurements tend to be about 10% less than a duplex derived measurement for stenoses <80%. (e.g., 65% reduction by duplex will only measure about 55% by NASCET). but in a large bulb, a 50% duplex reduction may be only 10% by NASCET.

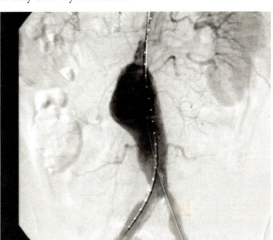

Fig. 47-17: *Fusiform aortic aneurysm by digital subtraction angiography*

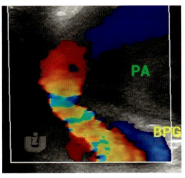

Fig. 47-18: *Color image of pseudoaneurysm neck off the bypass graft, pre-repair*

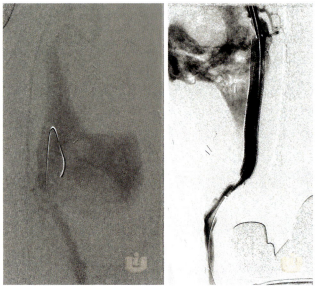

Fig. 47-19: Angiogram images of a pseudoaneurysm off a bypass graft pre-repair (left) and post-repair (right)

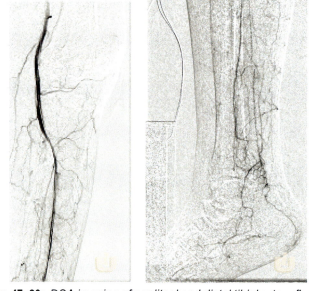

Fig. 47-20: DSA imaging of popliteal and distal tibial artery flow

Venogram

There are two types of venograms, ascending and descending. They are no longer used as screening studies and have mostly been replaced by duplex ultrasound imaging. During this invasive angiographic imaging technique, a radio-opaque contrast material is injected into the veins with a needle.

Descending Venography

Descending venography is used to assess for chronic venous insufficiency. The contrast is injected into the common femoral vein (or into a superficial vein in the upper extremity). On the x-ray film, the contrast in the veins either:
- Returns to the heart (indicating that valves are competent)
- Appears to "pool" in the extremity (indicating that valves are incompetent)

Ascending Venography

Ascending venography is used to image the veins of patients with suspected deep venous thrombosis (DVT), venous malformations, venous aneurysm and incompetent perforators. Contrast material is injected into a vein on the dorsum aspect of the foot or a segment distal to the area of interest.

- If intravenous thrombus is present, there will be partial or complete lack of contrast material that appears as a deficit on the x-ray image.
- Contrast helps highlight the dilated size of the vein in cases of venous aneurysm.
- Venous malformation will be highlighted on the image as an area with larger diameter veins that often appear "tangled."

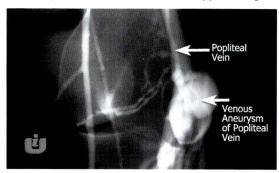

Fig. 47-21: Venography image of a popliteal vein aneurysm

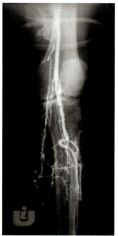

Fig. 47-22: Popliteal and tibial veins on venogram

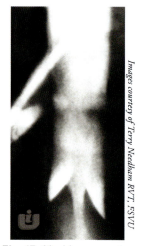

Fig. 47-23: Venous valve on descending venogram

Images courtesy of Terry Needham RVT, FSVU

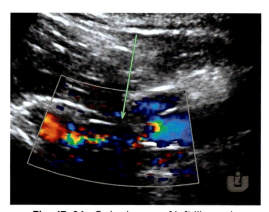

Fig. 47-24: Color image of left iliac vein stent with partial thrombosis

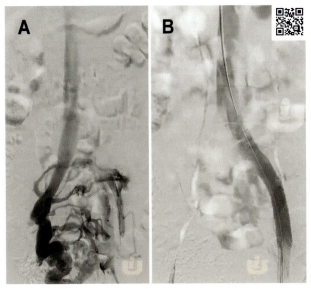

Fig. 47-25: *Cine loop using fluoroscopy with contrast (A) pre-stent demonstrating the absence of filling of the left CIV. (B) post-stenting filling.*

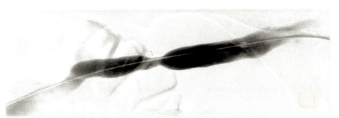

Fig. 47-26: *Venogram of stented left iliac vein with partial thrombosis*

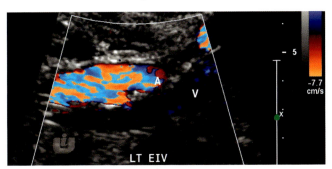

Fig. 47-27: *Occluded left iliac vein stent by color duplex*

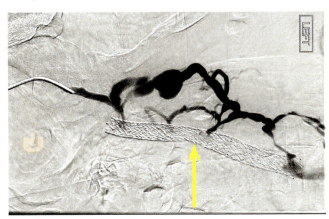

Fig. 47-28: *Imaging of an occluded left iliac vein stent using venography*

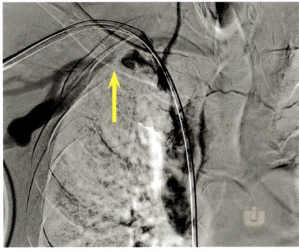

Fig. 47-29: *Innominate vein stenosis on venography*

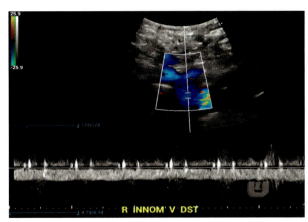

Fig. 47-30: *Continuous venous Doppler waveform pattern in the distal innominate vein from Fig. 47-29.*

Digital Subtraction Venography (DSV)

DSV may be used to obtain a more intense image of the veins. Bones and tissue are digitally subtracted, allowing the veins to be seen with greater clarity and detail.

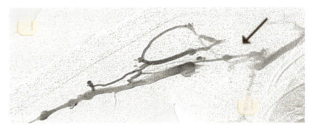

Fig. 47-31: *Digital subtraction venography*

Indications

- Deep vein thrombosis (DVT)
- Venous insufficiency
- Venous stenosis
- Adjunct imaging during venous thrombolysis
- Venous anomalies
- Venous vascular malformation
- Venous hypertension
- Venous aneurysm
- Vein mapping (preoperative planning)

Contraindications/Limitations
- Active cellulitis (involving the extremity to be imaged)
- Allergy to iodinated contrast agent
- Renal impairment
- Antiplatelet/blood thinning medication
- Coagulopathy
- Extreme anxiety
- Inability to lie still/flat

Intravascular Ultrasound

Intravascular Ultrasound (IVUS) is a medical imaging modality using a specially designed catheter with a miniaturized ultrasound transducer attached to the distal end of the catheter. The proximal end of the catheter is attached to computerized ultrasound equipment. It allows for the use of ultrasound technology to see from inside blood vessels, through the surrounding blood column, visualizing the endothelium (inner wall) of blood vessels.

IVUS is typically used in conjunction with arteriogram/venogram with the intent to treat significant lesions if they are identified. An example of treatment would be Percutaneous Transluminal Angioplasty (PTA).

Vessel access is obtained using ultrasound guidance. A needle is inserted into the vessel and a guide wire is introduced. A sheath is inserted into the vessel to allow for introduction of the IVUS catheter

Contraindications/limitations
- Obesity
- Severe edema
- Inability to lie still
- Inability to be anticoagulated

Arterial

IVUS is able to provide luminal cross-sectional measurements of the arteries and accurate information about lesion morphology such as: true vessel diameter, wall thickness/layers, the length, shape, and volume of a lesion, position of the lesion within a lumen (concentric or eccentric), type of lesion (fibrous, necrotic, calcified and mixed), presence and extent of plaque ulceration, arterial dissection or intimal flap and volume of thrombus. The information obtained may guide the choice of the appropriate PTA method, assist in the accurate deployment of an endovascular device, and check the efficiency of the procedure.[15]

Indications
- Peripheral vascular disease (PVD)
- Claudication (lower extremity pain with ambulation due to arterial insufficiency)
- Rest pain (lower extremity/foot pain due to arterial insufficiency which is exacerbated when the patient lies down and relieved by dependency relieved by dependency

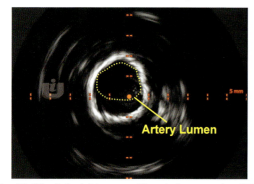

Fig. 47-32: *Arterial lumen without plaque using IVUS*

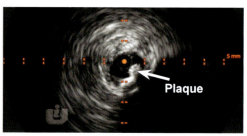

Fig. 47-33: *Arterial lumen with plaque*

Venous

IVUS of the vein is useful for the morphologic diagnosis of iliac venous outflow obstruction and is an invaluable tool in the accurate placement of venous stents after venoplasty. IVUS can accurately determine lumen size including cross sectional area stenosis. It identifies intraluminal lesions, wall thickness, delineates diseased or compressed vein segments, identifies the confluence of the iliac vein and IVC, identifies normal vein segments for landing sites of stents and helps estimate the stent diameter needed for a vein.[14]

Indications
- Suspicion of DVT
- Edema/swelling (especially when unilateral)
- Limb pain/tenderness
- Ulceration (venous or arterial)
- Discoloration in the gaiter area
- Iliac vein compression indicated during noninvasive testing

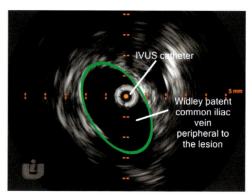

Fig. 47-34: *Visualization of the widely patent lumen of the peripheral left CIV using IVUS.*

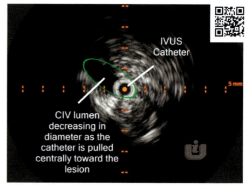

Fig. 47-35: *Visibly narrowed left CIV lumen as the catheter is moved centrally toward the lesion.*

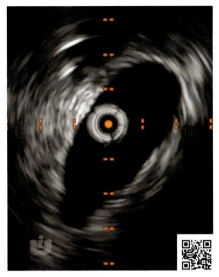

Fig. 47-36: *Cine loop of IVUS visualizing the Lt CIV post stenting.*

Arteriovenous Fistula (AVF) for Hemodialysis

IVUS of an AVF is particularly helpful when assessing the central vessels for stenosis in the cephalic arch and subclavian-innominate vein transition. Bands of connective tissue, intraluminal fibrotic strands, and/or dissections are well appreciated in the central and peripheral vessels using IVUS. This modality can also aid in differentiating between intimal hyperplasia and mural thrombus.[13]

Indications
- Abnormal HD access function
  - Difficult cannulation
  - Thrombus aspiration
  - High dynamic venous pressure (>200mmHg at 200ml/min)
  - Prolonged recirculation time (15%)
  - Unexplained urea reduction ratio
- Clinical signs/symptoms of HD access problems include:
  - Access collapse (inadequate arterial inflow)
  - Pulsatility (post-decannulation bleeding)
  - Loss of thrill/bruit
  - Graft-associated mass (infiltration, aneurysm, pseudoaneurysm)
  - Distal arm ischemia (sensory/motor)

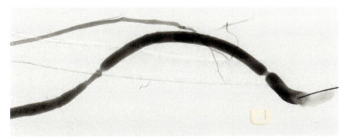

Fig. 47-37: *Venogram of an arteriovenous hemodialysis access with an outflow venous stenosis*

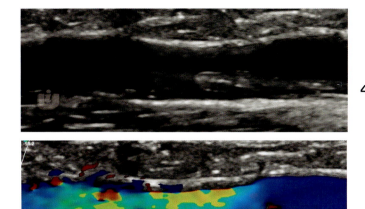

Fig. 47-38: *B-mode and color images of an arteriovenous hemodialysis access outflow vein stenosis*

VQ Scan

A VQ scan is a scintigraphic nuclear diagnostic technique that detects radiation emitted from radioactive tracers that are inhaled and injected intravenously, constructing a physiologic map of the lungs, representing air and blood flow patterns. The primary utilization of the scan is to help diagnose thrombus that has travelled to the lungs, known as a *pulmonary embolus*. The test is comprised of two nuclear scans that can be performed simultaneously or one after the other. The first part of the exams is known as the *ventilation scan* and the second is the *perfusion scan*.

If the results of the VQ scan are normal, there is a low probability for PE. Abnormal scans mean there may be a clot in the lungs. When the results are read as "intermediate probability" additional testing may be necessary. "High probability" suggests an 80-100% chance of a PE.[1]

Ventilation Scan

For a few minutes a radio-isotope labeled aerosol will be inhaled into the lungs through a non-rebreathing mask. The inhaled micro aerosol particles extend to the distal most aspects of the lungs. A nuclear scan using a gamma camera is then used to identify the areas of the lungs that are not receiving any or adequate air. Scans at different angles are obtained. The scan has three phases: initial breath, equilibrium and washout.

Perfusion Scan

An intravenously injected radioactive contrast travels throughout the lungs illuminating areas that are not receiving any or adequate blood flow. Similarly, a nuclear scan is performed where multiple images of the patient's chest are taken at different angles.

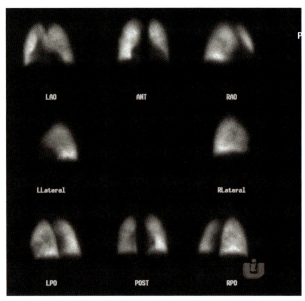

Fig. 47-39: *Normal VQ scan.*

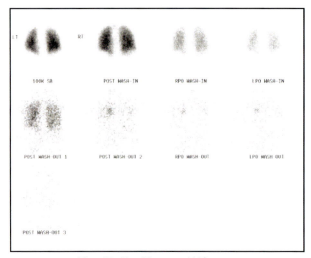

Fig. 47-40: *Abnormal VQ scan*

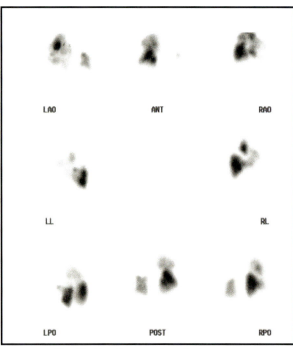

Fig. 47-41: *Abnormal perfusion scan.*

The ventilation images show a uniform distribution of activity on single-breath and wash-in images. There is abnormal Xe-133 retention during the wash-out phase focally in the right upper lung zone.

The perfusion images show multiple medium and large sized segmental defects which in sum make this a high probability examination for pulmonary embolism. These include the right upper posterior segment, and the left upper anterior and apical posterior segments as well as the left lower anterior medial basal segment and lateral basal segment.

IMPRESSION: High probability examination for pulmonary embolism.

Fig. 47-42: *Official report for abnormal VQ and perfusion images in Figs 47-40 and 47-41.*

Indications

- When CTPA for suspected PE is contraindicated or inconclusive
- Identification of chronic or acute PE
- Determining PE resolution
- Pregnancy with PE suspicion and normal chest radiograph
- Congenital pulmonary diseases
- Congenital cardiac diseases
- To confirm the presence of bronchopleural fistulae
- To evaluate the cause of pulmonary hypertension
- Evaluation of lung transplant
- Measuring lung function (preoperative/monitoring)

Contraindications/Limitations

- Potential fetal exposure: risk verses benefit should be assessed. A low-dose, perfusion-only imaging technique may be indicated.
- Lactating patients should stop breast-feeding for 24-hours after scan.

Table 47-1: Pioped Criteria (Prospective Investigation of Pulmonary Embolism Diagnosis)

The prospective investigation of pulmonary embolism diagnosis (PIOPED) criteria states ranges for diagnosing the likelihood of a pulmonary embolism (PE) by VQ scan:

Probability	Likelihood of PE
High	80-100%
Intermediate	20-80%
Low	0-20%

Source: Medoff, B. (9-13-2008). Pulmonary ventilation/perfusion scan-overview. Retrieved from http://www.umm.edu/ency/article/003828.htm

Table 47-2: Clinical Prediction Criteria for Pulmonary Embolism

Condition	# Points Assigned
Clinical DVT symptoms	+ 3
Alternative diagnosis as likely or more than DVT	+ 3
Heart rate >100 beats/min	+ 1.5
Major surgery/trauma within past 4 weeks	+ 1.5
History of DVT/PE	+ 1.5
Hemoptysis	+ 1
Malignancy	+ 1
Interpretation of risk according to point total:	
High	≥ 6 pts
Moderate	2 - 6 pts
Low	≤ 2 pts

Source: Line JA, Wells PS. (2003). Methodology for a rapid protocol to rule out pulmonary embolism in the emergency department. Annal Emerg Med; 42:266-275.

D-dimer

D-dimer is an adjunct intravenous blood test that is used to help rule out abnormal blood clotting, however it is not used independently to confirm a diagnosis. The test identifies the presence and the amount of a protein-product in the blood called *D-dimer*. The moment the clotting cascade is activated and thrombus formation occurs, the body begins to slowly break down the protein releasing the protein fragment into the blood. An enzyme called *plasmin* dissolves the thrombus into small pieces for removal. The thrombus is partly made up of threads of cross-linked fibrin. As the thrombus lyses, the subsequent fibrin fragments are called *fibrin degradation products (FDP)* and one of the final products is D-dimer. The level of D-dimer detected is dependent on the amount of cross-linked fibrin that is lysed; as thrombus formation increases, D-dimer production is higher.

The D-dimer blood test is low cost, easy to obtain and can be an initial screening for deep vein thrombosis and venous thromboembolism (VTE). When a positive D-dimer test is combined with a high clinical probability for DVT, further imaging tests are obtained (e.g., venous ultrasound exam, CT, direct pulmonary angiography or ventilation-perfusion scan). Elevated D-dimer levels are also seen in other conditions that cause the production and dismantling of fibrin (not just DVT).

- A D-dimer value is reported in units of parts per million (ng/ml or ug/ml).
- D-dimer is also known as fragment D-dimer and fibrin degradation fragment.
- Fibrinolytic activity in the blood reflects the breakdown of fibrin.
- D-dimer test results can be used as a predictive value for active blood clotting, therefore an elevated level suggests blood clot formation, where as a low level (within normal range value) indicates there is likely no significant activity of blood clot formation in the body.
- A normal D-dimer result, indicating lack of fibrinolytic activity is more useful than a positive D-dimer value. See the "Limitation" section.
- Following an initial encounter of unprovoked DVT and treatment of at least 6 months, a D-dimer test can be helpful in predicting the likelihood of a recurrent venous thrombosis.

Fig. 47-43: *D-dimer lecture*

- D-dimer levels can also be measured while a patient is on anticoagulant therapy. If normal, the anticoagulants can be stopped and the test may be repeated in 30 days. If the test result remains normal, the risk of recurrent thrombosis is low (about 3% per year). If the test result is positive, the risk of reoccurrence is > 10% per year. The test should be repeated in 3 months.

Indications

Suspicion of DVT
- Lower/upper extremity or tenderness
- Lower/upper extremity swelling or edema
- Lower/upper extremity discoloration
- Disseminated intravascular coagulation (DIC)- a rare, but serious condition where blood vessels clot throughout the body

Suspicion of PE
- Acute shortness of breath or labored breathing
- Lung-related chest pain
- Rapid heart rate
- Acute coughing with or without hemoptysis
- Fainting
- Stroke

Contraindications/Limitations

Note: Patients may have elevated D-dimer levels due to conditions other than DVT such as:

- Trauma
- Infection
- Recent surgery
- Heart attack
- Some cancers
- Liver disease (fibrin will not clear)
- High rheumatoid factor, trauma
- Pregnancy
- Advancing age

Caprini DTV Risk Score

The Caprini Risk Score assesses DVT risk with questions that divide patients into low, moderate, and high risk. Perform the assessment at **caprinirickscore.org**

REFERENCES

1. Medoff, B. (9-13-2008). Pulmonary ventilation/perfusion scan-overview. Retrieved from http://www.umm.edu/ency/article/003828.htm.
2. Dunn KL, Wolf JP, Dorfman DM, Fitzpatrick P, Baker JL, Goldhaber SZ. (2002). Normal D-dimer levels in emergency department patients suspected of acute pulmonary embolism. *J Am Coll Cardiology,* 40, 1475-1478.
3. American Association for Clinical Chemistry. (June 18, 2010) *D-dimer.* Retrieved from http://www.labtestsonline.org/understanding/analytes/d_dimer/test.html
4. Wells PS, Anderson DR, Rodger M, et al. (2003). Evaluation of D-dimer in the diagnosis of suspected deep-vein thrombosis." *N. Engl. J. Med.* 349 (13): 1227–35.
5. Kutinsky H, Blakely S, Roche V. (1999). Normal D-dimer levels in patients with pulmonary embolism. *Arch Intern Med,* 159, 1569-1572.
6. RadiologyInfo.org (March 15, 2010). Retrieved from http://www.radiologyinfo.org
7. Medical Journal of Australia.www.mja.com.au/public/issues/180_11_070604/dic10124_fm.html
8. McKenzie J, Goergen, S. (2017, Sept. 15). Computed Tomography (CT). Inside Radiology. https://www.insideradiology.com.au/
9. computed-tomography-hp/
10. Berger A. (2002). Magnetic resonance imaging. BMJ (Clinical research ed.), 324(7328), 35. https://doi.org/10.1136/bmj.324.7328.35
11. Cronenwett, J.L. (2014). Venography. In Rutherford Vascular Surgery (8th ed., pp. 307-311). Philadelphia. Elsevier Saunders
12. Bradley, A.M., Loscalzo, J. (2007) The Role of Platelets in Fibrinolysis. Science Direct. https://www.sciencedirect.com/topics/medicine-and-dentistry/fibrinolysis#:~:text=Fibrinolysis%20describes%20the%20process%20of,trauma%20or%20in%20pathological%20thrombosis.
13. Mirza H, Hashmi MF. Lung Ventilation Perfusion Scan (VQ Scan) [Updated 2020 Oct 24]. In: StatPearls [Internet]. Treasure Island (FL): StatPearls Publishing; 2021 Jan-. Available from: https://www.ncbi.nlm.nih.gov/books/NBK564428/
14. Philips Volcano. (2017, June). The Value of Intravascular Ultrasound Use in Hemodialysis Arteriovenous Access. A panel of experts addresses how and why clinicians today are increasingly reaching for IVUS during AV access evaluations. With Bart Dolmatch, MD; Rick de Graaf, MD, PhD; Jeffrey E. Hull, MD; and Edward Pavillard, MD. Endovascular Today. https://evtoday.com/articles/2017-june/the-value-of-intravascular-ultrasound-use-in-hemodialysis-arteriovenous-access
15. Neglén, P., & Raju, S. (2002). Intravascular ultrasound scan evaluation of the obstructed vein. Journal of vascular surgery, 35(4), 694–700. https://doi.org/10.1067/mva.2002.121127.)
16. Romaric, L., Falvo, N., Galland, C., Fréchier, L., Ledan, F., Midulla, M., Chevallier, O. (2020). Intravascular Ultrasound in the Endovascular Treatment of Patients With Peripheral Arterial Disease: Current Role and Future Perspectives. Frontiers in Cardiovascular Medicine, 7, 1-8. https://www.frontiersin.org/article/10.3389/fcvm.2020.551861. DOI=10.3389/fcvm.2020.551861

RESOURCES
48. Vascular Pharmacology

Aneurysm

- The main treatment is corrective surgery.
- Antihypertensives are sometimes used to control blood pressure and enlargement of the aneurysm.

Aortic Coarctation

- Antihypertensives are often used before and after surgery to control blood pressure.
- Infants may receive prostaglandin E1 (alprostadil) to help keep the ductus arteriosus open to serve as a bypass until the coarctation is repaired.

Arterial Dissection

- Although some patients may require surgery, medical management for Type B aortic dissection is standard.
- Anti-impulse therapy often uses IV esmolol or labetalol to decrease the rate of rise of left ventricular pressure (dP/dt)
- Afterload reduction agents with nitropresside or Nicardipine to reduce *afterload* (the amount of pressure the heart needs to exert) if blood pressure is still too high.
- Management with an anticoagulant can involve heparin.
- Analgesia for pain control

Arteritis *(see Vasculitis)*

Atherosclerosis

There is no direct treatment, just management of risk factors.

For patients with hyperlipidemia

- Statins
- Niacin
- Cholesterol absorption inhibitors
- PCSK9 inhibitors
- Fibrates
- Bile acid resins
- Omega-3-acid ethyl esters
- Nicotinic acid

For diabetic patients:

- Sulfonylureas
- Meglitinides
- Biguanides
- Thiazolidinediones
- Alpha-glucosidase inhibitors
- Insulin
- Dipeptidyl peptidase 4 (DPP-4) inhibitors
- Glucagon-like peptide 1based therapies
- Incretin mimetics
- Amylin analogues

For hypertensive patients:

- Diuretics
- Beta blockers
- ACE inhibitors
- ARBs (angiotension receptor blockers)
- CCBs (calcium channel blockers)
- Alpha blockers
- Central alpha agonists
- Direct renin inhibitors

Other agents used to manage patients with atherosclerosis include:

- Aspirin
- Clopidogrel
- Dipyridamole
- Cilostazol
- Direct oral anticoagulants
- Warfarin
- Direct thrombin inhibitors
- Thrombolytics
- Steroids

Carotid Body Tumor

Treatment is surgical

Cerebrovascular Events (TIA/Stroke)

- If blood pressure is too high, IV Labetalol is first-line treatment.
- Alteplase is the only FDA-approved thrombolytic for stroke.
- No antiplatelets or anticoagulants should be given for 24 hours.
- May use heparin or low molecular weight heparin (LMWH) for VTE (venous thromboembolism) prophylaxis after 48 hours.
- For non-cardioembolic stroke, antiplatelets are recommended for secondary prevention.
- For cardioembolic stroke, ASA is recommended for low-risk patients, and warfarin for high-risk patients for secondary prevention.
- For ischemic stroke, Factor VIIa is somctimes used, but there is a lack of evidence of efficacy.
- Supportive care is often the only treatment, including:
  - » Blood pressure control
  - » VTE prophylaxis
  - » Seizure prophylaxis
  - » Reduction of ICP

Fibromuscular Dysplasia

- Daily aspirin is generally considered first-line treatment.
- Plavix or Aggrenox can be substituted/added as necessary.

Iliac Vein Compression Syndrome
(previously May-Thurner Syndrome)

Prescribed medications include those to treat venous thrombosis.

Table 48-1: Anticoagulants and Thrombolytics

Class	Agents
Anticoagulants (clot prevention)	Warfarin
Thrombolytics (clot treatment)	Streptokinase, Urokinase, Anistreplase, Alteplase, Reteplase, Tenecteplase

Lymphedema

- Diuretics have been used somewhat successfully, but the oncotic pressure of lymph quickly causes recurrence of edema.
- Benzopyrones have also been used, but are no longer recommended.
- Refractory pain can be managed with analgesics, concomitant TCA, corticosteroids, anticonvulsants, and local anesthetics.

Mesenteric Ischemia

- The vasodilator papaverine is often given if the condition is discovered during angiography, or during and after surgery to repair this condition.
- Heparin, warfarin, and thrombolytics are often used to treat and prevent clot formation.

Neointimal Hyperplasia

- The current treatment regimen involves the placement of drug-eluding stents.

Phlegmasia Alba or Cerulea Dolens
(see Venous Thromboembolism)

Popliteal Artery Entrapment Syndrome

No drug therapy indicated unless thrombus is present. If present, options include:
- Streptokinase
- Reteplase
- Anistreplase
- Tenecteplase
- Alteplase

Popliteal Cystic Disease

- Pharmaceutical treatment is strictly supportive, likely corticosteroids.

Portal Hypertension

- Primary prophylaxis is with non-selective betaadrenergic blockers. Agents include:
  » Propranolol
  » Nadolol
- For acute variceal bleeding:
  » Somatostatin
  » Octreotide
  » Vasopressin

Postphlebitic Syndrome/Venous Insufficiency

- There is no indication for pharmacologic treatment of postphlebitic syndrome.
- Proper anticoagulation after VTE may prevent the onset of the condition.

Pseudoaneurysm

- Preliminary evidence suggests that sonographically-directed percutaneous injection of thrombin is safe and effective.
  » Overall success rate of 96%
  » Usual dose of 1-5 mL of thrombin

Raynaud's Syndrome

- Medications may be prescribed to dilate blood vessels.

Table 48-2: Pharmacological Agentsused for Raynaud's

Class	Agents
Dihydropyridine calcium channel blockers	Nifedipine, amlodipine, felodipine, isradipine
Angiotensin receptor antagonist	Losartan
Selective serotonin reuptake inhibitor	Fluoxetine
Alpha adrenergic antagonists	Prazosin
Prostaglandins	Epoprostenol, alprostadil

Alternatives include: nitroglycerin ointment and pentoxifylline

Renovascular Hypertension

- This condition is often treated surgically.
- Renal function may deteriorate even with controlled blood pressure. Agents often used include:
  » ACEIs (angiotensin-converting enzyme)- first line management
  » CCBs (slightly less effective but safer)

Subclavian Steal Syndrome

- No pharmacological treatment is known to be of value in the treatment of this syndrome.

Superior Vena Cava Syndrome

- Diuretics are often used to reduce the pressure on the vena cava. Furosemide is most commonly used.
- Steroids are sometimes used to decrease the swelling of any tumors exerting pressure.
- Anticoagulants and thrombolytics are used to treat and prevent clot formation.

Thoracic Outlet Compression Syndrome

Anti-inflammatory, pain medication and muscle relaxants are commonly prescribed.

Table 48-3: Anti-inflammatory Agents

Class	Agents
NSAIDS	ASA, naproxen, IBU, diclofenac
Anticoagulant	Warfarin
Muscle relaxants	Baclofen, carisoprodol, cyclobenzaprine

Alternatives include:
Nerve block and thrombolytics for acute blockage

Varicose Veins

- Sclerotherapy is the standard treatment.
- Additional agents include:
  - » Sotradecol
  - » Scleromate
  - » Polidocanol (not FDA approved for use in the U.S.)

Vasculitis

- Standard treatment is corticosteroids, including prednisone and methylprednisone.
- Controversial agents include non-steroidal anti-inflammatory drugs (NSAIDs), azathioprine, cyclophosphamide, dapsone, methotrexate.

Venous Thromboembolism/Pulmonary Embolism

- Empiric treatment should be started in all patients with suspected DVT or PE.
- "Unfractionated heparin" (UFH, class = antithrombotic) and subqutaneous low-molecular weight heparin (LMWH) are common drugs used in treatment.
- Initially give IV UFH or Sub-Q (injection into the fatty tissue) of LMWH and overlap with warfarin therapy.
- LMWH (e.g., Enoxaparin, Dalteparin, Tinzaparin, Lovenox) should be stopped once patient is on therapy for at least 5 days and INR >2 for 24 hours.
- Warfarin (class = anticoagulant) should be continued for a minimum of 3 months.
- Fondaparinux is an agent of the drug class, factor X inhibitor.

REFERENCES

1. Third Report of the Expert Panel on Detection, Evaluation, and Treatment of High Blood Cholesterol in Adults. Sept 2002. JAMA. www.nhibi.nih.gov. Accessed 13 Nov 2009.
2. The Seventh Report of the Joint National Committee on Prevention, Detection, Evaluation, and Treatment of High Blood Pressure. 21 May 2003. JAMA. www.nhibi.nig.gov. Accessed 13 Nov 2009.
3. Aneurysm. www.mayoclinic.org. Accessed 10 Oct 2009.
4. Pazzullo JA, Dupuy DE, Cronan JJ. Percutaneous injection of thrombin for the treatment of pseudoaneurysm after catheterization. AJR 200; 175:1035-1040.
5. Vega, Jose MD. Arterial dissection and stroke.
6. Moon, Marc MD. Approach to the treatment of aortic dissection. Surgical Clinics of North America. 2009 Aug 89(4): 869-93.
7. Schmidt, WA. Current diagnosis and treatment of temporal arteritis. Current Treatment Options in Cardiovascular Medicine. 2006 April; 8(2): 125-51.
8. Drug therapy of temporal arteritis and polymyalgia rheumatica. DRUGDEX Consults.
9. Wigley, Frederick M. Reynaud's Phenomenon. NEJM. 2002 Sept; Vol 347: 1001-8.
10. Coarctation of the aorta. www.mayoclinic.org. Accessed 1 Nov 2009.
11. Wright LB, Matchett JW, Cruz CP, et al. Popliteal artery disease: diagnosis and treatment. RadioGraphics. 2004 March; 24(2):467-79.
12. Drug Facts and Comparisons
13. Popliteal Cystic Disease. www.mayclinic.org. Accessed 29 Sept 2009.
14. Adams, HP, del Zoppo G, Alberts MJ et al. Guidelines for the early management of adults with ischemic stroke. Stroke 2007;38:1655-1711.
15. Adams RJ, Albers H, Alberts MH et al. Update to the AHA/ASA recommendations for the prevention of stroke in patients with stroke and transient ischemic attack. Stroke 2008;39:1647-52.
16. Sahid MS, Hamilton G, Baker DM. A Multicenter review of carotid body tumor management. European Journal of Vascular and Endovascular Surgery. 2007 Aug 34(2): 127-30.
17. Wilson, James. Fibromuscular dysplasia: treatment & medication. The Fibromuscular Dysplasia Society of America. www.fmdsa.org. Accessed 3 Nov 2009.
18. McIntrye, Keneth. Subclavian Steal Syndrome. Medscape. www.medscape.com. Accessed 3 Nov 2009.
19. Schachner T, Steger C, Heiss S et al. Paclitaxel treatment reduces neointimal hyperplasia in cultured human saphenous veins. European Journal of Cardio-Thoracic Surgery. 2007 Dec; 32(6):906-11.
20. Chronic venous insufficiency and postphlebitic syndrome. The Merck Manual. www.merck.com. Accessed 3, Nov 2009.
21. Shebel ND, Whalen CC. Diagnosis and management of iliac vein compression syndrome. J Vasc. Nurs. 2005 Mar; 23(1):10-17.
22. Antithrombotic and thrombolytic therapy, 8th Ed: ACCP Guidelines. Accessed 01 Oct 2009 Drug Facts and Comparisons
23. Bhalla A, D'Cruz S, Lehl SS, Singh R. Renovascular hypertension - its evaluation and management. JIACM 2003; 4(2): 139-46.
24. Acute Mesenteric Ischemia. The Merck Manual Online. www.merck.com. Accessed 12 Nov 2009. Depiro seventh edition.
25. Tajani S, Sanoski C. Davis's Pocket Clinical Drug Reference. 2009 F.A. Davis Company.
26. Harris SR, Hugi MR, Olivotto IA, et al. Clinical practice guidelines for the care and treatment of breast cancer: 11. Lymphedema. CMAJ 2001 Jan 23; 154(2):191-9.

Table 48-4: **Recommendations for Treatment of DVT and PE**				
Caprini Score	**Risk**	**VTE Incidence**	**Recommended Prophylaxis**	**Duration**
0 - 2	Very low to low	<1.5%[1]	Early ambulation, IPC	During hospitalization
3 - 4	Moderate	3%[1]	LMWH; UFH; or IPC. If high bleeding risk, IPC until bleeding risk diminishes.	At least 5 - 7 days
5 - 8	High	6%[1]	LMWH + IPC; or UFH + IPC. If high bleeding risk, IPC until bleeding risk diminishes.	At least 5 - 7 days*
>8	Very high	6.5 to 18.3%[2,3,4]	LMWH + IPC; or UFH + IPC. If high bleeding risk, IPC until bleeding risk diminishes.	Consider extended prophylaxis (e.g., 14-30 days)

Abdominal or pelvic surgery for cancer should receive extended VTE prophylaxis with LMWH x 30 days.[1]

IPC = intermittent pneumatic compression

LMWH = low molecular weight heparin

UFH = unfractionated heparin

1. Gould MK, Garcia DA, Wren SM, et.al. Prevention of VTE in nonorthopedic surgical patients: antithrombotic therapy and prevention of thrombosis, 9th ed: Americal College of Chest Physicians Evidence-Based Clinical Practice Guidelines. Chest. 2012; 141(2)(Suppl): e227S-e277S.

2. Bahl V, Hu HM, Henke PK, et.al. A validation study of a retrospective venous thromboembolism risk scoring method. Ann Surg. 2010; 251(2): 344-350.

3. Pannucci CJ, Bailey SH, Dreszer G, et.al. Validation of the Caprini risk assessment model in plastic and reconstructive surgery patients. J Am Coll Surg. 2011 January; 212 (1): 101-112.

4. Shuman AG, Hu HM, Pannucci CJ, et al. Stratifying the risk of venous thromboembolism in otolaryngology. Otolaryngology - Head and Neck Surgery 2012;146:719-724

Reprinted with permission from J. A. Caprini, MD.

RESOURCES
49. Testing Optimization

Purpose
Optimizing your image is a way of putting your stamp of approval on a study. Many factors come together in image optimization. General optimization techniques include:
- Ensure the comfort of your patient in terms of environment and positioning. Results of certain vascular studies, such as preoperative vein mapping, can be directly related to environment and patient comfort.
- Choose the transducer which is most appropriate for the study.
  » Abdominal studies should be performed using a lower frequency transducer, such as a curved transducer.
  » Evaluate the patient's body habitus as well identifying any swelling or edema in the extremities, as this could lead to the use of lower frequency transducers.

Optimization of Settings
- **Depth**: The depth of the image is shown by the markers on the side of the screen.
  » The vessel or structure of interest should be adjusted to the center of the screen eliminating any excess space above or below the image.
  » The depth is directly related to the pulse repetition period (PRP).

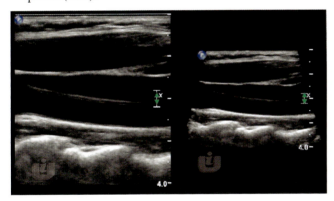

Fig. 49-1: *Decreased depth*   Fig. 49-2: *Increased depth*

Note: decreasing the depth improves the resolution of the vessel

- **Gain**: The gain adjusts the overall "brightness" of the image.
  » The gains need to be adjusted appropriately to demonstrate the area of interest without obscuring the image with too many echoes.

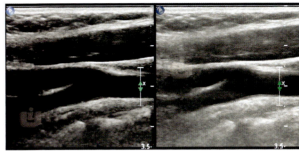

Fig. 49-3: *Appropriately adjusted gain on the left and high gain on the right (sometimes referred to as over gaining) which can obscure the image.*

- **Time gain compensation (TGC)**: The TGC allows for adjustment of different reflecting echoes at different depths and in return produces an image that is consistent in appearance.
  » Careful attention should be taken not to eliminate low-level echoes, resulting in elimination of soft/homogeneous appearing plaque.
  » The TGC controls aid in creating a uniform brightness from top to bottom in the image.

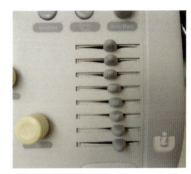

Fig. 49-4: *Typical TGC controls on a duplex machine*

- **Focus (focal zones)**: The focal zone(s) should be placed beside the vessel or structure of interest.
  » This is the point at which the ultrasound beam becomes the most intense.
  » This feature is adjustable so it can "focus" on a particular point in the image and provide the highest quality detail possible. *(Fig. 49-5)*

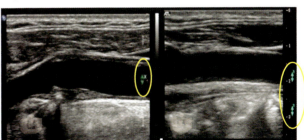

Fig. 49-5: *The focal zone(s) are usually placed just below or next to the structure of interest*

Image courtesy of Philips Healthcare

Active Gains

Active gains include color/power Doppler and spectral Doppler.

- **Color Doppler:** Color should fill the lumen of the vessel or structure without "bleeding" outside of the vessel.
    » Adjusting the wall filter can eliminate any low frequency Doppler shifts outside the vessel wall.
    » It is important to be able to visualize any intralumenal wall irregularities that may be present.
    » It may be necessary to decrease the scale to fill in low flow state vessels or increase the scale in areas of higher velocities.
    » While it is important to eliminate excess color outside the vessel wall, it is equally important to ensure the lumen of the vessel fills with color. *(Fig. 49-6)*
    » If the lumen is not filling with color, it could be suggestive of obstruction. Consider using power Doppler (color angio) to evaluate for low flow states or occlusions.

Spectral Doppler should also be used to determine an obstruction.

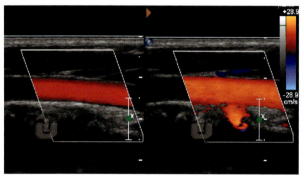

Fig. 49-6: *Color should fill the vessel lumen (left image) without spilling out the vessel wall (right image)*

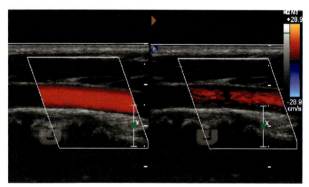

Fig. 49-7: *Color fills the vessel lumen on the left. Having the color gain set too low causes poor color filling within the vessel lumen (right)*

- **Spectral Doppler:** It is important to demonstrate the silhouette of the Doppler waveform. Over-gained waveforms can overestimate the velocity as under-gained waveforms can underestimate the velocity. *(Figs. 49-8 and 9)*

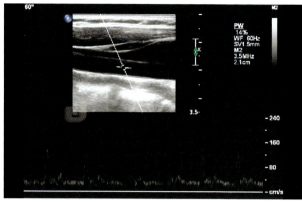

Fig. 49-8: *Under-gained Doppler waveforms are difficult to measure.*

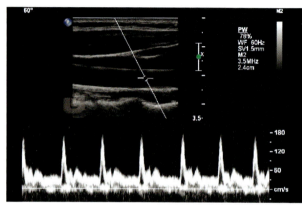

Fig. 49-9: *Over-gained Doppler waveform creates spectral broadening and can over estimate velocities.*

- Aliasing occurs when the sampled velocity is too high in comparison to the setting of the scale.
    » The Doppler waveform appears at the bottom of Doppler scale, in turn making the measurement inaccurate. *(Fig. 49-10)*
    » The scale needs to be increased to allow for the higher velocities in order to eliminate aliasing.
    » Adjusting the baseline is also another option.

HINT: In many cases where aliasing occurs, a combination of increasing the scale and adjusting the baseline is necessary to optimize the spectral waveform.

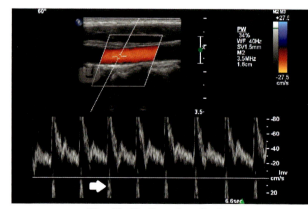

Fig. 49-10: *Doppler aliasing*

- **Frame rate**: A desirable image has a higher frame rate which increases the temporal resolution. Frame rate is affected by multiple factors:
  » Focal zones
  » Color box
  » Sector width of the image
  » Depth

Multiple frame rates, larger color boxes, increased depth and width of the image will slow down the frame rate. Try to reduce as many of these as possible.

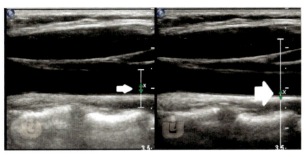

Fig. 49-11: *One, smaller focal zone*

Fig. 49-12: *Multiple, larger focal zones*

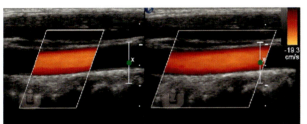

Fig. 49-13: *Narrow color box/sector width*

Fig. 49-14: *Wider color box/sector width*

- **Compression** alters the appearance of the B-mode image allowing it to be in range of the human eye.
  » Compression is adjustable by the sonographer.
  » An image with higher compression demonstrates more shades of grey.
  » An image with lower compression demonstrates less shades of grey.

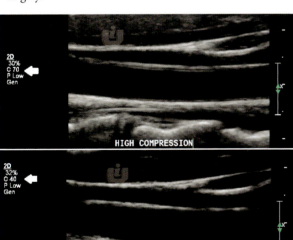

Fig. 49-15: *Examples of high and low compression*

- **Doppler angle**: The Doppler cursor should be placed in the middle of the vessel and be parallel to the flow within the vessel.
- **Angle of the color Doppler box**: Due to the cosine of the angle, correct steering of the color box will ensure maximum color fill. *(Fig. 49-16)*
  » The cosine of the angle is in reference to the beam of the ultrasound and the blood flow.
  » Incorrect steering of the color box prevents complete color fill of the vessel lumen. *(Figs. 49-17 and 18)*

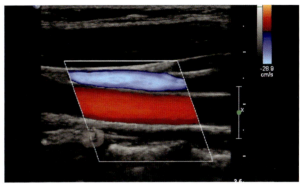

Fig. 49-16: *Correct steering of the color box optimizes color filling.*

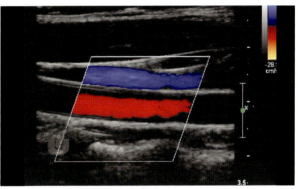

Fig. 49-17: *Suboptimal color flow noted when the color box angle is poorly optimized.*

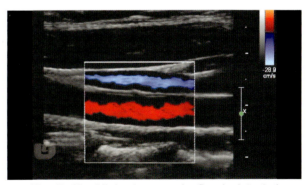

Fig. 49-18: *Minimal or no color flow is detected when the color box is perpendicular to flow.*

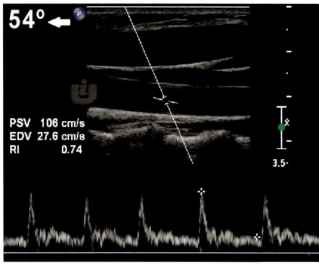

Fig. 49-19: *Doppler angle <60°: Velocity underestimated*

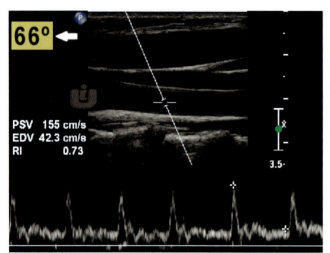

Fig. 49-20: *Doppler angle >60°: Velocity overestimated*

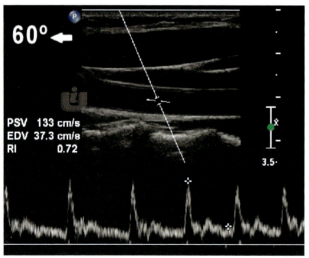

Fig. 49-21: *Doppler angle at 60°: Optimal velocity*

Points to Remember

- Be familiar with your ultrasound machine and its capabilities, this is essential to optimize the image. The ultrasound machine is only as useful as you make it.
- A brief, initial evaluation of your patient and decisions about what type of transducer and examination presets will be used are the first few steps in ensuring an optimal study.
- Prior to capturing each image, perform a quick run through, evaluating each of the settings. This will help optimize your images.
- Capturing an accurate velocity is one of the most important components in vascular ultrasound.
- Remain perpendicular to your vessel when scanning in B-mode.
- Try to keep the sample volume gate at 1.5–2mm and the sample gate centered in a normal lumen whenever possible.
- If there are reverberations throughout the vessel, change the color gain.
- Adequate color flow in the vertebral arteries may be difficult. Try the following adjustments:
  » Increase the color gain
  » Decrease the color scale
  » Increase the color gate
  » Increase the color filter
- A quality image of the distal SFA can be difficult to obtain. Try "harmonics" to make the vessel stand out. Enlarge the image and create a smaller color box. Apply pressure to omit any venous flow interference.
- The subclavian artery can also be difficult to image:
  » Recall your anatomy. The mid subclavian vessels run underneath the clavicle bone. Start with the transducer at the clavicular area (supraclavicular is suggested).
  » Begin with the transducer in sagittal and with the notch towards the head. The opposite end of the transducer should touch the clavicle.
  » Using enough gel, a longitudinal view of both the proximal and distal subclavian vessels can often be visualized in a single image.
- If you are not getting adequate color flow through a vessel, try the following adjustments:
  » Turn up the gain. Increase all the way up till you see color "speckles" and decrease from there.
  » Decrease the scale (especially for calf veins)
  » Decrease the frequency
  » Increase the color filter
  » Increase the size of the color gate
  » Change transducers (use an abdominal transducer for difficult/obese patients)
  » Place the patient in reverse Trendelenburg while imaging lower extremity veins

REFERENCES

1. Non Invasive Vascular Diagnostics, *A Practical Guide to Therapy*, 2nd Edition, Ali F. AbuRahma MD, FACS, FRCS, RVT, RPVI, John J Bergan MD, FACS, Hon FRCS; Springer-Verlag London Limited 2007; ISBN-13: 978-1-84628-446-5; Pg 262 graft surveys
2. Vascular Technology, *An Illustrated Review*, 3Rd Edition, Claudia Rumwell RN, RVT, FSVU, Michalene McPharlin RN, RVT, FSVU, Davies Publishing, Inc 2006, ISBN-0-941022-69-2
3. Understanding Ultrasound Physics, 3rd Edition, Sidney Edelman, Ph.D., Copyright 2007, ISBN 0-9626444-4-7

RESOURCES
50. Math Used in Sonography

Math Symbols

SYMBOLS	MEANING	EXAMPLE
+	Add to	5 + 5 = 10
-	Subtract from	9 – 5 = 4
x	Multiply	4 x 2 = 8
*	Multiply	4 * 2 = 8
( )	Multiply	4 (2) = 8
·	Multiply	4 · 2 = 8
÷	Divide by	8 ÷ 2 = 4
/	Divide by	8 ÷ 2 = 4
=	Equal to	5 = 5
≠	Not equal to	5 – 4 ≠ 8 - 2
±	Plus or minus (answer may deviate in a certain range)	The results of the study showed 36% ± 2% of those examined.
∞	Infinity	Never ending string of numbers
≈	Approximately/almost equal to	5.24 + 5.66 ≈ 11
~	Approximately/almost equal to	5.24 + 5.66 ~ 11
>	Greater than	8 >2
<	Less than	4 <9
≤	Less than or equal to	In 6 ≤6 the number to the left may be less than (<) or equal to (=) to the number on the right
≥	Greater than or equal to	In 6 ≥6 the number to the left may be greater than (>) or equal to (=) the number on the right
μ	Micro (millionth)	The speed of sound through soft tissue is 1.54mm/μs.
π	Pi	3.14
λ	Lambda	Wavelength (λ) = c/f
:	Colon	The ratio of females to males in the class is 4:1
Δ	Change	ΔP = change in pressure
∝	Proportional to	Power is proportional to amplitude^2

Order of Operations

A specific order of operations must be followed when multiple techniques are used to solve a problem:

The acronym PEMDAS (Please Excuse My Dear Aunt Sally) is often used to remember the order of operations.

Parenthesis (solve all portions of the equation in parenthesis first).
Exponents (solve all portions of the equation containing exponents next).
Multiplication and **D**ivision (working left to right, solve all portions of the equation that use multiplication and division next).
Addition and **S**ubtraction (working left to right, solve all portions of an equation using addition and subtraction next).

Example
$4^2 + (2 \times 6) + 9 – 6 =$
$4^2 + 12 + 9 – 6 =$
$16 + 12 + 9 – 6 =$
$37 – 6 =$
$37 – 6 = 31$

Additional Example
The equation $4v^2$ refers to a simplified calculation to determine pressure:
$4v^2$ if v = 2, then the calculation is as follows:
$4 \times 2^2 = 4 \times 4 = 16$ (correct answer)

If the order of operations was not followed and multiplication was performed first instead of calculating exponents, the result would be dramatically different.

$4 \times 22 \neq 82 = 64$ (incorrect answer)

If the order of operations are not followed, the calculation will produce an incorrect answer.

Variables

- Symbols (usually letters) are used to represent a value.
- When variables are placed next to a number, it implies multiplication should be performed.

Example: 4a = 4 x a

Distributive Property
When expressions use more than one math function, it can be viewed or solved in more than one way.

Example: a (b + c) = ab + ac
If we assign each variable a value: a = 2, b = 3, c = 7

2 (3 + 7) = (2) (3) + (2) (7)

2 (10) = 6 + 14

20 = 20

Integers

Adding Integers

When adding positive and negative integers, there are a certain set of rules to follow.

- When adding similar signs, add the absolute values and give the result using the same sign.

  Examples: (+4) + (+4) = 8
  (-4) + (-4) = -8
  (-4) + (-2) = -6

- When adding opposite signs, subtract the smaller value and use the sign from the larger integer.

  Examples: (+5) + (-2) = 3
  (+4) + (-4) = 0

Additional Example: If a brachial pressure is measured at 120mmHg and hydrostatic pressure is estimated at -30mmHg, what is the measured pressure? Using the equation:

circulatory pressure + hydrostatic pressure = measured pressure

(+120mmHg) + (-30mmHg) = 90mmHg

Subtracting Integers

When subtracting integers, add "its opposite":

  Examples: (-7) – (+2) = -9 (add "negative" 2 to the negative 7)

  Two negatives combined make a positive:

  (-6) – (-6) = 0 (add "positive" 6 to the negative 6)

  (+4) – (-6) = 10 (add "positive" 6 to the positive 4)

Multiplication and Division of Integers

When multiplying or dividing positive and negative integers:

A positive (+) and positive (+) will result in a positive (+) number

Example: (+ 4) divided by (+ 2) is equal to (+ 2)

A positive (+) and negative (-) will result in a negative (-) number

Example: (+ 4) multiplied by (- 4) is equal to (-16)

A negative (-) and negative (-) will result in a positive (+) number

Example: (- 4) multiplied by (- 4) is equal to (+ 16)

When multiplying the same sign, the answer is positive. When the signs are different, the result will be negative.

Fractions

- Any whole number can be treated as a fraction.
- May be written several different ways:

number ÷ number   or   number / number

- Any number divided by 1 will equal the original number.

  Examples: 25/1 = 25   6/1 = 16

- Zero divided by any number is zero.

  Examples: 0/25 = 0   0/16 = 0

- Any number divided by itself equals 1.

  Examples: 25/25 = 1   16/16 = 1

Fractions may be reduced by dividing the numerator and denominator by the same number (any common denominator that can divide into both numbers). "Simplifying fractions" is a function that reduces or makes the fraction as simple as possible.

Example:

Both the numerator and denominator can be divided by 5

  5/10 = 1/2

  because 5 divided by 5 equals 1
  and 10 divided by 5 equals 2

Multiplying fractions: when multiplying fractions, both numerator and denominator are multiplied.

Example: $\dfrac{5}{8} \times \dfrac{2}{5} = \dfrac{10}{40} = \dfrac{1}{4}$

"Cancelling out" is a shortcut that can also be used to reduce fractions, when the numerator and denominator are the same, cancel out both variables.

Example: $\dfrac{\cancel{5}}{8} \times \dfrac{2}{\cancel{5}} = \dfrac{2}{8} = \dfrac{1}{4}$

Although cancelling out is a shortcut, it does not change the answer that would have been given if the expanded work was completed as referenced below:

Expanded work shown:

$$\dfrac{5 \times 2}{8 \times 5} = \dfrac{5 \times 2}{8 \times 5}$$

$$\dfrac{5 \times 2}{8 \times 5} = \dfrac{2 \times 5}{8 \times 5}$$

$$\dfrac{2 \times \cancel{5}}{8 \times \cancel{5}} = \dfrac{2 \times 1}{8 \times 1}$$

$$\dfrac{2 \times 1}{8 \quad 1} = \dfrac{2}{8}$$

$$\dfrac{2}{8} = \dfrac{1}{4}$$

Conversions

Fraction and Decimal Conversions

To convert a fraction to a decimal, divide the numerator by the denominator.

  Example: ½ =1 ÷ 2 = 0.5

- To convert a decimal to fraction, use the place value to create a fraction, then reduce if necessary.

  Examples: 0.5 = 5/10   5/10 = ½
  0.75 = 75/100   75/100 = ¾

  (reduced by the common denominator of 25)

- When converting to a fraction, the denominator can usually be reduced since it is based on a system of tens.

If the conversion is done correctly, the resulting decimal will equal less than 1 when the numerator is less than the denominator. If the numerator is greater than the denominator, the resulting conversion will be >1.

Math Used in Sonography

Table 50-1: Fraction to Decimal Conversion/Equivalent

1/10	.1	3/5	.6
1/8	.125	5/8	.625
1/6	.16666…	2/3	.666…
1/5	.2	7/10	.7
1/4	.25	3/4	.75
3/10	.3	4/5	.8
1/3	.3333…	5/6	.8333…
3/8	.375	7/8	.875
2/5	.4	9/10	.9
1/2	.5	1/1	1

Example:

ABI (ankle-brachial index) = $\frac{\text{Highest ankle pressure}}{\text{Highest brachial pressure}}$

If the ankle pressure is measured at 105mmHg and the brachial pressure is measured at 120mmHg, the ABI equation will produce a fraction of 105/120. ABIs are reported in the form of a decimal, so a conversion is necessary. 105 divided by 120 yields a decimal conversion of .875 (Rounded to .88).

Metric Conversions

The metric system is used to represent weight (grams), distance (meters), area (square meters), and volume (liters).
- Units can be further expressed as larger or smaller numbers simply by adding a prefix (e.g., centi-, kilo-). The prefixes used in the metric system change the place value of the decimal.
- Movement of the decimal changes the value of a number by factors of ten.

Example: **1 kilometer = 1000 meters**

Kilo stands for 1000. In this case, it is necessary to move the decimal 3 placements. Three decimal placements to the right increases any number by a thousand (add three 0s).

Table 50-2: Prefix Definitions

Mega- (M)	million	(1,000,000)	10^6
Kilo- (k)	thousand	(1,000)	10^4
Hecto- (h)	hundred	(100)	10^2
Deka- (da)	ten	(10)	10^1
Deci- (d)	one-tenth	(.1) = 1/10	10^{-1}
Centi- (c)	one-hundredth	(.01) = 1/100	10^{-2}
Milli- (m)	one-thousandth	(.001) = 1/1000	10^{-3}
Micro- (µ)	one-millionth	(.000001) = 1/1000000	10^{-6}

- It may be necessary to convert from one unit to another. Consider the prefix and move the decimal the correct number of places.

Example: The difference from kilo to mega is 3 decimal places. Conversion from a smaller unit (kilo) to a larger unit (mega), means the decimal will move 3 places to the right (so add three 0s).

1000 kilo = 1 mega
(kilo means a thousand, so 1000 kilo is equal to 1000 x 1000 or 1,000 x 1,000 = 1,000,000 or 1 mega (multiplying by 1000 = adding 3 zeros to the right)

Practice examples: When the ultrasound machines measures in a different unit than needed for an exam report, measurements have to be converted.

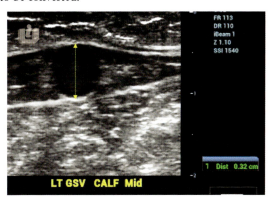

Fig. 50-1: *GSV diameter measured in cm by the ultrasound machine. The reported diameter needs to be converted to mm.*

Centi is a hundredth and milli is a thousandth. There is one decimal place difference between the two. Determine which way to move the decimal: left or right. Since the conversion is from a larger to smaller number, the resulting number will be larger.

0.32cm = 3.2mm

Differences in Prefixes

When converting from a smaller to larger prefix, the resulting number will be smaller.

centi = 0.01
milli = 0.001
mm < cm (1/1000 is smaller than 1/100)
100mm = 100 X .001 (milli = .001) = 0.1 meters
10cm = 10 X .01 (centi = .01) = 0.1 meters
(If the conversion was done properly, they should be equal)

Temperature Conversion

- The formula to convert Fahrenheit to Celsius:
  C = (F - 32) x 5/9
- From Celsius to Fahrenheit: **F = 9/5 C + 32**

Table 50-3: American-Metric Conversion

American unit	Metric equivalent unit
2.2 lbs (pounds)	1 kilogram
1 lb (pound)	0.454 kilogram
1 inch	2.54 centimeters
0.394 inches	1 centimeter
1 mile	1.61 kilometers
0.62 mile	1 kilometer

Exponents

- Exponential notation is used to express numbers that are multiplied by themselves. It is a kind of shorthand that is used in mathematics to represent large numbers.

Example: 10^2 = 10 X 10
10^4 = 10 X 10 X 10 X 10

- **Multiplication of exponents**: When exponents have the same base number, the exponents are simply added together. This technique can also be used when the two exponents have the same variable.

Example: 10^4 x 10^2 = 10^6

Example: a^4 x a^2 = a^6

- **Dividing exponents**: When exponents have the same base number, the exponents are simply subtracted. This technique can also be used when the two exponents have the same variable.

Example: $10^5 \div 10^2 = 10^3$

Example: $a^5 \div a^2 = a^3$

- A negative exponent is equivalent to the inverse of the number with a positive exponent.

Example: $a^{-3} = 1 \div a^3$
$10^{-3} = 1 \div 10^3$
$10^{-6} = 1 \div 10^6$

- Any number with an exponent to the power of 0 will equal 1.

Example: $5^0 = 1$

Formulas

- Area reduction versus diameter reduction calculations will yield different percentages of change.

Example: 50% diameter reduction = 75% area reduction

Proportionality

Proportionality refers to how variables are related in any equation if a change is made to one variable.

Direct: In a direct relationship, when one factor or variable is manipulated, another is affected in the same way.

Example: $A = \dfrac{B}{C}$

B is directly proportional to A. If A increases, so will B.

If the numerator (B) is increased, the sum (A) will also be increased.

- **Inverse:** In an inverse or opposite relationship, when one factor or variable is manipulated, another is affected in the opposite way.

Example: $A = \dfrac{B}{C}$

Since C is inversely proportional to A, if A increases C will decrease.

When approaching equations, the sum and the denominator are inversely proportional. If the denominator (C) is increased, the sum (A) will be decreased.

Additional Examples:

$$\uparrow A = \dfrac{B\uparrow}{C} \qquad \downarrow A = \dfrac{B\downarrow}{C} \qquad \downarrow A = \dfrac{B}{C\uparrow} \qquad \uparrow A = \dfrac{B}{C\downarrow}$$

$$5 = \dfrac{10}{2}$$

If 10 is increased to 20, the resulting effect to 5 will be to increase to 10 (directly proportional)

$$10 = \dfrac{20}{2}$$

Linear Versus Non-Linear Proportionality

Linear
If two variables have linear proportionality, each variable is affected the same way.

I = P/A

I (intensity), P (power), A (area).

Power is proportional to intensity.

Example: If power is increased, intensity is also increased. If power is decreased, intensity is also decreased.

If power is increased by a factor of 2, intensity is increased by a factor of 2. If power is decreased by a factor of 2, intensity is decreased by a factor of 2.

Non-linear
If two variables have non-linear proportionality, each variable is not affected the same way.

Example: Power is proportional to amplitude squared. If amplitude is increased by a factor of 2, power is increased by a factor 2^2 or a factor of 4. Both variables are affected, but not equally (non-linear).

Decibels

- Decibels are used commonly in word problems when describing a change in power or intensity.

Example: Initial power is 2 watts. If the power is increased by a factor of 16, what is the change in decibels?

To calculate a decibel gain, divide the final power by the initial power and calculate the log of this ratio, then multiply by 10. The formula used to calculate a dB gain: [9]

$$dB = 10 \times \log(P_2/P_1)$$

dB is the decibel gain (decibels)
P_2 (final power level (watts))
P_1 (initial power level (watts))

Increasing 2 watts by a factor of 16 equals a final power of 32 watts.

dB = 10 x log(32 ÷ 2)

dB = 10 x 1.20411998266

dB = 12.0 (rounded number) = +12dB

Example: Calculate the final power for the example above:

Since a 12 dB change instructs to multiple by 16 (see Decibel Chart Table 50-4), 2 watts x 16 = 32 watts

Example: Use Table 50-4 to calculate final power if an initial 5 watts was increased by 12dB.

5 watts x 16 = 80 watts

Intensity example: Use Table 50-4 to calculate final intensity if the initial intensity = 8w/cm² decreases in intensity decreases by 6 dB.

2.8w/cm² ÷ 4 = 2w/cm²

Use multiplication when increasing by a factor.
Use division when decreasing by a factor.

Table 50-4: Decibel Chart

Decibel change	Meaning or instruction
3 dB	Multiply by 2 (increase by a factor) or divide by 2 (decrease by a factor)
6 dB	Multiply by 4 (increase by a factor) or divide by 4 (decrease by a factor)
9 dB	Multiply by 8 (increase by a factor) or divide by 8 (decrease by a factor)
10 dB	Multiply by 10 (increase by a factor) or divide by 10 (decrease by a factor)
12 dB	Multiply by 16 (increase by a factor) or divide by 16 (decrease by a factor)
15 dB	Multiply by 32 (increase by a factor) or divide by 32 (decrease by a factor)
20 dB	Multiply by 100 (increase by a factor) or divide by 100 (decrease by a factor)
30 dB	Multiply by 1,000 (increase by a factor) or divide by 1,000 (decrease by a factor)
40 dB	Multiply by 10,000 (increase by a factor) or divide by 10,000 (decrease by a factor)
50 dB	Multiply by 100,000 (increase by a factor) or divide by 100,000 (decrease by a factor)

Cosine

Table 50-5: Commonly Used Cosines

Cos (0°)	1
Cos (30°)	0.87
Cos (45°)	0.71
Cos (60°)	0.50
Cos (90°)	0

Cosine angles are used when calculating frequency shifts.

Example: $f_{Dop} = \dfrac{2 f_o\ v\ cos\ (\theta)}{c}$

Doppler Shift = $\dfrac{2\ (speed\ of\ blood)\ (operating\ frequency)\ cos\ (\theta)}{propagation\ speed}$

Table 50-6: Circular Formulas

Area	πr^2
Area reduction*	(%) = $(1 - \pi r_2^2 \div \pi r_1^2)$ x 100
	r_1 represents true lumenal radius of the native vessel
	r_2 represents residual lumenal radius of the narrowed lumen
Circumference	$2 \pi r$
Diameter	$2 r$
Diameter reduction*	(%) = $(1 - D_2 \div D_1)$ x 100
	D_1 represents the true lumenal diameter of native vessel
	D_2 represents the residual lumenal diameter of narrowed lumen
Volume	$4 \div 3 \pi r^3$

Manipulating Equations

To separate a variable, utilize division or multiplication to isolate the variable to one side of the equation.

Whatever you do to one side of the equation,
you MUST do to the other side.

Example
Given the equation:

A = B ÷ C

To isolate B, multiply each side by C

C x A = (B ÷ C) x C

Since the C's cancel themselves out on the right side, the equation is now:

C x A = B or B = C x A

To isolate C in the equation:

B = C x A

Divide each side by A

B ÷ A = (C x A) ÷ A

Since "A" cancels out, the equation is:

B ÷ A = C

Example: To manipulate an equation utilizing addition and subtraction:

8A − 2 = 30

Isolate variable A: add 2 to each side to isolate 8A:

(2 +) 8A − 2 = 30 (+ 2)

The +2 and -2 on the left side of the equation equal zero:

8A = 32

Isolate A by itself, divide each side by 8.

$\dfrac{8A}{8} = \dfrac{32}{8}$ (8/8 cancels out)

$A = \dfrac{32}{8}$ or   A = 4

Table 50-7: Additional Formulas

Reynolds Number	$Re = \dfrac{V\rho 2r}{\eta}$ Reminder: The Reynolds number is considered "dimensionless"(no unit of measure). A Reynolds number >2000 is an indication of flow disturbance (turbulence).	Re = Reynolds number V = velocity ρ = density of fluid r = radius of vessel η = viscosity of fluid within the vessel
Resistance equation Reminder: Changes in radius will have the greatest effect on resistance.	$R = \dfrac{8\,L\,\eta}{\pi\,r^4}$	R = resistance L = length of the vessel r = radius of vessel π = 3.14 η = viscosity of fluid
Attenuation coefficient for soft tissue	$\approx .5$ dB/cm/MHz	
Nyquist limit	$\dfrac{\text{pulse repetition frequency (PRF)}}{2}$	
Doppler equation	$f_{Dop} = \dfrac{2\ fo\ v\ \ \cos(\theta)}{c}$	
The Doppler equation may also be seen as	$\dfrac{2\ (\text{speed of blood})\ (\text{operating frequency})\ \cos(\theta)}{\text{propagation speed}}$	
Change in pressure (simplified equation)	volume flow x resistance	
Ohm's law	voltage = current x resistance	
Measured pressure	circulatory pressure + hydrostatic pressure	Note: hydrostatic pressure is 0mmHg at heart level
Poiseuille's law	$Q = \dfrac{\Delta P\ \pi\ r^4}{8\,L\,\eta}$	Q = volume flow ΔP = change in pressure $(P_1 - P_2)$ r = radius L = length of vessel η = viscosity of fluid π = 3.14
Simplified Bernoulli equation	Pressure (mmHg)= $4v^2$	When calculating a change in pressure, Δ Pressure(mmHg)= $4(v_2^2 - v_1^2)$
Ankle-brachial index (ABI)	$\dfrac{\text{highest ankle pressure}}{\text{highest brachial pressure}}$	

REFERENCES

1. Bello I. (2006). Introductory Algebra, A Real-World Approach 2nd edition. McGraw Hill.
2. Hutchison,Bergman B, Baratto. (2005). Basic Mathematical Skills with Geometry 6th edition. McGraw Hill.
3. Slater, TJ. (2002). Basic College Mathematics 4th edition. Pearson/Prentice Hall.
4. Shulte AP, Peterson RE, (1986). Preparing to use Algebra 4th edition. Laidlaw Brothers.
5. Kime LA, Clark J, Michael BK. (2005). Explorations in College Algebra 3rd Edition. John Wiley & Sons, Inc.
6. Smith KJ. (2006). Mathematics: Its Power and Utility. Thomson Brooks/Cole..
7. Edelman, SK. (2005). Understanding Ultrasound Physics. ESP Ultrasound.
8. Miele FR. (2006). Ultrasound Physics and Instrumentation Vol.1 & 2. Pegasus Lectures Inc.
9. Calculator Academy Team. 2023, July 27. DB Gain Calculator. Calculator Academy. https://calculator.academy/db-gain-calculator.

RESOURCES
51. Statistics

Rationale

One of the main objectives for any non-invasive vascular laboratory is to provide accurate test results. Physicians expect that a positive exam truly means that their patient has disease and a negative exam truly means the patient has no significant disease. Exams should also have a high degree of reliability and repeatability.

Regular, ongoing correlations by the non-invasive lab with gold standard procedures ensure the highest quality of service to patients and their referring physicians.

Definitions

- **Gold standard**: A well accepted standard used during the comparison of diagnostic information derived from the non-invasive vascular lab exam. Examples of gold standard exams include, but are not limited to:

  » **Peripheral arterial:** Angiograms, CT scans, operative findings, MRA, surgical pathology reports

  » **Extracranial/intracranial:** CT scans, angiography

  » **Peripheral venous:** Venograms, repeat non-invasive exams, MRV

  » **Visceral:** CT scans, angiography

Terms used in accuracy studies

Positive and negative levels of disease must be defined to determine true and false, positive and negative comparisons. Positive exams can be defined by a Lab in broad terms (e.g., significant findings equal >50%) or Labs may adopt more specific ranges and category definitions (e.g., 50-69%, 60-69%, 70-79%, etc.).

Consider how your correlative exams will be interpreted and whether there could be any significant issues with comparisons. For instance, if a positive non-invasive carotid is any exam with a stenosis >50% (including occlusions) and a CTA shows a 40% stenosis, the duplex would correlate as a false positive non-invasive exam. Though both exams demonstrate disease, the degree by CTA is considered "not significant," since the stenosis is < 50%. Separate correlations can be done for differing levels of disease, e.g., >50%, >70%, or 80-99%, etc.

- **True positive (TP)**: Significant disease is present by both the gold standard and the non-invasive exam.

- **True negative (TN)**: No significant disease present by either the gold standard or the non-invasive exam.

- **False positive (FP)**: Although significant disease is suggested by the non-invasive exam, the gold standard detected no significant disease.

- **False negative (FN)**: No disease was suggested by the non-invasive exam, though the gold standard indicated significant disease was present.

- **Sensitivity**: The ability of the non-invasive exam to detect disease.

- **Specificity**: The ability of the non-invasive exam to detect the lack of disease.

- **Positive predictive value (PPV)**: How often any positive non-invasive exam truly indicates the presence of significant disease.

- **Negative predictive value (NPV)**: How often a negative non-invasive exam is found to be truly negative by the gold standard.

- **Overestimation**: The non-invasive exam suggested disease or a disease category that was greater than diagnosed by the gold standard.

- **Underestimation**: The non-invasive exam graded the disease in a lower category than the gold standard.

- **Sample size (n)**: The number of examinations used in analysis.

Formulas

- **Sensitivity** $= \dfrac{\text{True Positive non-invasive exams}}{\text{All positive gold standard exams}}$

- **Specificity** $= \dfrac{\text{True Negative non-invasive exams}}{\text{All negative gold standard exams}}$

- **PPV** $= \dfrac{\text{True Positive non-invasive exams}}{\text{All positive non-invasive exams}}$

- **NPV** $= \dfrac{\text{True Negative non-invasive exams}}{\text{All negative non-invasive exams}}$

- **Overall accuracy (OA)** $= \dfrac{\text{TP + TN}}{\text{TP+TN+FN+FP}}$

Protocol for Gathering Statistical Correlation

The non-invasive exam should have been performed before the gold standard test for the most honest comparison.

- Use all results regardless of agreement with the non-invasive exam to eliminate bias. Test results should not be altered after review of the correlating examination. Instead, concentrate on how to improve testing methods for the future. In addition, keep a list of uninterpretable non-invasive exams.

- Each laboratory should have a written policy outlining the procedure used to collect data, frequency of analysis, personnel responsible and how results are disseminated to staff.

- Gather data throughout the year to be used for quality assurance (QA) analysis.

  » Keep logs of all results. Keeping a list of abnormal results only will skew the data. Normals exams are important to identify and are comparable too. They may improve statistics.

Be sure that no surgical or therapeutic procedures were performed between the non-invasive and gold standard exams.

  » Determine if any patients tested by a non-invasive exam were also referred for a correlating exam.

Date	Name	1st TECH Venous Right Leg	1st TECH Venous Left Leg	2nd TECH Venous Right Leg	2nd TECH Venous Left Leg	Agree? Yes/No RIGHT	Agree? Yes/No LEFT	Comments
	DVT/SVT							
	CVI							
	DVT/SVT							
	CVI							
	DVT/SVT							
	CVI							

Fig. 51-1: *Sample log for the repeat venous examination method of correlation*

» Options specifically for venous correlations include gathering information about a patient's clinical outcome, or designating 1-2 days throughout the month as "repeat exam" days.

- On these days, two technologists will scan the patient during their visit and a third technologist will compare the results.
- The first technologist/sonographer performs the exam and writes a preliminary report.
- The second technologist/sonographer repeats the examination without knowing the results of the first examiner's work. The second examiner should write their own preliminary results.
- Designate a third person to compare both results and log agreement/disagreement.

» Consider combining QA data for upper and lower extremity venous exams in order to reach the minimum accreditation requirements for numbers of limbs necessary for correlation.

- Consider engaging all technologists in the ongoing quality assurance initiative in your lab. Rotate who maintains the logs, collects the correlating studies and calculates the statistics each year. This enables the team to have a greater appreciation for the QA process and accuracy of their work.
- Different radiologists or interpreting physicians within the same institution may use different methods for measuring stenosis (on an angiogram for example). Different percent stenosis may be calculated on an imaging study depending on whether the observer used the distal ICA or residual lumen at the point of stenosis. Ensure that the same method is used for interpretation before studying QA and exam accuracy. [1]
- Case Peer Review by a second interpreting physician is another opportunity to correlate reporting methods, document technical adequacy, interpretation accuracy and final report completeness.

CPT charge reports can be a useful tool to identify which patients have had a study that can be used for correlation.

Statistical Correlation

It is important to account for any false negative or false positive results in the vascular lab in order to improve the quality of testing.

- Statistical analysis can also be calculated for each modality used in a particular area of testing. For example, QA data can be generated for segmental pressures, volume pulse recording and arterial duplex separately. This may provide insight into which modality is the most reliable in your laboratory.

- Each aspect of the diagnostic criteria used can also be analyzed. For example, carotid QA may include accuracy calculations for:
  » B-mode image
  » ICA peak systolic velocity
  » ICA end-diastolic velocity
  » ICA/CCA peak velocity ratio
  » ICA/CCA end diastolic velocity ratio

- The time frame between the non-invasive exam and the gold standard may need to be less than 3-4 months when rapidly progressing disease is involved (e.g., transcranial imaging for vasospasms).[2]

The acceptable time frame between the non-invasive test and the gold standard is typically no more than 3-6 months.

- 2 x 2 table or chi-square tables are helpful when organizing data and calculating accuracies. Typically, the gold standard can be plotted along the x-axis and the non-invasive exam can be plotted along the y-axis:

		Gold Standard Test Results	
		+	−
Non-invasive Test Results	+	True Positive (TP)	False Positive (FP)
	−	False Negative (FN)	True Negative (TN)

Practical Consideration for Statistical Calculations

Question: Why is the overall accuracy (OA) lower for predicting disease at the aortoiliac level compared to the femoropopliteal segment?

Considerations: The femoropopliteal segment is imaged directly using duplex scanning. Common femoral artery waveforms alone are all that is considered when predicting aortoiliac disease.

Possible solutions: Add additional testing, such as volume pulse recording, to gather supporting evidence of aortoiliac obstruction. Add direct imaging of the aortoiliac segment to look for stenosis/occlusion and recalculate to see if accuracies improve. You may consider better ways to interpret the common femoral using duplex.

When using several gold standards to assess accuracy for a given exam calculate sensitivity, specificity, PPV, NPV and OA for each exam separately rather than combining gold standards (e.g., assess duplex vs. CT scan and duplex vs. angiography separately).

Patient Name	Medical Record #	Side	Date of Vascular Lab Studies	B-Mode Diameter Reduction	PSV	EDV	% Stenosis in conclusion	Date of CTA	CTA Results	Correlation	Notes
Smith, McKenzie	12345798	R	12/30/2008		61	25	0-49%	1/2/2009	No stenosis	TN	
Smith, McKenzie	12345798	L	12/30/2008		98	34	0-49%	1/2/2009	No stenosis	TN	
Thomas, Tom	9876541	R	1/23/2009		80	42	0-49%	1/25/2009	No stenosis	TN	
Thomas, Tom	9876541	L	1/23/2009	82%	422	223	80-99%	1/25/2009	80-90% stenosis	TP	
Manning, Ted	7095312	R	7/7/2009	64%	202	51	50-79%	7/16/2009	50% stenosis	TP	
Manning, Ted	7095312	L	7/7/2009		40	4	0-49%	7/16/2009	40% stenosis	TN	
Kromer, Blair	7772213	R	4/16/2009		273	76	50-79%	4/16/2009	Heavily calcified	FP	When CT was remeasured a 73% stenosis was found in the RICA and this correlates with duplex findings
Kromer, Blair	7772213	L	4/16/2009		261	65	50-79%	4/16/2009	Heavily calcified	FP	When CT was remeasured a 54% stenosis was found in the LICA and this correlates with duplex findings

Fig. 51-2: *Excerpt from a QA log for the year*

Practical Examples of Statistical Calculations

Question: How accurately did our lab identify carotid stenosis in the 50-79% range?

Solution: The question is best answered with the percent agreement plotted on a matrix.

150 carotid arteries scanned during the year were found to have a corresponding CT scan on record at our hospital. The results of the non-invasive and CT scans for each carotid were plotted onto a matrix. The various ranges of carotid disease used in this particular institution were considered; (0-49%) (50-79%) (80-99%) and (100%).

Duplex \ CT Scan	0-49%	50-79%	80-99%	100%
0-49%	136	0		
50-79%	2	6		
80-99%		1	3	
100%				2

0% underestimated
98% agreement
2% overestimated

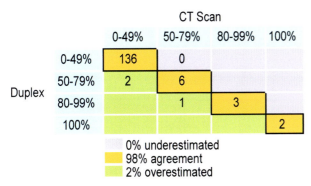

Fig. 51-3: *Expanded version of a 2 x 2 table used to tabulate TN, TP, FP and FN*

The total number of TP, TN, FP and FN were calculated:

Gold Standard Test Results

Non-invasive Test Results	+	–
+	True Positive 11 cases	False Positive 3 cases
–	False Negative 0 cases	True Negative 136 cases

TN = 136 TP = 11 FP = 3 FN = 0

Using these values in the statistical formulas for sensitivity, specificity, PPV, NPV and OA, the following percentages were calculated:

$$\textbf{Sensitivity} = \frac{\text{TP}}{\text{All positive CT scans}} = \frac{11}{11+0} \text{ x } 100 = 100\%$$

$$\textbf{Specificity} = \frac{\text{TN}}{\text{All negative CT scans}} = \frac{136}{136+3} \text{ x } 100 = 98\%$$

$$\textbf{PPV} = \frac{\text{TP}}{\text{All positive duplex scans}} = \frac{11}{11+3} \text{ x } 100 = 79\%$$

$$\textbf{NPV} = \frac{\text{TN}}{\text{All negative duplex scans}} = \frac{136}{136+0} \text{ x } 100 = 100\%$$

$$\textbf{OA} = \frac{\text{TN}+\text{TP}}{\text{TP}+\text{TN}+\text{FN}+\text{FP}} = \frac{136+11}{136+11+3+0} \text{ x } 100 = 98\% \text{ OA}$$

Question: Of all the stenoses in the 80-99% range, what is the most predictable peak systolic velocity (PSV) to indicate the presence of disease ≥80%?

Solution: There are commercial software programs available for biomedical researchers which use ROC (receiver operating characteristic) curve analysis that can help determine the most accurate velocity to use for diagnosing disease in a certain patient population, establishing a new threshold for your lab.

Reporting on QA Studies

- Calculating accuracy statistics is fairly useless without subsequent analysis, discussion, and action plans to improve accuracy. Regular meetings/discussions should occur.
  - » Meeting minutes and attendance should be kept and agenda items should include, but are not limited to: [2]
    - Discussion of QA results
    - Discussion of any discrepancies (e.g., FP or FN exams)
    - Review of challenging cases
    - Discussion of QA issues identified within the laboratory
- A goal for percent agreement should be at least 70% for any given exam.[2]
- Accurate diagnosis by "level of disease" (aortoiliac, versus, femoropopliteal versus infrapopliteal versus multilevel disease) can be a useful analysis.
- After correlations are completed, it is important to find ways to improve any areas of concern.

Reporting Example:

Accuracy for hemodynamically significant arterial obstruction using angiograms:

TN = 33

TP = 64

FN = 0

FP = 6

$$\text{Sensitivity} = \frac{TP}{TP+FN} = \frac{64}{64 + 0} \times 100 = 100\%$$

$$\text{Specificity} = \frac{TN}{FP+TN} = \frac{33}{6 + 33} \times 100 = 85\%$$

$$\text{Positive Predictive Value} = \frac{TP}{TP + FP} = \frac{64}{64 + 6} \times 100 = 91\%$$

$$\text{Negative Predictive Value} = \frac{TN}{TN + FN} = \frac{33}{33 + 0} \times 100 = 100\%$$

$$\text{OA} = \frac{TP+TN}{TP +TN + FP + FN} = \frac{64 + 33}{64 + 33 + 6 + 0} \times 100 = 94\%$$

Accuracy using Infused CTs:

TN=40

TP=0

FN=0

FP=5

$$\text{Sensitivity} = \frac{TP}{TP+FN} = \text{Not applicable. No data.}$$

$$\text{Specificity} = \frac{TN}{FP+TN} = \frac{40}{5 + 40} \times 100 = 89\%$$

$$\text{Positive Predictive Value} = \frac{TP}{FN+FP} = \text{Not applicable}$$

$$\text{Negative Predictive Value} = \frac{TN}{TN+FN} = \frac{40}{40 + 0} \times 100 = 100\%$$

$$\text{OA} = \frac{TP+TN}{TP+TN+FP+FN} = \frac{0 + 40}{0 + 40 + 5 + 0} \times 100 = 89\%$$

Carotid Quality Assurance Report

METHOD: Carotid exams are correlated with CTA and MRAs. The CTA and MRA's must be performed within six months of the non-invasive vascular study. The CTA and MRA reports are compared to the non-invasive carotid duplex exams. The results are entered on a log sheet. True positive and negative, false positive and negative, sensitivity and specificity, positive and negative predictive values and overall accuracy are calculated.

Data Source: Vascular Laboratory

Sample Size: Available CTA and MRA

Frequency: Yearly

Staff Member(s) Responsible: Mary Buzzeo, BS RVT and Gail Santopadre, RVT

626 carotids performed by the non-invasive vascular laboratory this year. 257 carotid ultrasounds were able to be compared with CTAs and MRAs.

Accuracy using CTA and MRA:

TP = 55	TN = 184	FN = 10	FP = 8

Fig. 51-4: *Sample QA Report*

REFERENCES

1. Gerlock AJ. (1988). Accuracy of measurement determinations. In Application of Non-invasive Vascular Techniques. (526-530). W.B. Saunders Company.
2. Intersocietal Commission for the Accreditation of Vascular Laboratories. ICAVL standards for accreditation in non-invasive testing. Retrieved from http://icavl.org/icavl/standards/2010_ICAVL_Standards.pdf (accessed 1/8/12).

ADDITIONAL REFERENCES

Hayes AC. "Calculation and implication of accuracy measurements." Bruit. 9:178-182, July 1985.
Lambeth A. "Statistics in the vascular laboratory" Bruit. 6:47-48, June 1982.

RESOURCES
52. Measurements and Calculations

The most common measurements calculated are summarized in this chapter for quick reference. Some of the measurements covered such as velocity ratio and diameter reductions are used in multiple vascular exams. The last section of the chapter provides reminders for measuring different atypical waveforms.

Lower Extremity Arterial

When narrowing of the arterial lumen reaches a critical level, distal arterial flow and pressure decrease significantly. Ankle and toe brachial indices define the resulting decrease in blood flow to the extremity at the ankle level.

Ankle Brachial Index (ABI)

$$ABI = \frac{\text{Ankle pressure}}{\text{Higher brachial pressure}}$$

Toe Brachial Index (TBI)

$$TBI = \frac{\text{Toe pressure}}{\text{Higher brachial pressure}}$$

Table 52-1: Disease Categorization for ABI and TBI

ABI		TBI
≥1.0	Normal	>0.70
0.90-<1.0	Mild	0.60-0.69
0.50-0.90	Moderate	0.59-0.40
0.30-0.50	Severe	<0.39
<0.30	Critical	-

ABI Data Source: Modified from AbuRahma AF. (2000). Segmental Doppler pressures and Doppler waveform analysis in peripheral vascular disease of the lower extremities. In AbuRahma AF, Bergan JJ (Eds). Non-invasive Vascular Diagnosis. (213-229). London: Springer. TBI Data Source: Internally validated at the University of Chicago Medicine Vascular Laboratory

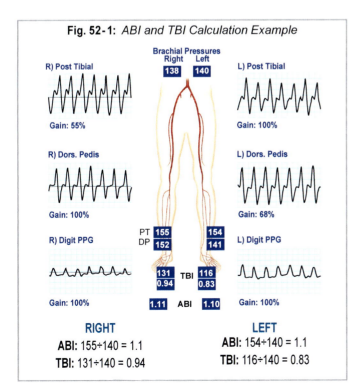

Fig. 52-1: *ABI and TBI Calculation Example*

RIGHT: ABI: 155÷140 = 1.1; TBI: 131÷140 = 0.94

LEFT: ABI: 154÷140 = 1.1; TBI: 116÷140 = 0.83

Lower Extremity Segmental Pressures

Segmental pressures define the level of disease by comparing the limb and brachial pressures from one level to the next. A pressure gradient (pressure difference) of 20-30mmHg indicates a significant stenosis or occlusion between cuff levels. Higher gradients most likely represent an occlusion, rather than a stenosis. Doppler waveforms from the lower extremity arteries normally demonstrate a high resistance waveform pattern, whereas waveforms distal to a significant obstruction typically reflect a low resistance configuration.

$$\text{Segmental pressure} \over \text{Higher brachial pressure}$$

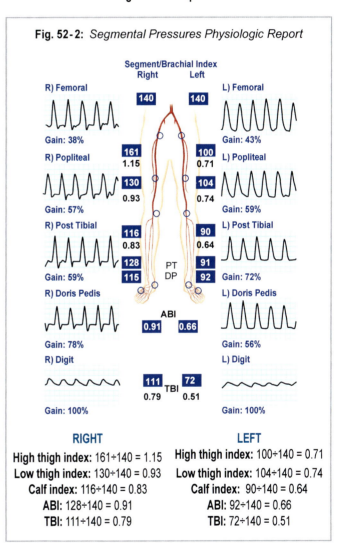

Fig. 52-2: *Segmental Pressures Physiologic Report*

RIGHT:
High thigh index: 161÷140 = 1.15
Low thigh index: 130÷140 = 0.93
Calf index: 116÷140 = 0.83
ABI: 128÷140 = 0.91
TBI: 111÷140 = 0.79

LEFT:
High thigh index: 100÷140 = 0.71
Low thigh index: 104÷140 = 0.74
Calf index: 90÷140 = 0.64
ABI: 92÷140 = 0.66
TBI: 72÷140 = 0.51

Exercise and Stress Ankle Brachial Indices (ABIs)

Upon exercise, an individual's distal vascular bed vasodilates, decreasing resistance and increasing blood flow in response to the demand. If a patient cannot exercise, the reactive hyperemia technique is an alternative means of increasing blood flow in order to elicit a pressure gradient that might not be present at rest. The ankle pressure will decrease in the presence of increased flow demands and a significant arterial obstruction.

Calculate the change in ABI pre/post exercise:

% pressure drop = (1 - (post exercise pressure ÷ resting pressure)) x 100

Table 52-2: Diagnostic Criteria for Post-Treadmill Exercise Ankle-Brachial Indices and Recovery Times

Recovery Time	Classification
<3 minutes *	Normal
2-6 minutes **	Single-level disease
6-12 minutes **	Multi-level disease
>15 minutes **	Severe occlusive disease

* The post-exercise systolic ankle pressure drops <20% compared to the resting systolic pressure.

** The post-exercise systolic ankle pressure drops >20% compared to the resting systolic pressure.

Source: Modified from Strandess DE, Zierler RE. (1993). Exercise ankle pressure measurements in arterial disease. In Bernstein EF (Ed.), Vascular Diagnosis (54 553). St. Louis: Mosby.

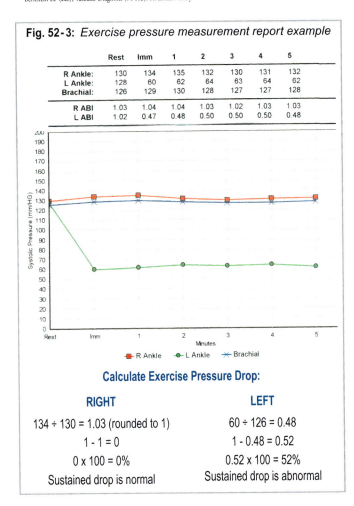

Fig. 52-3: *Exercise pressure measurement report example*

Calculate Exercise Pressure Drop:

RIGHT	LEFT
134 ÷ 130 = 1.03 (rounded to 1)	60 ÷ 126 = 0.48
1 - 1 = 0	1 - 0.48 = 0.52
0 x 100 = 0%	0.52 x 100 = 52%
Sustained drop is normal	Sustained drop is abnormal

Upper Extremity Arterial

Non-invasive physiological tests compare the systolic pressure at the level of the wrist and brachial artery to the systolic pressure at the level of the digits in the hand and detect arterial pulsations in the terminal portions of the digits (PPG). A pressure gradient (pressure difference) of 20-30mmHg indicates a significant stenosis or occlusion between cuff levels.

Wrist Brachial Index (WBI)

$$WBI = \frac{\text{Higher wrist pressure}}{\text{Higher brachial pressure}}$$

Digital Brachial Index (DBI)

$$DBI = \frac{\text{Digit pressure}}{\text{Higher brachial pressure}}$$

Table 52-3: Diagnostic Criteria for WBI and DBI

WBI		DBI
≥1.0	Normal	>0.70
0.9 to <1.0	Mild	0.60-0.69
0.5 - 0.9	Moderate	0.59-0.40
0.30 - 0.5	Severe	<0.39
<0.30	Critical	

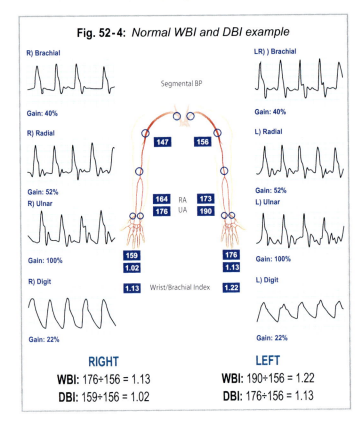

Fig. 52-4: *Normal WBI and DBI example*

RIGHT
WBI: 176÷156 = 1.13
DBI: 159÷156 = 1.02

LEFT
WBI: 190÷156 = 1.22
DBI: 176÷156 = 1.13

Penile Arterial Penile

Penile Brachial Index (PBI)

Non-invasive physiological testing which compares systolic blood pressures to evaluate the penile arterial system.

$$PBI = \frac{\text{Penile Pressure}}{\text{Higher Brachial Pressure}}$$

Table 52-4: Diagnostic Criteria for Penile Brachial Index (PBI)

Disease Category	PBI
Normal	>0.75
Marginal	0.6 - 0.74
Abnormal	<0.60

Source: Modified from Zierler RE, Sumner DS. (2005). Physiologic assessment of peripheral arterial occlusive disease. In Rutherford Vascular Surgery 6th edition. (197-222). Philadelphia. Elsevier Saunders

Calculation example:

RIGHT	LEFT
Brachial pressure: 128mmHg	Brachial pressure: 132mmHg
Cavernosal pressure: 91mmHg	Cavernosal pressure: 95mmHg
PBI: 91 ÷ 132 = 0.69	PBI: 95 ÷ 132 = 0.72

Velocity Ratio

Calculated by dividing the maximum PSV (peak systolic velocity) of the stenosis into the PSV of the proximal segment of the vessel:

$$Vr = \frac{\text{Maximum PSV}}{\text{Pre-stenotic PSV}}$$

For increased accuracy when assessing disease, measure B-mode reductions whenever possible and consider together with Doppler velocity ratios.

Table 52-5: Velocity Ratio vs. Diameter Reduction

Velocity Ratio	Diameter Reduction
<2.1	<50%
2.1 – 4.1	50 – 74%
>4.1	>75%

Source: Cossman DV, Ellison JE, et al (1989). Comparison of contrast arteriography to arterial mapping with color flow duplex imaging in the lower extremity The Journal of Vascular Surgery, Nov; 10(5):522-8; discussion 528-9.

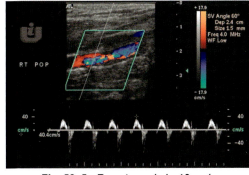

Fig. 52-5: *Pre-stenosis is 40cm/s*

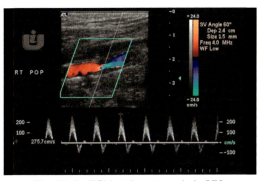

Fig. 52-6: *PSV at the stenosis is 276.*

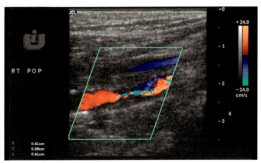

Fig. 52-7: *Calculated ~ 78% diameter reduction (DR) at stenosis*

Calculation of velocity ratio:

276 ÷ 40 = 6.9

78% DR and Vratio of 6.9 both suggest >75% stenosis

Lumenal Reduction

Lumenal reductions are reported using area and diameter reductions to communicate a percent stenosis calculation. Diameter reduction measurements are typically measured in the longitudinal plane and should only be used in conjunction with peak systolic velocity measurements. Area reductions are measured from a transverse view. Diameter and area reduction tools may prove extremely useful in cases of arrhythmias and irregular PSV when velocities are less reliable.

Diameter Reduction

$= 1 - (d \div D) \times 100$

Cross Sectional (Area Reduction)

$= 1 - (d^2 \div D^2) \times 100$

where D= true lumen, d= residual lumen

Lumenal reduction calculation examples:

Diameter reduction	Area reduction
D = 0.41	D = 0.41
d = 0.09	d = 0.09
1 - (0.09 ÷ 0.41) x 100	1 - (0.09^2 ÷ 0.41^2) x 100
0.09 ÷ 0.41 = 0.22	(0.0081 ÷ 0.1681) = 0.048
1 - 0.22 = 0.78	1 - 0.048 = 0.95
0.78 x 100 = 78%	0.95 x 100 = 95%

Pulsatility Index (PI)

Provides information regarding the resistance in distal vascular beds. It is expected that the ratio increases from the central to peripheral arteries.

$$PI = \frac{PSV - EDV}{MV}$$

PSV = peak systolic velocity
EDV = end diastolic velocity
MV = mean velocity

Table 52-6: Pulsatility Index and Resistance Relationship

Higher Pulsatility Index	↑ Increased Vascular Resistance
Lower Pulsatility Index	↓ Decreased Vascular Resistance

Peripheral Venous

Venous Insufficiency

Reflux means to "flow backward." Venous reflux is venous flow moving in the wrong direction, either away from the heart or from the deep to the superficial system through the perforating veins.
- Duplex ultrasound can identify the presence, exact location, extent, and severity of venous reflux.
- Evaluated by measuring the time in seconds for the purpose of assessing reflux for significance

Table 52-7: Diagnostic Criteria for Venous Reflux by Duplex

System	Normal	Abnormal
Superficial	<0.5 seconds	>0.5 seconds
Deep	<1 second	≥1 second
Perforators	<0.5 seconds	≥0.5 seconds

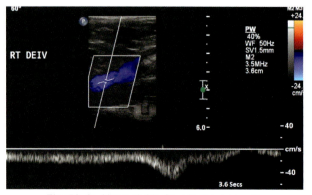

Fig. 52-8: *Normal: No flow in the opposite direction suggests no venous insufficiency*

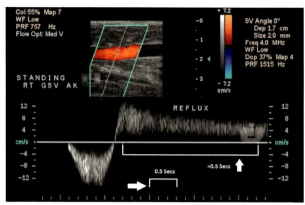

Fig. 52-9: *Significant venous insufficiency indicated by flow reversal above the baseline when the patient is standing*

Venous Refill Time (VRT)

Measurement reflecting volume changes (venous emptying and filling) as a result of the calf muscle pump in the leg.
- ≥20s is considered normal; legs completely empty and the veins refill by the arterial system within normal limits.
- <20s is associated with chronic venous insufficiency (CVI). The calf veins do not empty properly due to venous obstruction and incompetent venous valves allow for retrograde flow (back flow).

Table 52-8: Venous Refill Time (VRT)

Normal	Abnormal
≥20 seconds	<20 seconds

Renal

Renal Aortic Ratio (RAR)

The renal to aortic ratio may provide additional information and can be useful when the B-mode information does not match the increased systolic velocities.

$$RAR = \frac{\text{Highest renal artery PSV}}{\text{Highest PSV in the suprarenal abdominal aortic segment}}$$

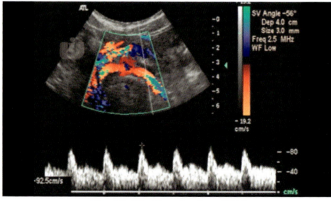

Fig. 52-10: *Renal artery PSV*

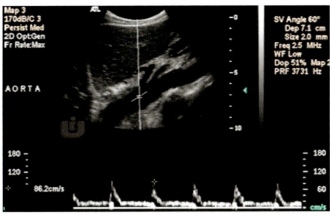

Fig. 52-11: *Suprarenal aortic PSV*

Calculation example (using Figs. 52-10 and 52-11):

93 ÷ 86 = **1.1** categorizing the RAR as normal

Table 52-9: **Diagnostic Criteria for Disease According Renal-to-Aortic-Ratio (RAR)**		
<3.5	Normal	<60% Diameter Reduction
>3.5	Abnormal	>60% Diameter Reduction

Resistive Index (RI)

Measures the resistance to arterial flow within the renal vascular bed. The RI provides information regarding the presence of intrinsic kidney disease. It is calculated considering the velocities within the kidney:

$$RI = \frac{PSV - EDV}{PSV}$$

Table 52-10: **Resistive Index (RI)**	
<0.70	Normal
0.70 – 0.80	Indeterminate
>0.80	Abnormal

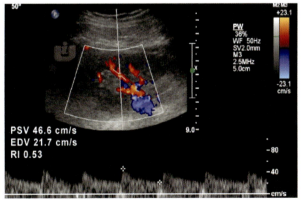

Fig. 52-12: *Intrarenal arterial spectral tracing*

Calculation example:

(47 - 22) ÷ 47 = **0.53**

Categorizing the renovascular resistance as normal

End-diastolic-ratio (EDR)

Provides additional information regarding the arterial resistance within the kidney.

$$EDR = \frac{End\ Diastolic\ Velocity}{Peak\ Systolic\ Velocity}$$

Table 52-11: **Interpretation of End-Diastolic Ratio (EDR)**	
>0.2	Normal
<0.2	Abnormal: Indicates an increase in resistance within the kidney

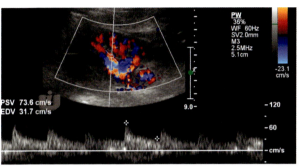

Fig. 52-13: *Normal intrarenal arterial spectral waveform*

Calculation example:

32 ÷ 74 = **0.43**

categorizing the EDR ratio as normal

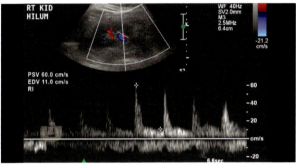

Fig. 52-14: *Abnormal intrarenal arterial spectral waveform*

Calculation example:

EDR = 11 ÷ 60 = **0.18**

you can also calculate the RI using this image, RI = 63 - 11/63 = 82%

Note: An EDR of 18% and RI of 82% both suggest kidney abnormality

Extracranial Cerebrovascular

ICA/CCA Ratio

The ICA/CCA ratio may provide additional information and can be useful when the B-mode information does not match the increased systolic velocities.

$$ICA/CCA\ ratio = \frac{Maximum\ PSV\ from\ the\ ICA}{PSV\ from\ the\ mid/distal\ CCA}$$

The ICA/CCA ratio may be unreliable if significant CCA disease is present.

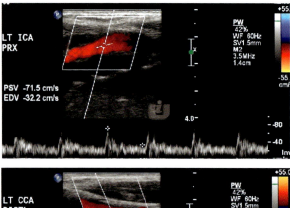

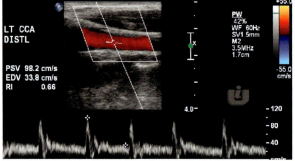

Fig. 52-15: *Normal PSV of an internal and common carotid artery*

Calculation example: 72 ÷ 98 = 0.73

categorizing the ICA/CCA ratio as <2 (<50% DR)

Table 52-12: Ratio Correlation to Diameter Reduction

ICA/CCA Ratio	Diameter Reduction
<2	<50%
2-4	50-69%
>4	70-99%

Hemodialysis AVF/Prosthetic Graft

Two calculations used in a hemodialysis duplex exam are velocity ratios and volume flow. Velocity ratios indicate whether there is a significant stenosis in the graft/fistula and volume flow measurements suggest whether there is an adequate amount of flow moving through the access.

$$\text{AVF/AVG velocity ratio} = \frac{\text{PSV }(V_2)\text{ distal}}{\text{PSV }(V_1)\text{ proximal ratio}}$$

Table 52-13: Diagnostic Criteria for Hemodialysis AVF

Hemodynamically significant stenosis (arterial inflow or venous outflow)	>2
Hemodynamically significant stenosis at the anastomosis	>3
Occlusion	Absent signal

Table 52-14: Diagnostic Criteria for Prosthetic Hemodialysis Graft (AVG)

Location/Disease	Ratio/Velocity
Within Normal Limits (0-49% Stenosis)	<2
Hemodynamically Significant (50-74%)	>2
Hemodynamically Significant (>75%)	>3
Venous Anastomosis	>400 cm/s
Occlusion	–

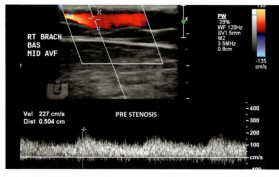

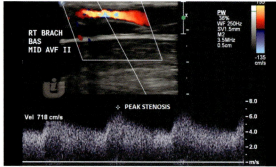

Fig. 52-16: *PSV in a Hemodialysis AVF used to calculate a velocity ratio*

Calculation example: 718 ÷ 227 = 3.2

categorizing the ratio as a hemodynamically significant stenosis

Volume Flow

Activate the "time average maximum" measurement or its equivalent on the duplex scanner and the machine will perform the volume flow calculation. Make sure to set up the calculation properly by sampling a straight, non-tapering segment of the access. Next place the calipers perpendicular to the vessel wall and open the Doppler gate to include the entire width of the vessel. Measure 1-3 cycles (PSV to PSV or EDV to EDV) on the spectral tracing to obtain volume flow (mL/min).

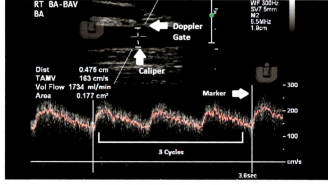

Fig. 52-17: *Volume flow*

Measurement of Volume Flow (VF)

VF (mL/min) = Cross-sectional area x mean velocity x 60

where *Cross-sectional area (cm²) = π d²/4*

d = diameter

REFERENCES

1. Non Invasive Vascular Diagnostics A Practical Guide to Therapy, 2nd Edition
2. Ali F. AbuRahma MD, FACS, FRCS, RVT, RPVI John J Bergan MD, FACS, Hon FRCS
3. Springer-Verlag London Limited 2007 Pg 262 graft surveys (mean velocity for failing graft)
4. Rumwell C., McPharlin, M. Vascular Technology An illustrated review 3rd Edition, Davies Publishing, Inc 2006
5. Edelman, S, Understanding Ultrasound Physics, 3rd Edition. Vortex Communications 2007

RESOURCES
53. Glossary

Printed with permission from the Society of Vascular Ultrasound. This glossary has been updated from Terminology for the Vascular Ultrasound Technologist/Sonographer www.svu.org

Acknowledgements The *Glossary of Terms* for the Vascular Technologists as first compiled in 1983 by the Education Committee of the then Society of Non-Invasive Vascular Technology, Mary Jane Pomajzl, Chair. The Glossary has since been updated three times. The second edition was published in 1989 under the direction of Paula A. Heggerick, RDMS RVT FSVU, Chair, SVT Publication Committee. The third edition was published in 1995; Joanne E. Drago, LPN RVT, Chair. The fourth edition was revised and updated in 2001 due to the efforts of Jean White, RVT, Chair, and Allene Woodley, RN RVT; Joanne Spindell, RVT RDCS; Paula Gehr, RVT; Cathy Brown, BSCVN RN RVT RDCVS; and Michael Sampson, RVT. This fifth edition has been revised and updated in 2005 due to the efforts of Products Committee Chair Michel Comeaux, RN RVT RDMS FSVU; Tom Baer, MBA RVT RDMS RDCS; Debbie Pirt, AS RVT; William Harkrider, MD RVT; and Bill Zang, BS RVT RDMS.

A

Abduction Away from the midline, opposite of adduction.

Abscess A localized collection of pus surrounded by inflamed tissue.

Acoustic shadow Loss of acoustic properties of targets lying behind an attenuating structure. In the arteries, the most common cause of acoustic shadowing is calcified plaque (see calcification).

Acute Short, severe symptoms of sudden onset or short duration.

Adduction Drawing toward the midline.

Adventitia The outermost layer of a vein or an artery.

Aliasing A phenomenon associated with pulsed Doppler; Doppler shift in a negative direction occurs when the Doppler shift exceeds half the pulse repetition frequency.

Alignment sign Distinguishes the Anterior Saphenous Vein from the Great Saphenous Vein. The ASV is seated anterior and lateral to the GSV, aligning itself over the deep vessels.

Allen test A test performed to check the continuity of the palmar arch normally supplied by both the radial and ulnar arteries. The test may be performed using a Doppler or PPG.

Ambulatory phlebectomy (also known as phlebectomy, microphlebectomy, or stab avulsion) A technique to remove varicose veins. In this procedure, several tiny cuts (incisions) are made in the skin through which the varicose vein is removed.

Amplitude The maximum variation in an acoustic variable. It is the difference between the average value and the maximum value of an acoustic variable. Units used with amplitude coincide with the acoustic variable used.

Amputation The cutting off (traumatic or surgical) of all or part of an appendage.

Anastomosis The natural or surgically-created communication between blood vessels or prosthetic graft and blood vessel as in a bypass graft. Anastomosis can then be referred to as proximal or distal.

Anechoic Describes the property of being echo-free or without echoes (i.e., fluid-filled cyst).

Angiogram A series of x-rays taken of a blood vessel following the injection of a radiopaque substance into the vessel (arteriogram).

Angioplasty Dilation of an artery by a balloon tipped catheter. Often referred to as percutaneous transluminal angioplasty (PTA).

Ankle-brachial index (ABI) The ratio of ankle systolic pressure to highest arm systolic pressure. The numerical index serves as an indicator of arterial insufficiency. Normal value is 1.0 or greater; the ratio decreases as arterial insufficiency increases. Usually referred to as ABI.

Antecubital fossa A triangular area located at the bend of the elbow that contains the cephalic, median cubital and basilic veins.

Antegrade Proceeding toward.

Antegrade flow Proceeding towards or forward. Opposite of retrograde or reversed.

Anterior Situated in the frontal plane, in the front of.

Anticoagulant Substances which prohibit or delay the normal blood clotting mechanism, e.g., Coumadin and heparin.

Aorta The main trunk of the arterial system with its origin off the surface of the left ventricle. It is usually described in several portions, the ascending.

Aplasia Indicates the lack of development of a vein or of a segment of a vein. The vein is present but diminutive in size. Its structure is similar to the embryo.

Aplastic Not exhibiting growth or change in structure.

Arrhythmia Abnormal heart rhythm.

Arterial inflow Pertaining to blood flow into the lower extremities proximal to the level of the common femoral arteries.

Arterial insufficiency Reduction in blood flow within the arterial system. Inadequate blood flow results in hypoxia; the symptoms produced by arterial insufficiency vary with the end organ site.

Arterial occlusion Complete blockage of an artery.

Arterial outflow Normally pertaining to the medium size blood vessels, common femoral through the popliteal. Outflow could also pertain to the vessels carrying blood away from a bypass graft.

Arterial runoff The infra-popliteal vessels (tibial and distal vessels).

Arterial ulceration A local defect or excavation which is produced by sloughing of inflammatory necrotic tissue.

Arteriography A radiologic procedure in which an opaque substance is injected into an artery and subsequent x-ray films are taken in order to visualize the arterial system.

Arteriole A minute artery whose distal end leads to a capillary.

Arteriovenous malformation congenital anomalies resulting from faulty development of arterial, capillary, venous or lymphatic structures or any combination thereof. These lesions are thought to be present from birth and do not represent neoplasms.

Artery Any of the blood vessels which carry blood from the heart to the other parts of the body. With the exception of the pulmonary and umbilical arteries, arteries transport oxygenated blood.

Artifact In ultrasound usage, refers to an echo which does not correspond to a real target. In general, refers to any artificial finding which may resemble the expected findings. artifacts may be intrinsic, e.g., reverberation or extrinsic.

Ascites Accumulation of serous fluid in spaces between tissues and organs in the abdominal cavity.

Atherosclerosis Disease of the arterial intima, characterized by intimal proliferation (hyperplasia), deposition of fatty substances and luminal reduction.

Attenuation Reduction in amplitude and intensity as a sound wave passes through a medium. Factors contributing to attenuation include absorption, reflection, refraction, and scattering.

Augmentation To cause to augment or increase. When used in conjunction with Doppler examinations of the venous or cerebral systems, refer to the increased flow velocity which is noted after one or more compression/ release maneuvers.

Avalvulia An absence of valves in the venous trunks of one or more extremities.

B

Basilic vein Large vein on the inner side of the arm (medial), near the brachial veins, a superficial vein.

Bi-directional Doppler A Doppler instrument capable of determining whether the frequency of the Doppler shift is above or below the transmission frequency, permitting determination of blood flow towards or away from the transducer.

Bifurcation That location where an artery branches; a frequent site of atherosclerosis.

Bilateral On both sides.

Biphasic Having two phases or variations having a forward and reverse component.

Blood pressure (BP) Pressure within the arterial system, quantified in millimeters of mercury (mm Hg); includes systolic pressure (during heart contraction), diastolic pressure (during cardiac relaxation) or mean blood pressure. Blood pressure is usually expressed as systolic over diastolic pressure.

Brachial veins A paired set of veins which accompany the brachial artery. They are formed at the elbow by the confluence of the radial and ulnar veins. They drain the same area that the brachial artery supplies.

Brachiocephalic (Innominate) Right artery arising from the arch of the aorta dividing into the right subclavian and right common carotid arteries.

Bradycardia Abnormally low heart rate, generally less than 60 beats per minute.

Budd-Chiari syndrome Venous outflow obstruction or occlusion, located at any level from the hepatic venules to the inferior vena cava (IVC), associated with ascites and liver failure.

C

Calcification Deposition of calcium salts within an organic substance causing hardening. Medial calcification is known as Monckeberg's sclerosis. Arterial calcification hampers Doppler ultrasonic evaluation of blood flow because of the high reflectivity of calcium. Calcified structures have a higher acoustic impedance than the surrounding tissues.

Caprini Risk Score An online assessment that divides patients into low, moderate, and high risk for DVT. capriniriskscore.org

Caval Pertaining to the vena cava.

Caudad In a direction toward the feet (or tail), the opposite of cephalad.

CEAP (Clinical-Etiology-Anatomy-Pathophysiology) A classification system for chronic venous disease.

Cellulitis Inflammation of cellular or connective tissue. An infection in or close to the skin is usually localized by the body defense mechanisms.

Central Areas at or near the center of the body.

Cephalad Toward the head.

Cephalic Cranial; superior in position.

Cephalic vein A superficial vein that ascends from the dorsal aspect of the radial border of the forearm, to the anterior surface and subcutaneously up the arm and ends in the axillary vein near the clavicle. Frequently used for arteriovenous fistula formation for dialysis access.

CHIVA The French acronym for "Cure conservatrice et Hemodynamique de l'Insuffisance Veineuse en Ambulatoire" (Conservative and Hemodynamic treatment of Venous Insufficiency in the Office). It is a saphenous-sparing therapeutic approach to lower limb chronic venous disease (CVD) based on hemodynamic concepts proposed by Claude Franceschi in 1988.

Cirrhosis A chronic disease of the liver; dense connective tissue forms, liver cells cease to function.

Claudication Literally, "to limp" symptoms associated with arterial insufficiency of the extremity; intermittent leg pain (ache, cramp, etc.) brought on by exercise and relieved by rest.

Coagulate To become clotted or congealed.

Coagulation To change from a fluid to a semi solid mass.

Coalesce To fuse; to run or grow together.

Coapt To meet or join. When performing a venous duplex exam, with light transducer pressure, the walls of normal veins collapse and come together.

Collateral circulation An alternate, natural circulatory pathway. When there is interference in the arterial supply because of obstruction, communicating channels develop to accommodate blood flow. The peripheral resistance of the collateral vessels is higher because of the smaller diameter of the vessels.

Compartment syndrome This syndrome occurs when increased pressure in the noncompliant fascia compromises circulation and neuromuscular function in that anatomic space.

Competence In the normal vein no retrograde flow is detected, either with Valsalva maneuver, with proximal compression, or with the release of distal compression. Absence of retrograde flow confirms adequate venous valve closure.

Compression The act of pressing or squeezing; the condition of being pressed together.

Confluence A flowing or meeting together; a joining.

Congenital Present at birth.

Congestive heart failure (CHF) A chronic cardiac condition in which the heart is unable to maintain adequate output of blood resulting in congestion of blood in the veins and other organs of the body.

Constriction The narrowing of a vessel opening.

Continuous flow In abnormal veins the respiratory phasicity is lost, resulting in a steady flow signal. When coupled with very low velocity, continuous flow indicates proximal (except in the Portal system) obstruction that is preventing the normal fluctuations in flow that occurs during respiration. It is not always possible to distinguish between extrinsic vein compression and intrinsic obstruction (DVT), most especially in the iliac segments.

Continuous wave Doppler (CW) A Doppler which uses separate transmitting and receiving piezoelectric crystals, each operating without interruption. The reflected sound waves are processed continuously.

Contralateral On the opposite side.

Cord A string like structure. A firm elongated structure consistent with a thrombosed vein.

Coronary artery bypass surgery Surgical establishment of a shunt that permits blood to travel from the aorta to a branch of the coronary artery at a point past an obstruction.

Costoclavicular Pertains to the ribs and the clavicle.

Coumadin anticoagulant One of a group of natural and synthetic compounds that antagonize the biosynthesis of vitamin K dependent on coagulation factors in the liver.

Cramp Spasmodic muscle contraction; term often used by patients to describe claudication pain.

Cuff artifact Refers to abnormally high pressures associated with the use of cuffs which are proportionately too narrow for the limb they are encircling.

Cyanosis A slight bluish, grayish, slate like or dark purple discoloration of the skin caused by reduced amounts of hemoglobin in the blood. Etiology a deficiency of oxygen.

Cyst A closed sac or pouch, with a definite wall, contains fluid, semi fluid, or solid material. A simple cyst is usually spherical, with echo enhancement posterior to cyst. Complex cysts can have internal debris and septations.

D

D-Dimer Formed as fibrin is broken down. Positive levels are suggestive of a thrombotic event such as deep vein thrombosis or pulmonary embolism. Negative levels can virtually rule out the presence of DVT or PE, sparing the patient further expensive, uncomfortable and/or invasive testing

Deceleration A decrease in velocity.

Decubitus, lateral Refers to a patient lying on their side.

Deep vein thrombosis (DVT) Obstruction of the deep veins by blood clot. DVT is a non-inflammatory process. The possibility of the loosely attached thrombus dislodging is always present. DVT can lead to valvular destruction, post-phlebitic syndrome, and pulmonary embolism.

Dependent rubor Abnormal redness noted of the toes (filling of the small vessels) and forefoot when the leg is in the dependent position. This is usually noted in patients with severe occlusive disease.

Depth of penetration That depth wherein echoes are no longer detectable; a function of the operating frequency of the transducer.

Dermatitis Inflammation of skin evidenced by itching, redness, and various skin lesions.

Diaphragm A musculomembranous wall separating the abdomen from the thoracic cavity. It contracts and expands with respiration.

Digit A toe or finger.

Dilatation A vessel is stretched beyond normal dimensions.

Dissection Separation of tissues; usually surgically (see aneurysm, dissecting).

Disseminated intravascular coagulation (DIC) A pathological form of coagulation that is diffuse rather than localized. The process damages rather than protects the area involved, and several clotting factors are consumed to such extent that generalized bleeding may occur.

Distal Farthest from the center from medial line, or from the trunk; opposite of proximal.

Doppler A diagnostic instrument which emits an ultrasonic beam into the body. This ultrasound is reflected back from moving structures within the body at a frequency higher or lower than this transmitted frequency (Doppler shift). This shift is amplified and presented as a sound or graphic (chart) display.

Doppler angle The angle between the direction of propagation of the ultrasound and the direction of flow. As an approximation, the angle between the axis of the ultrasound beam and the axis of the vessel lumen is generally used.

Doppler effect Observed frequency change of reflected sound due to reflector movement to the source or the observer.

Doppler shift The frequency shift created between the transmitted frequency and received frequency by an interface moving with velocity at an angle to the sound source.

Dorsal Indicating a position toward the rear part, pertaining to the back opposed to ventral.

E

Ecchymosis A skin discoloration consisting of large irregularity formed hemorrhagic areas.

Echo Reflection of acoustic energy.

Echogenic The acoustic property of a medium which renders it capable of producing echoes.

Ectatic Distended or stretched.

Edema A local or generalized condition in which the body tissues contain an excessive amount of tissue fluid.

EHIT Endothermal Heat-Induced Thrombosis is defined as propagation of a thrombus from a superficial vein into a deeper vein. It is generally considered clinically insignificant if the thrombus does not propagate to the deep venous system.

Embolectomy Removal of an embolus from a vessel.

Embolism An obstruction in a vessel from a foreign substance or blood clot.

Embolus A mass of undissolved matter present in a blood or lymphatic vessel and carried there by the blood or lymph current.

E Point An ultrasound marker of the great saphenous vein, found 3-5cm below the saphenofemoral junction where it crosses superficially over the adductor longus muscle. This marker was named "E Point" because it is easy to identify the great saphenous vein at this point.

Erythema Reddening of the skin.

Erythrocyte A mature red blood cell (RBC) or corpuscle.

Esophageal varices Varicosities of the branches of the azygos vein that anastomose with the tributaries of the portal vein in the lower esophagus; occurs in patients with portal hypertension.

Etiology Study of the causation of disease.

Extravasation Discharge or escape, as of blood or other substance from within a vessel into the tissue.

Extrinsic Originating from without, opposite of intrinsic.

Eye Sign The B-mode identification of the great saphenous vein.

F

False aneurysm See aneurysm, pseudo.

False negative rate Rate at which a diagnostic test produces negative results when disease is actually present. False Neg. Rate = FN × 100 = % TP + FN FN = false negative, TP = true positive False positive rate Rate at which a diagnostic test produces positive results when disease is not present.

False positive rate The rate at which a diagnostic test produces positive results when disease is actually not present. FP × 100 = % TN + FP TN = true negative, FP = false positive.

Fascia A band or sheet of connective tissue, that surrounds, encloses, and separates muscles, vessels and nerves.

Field of view That plane seen by specific ultrasound transducer.

Fistula, arteriovenous Communication between an artery and a vein. It may be congenital, traumatic, or surgically created for dialysis access.

Frequency Number of cycles per unit of time (usually seconds); expressed in Hertz (Hz) l Hz = 1 cycle per second, Kilohertz (KHz) l KHz = 1,000 Hz, or Megahertz (MHz) l MHz = 1,000,000 Hz or 1,000,000 cycles per second.

G

Gain The ratio of output to input in an amplifying system.

Gaiter area zone The region of the medial lower leg just above the ankle. It is this area where signs of venous stasis are most evident.

Gangrene Tissue death, usually as a result of inadequate blood supply; occasionally due to infection. Lack of blood supply may be due to atherosclerosis, embolism, spasm, frostbite, tourniquets, etc.

Gastrocnemius That large muscle of the posterior portion of the lower leg that propels venous blood up the leg as it contracts. Commonly referred to as the calf muscle pump, this superficial muscle extends the foot and helps to flex the knee.

Genicular Venous Plexis The term genicular venous plexus (plexus venosus genicularis) should replace the term genicular veins. At the knee, deep veins do not correspond exactly to the branches of the popliteal artery (articular arteries). They are arranged in a complex plexus of interconnecting veins.

Grayscale A display format in which the intensity information is recorded as changes in brightness. Also known as B-mode.

Great saphenous vein (GSV) One of the two major superficial veins of the lower limb. It originates on the dorsum of the foot, ascends medially along the calf and thigh, and drains into the common femoral vein. It is the longest vein in the body and is the vessel of choice for lower extremity bypass procedures and is also used for coronary artery bypass.

H

Hemangioma A tumor, growth, or abnormal mass composed of blood vessels.

Hematoma A blood-filled swelling.

Hemodynamics Pertaining to the physical principles governing blood flow (i.e., blood pressure, blood flow, vascular volumes, heart rate, ventricular function).

Hemoglobin The iron containing pigment of the red blood cells. Its function is to carry oxygen from the lungs to the tissues. The amount of hemoglobin in the blood averages 14-16 grams per 100ml.

Hemorrhage Escape of blood from a vessel (arterial or venous). Abnormal bleeding.

Heparin Substance used to inhibit coagulation of blood; frequently used in the treatment of deep venous thrombosis.

Hepatic veins Drain blood flow from the liver into the inferior vena cava. There are three main veins, the left, middle and the right.

Hepatofugal flow Directed or flowing away from the liver.

Hepatopetal flow Directed or flowing toward the liver.

Heterogeneous Of different kind or species; used in ultrasound to describe sonographic characteristics of atherosclerotic plaque; opposite of homogeneous.

Homan's sign Pain in the calf muscle resulting from passive dorsiflexion of the foot. Is sometimes indicative of deep venous thrombosis; of limited accuracy.

Homogeneous Uniform in structure, of the same composition.

Hunter's canal A triangular space lying in the distal thigh beneath the sartorius muscle and between the adductor longus and the vastus medialis muscle. It is at this location that the femoral vessels and the saphenous nerve are transmitted.

Hydrostatic pressure A pressure created in a fluid system, such as the circulatory system.

Hyperechoic Producing echoes of higher amplitude than normal for the surrounding medium.

Hyperemia Increased blood in an area. May be active, i.e., caused by increased flow or passive, i.e., increased flow that occurs in response to a previous restriction of flow.

Hypertension Abnormally elevated blood pressure may be essential (etiology unknown) or secondary to another condition (e.g., renal disease, pregnancy). Although there is no universal agreement, l40 systolic and 90 diastolic are considered the upper limits of normal. Control of hypertension is an important consideration; some sequelae of hypertension include stroke, small vessel damage, and congestive heart failure.

Hypoechoic Producing echoes of lower amplitude than normal for the surrounding medium.

Hypoplasia Indicates the incomplete development of a vein or of a segment of a vein. It is less severe in degree than aplasia, and the hypoplastic vein has a reduced caliber with a normal structure.

Hypoplastic Incomplete or underdevelopment of a tissue or organ.

Hypotension Abnormally low blood pressure; may be primary, secondary, or postural.

Hypovolemia Decreased blood volume.

Hypoxia Diminished oxygen content in the tissues.

I

Iliac vein Formed by the confluence of the internal iliac vein which drains the pelvis and the external iliac vein which is a continuation of the common femoral vein. The right and left common iliac veins unite to form the inferior vena cava.

Incompetent Unable to perform natural function. Used to refer to venous valves which no longer close completely, permitting blood to flow in a backward direction.

Inflow obstruction Arterial blood flow is severely restricted due to a proximal obstructing lesion.

Inferior Lower than, beneath.

Inferior mesenteric vein (IMV) Is usually small in size and runs to the left of the superior mesenteric vein to join the splenic vein.

Inferior vena cava (IVC) Originates from the confluence of the right and left iliac veins terminating in the right atrium of the heart.

Infrapopliteal Located below the popliteal artery or popliteal space.

Inguinal ligament A fibrous band extending from the anterior superficial iliac spine to the pubis tubercle in the groin.

Innominate vein Formed by the confluence of the internal jugular with the subclavian vein.

Intermittent Occurring at intervals, not constant. Used when describing claudication.

Internal Inside, opposite of external.

Intima Innermost layer of a vein or an artery; comprised of an endothelial lining, a thin layer of connective tissue, and an internal elastic membrane.

Ipsilateral On the same side, opposite of contralateral.

Ischemia Deficient local blood supply to body tissues; due to obstruction of arterial inflow. Symptoms of ischemia include coldness, pallor, pain, impairment of function and ultimately tissue necrosis (gangrene).

J

Jugular vein Major neck vein subdivided into anterior, external, and internal jugular veins bilaterally.

Jugular vein anterior Originates from the veins draining the lower jaw, descends anteriorly, and terminates in the external jugular vein.

Jugular vein external Drains the exterior of the cranium and deep parts of the face, runs perpendicularly in the neck to empty into the subclavian, internal jugular, or brachiocephalic vein.

Jugular vein internal Continues from the transverse sinus at the base of the skull, runs vertically in the neck to unite with the subclavian vein to form the brachiocephalic vein.

K

Klippel-Trenaunay Syndrome A rare disorder that is present at birth (congenital) and is characterized by a triad of cutaneous capillary malformation ("port-wine stain"), lymphatic anomalies, and abnormal veins in association with variable overgrowth of soft tissue and bone.

L

Lamina A thin layer.

Laminar flow Blood flowing in thin layers in a streamline direction parallel to the vessel wall. The highest velocities are at center stream; slowest along the wall. In laminar flow, red blood cells tend to migrate toward center stream, leaving the less viscous plasma along the wall.

Lateral Away from the mid-line, to the side.

Ligate To tie off, e.g., to tie off a blood vessel at surgery.

Linear Relating to, consisting of, or resembling a line. Linear transducer; multiple elements arranged in a line.

Lipid A broad group of chemicals that include steroids, fats, and waxes characterized by their insolubility in water.

Longitudinal Along the path of a sound beam; or along a lengthwise course, as in a longitudinal scan. (Long axis, LAX)

Lumen The space inside a tube, blood vessel, or duct.

Lymph Transparent fluid, comprised of white blood cells (lymphocytes), conveyed in the lymphatic vessels.

Lymphangitis Inflammation of a lymph vessel.

Lymphedema Fluid retention in the tissues as a result of obstruction in the lymphatic system. Can present symptoms similar to deep venous thrombosis.

Lymphoceles Fluid collections, which result from lymphatic leakage from, disrupted channels along the iliac vessels.

M

Maximum venous outflow Describes the maximum rate of venous emptying which occurs in a limb following rapid cuff deflation post venous occlusion.

Mean Midway between two points or measurements; the arithmetic average.

Media Middle layer of a vein or an artery.

Medial Toward the midline, opposite of lateral.

Median The middle number in a distribution, half of the numbers will be above and half of the numbers will be below it.

Median cubital vein Located in the antecubital fossa and crosses from the medial to the lateral side of the fossa and connects the basilic and cephalic veins.

Membrane A thin lining or covering.

Microphlebectomy (also known as phlebectomy, ambulatory phlebectomy, or stab avulsion) A technique to remove varicose veins. In this procedure, several tiny cuts (incisions) are made in the skin through which the varicosed vein is removed.

Morbidity The ratio of unhealthy individuals to the total population of a given group; a state of being sick/diseased.

Mortality The ratio or total number of deaths to the total number of a given group.

Mottling A condition that is marked by discolored areas.

Mural Refers to the wall of a cavity, organ, or vessel.

Muscle pump A mechanism to direct blood from the lower extremities towards the heart. The contracting muscles of the leg, especially the calf, act as a power source to propel the venous drainage collected in the soleal sinusoids. Competent valves prevent the reflux of blood. When the muscles relax, the space created in the now-emptied deep veins draws blood from the superficial veins into the deep system via the perforators.

N

Necrosis Localized tissue death; when due to arterial insufficiency is called ischemic necrosis; often used interchangeably with the term gangrene.

Negative predictive value The ability of a test to anticipate (predict) normal findings. Neg. Pred. Value = TN × 100 = % TN + FN TN = true negative, FN = false negative

Neointimal hyperplasia The narrowing of an endarterectomized artery by smooth muscle and fibrous overgrowth of the tissue layer that replaces the intima after surgery.

Neovascularization Recurrence through the growth of new vessels.

Neuropathy A functional disturbance or pathological change in the nervous system. Can be related to peripheral vascular disease in the diabetic patient, sensory, motor, autonomic, and mixed varieties.

Nocturnal Occurring during the night. May be used to describe rest pain which causes awakening from sleep.

Nondirectional A Doppler instrument which assesses flow, via frequency shift, without regard for direction of blood flow.

Nonocclusive Not totally obstructed.

O

Obstructive Raynaud's syndrome Episodic attacks of vasospasm resulting in the closure of small arteries and arterioles of the distal extremities in response to cold or stress with obstruction of the palmar and digital arteries.

Occlusion The complete closure of an opening, duct or vessel.

Ohm's law States that voltage equals current multiplied by resistance (impedance). Voltage = Current × Resistance This is the basis for strain gauge and impedance plethysmographic testing. When voltage and current are held constant, the changes in resistance can only be due to changes in limb volume.

Ostial Valve A valve located at the point of entry of a tributary. Ostial valves usually consist of a single cusp.

Overall accuracy Sum of true positive tests and true negative tests divided by the total number of tests performed.

Glossary 385

P

Pallor Abnormal paleness or lack of color in the skin.

Parasympathetic A division of the autonomic nervous system involved primarily with restorative functions. The parasympathetic nerves are derived from intracranial and sacral nerves and travel via the vagus nerves.

Paraná maneuver A slight push to the waist triggers an isometric contraction of the leg muscle propelling deep venous flow toward the popliteal vein without any ankle movement. Commonly used outside the United States.

Parietal valve A valve located within the lumen of a vein. Parietal valves are bicuspid, usually consisting of two cusps.

PASTE A Post Ablation Superficial Thrombus Extension into the common femoral vein as a consequence of endovenous treatment of the GSV with laser or radiofrequency.

Patency The state of being open. A venous characteristic assessed in the venous Doppler examination.

Patent Open, not occluded.

Pedal Pertaining to the foot as in pedal pulses, the pulses of the foot.

Perforating veins (communicating veins) Veins that cross the muscular fascia, connecting the superficial and deep venous systems.

Peripheral Areas away from the center of the body.

Peripheral vascular resistance That resistance (or impedance) to blood flow in the systemic arterial system. Resistance to blood flow is determined primarily by the caliber of small arterioles, i.e., the smaller the vessel the greater the resistance. Other factors affecting resistance include the length of the vessel and viscosity. It is vascular resistance which contributes to the brief period of flow reversal in the peripheral vessels.

Perivascular Surrounding a blood vessel.

Phasicity Normal venous flow increases and decreases in response to respiration. In a normal lower extremity, flow will diminish or cease with respiration. Phasicity is reversed in the upper extremity veins.

Phlebectomy (also known as microphlebectomy, ambulatory phlebectomy, or stab avulsion) A technique to remove varicose veins. In this procedure, several tiny cuts (incisions) are made in the skin through which a varicose vein is removed.

Phlebitis Inflammation of a vein.

Phlebography Radiologic procedure in which an opaque substance is injected into a vein; subsequent x-ray pictures are taken in order to visualize the venous system. Synonymous with venography.

Phlebolymphedema A mixed etiology swelling due to chronic venous insufficiency and lymphatic insufficiency. It is most commonly due to the inability of the lymphatic system to adequately drain the interstitial fluid that accumulates in severe chronic venous hypertension.

Phlebosclerosis refers to the thickening and hardening of the vein walls.

Phlebothrombosis Term used to describe occlusion of vein by clot in the absence of an inflammatory process (see deep venous thrombosis).

Phlegmasia Cerulea Dolens When DVT involves the major veins proximal to the inguinal ligament. Commonly referred to as iliofemoral thrombosis.

Photoplethysmograph (PPG) Infrared light is emitted from a transmitting diode and reflected back to a receiving diode; changes in red blood cell density associated with arterial pulsation are detected by the transducer. PPG detects changes in red blood cell volume; the signal output is in the form of a pulse wave form. PPG is used in a number of noninvasive diagnostic examinations; venous reflux plethysmography, supraorbital plethysmography, digital pressures, Allen's test, and thoracic outlet maneuvers.

Piezoelectric effect Changing of mechanical to electrical energy and vice versa.

Plantar Pertaining to the sole of the foot.

Plaque Generic term used to describe an atherosclerotic lesion. It can consist of platelets, fibrin, lipids, and calcium.

Plasma Fluid portion of the blood.

Platelet A round or oval disk, 1/3 to 1/2 the size of an erythrocyte found in the blood. Platelets number from 150,000 to 450,000 per cc. Platelets play an important role in blood coagulation, hemostasis and blood thrombus formation. When a vessel is injured, platelets adhere to each other and the edges of the injury and form a plug which covers the area. The plug or blood clot formed soon retract and stops the loss of blood.

Plethysmograph Any device, instrument, or transducer which measures volume changes in size or amount. Air plethysmography include volume pulse recordings.

Poiseuille's Law Q= P/R describes the relationship between flow (Q), pressure gradient (P), and resistance (R).

Portal hypertension Increased portal venous pressure, usually due to liver disease. Can cause the dilatation or thrombosis of the portal vein, superior mesenteric vein, splenic vein, and the formation of varices.

Portal system Consists of the portal vein, splenic vein, and inferior and superior mesenteric veins.

Portal vein (PV) Collects blood from the digestive tract and empties into the liver to be detoxified. Formed by the junction of the splenic vein and the superior mesenteric vein.

Positive predictive value The ability of a test to anticipate (predict) abnormal findings. Pos. Pred. Value = P × 100 = % TP + FP TP = true positive, FP = False positive

Posterior Refers to the back; or dorsal side of the body; opposite of anterior.

Postphlebitic syndrome Chronic venous insufficiency secondary to previous deep venous thrombosis. Venous thrombosis damages the valves and renders them incompetent. The physical signs include edema, stasis pigmentation changes, pain, and ulceration.

Prevait Presence of varices (residual or recurrent) after intervention

Prone Lying on the abdomen with the face downward, opposite of supine.

Prophylaxis Pertaining to any measures designed to prevent disease development.

Proximal Nearest to a point of reference. Opposite of distal.

Pseudoclaudication Term used to describe a syndrome of symptoms resembling claudication but not of a vascular origin. The most common etiology is neurogenic. Pseudoclaudication can be differentiated from true claudication by the nature of the presenting symptoms. The exercise-pain-rest-relief cycle is not present in pseudoclaudication.

Pulmonary embolus Embolus (blood clot, air, fat) which is carried through the venous system ultimately lodging in the pulmonary vasculature. PE is a serious and occasionally fatal complication of deep venous thrombosis.

Pulse repetition frequency (pulse repetition rate) The rate of repetition of pulses per unit time; in a pulsed system, the number of pulses generated every second. Not to be confused with frequency, PRF is the rate of pulse repetition.

Pulse volume recorder (PVR) Plethysmographic technique in which air-filled cuffs are placed segmentally on an extremity; changes in limb volume associated with arterial pulsation are translated in pulse waveforms. Alterations in the shape of the waveform at each level are associated with obstruction proximal to the cuff.

Q

Qualitative A non-objective measurement relating to quality; descriptive assessment of attributes, traits, or characteristics. Measurements in which an exact numerical value cannot be assigned; scales or grades can be used.

Quantitative An observable quantity which can be described in objective, measurable terms, i.e., numbers.

R

Radiography Generic terms referring to any type of x-ray procedure; venography, arteriography are two types of radiographic techniques.

Recanalization The formation of a new canal or channel of blood flow through an obstruction, such as blood clot or thrombus (deep vein thrombosis).

Reflux Backward flow. A characteristic noted on the venous Doppler examination during peripheral limb compression release maneuver; indicative of valvular dysfunction.

Renal veins Drain the kidney and empty into the inferior vena cava. The left renal vein is longer than the right renal vein.

Renovascular hypertension High blood pressure pertaining to or affecting blood vessels of the kidney, or hypertension produced by renal artery flow reducing stenosis or occlusion.

Rest pain A sign of severe arterial obstruction resulting in pronounced ischemia of an extremity. Arterial compromise is such that pain occurs at rest; often causing night-time wakefulness (due to recumbency and the reduced cardiac output of sleep). The pain is confined to the digit and dorsum of the foot and symptoms are relieved, in part, by dependency of the limb.

Retrograde Proceeding away from or backward; opposite of antegrade or forward.

Retrograde flow Blood flowing moving backwards or against the usual direction of flow.

Revascularization Varicose veins that recur in the saphenous compartment after a saphenous vein procedure.

Rouleaux Flow Stacks or aggregations of red blood cells (RBCs) that form because of the unique discoid shape of the cells.

S

Sagittal In the anterior-posterior plane of the body.

Sample volume With a pulsed Doppler system, describes the site of flow detection; size of the sample volume is determined by beam diameter and length of the ultrasound pulse (see pulsed Doppler, gate).

Saphenous vein There are two veins that serve as the principal superficial venous outflow, the great saphenous and small saphenous. The great saphenous vein runs from the foot to the groin where it joins with the common femoral vein. The small saphenous vein runs from the posterior lateral malleolus (lateral to the Achilles' tendon, near ankle) along the posterior leg and usually joins the popliteal vein in the space behind the knee.

Segmental blood pressures Obtaining blood pressure measurements at different levels of the upper or lower extremities, the comparison of pressure change across each segment of the limb in order to determine the level of occlusive disease.

Sensitivity The ability of a diagnostic technique to identify the presence of disease when disease is actually present. Sens. = TP × 100 = % TP + FN TP = true positive, FN = false negative.

Sequential bypass Arterial bypasses in series; a continuation and/or additional bypass performed to maintain patency of previous surgery.

Shunt A term used to describe a pathway other than the usual to divert blood from one point to another; may be a natural channel, i.e., an arteriovenous fistula or a surgically created channel, i.e., a bypass graft. In carotid endarterectomy a shunt is often used to divert blood from the common carotid artery to the internal system during the procedure. Shunt is synonymous with bypass.

Small saphenous vein (SSV) One of two major superficial veins of the lower limb. Originating on the lateral side of the foot, it extends along the posterior aspect of the calf. The termination of the SSV varies; terminations include the popliteal 2-4cm/s near knee crease, distal FV, or GSV (either directly or via a perforating vein).

Specificity The ability of a diagnostic technique to identify the absence of disease (normalcy) when no disease is actually present. Spec. = TN × 100 = % TN + FP TN = true negative, FP = false positive

Spectral analysis A method of analyzing and/or displaying the Doppler signal output. Spectral analysis, using a microprocessor, is capable of analyzing and displaying the complete range of frequencies in each waveform. This technique may be used with pulsed or continuous wave Doppler systems. Time is displayed on the horizontal axis, frequency on the vertical axis and amplitude of the signal by the intensity of the gray scale. Spectral analysis provides the most complete assessment of the Doppler waveform and is a useful technique for quantifying degree of arterial stenosis.

Splenic vein Collects blood from the spleen and part of the stomach and joins with the superior mesenteric vein to form the portal vein.

Spontaneity In normal veins flow occurs passively. It should be detectable in all major veins.

Stab Avulsion (also known as phlebectomy, microphlebectomy, or ambulatory phlebectomy) A technique to remove varicose veins. In this procedure, several tiny cuts (incisions) are made in the skin through which the varicosed vein is removed.

Stasis Refers to the stagnation of blood; cessation of normal blood flow. In the venous system of the lower extremity, stagnant blood flow as the result of immobility contributes to venous thrombosis. Stagnation of venous blood in the extremity because of valvular dysfunction (or post-phlebitic syndrome) results in pigmentation changes and ulceration.

Stent A tube made of metal or plastic that is inserted into a vessel or passage to keep it open and prevent closure due to a stricture or external compression.

Streptokinase A protein produced B-hemolytic streptococci. It is used as a thrombolytic agent; used topically on surface lesions or by instillation in closed body cavities to remove clotted blood.

Stricture A narrowing of a tube, usually due to scar tissue formation.

Subclavian vein The direct continuation of the axillary vein at the lateral border of the first rib, it passes medially to join the internal jugular vein and form the brachiocephalic veins bilaterally.

Superior mesenteric vein (SMV) Drains the cecum, transverse and sigmoid colon, and small bowel.

Superior vena cava (SVC) Returns blood from the head and neck, upper limbs and thorax, and is formed by the confluence of the two brachiocephalic veins (innominate veins).

Supine Lying on the back with face upwards, opposite of prone.

Sympathetic A division of the autonomic nervous system involved primarily with emergency responses and muscular activity. It is the sympathetic system which mediates homeostasis and vascular smooth muscle response, i.e., vasodilation and vasoconstriction.

Symptom A subjective manifestation of disease, e.g., pain.

Synechiae (Webbing) Organization and subsequent contraction of a thrombus leading to adherence of thrombus to the vein wall and spontaneous lysis of areas within the thrombus. A fibrous membrane may remain within the lumen of the vein.

Systole The contraction phase of the cardiac cycle.

T

Tachycardia Excessively rapid heart rate, usually over 100 beats per minute.

Thoracic outlet syndrome (TOS) A symptom complex associated with compression of the arteries, veins, or nerves of the upper extremity at the outlet from the thoracic cavity. Symptoms include numbness or pain of the arm associated with activity, elevation, or hyperabduction.

Thrombectomy Surgical removal of a blood clot from a vessel.

Thromboangiitis Clot formation within an inflamed vessel; Buerger's disease was referred to as thromboangiitis obliterans.

Thromboendarterectomy Surgical removal of a blood clot from within an artery.

Thrombogenic Capable of causing blood clotting.

Thrombolysis The breaking up of thrombus.

Thrombolytic Capable of disintegrating a blood clot. TPA, Streptokinase and Urokinase are used to dissolve clots. This agent acts by stimulating the conversion of plasminogen to plasmin (an enzyme which breaks down fibrin). Thrombolytic therapy is used successfully in the treatment of deep venous thrombosis, for acute arterial thrombosis, and graft occlusion.

Thrombophlebitis Inflammation of a vein with secondary thrombosis in the involved segment.

Thrombosis The formation of an intravascular blood clot formation.

Thrombus An intravascular blood clot; plural, thrombi.

Tibio-gastrocnemious Angle Sign Identifies the Great Saphenous Vein relative to the tibia and medial gastrocnemius muscle below the knee.

Tissue plasminogen activator (TPA) A generic term for a group of substances that have the ability to cleave to plasminogen and convert it to plasmin in its active form; it is used for therapeutic thrombolysis.

Transmetatarsal amputation Toe amputation (across the metatarsals).

Transverse Along the path of a sound beam; or along a cross-sectional course, as in a transverse scan. (Short axis, SAX)

Triphasic Having three phases or variations; forward flow in systole, brief reverse flow, and a third forward flow component (multiphasic).

Trophic Pertaining to nutrition; trophic changes on an extremity (e.g., nail thickening, atrophied skin) are the results of ischemia or lack of nutrition to the skin.

Tunica A coat; lining membrane, as in tunica intima, tunica media, tunica adventitia.

Turbulence The disruption of the normal laminar flow within a tube or vessel; disturbed blood flow in which whirls and eddies occur; usually due to obstruction to blood flow; a source of bruits.

U

Ulcer The most common type of ulcer is a venous ulcer caused by chronic venous disorders. The venous ulcers are typically shallow with granulation tissue and fibrin and are located in the gaiter area over the media malleolus.

Unilateral Pertaining to one side.

V

Valsalva maneuver Forced expiration against the closed glottis impeding blood flow through the pulmonary capillary bed and increasing intrathoracic pressure. This maneuver impedes venous return and is used in the venous Doppler examination to assess venous flow and valvular competency.

Valve A membrane within a tube or vessel allowing flow to move in one direction only. The venous valves are bicuspid and open towards the heart to prevent reflux. Damaged or incompetent valves allow retrograde venous flow.

Varices Enlarged tortuous vessel; the vessels can be veins or lymphatic vessels.

Varicocele Varicosity of the veins of the spermatic cord. A common cause of infertility in the male. Diagnosis can be made by palpation or (in subclinical presentation) by Doppler ultrasound. Venous reflux during Valsalva maneuver is found in the presence of varicocele.

Varicose veins Veins that are distended, lengthened, and tortuous. The superficial veins (saphenous veins) of the legs are most commonly affected. There is an inherited tendency to varicose veins (primary) but obstruction to blood flow or incompetent valves, which permit backflow of venous blood (secondary), also may be responsible.

Vascular Pertaining to the blood vessels.

Vasculogenic Of a vascular origin.

Vasoconstriction Narrowing of the vessel lumen caused by contraction of the muscular vessel wall.

Vasodilation Enlarging of the vessel wall caused by relaxation of the muscular vessel wall.

Vasospasm Spasmodic constricting of a vessel wall.

Vein A blood vessel which conveys blood from the capillaries back to the heart. Veins are composed of three layers, intima, media, and adventitia. The media of the vein is less muscular than an artery. Veins are more compliant than arteries and are equipped with one-way valves to prevent reflux of blood.

Velocity Speed of an acoustic wave per unit time in a specific direction.

Vena cava filter A device placed in the IVC to catch emboli and prevent them from getting to the lungs.

Venography A radiographic procedure in which an opaque substance is injected into the veins. Subsequent x-ray pictures are taken for the purpose of visualizing the venous system (see phlebography).

Venous Pertaining to the veins.

Venous air embolism An air bubble which may enter the venous system during any surgical procedure in which the surgical site is above the level of the right atrium. Doppler ultrasound is the most sensitive method of detection of air emboli in the right atrium.

Venous Aneurysm A localized dilation of a venous segment, with a caliber increase 50% compared with normal.

Venous insufficiency Condition in which faulty or damaged venous valves permit retrograde or backward flow of blood. Stagnant venous blood in the lower extremity may result in pigmentation changes, edema, pain, and ulceration (see post phlebitic syndrome).

Venule A small vein.

Virchow's triad The three mechanisms of thrombosis, injury to the vessel wall, decrease in blood flow (stasis), and blood hypercoagulability.

Viscosity Resistance of a fluid to flow when a pressure is applied.

W

Waveform A curve or undulation traced by a recording device and reflecting alterations in electrical activity; the shape of a wave on a graph (see triphasic).

Webbing (Synechiae) Organization and subsequent contraction of a thrombus leading to adherence of thrombus to the vein wall and spontaneous lysis of areas within the thrombus. A fibrous membrane may remain within the lumen of the vein.

X

Xiphoid process The pointed part of cartilage located at the lower end of the sternum.

Prefixes

sub-	below (subacute)
supra-	above (supraorbital)
tachy-	apid (tachycardia)
thermo-	temperature (thermography)
thrombo-	blood clot (thrombophlebitis)
trans-	across (transverse)
ultra-	from, beyond, to above (ultrasound)
uni-	one (unidirectional)
vaso-	vessel (vasospasm)

Suffixes

-algia	pain (causalgia)
-ectomy	removal of (thrombectomy)
-emia	blood (anemia)
-esthesia	sensation (parasthesia)
-genesis	origin (thrombogenesis
-genic	causation (vasculogenic)
-graphy	writing (plethysmography)
-itis	inflammation (arteritis)
-logy	study of (physiology)
-meter	measure (manometer)
-otomy	opening (arteriotomy)
-ous	like (atheromatous)
-pathy	disease (cardiopathy)
-penia	lack of (thrombocytopenia)
-phagia	swallowing (dysphasia)
-phasia	speech (aphasia)
-plegia	paralysis (paraplegia)
-rhage	burst forth (hemorrhage)
-sonic	sound (ultrasonic)
-stasis	stagnation (hemostasis)

Acronyms

A

AAA	Abdominal Aortic Aneurysm
ASV	Anterior Saphenous Vein (formerly Anterior Accessory Saphenous Vein)
ABI	Ankle-Brachial Index
ACAS	Asymptomatic Carotid Atherosclerosis Study
ACC	American College of Cardiology
ACR	American College of Radiology
AEUS	American Emergency Ultrasonographic Society
AFB	Aortobifemoral Bypass
AHA	American Hospital Association
AI	Acceleration Index
AIUM	American Institute of Ultrasound in Medicine
AJV	Anterior Jugular Vein
AKA	Above Knee Amputation
AK	Above Knee
AMA	American Medical Association
AP	Ambulatory Phlebectomy
AP	Anterior Posterior
APG	Air Plethysmography
ARDMS	American Registry of Diagnostic Medical Sonography
ARRT	American Registry of Radiologic Technologists
ASE	American Society of Echocardiography
ASN	American Society of Neuroimaging
ASRT	American Society of Radiologic Technologists
ASVAL	Ambulatory Selective Varices Ablation under Local Anesthesia
ATA	Anterior Tibial Artery
ATA	Anterior Tibial Artery
AT	Acceleration Time

ATCV	Anterior Thigh Circumflex Vein
ATV	Anterior Tibial Vein
ATVs	Anterior Tibial Veins
AVA	American Vascular Association
AV	Arteriovenous
AVF	Arteriovenous Fistula
AVG	Arteriovenous Graft
AVIR	Association of Vascular and Interventional Radiographers
AVM	Arteriovenous Malformation
AVP	Ambulatory Venous Pressure
AVVQ	Aberdeen Varicose Vein Questionnaire
AXV	Axillary vein

B

BsV	Basilic Vein
BCV	Brachiocephalic Vein
BKA	Below Knee Amputation
BK	Below Knee
BMI	Body Mass Index
BP	Blood Pressure
BrA	Brachial Artery
BrVs	Brachial Veins
BUN	Blood Urea Nitrogen

C

CAAHEP	Commission on Accreditation of Allied Health Education Programs
CABG	Coronary Artery Bypass Graft
CABG	Coronary Artery Bypass Graft
CAC	Carrier Advisory Committee
CAD	Coronary Artery Disease
CAS	Carotid Artery Stenting
CBD	Common Bile Duct
CCA	Common Carotid Artery
CCI	Cardiovascular Credentialing International
CDI	Color Doppler Imaging
CDT	Complex/Complete Decongestive Therapy
CEA	Carotid Endarterectomy
CEAP	Clinical, Etiologic, Anatomic, Pathophysiology
CFA	Common Femoral Artery
CFV	Common Femoral Vein
CHF	Congestive Heart Failure
CHIVA	Cure conservatrice et Hemodynamique de l'Insuffisance Veineuse en Ambulatoire – Outpatient Hemodynamic Correction of Venous Insufficiency
CIA	Common Iliac Artery
CIV	Common Iliac Vein
CMD	Carrier Medical Director
CME	Continuing Medical Education units
CMS	Centers for Medicare and Medicaid Services
CMV	Congenital Venous Malformation
COPD	Chronic Obstructive Pulmonary Disease

CQU	Coalition for Quality in Ultrasound
CREST	Carotid Revascularization Endarterectomy vs. Stenting Trial
CRP	C-Reactive Protein
CTA	Computed Tomography Angiography
CT	Computed Tomography
CTV	Computed Tomography Venography
CVA	Cerebrovascular Accident
CV	Cephalic Vein
CVD	Chronic Venous Disease/Disorder
CVI	Chronic Venous Insufficiency
CVM	Congenital Venous Malformation
CW	Continuous Wave

D

DBI	Digit-Brachial Index
DC	Distal Calf
DES	Drug Eluting Stents
DFV	Deep Femoral Vein
DHHS	Dept. of Health and Human Services
DIC	Disseminated Intravascular Coagulation
DOL	Dept. of Labor
DPA	Dorsalis Pedis Artery
DPV	Dorsalis Pedis Vein
DT	Distal Thigh
DUS	Duplex Ultrasound
DVI	Deep Venous Insufficiency
DVS	Deep Venous System
DVT	Deep Vein Thrombosis

E

EAA	Endovenous Adhesive Ablation
EC-IC	Extracranial To Intracranial Bypass
ECA	External Carotid Artery
EDV	End-Diastolic Velocity
EF	Ejection Fraction
EFIT	Endovenous Foam Induced Thrombus
EGIT	Endovenous Glue Induced Thrombus
EHIT	Endothermal Heat Induced Thrombosis
EIA	External Iliac Artery
EJV	External Jugular Vein
ESRD	End Stage Renal Disease
EVA	Endovenous Ablation
EVAR	Endovascular Aneurysm Repair
EV	Ejection Volume
EVLA	Endovenous Laser Ablation
EVLT	Endovenous Laser Treatment

F

FA	Femoral Artery
Fem-pop	Femoropopliteal
FEVAR	Fenestrated Endovascular Aortic Aneurysm Repair
FMD	Fibromuscular Dysplasia
FP	Femoropopliteal
FV	Femoral Vein

G

GA	Gastric Artery
GCA	Giant Cell Arteritis
GI	Gastrointestinal

GSV	Great Saphenous Vein
GV	Gastric Vein
GV	Gonadal Vein
GVP	Genicular Venous Plexus
GVs	Gastrocnemius Veins

H

HA	Hepatic Artery
HBP	High Blood Pressure
HCT	Hematocrit
HD	Hemodialysis
HDL	High-Density Lipoprotein
HGB	Hemoglobin
HHD	Hand-held Doppler
HHS	Hypothenar Hammer Syndrome
HIPAA	Health Insurance Portability and Accountability Act of 1996
HIT	Heparin-Induced Thrombocytopenia
HITT	Heparin-Induced Thrombocytopenia with Thrombosis
HTN	Hypertension
HV	Hepatic Vein
Hz	Hertz

I

IAC	Intersocietal Accreditation Commission (accredits Vascular and Echocardiography Laboratories)
ICA	Internal Carotid Artery
ICS	Iliac Compression Syndrome
IDTF	Independent Diagnostic Testing Facility
IGV	Inferior Gluteal Vein
IIA	Internal Iliac Artery
IIV	Internal Iliac Vein
IJV	Internal Jugular Vein
IMA	Inferior Mesenteric Artery
IMT	Intimal Medial Thickness
IMV	Inferior Mesenteric Vein
IntSvs	Intersaphenous veins
InV	Innominate Vein
IPV	Incompetent Perforating Vein
IVC	Inferior Vena Cava
IVUS	Intravascular Ultrasound

J

J	Joule
JDMS	Journal of Diagnostic Medical Sonography
JRC-CVT	Joint Review Committee on Education in Cardiovascular Technology
JRC-DMS	Joint Review Committee on Education in Diagnostic Medical Sonography
JVU	Journal for Vascular Ultrasound

K

| KHz | Kilohertz |
| KTS | Klippel-Trenaunay Syndrome |

L

LASER	Light Amplification by Stimulated Emission of Radiation
LCD	Local Coverage Determination
LDS	Lipodermatosclerosis

LEED	Linear Endovenous Energy Density
LE	Lower Extremity
LGVs	Lateral Gastrocnemius Veins
LLE	Left Lower Extremity
LMRP	Local Medical Review Policy
LMV	Lateral Marginal Vein
LMWH	Low-Molecular-Weight Heparin
LNVN	Lymph Node Vein Network
LRV	Left Renal Vein
LVS	Lateral Venous System

M

MALS	Median Arcuate Ligament Syndrome
MAV	Median Antebrachial Vein
MC	Mid-Calf
MCV	Median Cubital Vein
MedPAC	Medicare Payment Advisory Commission
MGVs	Medial Gastrocnemius Veins
MHz	Megahertz
MI	Myocardial Infarction
mmHg	Millimeters of Mercury
MMV	Medial Marginal Vein
MRA	Magnetic Resonance Angiography
MRI	Magnetic Resonance Imaging
MRV	Magnetic Resonance Venography
MSD	Musculoskeletal Disorder
MT	Mid-Thigh
MV	Medial Vein of forearm
MVO	Maximum Venous Outflow

N

NAA	National Aneurysm Alliance
NASCET	North American Symptomatic Carotid Endarterectomy Trial
NIVLs	Nonthrombotic Iliac Vein Lesions

O

OSHA	Occupational Safety & Health Administration
OV	Ovarian Vein

P

PAD	Peripheral Arterial Disease
PAGSV	Posterior Accessory Great Saphenous Vein
PASTE	Post Ablation Superficial Thrombus Extension
PBI	Penile Brachial Index
PC	Proximal Calf
PCRM	Peripheral Compression Release Maneuver
PEP	Pelvic Escape Points
PE	Pulmonary Embolus
PerA	Peroneal Artery
PerVs	Peroneal Veins
PeVD	Pelvic Venous Disorders
PFV	Profunda Femoral Vein
PICC	Peripherally Inserted Central Catheter
PI	Pulsatility Index
POP	Popliteal
PopV	Popliteal Vein
PPG	Photoplethysmography
PPV	Pathologic Perforating Vein
PREVAIT	PREsence of Varices (residual or recurrent) After InTervention

PRF	Pulse Repetition Frequency
PRG	Phleborheography
PSV	Peak-Systolic Velocity
PTA	Percutaneous Transluminal Angioplasty
PTA	Posterior Tibial Artery
PTCV	Posterior Thigh Circumflex Vein
PTFE	Polytetrafloroethylene
PT	Proximal Thigh
PTS	Post Thrombotic Syndrome
PTV	Posterior Tibial Vein
PTVs	Posterior Tibial Veins
PVD	Peripheral Vascular Disease
PVE	Popliteal Vein Extrinsic Positional Obliteration Syndrome
PV	Portal Vein
PVR	Pulse Volume Recording
PVs	Perforating Veins

Q

QoL	Quality of Life

R

RadA	Radial Artery
RadVs	Radial Veins
RA	Renal Artery
RAR	Renal Aortic Ratio
RAS	Renal Artery Stenosis
RDCS	Registered Diagnostic Cardiac Sonographer
REVAS	REcurrent Varices After Surgery
RFA	Radio Frequency Ablation
RIND	Reversible Ischemic Neurological Deficit
RI	Resistive Index
RLE	Right Lower Extremity
ROUB	Registered Ophthalmic Ultrasound Biometrics
RRV	Right Renal Vein
RSD	Reflex Sympathetic Dystrophy
RVF	Residual Volume Fraction
RV	Renal Vein
RVS	Registered Vascular Specialist
RVT	Registered Vascular Technologist

S

SA	Splenic Artery
SAV	Superficial Accessory Vein
SCIV	Superficial Circumflex Iliac Vein
ScP	Sciatic Perforator
SC	Saphenous Compartment
SCV	Subclavian Vein
SDMS	Society of Diagnostic Medical Sonography
SEPS	Subfascial Endoscopic Perforator Surgery
SEP	Superficial External Pudendal
SEPV	Superficial Epigastric Vein
SFJptv	Sapheno-femoral Junction pre-terminal valve
SFJ	Saphenofemoral Junction
SFJtv	Sapheno-femoral Junction terminal valve
SIEV	Superficial Inferior Epigastric Vein
SIR	Society of Interventional Radiology
SMA	Superior Mesenteric Artery
SMV	Superior Mesenteric Vein

SolV	Soleal Vein
SPJ	Saphenopopliteal Junction
SplV	Splenic Vein
SSV	Small Saphenous Vein
SVC	Superior Vena Cava
SVI	Superficial Venous Insufficiency
SVMB	Society for Vascular Medicine and Biology
SVN	Society for Vascular Nursing
SV	Splenic Vein
SVS	Society for Vascular Surgery
SVT	Superficial Vein Thrombosis
SVU	Society for Vascular Ultrasound

T

TAVR	Transcatheter Aortic Valve Replacement
TBI	Toe-Brachial Index
TCD	Transcranial Doppler
TCPO2	Transcutaneous Pulse Oximetry
TE-SSV	Thigh Extension of the Small Saphenous Vein
TE	Thigh Extension
TEVAR	Thoracic Endovascular Abdominal Aortic Aneurysm Repair
TGC	Time Gain Compensation
TIA	Transient Ischemic Attack
TMA	Transmetatarsal Amputation
TOS	Thoracic Outlet Syndrome
TPA	Tissue Plasminogen Activator
TV	Terminal Valve

U

UA	Ulnar Artery
UE	Upper Extremity
UGFS	Ultrasound Guided Foam Sclerotherapy
UGS	Ultrasound Guided Sclerotherapy
USPSTF	United States Preventative Services Task Force
US	Ultrasound
UVs	Ulnar Veins

V

VA	Vertebral artery
VCSS	Venous Clinical Severity Score
VCT	Valve Closure Time
VDF	Vascular Disease Foundation
VertV	Vertebral Vein
VFT	Venous Filling Time
VM	Venous Malformation
VPR	Volume Pulse Recording
VTE	Venous Thromboembolism
VVs	Varicose Veins
VV	Varicose Vein
VV	Venous Volume

W

WRMSDs	Work Related Musculoskeletal Disorders

54. Index

A

Acceleration index 279, 283, 387

Abdominal aortic aneurysm 73, 75, 77, 112, 146, 163, 249, 251, 254, 258, 260-261, 268, 294-295

Adventitial cystic disease 74, 90, 97, 163

Anatomy *(See arterial anatomy, venous anatomy)*

Aneurysm 8, 45, 65-66, 68, 74-77, 80, 86, 89-90, 92, 94, 96-97, 101, 104, 111-112, 116-119, 129, 131-132, 137, 142, 146, 155-156, 162-164, 166, 170, 173, 178, 181, 185, 187, 191, 198, 206, 234, 241, 243, 249-254, 257-258, 260-263, 265-273, 275, 287-291, 294-295, 303, 306, 314, 316, 321-322, 351-353, 355, 358, 360, 382-383, 387-
see abdominal aortic aneurysm
bilobed 74
fusiform aneurysm 74
pseudoaneurysm 46, 65, 74, 77, 89-90, 94, 97-98, 100-101, 104, 132, 137, 146, 155, 162, 164, 170, 173, 181, 185, 191, 251, 254, 258, 260, 269, 278, 284-286, 303, 306, 313-320, 351-352, 355, 359-360
saccular aneurysm 74-76, 163, 260

Anterior cerebral artery 4, 8, 82, 118

Anterior communicating artery 7-8

Anterior tibial artery 25-26, 156, 387

Anterior tibial vein 388

Aorta 11-17, 25, 34-35, 42, 47, 49, 74-77, 80, 86, 89, 93, 95-97, 156, 164, 220, 225, 227, 233, 249-254, 256-257, 260-262, 265, 268-274, 277, 287-292, 335-336, 350, 360, 381-382

Aortic coarctation 77, 97, 249, 358

Aortic insufficiency 335

Aortic regurgitation 106, 128, 335-336, 341

Aortic stenosis 76, 334-335, 341

Ankle brachial index (ABI) 141, 155, 164, 367, 370, 375, 132, 134-135, 140-142, 151-153, 155-156, 164, 168, 171-172, 175, 258-259, 318, 320, 367, 370, 375-376, 381, 387

Arterial anatomy 1-32
abdominal 15-17
extracranial 1-6
intracranial 1, 6-9
lower extremity 25-26
renal 11-12, 15-17
upper extremity 31-32

Arterial dissection

Arterial dissection 77-78, 81, 100, 111, 130, 163, 192, 258, 270, 275, 287, 295, 354, 358, 360

Arteriomegaly 162, 191, 258

Arteriovenous fistula 61, 63-64, 66, 71, 87, 132, 137, 155, 162, 174, 177, 185, 191, 197, 207, 213, 225, 242, 244, 269, 273, 277-278, 284, 287, 296, 303-306, 308, 310, 313, 315, 320, 355, 382, 386, 388
hemodialysis access 248, 303, 306, 314-315, 355

Arteritis *(also see Vasculitis)* 65, 76, 83, 85-86, 91, 93-97, 102, 106, 111-112, 130, 137, 146, 173, 177, 181, 185, 287, 358, 360, 387-388

Atherosclerosis 35, 50, 65, 72-74, 78-81, 86-88, 90-94, 96, 98, 100, 112-113, 115-116, 118, 130, 132, 137, 142, 146, 155, 164, 173, 176-177, 181, 185, 243, 249-250, 260-261, 268-270, 277, 287, 303, 321, 358, 381, 383, 387

Augmentation 37, 39-40, 131, 144, 202-206, 218, 222-224, 228, 233, 235-237, 240, 246-248, 307-309, 318, 325, 345-346, 381

Axillary artery 31, 66, 73, 89, 94-95, 174-175, 185-186, 250, 303, 317, 323

Axillary vein 27-28, 30, 236-237, 307-309, 323, 325, 382, 386, 388

B

Basilar artery 7-8, 82, 118-119, 125

Basilic vein 27-28, 165, 236, 244, 303, 381, 388

Behcet's disease 96

Bernoulli Principle 54

Bigeminy 341

Blunt flow (plug flow) 49

Brachial artery 31, 44, 85, 89, 132-133, 139, 146-147, 152, 173-174, 176-177, 179, 182, 185-187, 190-191, 303, 317, 330, 376, 382, 388

Brachial vein 236, 238, 244,

Brachiocephalic (innominate) artery 2-3, 6, 27-28, 30-31, 77, 94, 107, 236-237, 241, 303, 325, 382, 384, 386, 388

Brachiocephalic vein 27, 30, 384, 388

Budd Chiari syndrome 296

Buerger's disease 91, 146, 149, 177, 180-181, 184, 386

C

Calf muscle pump 23, 38-39, 58, 67, 193-194, 209, 378, 383

Caprini DVT Risk Score 56, 207, 357, 382

Cardiac effects 72, 333-341
cardiac arrhythmias 334, 339
cardiac output 39, 86, 278, 292, 305, 334, 386

Carotid artery

Carotid artery 2-5, 8-9, 27-28, 31, 47-48, 50, 76, 82-85, 89, 97-98, 100-102, 106-107, 109, 112-115, 118-119, 125-126, 131, 317, 335, 339, 351, 380, 386, 388
common carotid artery 2-3, 9, 27-28, 31, 83-84, 98, 102, 107, 110, 113, 125, 335, 341, 380, 386, 388, 390
external carotid artery 3-4, 47, 84, 98, 101, 107, 351, 388
internal carotid artery 3-5, 8-9, 48, 50, 82, 85, 97-98, 100-102, 106-107, 113, 118-119, 126, 131, 388

Carotid intima media thickness testing 113-115

Carotid body tumor 84, 98, 101, 350, 358, 360

Carotid siphon 5-6, 118-119, 123

CEAP 55-56, 60, 71, 210, 382, 388

Cephalic vein 27-28, 30, 165, 236, 243-244, 303, 307-308, 382, 388

Cerebrovascular Events *(Transient Ischemic Attack, Stroke)* 81-84

Churg-Strauss angiitis 96

Circle of Willis 7-9, 116, 118

Cold immersion testing 181-184

Collateral flow 6-7, 53, 160, 292

Common carotid artery 2-3, 9, 27-28, 31, 83-84, 98, 102, 106, 113, 125, 335, 380, 386, 388

Compliance 35-37, 135, 140, 175, 189, 256, 266, 292, 332

Computed Tomography (CT) 59, 61-66, 69, 71, 73, 75, 77, 80-81, 83-86, 88-90, 92-94, 96, 101, 112, 115, 130-131, 135, 141, 145, 149, 154, 163, 172, 176, 180, 192, 207, 218, 225, 233, 242, 251, 257, 260-261, 266, 268, 276, 286, 290, 295, 302, 320, 326, 348-349, 357, 371-373, 388 131, 207, 233, 348, 357, 388,

Continuous wave (CW) Doppler 133, 138, 174, 179-180, 213, 322, 324, 330, 382, 386

Correlative testing modalities 348-357
angiography 62, 64-66, 71, 73, 75-77, 80-81, 83-86, 88-90, 92-94, 96, 130-131, 149, 180, 184, 286, 302, 320, 332, 348-349, 351, 357, 359, 371-372, 388-390
computed tomography (CT) 131, 207, 233, 348, 357, 388,
D-dimer blood test 348, 357
magnetic resonance imaging (MRI) 65-66, 69, 71, 76, 83-85, 89-90, 94, 96, 112, 115, 130, 207, 225, 242, 268, 286, 302, 332, 348-350, 357

venography 59, 61, 63-68, 72, 94, 197, 207, 213, 218, 232, 348-349, 351-353, 357, 385

VQ scan (ventilation/perfusion) 347, 355-357

D

Deep vein thrombosis 20, 60, 73, 207-208, 226, 242, 353, 357, 382, 385, 388

Digital 19, 26-27, 32, 66, 90-92, 94, 114, 130-133, 137, 142-143, 146-149, 155, 164, 173-175, 177-185, 310, 313, 321-322, 324, 351, 353, 376, 384-385

Dissection 61, 63-65, 73, 76-77, 81, 83, 86, 92, 96-98, 100, 111-112, 116-117, 119, 124, 130, 155, 163, 185, 192, 251-253, 258, 260, 262, 268, 270-272, 275, 278, 287-288, 295, 354, 358, 360, 382

Doppler equation 45

Dorsalis pedis artery 26, 138, 388

E

Edema 41, 55, 59, 61-63, 65, 68, 71, 155, 164, 193-194, 198-199, 202, 207-210, 214, 219-220, 225-226, 228, 234-235, 241-243, 261, 270, 275, 278, 281, 303, 306, 321, 339, 354, 357, 359, 361, 383, 385, 387

Effort thrombosis 241
(see thoracic outlet compression syndrome)

EHIT 216, 383, 388,

Embolism 63-64, 70, 72-73, 81, 86, 91-92, 117, 124, 132, 137, 146, 177, 198, 219, 234-235, 287, 321, 338, 357, 360, 382-383, 387

Endoleak 261-267

Energy 35, 42, 46, 49, 52-54, 215, 383, 385, 389

External carotid artery 3-4, 47, 84, 98, 101, 107, 351, 388

External jugular vein 28, 30, 384, 388

F

Femoral
common femoral artery 17, 25, 46, 89, 138, 156, 163-164, 303, 317, 372, 388
common femoral vein 20, 38-39, 59, 200, 202, 211, 216, 352, 383-386, 388
deep femoral artery 26, 89, 138, 156, 317
deep femoral vein 68, 200, 202, 388
femoral artery 17, 20, 25-26, 46, 63-64, 73, 75, 89, 132, 138, 142, 144, 155-156, 159, 162-165, 169-172, 215, 250-251, 260, 303, 317, 320, 372, 388

femoral vein 20-21, 24, 38-39, 59, 65, 68, 71, 200-202, 211, 216, 233, 303, 352, 383-386, 388-389

Fibromuscular dysplasia 76, 81, 83, 86, 92, 98, 100, 111, 116, 119, 146, 177, 185, 269, 273, 275, 358, 360, 388

G

Gastric artery 15-16, 388
Gastrocnemius artery 25
Gastrocnemius vein 204
Giant cell arteritis 91, 95-97, 112, 130, 388

H

Hemodynamics 33-54
Hemorrhage 72, 79-80, 83, 88-89, 96-97, 112, 116-117, 119, 124, 128, 130-131, 214, 277, 296, 351, 383, 387
  hemorrhagic stroke 81, 119
  intracerebral hemorrhage 80, 97, 119
  subarachnoid hemorrhage 80, 116-117, 119, 124, 128, 131, 351
Hepatic artery 12, 15-16, 48, 289, 293-294, 388
Hepatic vein 11-12, 89, 220, 296-299, 301-302, 388
  left hepatic vein 297
  middle hepatic vein 297
  right hepatic vein 220, 297, 302
Hepatoportal duplex 296
Heterogeneous 106, 204, 223, 239, 247, 257, 383
High resistance 47, 107, 128, 256, 266, 292, 328, 375
Homogeneous 106, 281, 310, 331, 361, 383
Hydronephrosis 278-279, 281, 286
Hydrostatic pressure 36, 38, 41-42, 44, 133-134, 138, 140, 147, 194, 209, 366, 383
Hyperplasia
  Neointimal and Intimal 88-89

I

Iliac
  common iliac artery 17, 20, 60, 75, 198, 250, 253-254, 258, 388
  common iliac vein 10, 20, 58, 60, 62, 198, 222, 228, 388
  external iliac artery 13, 17, 25, 73, 85, 89, 95, 257, 277, 279, 281-282, 317, 388
  external iliac vein 10, 20, 60, 222-224, 231, 280, 384
  internal iliac artery 17, 25, 328, 388
  internal iliac vein 10, 20, 230, 384, 388
Iliac vein compression 60, 63, 69, 72, 220, 228, 354, 358, 360
Image optimization 114, 361-364

Inferior mesenteric artery (IMA) 15-17, 86, 290-291, 293, 388
Inferior vena cava 10-11, 16, 20, 34, 37, 71, 199, 202, 219, 222-226, 228-229, 233, 260-261, 268, 271, 297, 382-385, 388
Innominate (see brachiocephalic artery)
Insufficiency 30, 35, 41, 44, 55, 57, 61, 67-68, 71-72, 86, 177, 193-194, 196-197, 208, 210, 212-214, 287, 327, 332, 335, 338, 344-345, 352-354, 359-360, 378, 381-382, 384-385, 387-390
Internal carotid artery 3-5, 8-9, 48, 50, 82, 85, 97-98, 100-102, 106-107, 113, 118-119, 126, 131, 388
Intimal Hyperplasia 88-89
Intracranial cerebrovascular testing 116-131
Internal jugular vein 27-28, 236-237, 301, 338-339, 386, 388

K

Kawasaki's disease 96
Kinetic energy 42, 54
Klippel-Trenaunay Syndrome 68-69

L

Laminar flow 48-49, 52, 310, 384, 387
Low resistance 47-48, 107-108, 135, 140, 159, 162, 167, 170, 176, 189, 257, 259, 267, 274, 281, 284, 292-293, 305, 311, 328, 331, 375
Lymphangiosarcoma 62
Lymphedema 41, 59, 61-63, 68, 71-72, 197, 207, 213, 225, 242, 359-360, 384
Lymphedema Tarda 61

M

Math 365-371
May-Thurner Syndrome (see Iliac Vein Compression)
Median arcuate ligament syndrome 86, 287, 289, 294, 389
Median cubital vein 28, 245, 384, 389
Mesenteric 11-12, 15-17, 47-48, 75, 85-87, 89, 95-97, 261, 267, 270-273, 287-295, 300, 302, 359-360, 384-386, 388-389
  acute mesenteric ischemia 85-87, 97, 287, 295, 360
  chronic mesenteric ischemia 85-86, 287, 295
  inferior mesenteric artery 15, 17, 86, 290-291, 293, 388
  Inferior mesenteric vein 11, 384, 388
  Ischemia 86
  superior mesenteric artery 11, 15-16, 48, 86, 270-272, 287, 290, 389
  superior mesenteric vein 11, 89, 302, 384-386, 389

Middle cerebral artery 4, 8, 82, 118, 131
Mitral regurgitation 337
Mitral stenosis 336-337
Moyamoya disease 83, 85, 98, 112, 117, 130

N

Neointimal hyperplasia 88, 104, 359-360, 384
Neurofibromatosis 76, 85, 92, 287
Nyquist limit 370

O

Ohm's law 370, 384
Ophthalmic artery 4-6, 9

P

Paget-Schroetter syndrome 241
Palmar arch 32, 142, 174, 179-180, 182, 185, 305, 381
Paraumbilical vein 297, 300, 302
Parvus tardus 53, 135, 141, 159, 170, 176, 190, 257, 267, 275, 283, 337, 341
Penile 327-332, 377, 389
  cavernosal artery 328-331
  dorsal artery 327-328
  dorsal vein 328, 330-332
  penile brachial index 377, 389
  urethral artery 328
Peripheral resistance 44, 382
Peroneal artery 26, 133, 138, 389
Pharmacology 35, 332, 358
Phlegmasia alba dolens 63, 198-199, 219-220, 226
Phlegmasia cerulea dolens 63, 198-199, 220, 226, 385
Photoplethysmography (PPG) 146, 177, 193, 197, 213, 310, 322, 389
  arterial 146-149, 177-180
  venous 193-197
Plaque 49-51, 66, 78-82, 94, 99-100, 104, 106-108, 113-115, 118, 124, 128, 132, 137, 142, 146, 155-157, 159, 167-168, 173, 177-178, 185, 187-189, 250, 252-253, 256, 270-273, 287-290, 292, 299, 307, 311, 322, 327, 354, 361, 381, 383, 385
Platelets 34-35, 70, 87, 198, 219, 234, 357, 385
Poiseuille's Law 44-45, 51, 150, 385
Polyarteritis nodosa 92, 96
Popliteal 19, 22, 24-26, 37, 46, 58-59, 68, 70-71, 73, 75, 80, 90, 97, 132, 138, 142-144, 155-157, 159, 162-164, 198-199, 201-202, 204, 206-207, 211, 216, 249, 352, 359-360, 381, 383-386, 389
  popliteal artery 25-26, 73, 75, 90, 97, 132, 138, 142-144, 155-158, 162-164, 359-360, 383-384

popliteal artery entrapment syndrome 90, 143, 359
popliteal cystic disease 73, 359-360
popliteal vein 19, 22, 59, 70-71, 198, 201-202, 204-207, 211, 216, 352, 385-386, 389
PORH 150, 152, 187, 192
Portal veins 11, 88, 296, 300
  hypertension 38-39, 41, 55, 57, 60, 62, 64-65, 67-68, 73, 76-78, 80-82, 86, 92-93, 97-98, 113, 117, 119, 132, 137, 142, 146, 155, 164, 173, 177, 185, 193-194, 203, 208-209, 214, 220, 225, 249, 260-261, 269-270, 277-278, 287, 296, 300, 302-303, 306, 327, 334, 353, 356, 359-360, 383, 385, 388
  left portal vein 11-12, 88, 297, 300
  main portal vein 11-12, 88, 297-300
  right portal vein 11, 88, 297-298, 300
  thrombosis 20, 24, 35, 40, 55-60, 63-67, 69-73, 75, 79-80, 86, 88-89, 91-92, 94, 96-97, 112, 116, 118, 132, 135, 137, 141-142, 145, 150, 154, 163-166, 172-173, 176, 192, 194, 197-199, 205, 207-208, 210, 213-214, 216-219, 223-226, 229, 233-235, 240-243, 248, 251, 254, 260-261, 268-270, 273, 275, 277-278, 283-284, 286-287, 292, 296, 299-300, 302-303, 305-306, 316, 319, 321-326, 328, 332, 350, 352-353, 357-358, 360
Portal Hypertension 64-65
Posterior cerebral artery 8, 82, 118
Posterior communicating artery 8, 82
Posterior tibial artery 26, 133, 138, 160, 389
Posterior tibial vein 389
Post occlusive reactive hyperemia 187
Potential energy 42, 54
Pressure gradient 35-37, 42-44, 51, 58-59, 119, 125, 140, 150, 173, 375-376
Produndapopliteal collateral index 139-140
Pseudoaneurysm 46, 65, 74, 77, 89-90, 94, 97-98, 100-101, 104, 132, 137, 146, 155, 162, 164, 170, 173, 181, 185, 191, 251, 254, 258, 260, 269, 278, 284-286, 303, 306, 313-320, 351-352, 355, 359-360
Pulmonary circulation 34
Pulmonary embolism 65, 70, 72, 198, 219, 234-235, 338, 357, 360, 382
Pulmonic stenosis 339

R

Radial artery 32, 89, 173-174, 179-180, 186, 190, 303, 317, 389

Red blood cells 34-35, 41, 43, 68, 146, 177, 181, 194, 209, 383-384, 386

Renal
renal aortic ratio 378, 389
renal artery 16-17, 85, 92-93, 95, 97, 269-284, 286, 350, 378, 385, 389
renal duplex 260, 268-269, 274, 276
renal Parenchyma 273
renal transplant duplex 277-278, 280
renal vein 11-12, 16, 62-63, 89, 92, 270, 272, 274-275, 277-281, 283-284, 385, 389

Renovascular hypertension 92, 97, 269, 359-360, 385
Repetitive trauma theory 73
Resistance equation 43-44
Resistive Index 273-274, 279-282, 284, 379, 389
Respiratory function 37
Reynolds number 52

S

Saphenous vein 20-24, 63-64, 66-68, 97, 165, 194, 197, 200, 209, 211, 214, 216, 242, 245, 247, 303, 381, 383, 386-389
great saphenous 19-24, 63-64, 66-68, 71-72, 165, 194, 196-197, 200, 202, 209, 214, 216, 243, 245, 247, 303, 318, 381, 383, 386-389
saphenofemoral junction 21-22, 24, 59, 67, 194, 197, 199-200, 202, 210-211, 213, 216, 245-246, 383, 389
saphenopopliteal junction 22, 59, 211, 245-246, 389
small saphenous 19, 21-24, 71, 165, 196-197, 199, 201-202, 211, 214, 216, 245-246, 386, 389
venous mapping 243, 246-247

Segmental pressures 137-140, 173-176, 258-259, 331, 372, 375
Soleal sinuses 19
Soleal veins 20, 72, 392
Spectral broadening 49, 51-52, 103, 107, 159-160, 167, 170, 189-190, 257, 259, 267, 275, 282-283, 293, 362
Splenic artery 15-16, 48, 289, 389
Splenic vein 11-12, 88-89, 296-297, 300, 384-386, 389
Statistics 371-374
accuracy 45, 114, 121, 159, 167, 170, 176, 189, 226, 307, 371-372, 374, 377, 383-384
false negative 140, 371-373, 383-384, 386
false positive 125, 129, 178, 229, 279, 371-373, 383, 385-386
gold standard 39, 63, 279, 371-373
negative predictive value 371, 384
positive predictive value 371, 385

sensitivity 24, 127, 132, 137, 146, 153, 173, 177, 181-182, 185, 228, 282, 317, 371-373, 386
specificity 282, 371-373, 386
true negative 371-373, 383-384, 386
true positive 371-373, 383-386

Stent 66, 76, 89-90, 95, 98, 105-106, 112, 124, 136, 141, 145, 147, 154, 156, 163-167, 169-171, 174, 176, 192, 226, 228-233, 250-251, 254-255, 257-266, 270, 273-274, 276, 286-287, 291, 296, 301-302, 320, 326, 352-354, 386
Stroke 35, 42, 69, 76, 79-83, 96-98, 112-113, 117-119, 125, 129-131, 142, 150, 199, 219, 234, 357-358, 360, 383
cardioembolic stroke 358
hemorrhagic stroke 80, 119
ischemic stroke 77, 80, 83, 97, 112, 118-119, 131, 358, 360
lacunar stroke 82
Subclavian 2-3, 6, 27, 30-32, 53, 61, 65-66, 71, 75-77, 93-96, 98, 102-103, 108, 112, 124, 129, 139, 142, 152, 173-174, 176, 178, 185-187, 190-192, 235-238, 240, 243-244, 251, 303, 306-309, 312, 321-325, 335, 359-360, 364, 382, 384, 386, 389
subclavian artery 2-3, 6, 31-32, 53, 65, 75, 77, 93-95, 98, 102, 108-109, 112, 142, 173-175, 185-187, 191, 251, 303, 322-324, 364
subclavian steal syndrome 93, 102, 105, 108, 139, 152, 176, 187, 191, 359-360
subclavian vein 27, 65-66, 94, 173, 178, 235-237, 240, 243, 303, 322-323, 325, 384, 386, 389
Superficial vein thrombosis 214, 389
Superior mesenteric artery (SMA) 15-16, 293
Superior vena cava 27, 30, 66, 72, 207, 225, 235, 241, 359, 386, 389
Superior vena cava syndrome 66-67, 235, 241, 359

T

Takayasu's arteritis 76, 85-86, 93, 95-96, 112, 287
Tandem lesions 53
TCD 116-122, 124-125, 127-131, 389
Thermal regulation 39
Thoracic Outlet Compression Syndrome 66, 94, 359
effort thrombosis 65, 94, 240-241, 322
Thrombosis 20, 40, 55, 57-60, 63-70, 72-73, 75, 79-80, 86, 88-89, 91-92, 94, 96-97, 112, 116, 118, 132, 135, 137, 141-142, 145, 150, 154, 163-166, 172-173, 176, 192, 194, 197-199, 207-208, 210, 213-214, 216, 218-219, 223-226,

229, 233-235, 240-243, 248, 251, 254, 260-261, 268-270, 273, 275, 277-278, 283-284, 286-287, 292, 296, 299-300, 302-303, 305-306, 316, 319, 321-326, 328, 332, 350, 352-353, 357-358, 382-389
acute 65-66, 69, 71-72, 77, 80, 85-88, 92, 95, 97, 118, 125, 128, 131-132, 136-137, 141-142, 145, 149-150, 154, 173-174, 176, 180, 192, 197, 199, 204-207, 213, 220, 223, 225, 228, 233, 239, 242-243, 247-248, 260, 275-278, 284-287, 295-296, 300, 314, 322, 325, 332, 336, 356-357, 359-360, 381, 386
chronic 24, 35, 38, 41, 44, 53-59, 62, 64, 67, 71-72, 74, 77, 80, 82, 84-86, 88, 119, 172, 193, 196-197, 204-205, 207-208, 210, 213-214, 216, 223, 225, 229, 233, 239, 247-248, 250, 260, 275, 277-278, 285-287, 289, 295-296, 300, 306, 334, 336, 342, 349, 352, 356, 360, 378, 382, 385, 387-388
Indeterminate 204-205, 223, 239, 247, 263, 282
TIA 69, 80-81, 83, 98, 112, 117-119, 199, 219, 234, 358, 389
Tibioperoneal trunk 19, 25-26, 156
TOS 65, 94, 321-326, 386, 389
Transcranial Doppler 9, 116, 120, 125, 128, 131, 389
Transient ischemic attack 81, 96, 98, 102, 118-119, 131, 199, 360, 389
Transmural pressure 37
Tricuspid stenosis 338
Tumescent 215-217
Turbulence 51-54, 100, 106-108, 111, 123, 127-129, 157, 159-160, 167, 170, 186-188, 190-191, 229, 231, 233, 254-257, 259, 265, 267, 272, 274-275, 280, 282, 288-294, 312, 319, 324, 387
Turbulent flow 49, 52, 70, 80, 113, 133, 137, 143, 147, 156, 159-160, 166, 174, 178, 185-186, 189, 249, 270, 278-279, 281, 284, 288, 305, 310, 316, 321-322

U

Ulnar artery 176, 179-180, 186-187, 389
Ulnar vein 237

V

Valsalva maneuver 40, 125, 129, 210-212, 233, 382, 387
Varicella zoster virus 85
Varicose veins 41, 55, 57, 59, 62, 64, 67-68, 71-72, 193-194, 197-199, 208-210, 213-214, 219, 226, 228, 230, 243, 360, 381, 384-387, 389
Vasa vasorum 34, 66, 74, 78, 83, 85, 92, 95-96, 101, 209, 251

Vascular disease
venous 55-72
arterial 73-97
Vasculitis *(also see arteritis)* 65, 68, 71, 83, 85, 91, 94-97, 102, 112, 116-117, 119, 130, 132, 137, 146, 173, 177, 181, 185, 197, 207, 213, 242, 249, 269, 358, 360
Vasomotor tone 36, 39, 53
Vasospasm 66, 85-86, 90-91, 94, 116-117, 119, 124, 126-128, 130-132, 137, 142, 146-147, 155, 173, 177-178, 181-182, 184-185, 287, 332, 384, 387
Velocity 33, 35, 42-43, 45-54, 70, 85, 87, 100, 102, 104, 106-109, 111-112, 114, 120, 122-129, 131, 154-157, 159-160, 162, 167-170, 185-191, 228-229, 233, 240, 254-259, 262-267, 271-275, 279, 281-283, 288, 292-294, 297, 299, 301-302, 305, 309, 311-313, 318, 323-325, 329, 331-334, 339, 341, 362, 364, 372-373, 375, 377, 379-383, 387-389
Venous ablation 59, 68, 197, 213-215
Venous anatomy 14, 18-19, 21, 24, 30, 71, 321
Venous hemodynamics 36, 44, 338
Venous insufficiency 30, 35, 41, 44, 55, 57, 61, 68-69, 71-72, 193-194, 196-197, 208, 210, 212-214, 327, 332, 344-345, 352-353, 359-360, 378, 382, 385, 387-389
Venous malformations 69
Venous mapping 243, 246-247
Venous refill time 196, 378
Venous stenosis 206, 219, 225, 240, 243, 325
Venous thrombosis 55, 57-59, 63-64, 66-67, 70-72, 86, 88, 94, 132, 135, 137, 141-142, 145, 150, 154, 163, 172-173, 176, 192, 194, 197-199, 207-208, 213-214, 218-219, 225, 233-235, 241-243, 248, 292, 299, 306, 321-326, 332, 352, 357-358, 383-386
Venous valves 13, 22-24, 30, 36, 38, 40, 58, 67, 71, 193-194, 196, 209-210, 235, 378, 384, 387
Vertebral artery 4, 6-8, 53, 82-84, 93, 98, 101-102, 108, 112, 119, 139, 152, 173, 176-177, 185, 187, 191-192, 389
Vertebral vein 30, 389
Viscosity 43, 52, 385, 387
volume flow 303, 310-313, 380
Volume pulse recording (VPR) 66, 94, 142-143, 322, 372, 389
Von Willebrand factor (vWF) 70

W

Wegener's granulomatosis 91, 96
White blood cells 34-35, 198, 219, 234, 384

(Woo whoo!! Just made it fit!)